Delivery of Molecules Using Nanoscale Systems for Cancer Treatment and/or Diagnosis

Delivery of Molecules Using Nanoscale Systems for Cancer Treatment and/or Diagnosis

Editors

Marina Santiago Franco
Yu Seok Youn

MDPI • Basel • Beijing • Wuhan • Barcelona • Belgrade • Manchester • Tokyo • Cluj • Tianjin

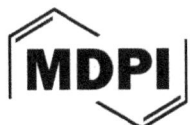

Editors
Marina Santiago Franco
Klinikum rechts der Isar,
Technical University of
Munich
Germany

Yu Seok Youn
School of Pharmacy,
Sungkyunkwan University
Korea

Editorial Office
MDPI
St. Alban-Anlage 66
4052 Basel, Switzerland

This is a reprint of articles from the Special Issue published online in the open access journal *Pharmaceutics* (ISSN 1999-4923) (available at: https://www.mdpi.com/journal/pharmaceutics/special_issues/nanoscale_cancer).

For citation purposes, cite each article independently as indicated on the article page online and as indicated below:

LastName, A.A.; LastName, B.B.; LastName, C.C. Article Title. *Journal Name* **Year**, *Volume Number*, Page Range.

ISBN 978-3-0365-4961-3 (Hbk)
ISBN 978-3-0365-4962-0 (PDF)

© 2022 by the authors. Articles in this book are Open Access and distributed under the Creative Commons Attribution (CC BY) license, which allows users to download, copy and build upon published articles, as long as the author and publisher are properly credited, which ensures maximum dissemination and a wider impact of our publications.

The book as a whole is distributed by MDPI under the terms and conditions of the Creative Commons license CC BY-NC-ND.

Contents

About the Editors vii

Marina Santiago Franco and Yu Seok Youn
Delivery of Molecules Using Nanoscale Systems for Cancer Treatment and/or Diagnosis
Reprinted from: *Pharmaceutics* **2022**, *14*, 851, doi:10.3390/pharmaceutics14040851 1

Cristiane M. Pinto, Laila S. Horta, Amanda P. Soares, Bárbara A. Carvalho, Enio Ferreira, Eduardo B. Lages, Lucas A. M. Ferreira, André A. G. Faraco, Helton C. Santiago and Gisele A. C. Goulart
Nanoencapsulated Doxorubicin Prevents Mucositis Development in Mice
Reprinted from: *Pharmaceutics* **2021**, *13*, 1021, doi:10.3390/pharmaceutics13071021 5

Karen Bolaños, Macarena Sánchez-Navarro, Andreas Tapia-Arellano, Ernest Giralt, Marcelo J. Kogan and Eyleen Araya
Oligoarginine Peptide Conjugated to BSA Improves Cell Penetration of Gold Nanorods and Nanoprisms for Biomedical Applications
Reprinted from: *Pharmaceutics* **2021**, *13*, 1204, doi:10.3390/pharmaceutics13081204 23

Laura Denise López-Barrera, Roberto Díaz-Torres, Joselo Ramón Martínez-Rosas, Ana María Salazar, Carlos Rosales and Patricia Ramírez-Noguera
Modification of Proliferation and Apoptosis in Breast Cancer Cells by Exposure of Antioxidant Nanoparticles Due to Modulation of the Cellular Redox State Induced by Doxorubicin Exposure
Reprinted from: *Pharmaceutics* **2021**, *13*, 1251, doi:10.3390/pharmaceutics13081251 39

Wen-Ying Huang, Chih-Ho Lai, Shin-Lei Peng, Che-Yu Hsu, Po-Hung Hsu, Pei-Yi Chu, Chun-Lung Feng and Yu-Hsin Lin
Targeting Tumor Cells with Nanoparticles for Enhanced Co-Drug Delivery in Cancer Treatment
Reprinted from: *Pharmaceutics* **2021**, *13*, 1327, doi:10.3390/pharmaceutics13091327 55

Giulia Vindigni, Sofia Raniolo, Federico Iacovelli, Valeria Unida, Carmine Stolfi, Alessandro Desideri and Silvia Biocca
AS1411 Aptamer Linked to DNA Nanostructures Diverts Its Traffic Inside Cancer Cells and Improves Its Therapeutic Efficacy
Reprinted from: *Pharmaceutics* **2021**, *13*, 1671, doi:10.3390/pharmaceutics13101671 75

Kyungmi Yang, Changhoon Choi, Hayeong Cho, Won-Gyun Ahn, Shin-Yeong Kim, Sung-Won Shin, Yeeun Kim, Taekyu Jang, Nohyun Lee and Hee Chul Park
Antigen-Capturing Mesoporous Silica Nanoparticles Enhance the Radiation-Induced Abscopal Effect in Murine Hepatocellular Carcinoma Hepa1-6 Models
Reprinted from: *Pharmaceutics* **2021**, *13*, 1811, doi:10.3390/pharmaceutics13111811 91

Adva Krivitsky, Sabina Pozzi, Eilam Yeini, Sahar Israeli Dangoor, Tal Zur, Sapir Golan, Vadim Krivitsky, Nitzan Albeck, Evgeny Pisarevsky, Paula Ofek, Asaf Madi and Ronit Satchi-Fainaro
Sulfonated Amphiphilic Poly(α)glutamate Amine—A Potential siRNA Nanocarrier for the Treatment of Both Chemo-Sensitive and Chemo-Resistant Glioblastoma Tumors
Reprinted from: *Pharmaceutics* **2021**, *13*, 2199, doi:10.3390/pharmaceutics13122199 107

Hanhee Cho, Man Kyu Shim, Suah Yang, Sukyung Song, Yujeong Moon, Jinseong Kim, Youngro Byun, Cheol-Hee Ahn and Kwangmeyung Kim
Cathepsin B-Overexpressed Tumor Cell Activatable Albumin-Binding Doxorubicin Prodrug for Cancer-Targeted Therapy
Reprinted from: *Pharmaceutics* **2022**, *14*, 83, doi:10.3390/pharmaceutics14010083 . . . . **127**

Lital Cohen, Yehuda G. Assaraf and Yoav D. Livney
Novel Selectively Targeted Multifunctional Nanostructured Lipid Carriers for Prostate Cancer Treatment
Reprinted from: *Pharmaceutics* **2022**, *14*, 88, doi:10.3390/pharmaceutics14010088 . . . . **141**

Woo Tak Lee, Johyun Yoon, Sung Soo Kim, Hanju Kim, Nguyen Thi Nguyen, Xuan Thien Le, Eun Seong Lee, Kyung Taek Oh, Han-Gon Choi and Yu Seok Youn
Combined Antitumor Therapy Using In Situ Injectable Hydrogels Formulated with Albumin Nanoparticles Containing Indocyanine Green, Chlorin e6, and Perfluorocarbon in Hypoxic Tumors
Reprinted from: *Pharmaceutics* **2022**, *14*, 148, doi:10.3390/pharmaceutics14010148 . . . . **163**

Artem A. Sizikov, Petr I. Nikitin and Maxim P. Nikitin
Magnetofection In Vivo by Nanomagnetic Carriers Systemically Administered into the Bloodstream
Reprinted from: *Pharmaceutics* **2021**, *13*, 1927, doi:10.3390/pharmaceutics13111927 . . . . **183**

Yu-Ling Yang, Ke Lin and Li Yang
Progress in Nanocarriers Codelivery System to Enhance the Anticancer Effect of Photodynamic Therapy
Reprinted from: *Pharmaceutics* **2021**, *13*, 1951, doi:10.3390/pharmaceutics13111951 . . . . **199**

Lucimara R. Carobeli, Lyvia E. de F. Meirelles, Gabrielle M. Z. F. Damke, Edilson Damke, Maria V. F. de Souza, Natália L. Mari, Kayane H. Mashiba, Cristiane S. Shinobu-Mesquita, Raquel P. Souza, Vânia R. S. da Silva, Renato S. Gonçalves, Wilker Caetano and Márcia E. L. Consolaro
Phthalocyanine and Its Formulations: A Promising Photosensitizer for Cervical Cancer Phototherapy
Reprinted from: *Pharmaceutics* **2021**, *13*, 2057, doi:10.3390/pharmaceutics13122057 . . . . **241**

Eliza Rocha Gomes and Marina Santiago Franco
Combining Nanocarrier-Assisted Delivery of Molecules and Radiotherapy
Reprinted from: *Pharmaceutics* **2022**, *14*, 105, doi:10.3390/pharmaceutics14010105 . . . . **269**

About the Editors

Marina Santiago Franco

Marina Santiago Franco, PhD, is a scientist at the Institute of Radiation Medicine at the Klinikum rechts der Isar, Technical University of Munich and a guest scientist at the Helmholtz Zentrum München (Germany). She studied Pharmacy (2011) at Universidade Federal de Minas Gerais (Brazil) and received her M.Sc. (2014) and PhD (2018) in Pharmaceutical Sciences from the same institution. Her scientific interests are centered on the development and characterization of lipid-based drug delivery systems co-encapsulating different agents for synergistic activity, as well as the investigation of radiobiological aspects of different radiotherapy modalities (high/low linear energy transfer and microbeams) for cancer treatment.

Yu Seok Youn

Yu Seok Youn, PhD, is a professor of the School of Pharmacy at Sungkyunkwan University. He graduated the pharmacy school in Sungkyunkwan University and received a Ph.D. degree in the topic of "site-specific PEGylation" in 2004. He worked as a postdoctoral fellow in the department of Pharmaceutics and Pharmaceutical Chemistry at the University of Utah from 2006 to 2007. He has worked as an assistant professor at the College of Pharmacy, Pusan National University, from 2007 to 2011, and moved to the School of Pharmacy, Sunkyunkwan University, in 2011. He has served as a major secretary of general/academic affairs in the Korean Society of Pharmaceutical Sciences and Technology (KSPST) since 2010. He has served as an editor of the Archives of Pharmacal Research (APR; SCI journal) in the pharmaceutics division (2014) and an editorial board member of the Journal of Controlled Release and Pharmaceutics (2021). He received a contribution award from the Korean-American Pharmaceutical Scientists Association (KAPSA) in 2015. His recent research focus is about targeted nanoparticles for cancer therapy, photoreactive inorganic nano/biomaterials, polymer conjugation technology for long-acting biopharmaceuticals, and oral/inhalation delivery systems.

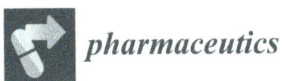

Editorial

Delivery of Molecules Using Nanoscale Systems for Cancer Treatment and/or Diagnosis

Marina Santiago Franco [1],* and Yu Seok Youn [2]

[1] Institute of Radiation Medicine (IRM), Department of Radiation Sciences (DRS), Helmholtz Zentrum München, 85764 Neuherberg, Germany
[2] School of Pharmacy, Sungkyunkwan University, 2066 Seobu-ro, Jangan-gu, Suwon 16419, Gyeonggi-do, Korea; ysyoun@skku.edu
* Correspondence: marina.franco@helmholtz-muenchen.de; Tel.: +49-89-3187-48767

Since clinical approval of the first liposomal formulation encapsulating a chemotherapeutic agent, nanoscale delivery systems have been a rapidly developing science. This Special Issue highlights the current advances and challenges in the broad theme of nanosystem development for the delivery of molecules to treat and/or diagnose tumors. A series of 10 original articles and 4 review articles written by researchers working in 11 countries were published. These publications provide the reader with a broad overview of some of the key strategies for nanocarrier design. These strategies are brought together by the wide compositional variety of these systems and the diversity of molecules that may be carried for functionalization strategies, codelivery, and combination with other treatment modalities.

Pinto et al. [1] reported the formulation of nanostructured lipid carriers containing doxorubicin (NLC–DOX). The formulation aims to prevent mucositis, one of the main recurring adverse effects of DOX. In an in vivo experiment, they demonstrated that NLC–DOX could attenuate DOX-induced mucositis in mice compared with DOX-free treatment. The formulation prevented morphological alterations, such as the shortening of crypt depth and villus height. Intestinal permeability was preserved, the expression of tight junctions increased, and inflammatory cytokines associated with mucositis were decreased in mice treated with NLC–DOX.

Bolaños et al. [2] prepared gold nanorods and gold nanoprisms coated with albumin functionalized with the cell-penetrating peptide octaarginine. When evaluated in vitro, improved internalization was observed for both nanoparticles coated with octaarginine-functionalized albumin compared to non-functionalized ones. These results validated the novel nanoconstructs as potential candidates for biomedical applications with improved biocompatibility and internalization.

López-Barrera et al. [3] developed chitosan-carrying-glutathione nanoparticles in combination with DOX. Glutathione, one of the primary endogenous antioxidants, is associated with redox state regulation. Therefore, the strategy aimed at reducing the oxidative stress induced by DOX, a key factor in its high toxicity. In vitro evaluation in two breast cancer cell lines suggested that the formulation reduces the oxidative stress induced by DOX interacting with reactive oxygen species, free radicals, or antioxidant enzymes. Additionally, they reported that the formulation increased caspase-3 activity, leading to apoptosis and impaired cell proliferation by decreasing Ki67 levels.

Huang et al. [4] designed hyaluronic-acid-based PEGylated nanoparticles to codeliver epigallocatechin-3-gallate (EGCG) and DOX. These nanoparticles were conjugated to fucoidan and D-alpha-tocopherylpoly(ethylene glycol) succinate for targeting P-selectin- and CD44-expressing gastric tumors. The authors demonstrated in vitro that the nanoparticles containing EGCG/DOX led to a better synergistic antiproliferation effect compared with the free combination of EGCG/DOX. This reflected a higher antitumor activity for the formulation in the orthotopic gastric tumor mouse model.

Citation: Franco, M.S.; Youn, Y.S. Delivery of Molecules Using Nanoscale Systems for Cancer Treatment and/or Diagnosis. *Pharmaceutics* 2022, 14, 851. https://doi.org/10.3390/pharmaceutics14040851

Received: 6 April 2022
Accepted: 11 April 2022
Published: 13 April 2022

Publisher's Note: MDPI stays neutral with regard to jurisdictional claims in published maps and institutional affiliations.

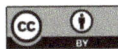

Copyright: © 2022 by the authors. Licensee MDPI, Basel, Switzerland. This article is an open access article distributed under the terms and conditions of the Creative Commons Attribution (CC BY) license (https://creativecommons.org/licenses/by/4.0/).

Vindigni et al. [5] designed aptamer-functionalized nanocages. The aptamer of choice was AS1411, which recognizes and binds specifically and with high affinity to nucleolin (a protein overexpressed on the surface of many tumor cells), inhibiting cell proliferation and inducing cell death. To enhance AS1411 stability and therapeutic efficacy, it was used to functionalize octahedral DNA nanocages. The aptamer acts as a selective tumor-targeting ligand when linked to the nanocages. The formulation presented high stability in serum and rapid and selective internalization in cancer cells. The anticancer activity was reported to be increased by over 200-fold compared with the free aptamer. Different intracellular trafficking for the formulation compared with the free aptamer was also reported.

Yang et al. [6] explored the ability of mesoporous silica nanoparticles (MSNs) to absorb biomaterials, such as antigens. They developed MSNs functionalized with (3-aminopropyl) triethoxysilane and investigated the potential of this formulation to deliver antigens to the tumor, enhancing the abscopal effect after radiotherapy. In vivo experiments in mice with bilateral hepatocellular carcinoma showed promising results, with a significant volume reduction in the non-irradiated tumor when radiotherapy+MSNs were combined in the primary tumor.

Krivitsky et al. [7] developed a sulfonated amphiphilic poly(α)glutamate nanocarrier as a delivery vehicle for siRNA targeting Plk1 genes to chemo-resistant glioblastoma tumors. The brain targeting ability of this formulation was improved by decorating it with sulfonate groups. These groups have a selective affinity towards P-selectin, a transmembrane glycoprotein overexpressed in glioblastoma. In vitro studies showed the potential of the formulation to be internalized by glioblastoma cells, leading to specific gene silencing and affecting its proliferation.

Cho et al. [8] prepared a nanostructured DOX prodrug consisting of an albumin-binding maleimide group, cathepsin-B-cleavable peptide (Phe-Arg-Arg-Gly), and DOX, designed to be activated in cathepsin-B-overexpressed tumor cells. It was demonstrated in vivo using breast tumor mice models that the formulation enhanced DOX accumulation in the tumor by passive targeting. It also induced potent antitumor efficacy due to the selective release of DOX from the formulation in the tumor cells. Furthermore, lower toxicity was observed towards normal tissues due to their low expression of cathepsin B, guaranteeing the formulation's safety.

Cohen et al. [9] developed PEGylated nanostructured lipid carriers (NLCs) decorated with a targeting ligand (Glu-Urea-Lys) to the prostate-specific membrane antigen. These NLCs were loaded with the anti-microtubule agent cabazitaxel. In their article, an extensive characterization of this formulation was presented, as well as its selective targeting, internalization, and growth-inhibitory activity in vitro against prostate cancer cells.

Lee et al. [10] formulated an in situ injectable multifunctional PEG hydrogel system to provide photodynamic, photothermal, and chemotherapeutic effects to hypoxic tumors. This system was prepared with (i) paclitaxel-bound albumin nanoparticles with chlorin-e6 (a photosensitizer)-conjugated bovine serum albumin and indocyanine green (a deep-penetrating NIR dye) and (ii) an albumin-stabilized perfluorocarbon nano-emulsion (to provide oxygen) in a PEG hydrogel. Under laser irradiation, the hydrogel induced hyperthermia as well as photodynamic cell death, while ultrasound irradiation triggered the release of oxygen. This allowed for the significantly enhanced killing of murine breast cancer cell spheroids in vitro, as well as suppressed tumor growth in 4T1 cell-xenograft mice.

Sizikov et al. [11] reviewed magnetofection, a delivery method for nucleic acids carried in magnetic nanoparticles under the guidance of a magnetic field. A special focus was given to the structure and coating of the magnetic nanocarriers developed so far. Possible ways to improve the technology, its challenges, and prospects were also discussed.

Yang et al. [12] provided a critical overview of the synergistic enhancement of photodynamic therapy (PDT) by combining it with the codelivery of molecules in nanocarriers. In this extensive review, nanocarriers used to codeliver combinations of different molecules, such as photosensitizers, photothermal agents, hyperthermia agents, scintillators/radionuclides, sonophotosensitizers, and chemotherapeutic agents, are reported.

On the other hand, the use of nanocarrier-assisted delivery in combination with PDT was the focus of the review article by Carobeli et al. [13]. Based on an extensive compilation of in vitro and in vivo data, this review highlights the potential of formulations of phthalocyanines as photosensitizers for different types of cervical cancer.

Finally, Gomes and Franco [14] reviewed the combination of nanocarrier-assisted molecule delivery and radiotherapy. Formulations designed to encapsulate molecules that improve the effects of radiotherapy on tumor cells, modulate the tumor microenvironment by relieving hypoxia, or boost the abscopal effect are described. The employment of radiotherapy to trigger molecule delivery from nanocarriers and the use of minibeam or microbeam radiotherapy as possibilities to modulate the enhanced permeability and retention (EPR) effect were also covered in this review.

Overall, the articles in this Special Issue highlight a very active field, and we expect to see an increasing number of nanocarriers reaching cancer clinical trials.

Author Contributions: Writing—original draft preparation, M.S.F.; writing—review and editing, M.S.F. and Y.S.Y. All authors have read and agreed to the published version of the manuscript.

Funding: This research received no external funding.

Conflicts of Interest: The authors declare no conflict of interest.

References

1. Pinto, C.; Horta, L.; Soares, A.; Carvalho, B.; Ferreira, E.; Lages, E.; Ferreira, L.; Faraco, A.; Santiago, H.; Goulart, G. Nanoencapsulated Doxorubicin Prevents Mucositis Development in Mice. *Pharmaceutics* **2021**, *13*, 1021. [CrossRef] [PubMed]
2. Bolaños, K.; Sánchez-Navarro, M.; Tapia-Arellano, A.; Giralt, E.; Kogan, M.J.; Araya, E. Oligoarginine Peptide Conjugated to BSA Improves Cell Penetration of Gold Nanorods and Nanoprisms for Biomedical Applications. *Pharmaceutics* **2021**, *13*, 1204. [CrossRef] [PubMed]
3. López-Barrera, L.D.; Díaz-Torres, R.; Martínez-Rosas, J.R.; Salazar, A.M.; Rosales, C.; Ramírez-Noguera, P. Modification of Proliferation and Apoptosis in Breast Cancer Cells by Exposure of Antioxidant Nanoparticles Due to Modulation of the Cellular Redox State Induced by Doxorubicin Exposure. *Pharmaceutics* **2021**, *13*, 1251. [CrossRef] [PubMed]
4. Huang, W.-Y.; Lai, C.-H.; Peng, S.-L.; Hsu, C.-Y.; Hsu, P.-H.; Chu, P.-Y.; Feng, C.-L.; Lin, Y.-H. Targeting Tumor Cells with Nanoparticles for Enhanced Co-Drug Delivery in Cancer Treatment. *Pharmaceutics* **2021**, *13*, 1327. [CrossRef] [PubMed]
5. Vindigni, G.; Raniolo, S.; Iacovelli, F.; Unida, V.; Stolfi, C.; Desideri, A.; Biocca, S. AS1411 Aptamer Linked to DNA Nanostructures Diverts Its Traffic inside Cancer Cells and Improves Its Therapeutic Efficacy. *Pharmaceutics* **2021**, *13*, 1671. [CrossRef] [PubMed]
6. Yang, K.; Choi, C.; Cho, H.; Ahn, W.-G.; Kim, S.-Y.; Shin, S.-W.; Kim, Y.; Jang, T.; Lee, N.; Park, H.C. Antigen-Capturing Mesoporous Silica Nanoparticles Enhance the Radiation-Induced Abscopal Effect in Murine Hepatocellular Carcinoma Hepa1-6 Models. *Pharmaceutics* **2021**, *13*, 1811. [CrossRef]
7. Krivitsky, A.; Pozzi, S.; Yeini, E.; Dangoor, S.I.; Zur, T.; Golan, S.; Krivitsky, V.; Albeck, N.; Pisarevsky, E.; Ofek, P.; et al. Sulfonated Amphiphilic Poly (α)glutamate Amine—A Potential siRNA Nanocarrier for the Treatment of Both Chemo-Sensitive and Chemo-Resistant Glioblastoma Tumors. *Pharmaceutics* **2021**, *13*, 2199. [CrossRef] [PubMed]
8. Cho, H.; Shim, M.K.; Yang, S.; Song, S.; Moon, Y.; Kim, J.; Byun, Y.; Ahn, C.-H.; Kim, K. Cathepsin B-Overexpressed Tumor Cell Activatable Albumin-Binding Doxorubicin Prodrug for Cancer-Targeted Therapy. *Pharmaceutics* **2021**, *14*, 83. [CrossRef] [PubMed]
9. Cohen, L.; Assaraf, Y.G.; Livney, Y.D. Novel Selectively Targeted Multifunctional Nanostructured Lipid Carriers for Prostate Cancer Treatment. *Pharmaceutics* **2021**, *14*, 88. [CrossRef] [PubMed]
10. Lee, W.T.; Yoon, J.; Kim, S.S.; Kim, H.; Nguyen, N.T.; Le, X.T.; Lee, E.S.; Oh, K.T.; Choi, H.-G.; Youn, Y.S. Combined Antitumor Therapy Using In Situ Injectable Hydrogels Formulated with Albumin Nanoparticles Containing Indocyanine Green, Chlorin c6, and Perfluorocarbon in Hypoxic Tumors. *Pharmaceutics* **2022**, *14*, 148. [CrossRef] [PubMed]
11. Sizikov, A.A.; Nikitin, P.I.; Nikitin, M.P. Magnetofection In Vivo by Nanomagnetic Carriers Systemically Administered into the Bloodstream. *Pharmaceutics* **2021**, *13*, 1927. [CrossRef]
12. Yang, Y.-L.; Lin, K.; Yang, L. Progress in Nanocarriers Codelivery System to Enhance the Anticancer Effect of Photodynamic Therapy. *Pharmaceutics* **2021**, *13*, 1951. [CrossRef] [PubMed]
13. Carobeli, L.R.; Meirelles, L.E.; Damke, G.M.Z.F.; Damke, E.; de Souza, M.V.F.; Mari, N.L.; Mashiba, K.H.; Shinobu-Mesquita, C.S.; Souza, R.P.; da Silva, V.R.S.; et al. Phthalocyanine and Its Formulations: A Promising Photosensitizer for Cervical Cancer Phototherapy. *Pharmaceutics* **2021**, *13*, 2057. [CrossRef] [PubMed]
14. Gomes, E.R.; Franco, M.S. Combining Nanocarrier-Assisted Delivery of Molecules and Radiotherapy. *Pharmaceutics* **2022**, *14*, 105. [CrossRef] [PubMed]

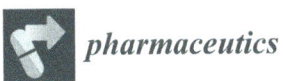

Article

Nanoencapsulated Doxorubicin Prevents Mucositis Development in Mice

Cristiane M. Pinto [1,†], Laila S. Horta [2,†], Amanda P. Soares [1,2,†], Bárbara A. Carvalho [3], Enio Ferreira [3], Eduardo B. Lages [1], Lucas A. M. Ferreira [1], André A. G. Faraco [1], Helton C. Santiago [2,†] and Gisele A. C. Goulart [1,*,†]

[1] Department of Pharmaceutics, Faculty of Pharmacy, Universidade Federal de Minas Gerais, Belo Horizonte 31270-901, MG, Brazil; crismp@ufmg.br (C.M.P.); ufmgamanda@gmail.com (A.P.S.); eduardoburgarelli@hotmail.com (E.B.L.); lucaufmg@gmail.com (L.A.M.F.); andre.faraco@gmail.com (A.A.G.F.)
[2] Department of Biochemistry and Immunology, Universidade Federal de Minas Gerais, Belo Horizonte 31270-901, MG, Brazil; laila.horta@yahoo.com.br (L.S.H.); heltonsantiago@icb.ufmg.br (H.C.S.)
[3] Department of General Pathology, Biological Science Institute, Universidade Federal de Minas Gerais, Belo Horizonte 31270-901, MG, Brazil; barbaraandradedecarvalho@yahoo.com.br (B.A.C.); eniofvet@hotmail.com (E.F.)
* Correspondence: gacg@ufmg.br or giseleacgoulart@gmail.com; Tel.: +55-31-3409-6993
† These authors contributed equally to this work.

Abstract: Doxorubicin (DOX), a chemotherapy drug successfully used in the therapy of various types of cancer, is currently associated with the mucositis development, an inflammation that can cause ulcerative lesions in the mucosa of the gastrointestinal tract, abdominal pain and secondary infections. To increase the safety of the chemotherapy, we loaded DOX into nanostructured lipid carriers (NLCs). The NLC–DOX was characterized by HPLC, DLS, NTA, Zeta potential, FTIR, DSC, TEM and cryogenic-TEM. The ability of NLC–DOX to control the DOX release was evaluated through in vitro release studies. Moreover, the effect of NLC–DOX on intestinal mucosa was compared to a free DOX solution in C57BL/6 mice. The NLC–DOX showed spherical shape, high drug encapsulation efficiency (84.8 ± 4.6%), high drug loading (55.2 ± 3.4 mg/g) and low average diameter (66.0–78.8 nm). The DSC and FTIR analyses showed high interaction between the NLC components, resulting in controlled drug release. Treatment with NLC–DOX attenuated DOX-induced mucositis in mice, improving shortening on villus height and crypt depth, decreased inflammatory parameters, preserved intestinal permeability and increased expression of tight junctions (ZO-1 and Ocludin). These results indicated that encapsulation of DOX in NLCs is viable and reduces the drug toxicity to mucosal structures.

Keywords: nanostructured lipid carriers; doxorubicin; mucositis

1. Introduction

Cancer incidence and deaths are increasing worldwide. According to the World Health Organization (WHO), the number of cancer deaths is expected to double between 2018 and 2040 [1]. Part of these deaths will be attributed to adverse events caused by the cancer treatment itself, or to the interruption of the treatment caused by such adverse events. One way to minimize these deaths and ameliorate the quality of life of patients is to develop treatments with improved efficacy and decreased toxicity. Among the efforts to improve cancer treatment, the encapsulation of active pharmaceutical ingredients (APIs) in nanocarriers, which can reduce the toxicity of the APIs used in cancer therapy, is one of the most studied options [2–4].

Mucositis, an inflammatory condition of the gastrointestinal tract (GIT) mucosa, is one of the most common and uncomfortable adverse reactions during cancer treatment, affecting at least 40% of patients. This condition can lead to ulcerative lesions, causing pain and discomfort to the patients, interfering directly in their quality of life and adherence to treatment. It can also lead to secondary infections and other complications, such as septicemia, due to increased GIT permeability [5–7].

Aiming to improve the safety of the treatment with chemotherapeutic agents, we proposed its encapsulation in nanostructured lipid carriers (NLCs), using doxorubicin (DOX) as a model. DOX is an API widely used in cancer therapy, being effective in treatment of several types of cancer, such as leukemia, Hodgkin's and non-Hodgkin's lymphomas and breast cancer [8]. To be used in the clinic, DOX is formulated as a hydrochloride salt dissolved in an aqueous solution for intravenous injection [9], being rapidly distributed into tissues [10,11].

Although DOX is subject to many studies, the mechanism of action is still considered unclear. It has been suggested that DOX can intercalate dsDNA and promote their break [12] and also impair the action of Topoisomerase II [12,13]. In addition, DOX has also been regarded as promoting oxidative stress when coupled with iron [14]. All of these mechanisms lead to DNA breakage or damage and inhibition of DNA and RNA synthesis, which compromise cell viability and induce a plethora of drug-associated adverse events, including cardiotoxicity and mucositis. These adverse events can lead to treatment interruption, in addition to increased treatment costs and mortality ratio [15–19]. The clinical approach to DOX-associated toxicities is updated regularly [20]. However, there is still a pressing need for fewer toxic drugs formulation and presentation. In order to circumvent the adverse effects of DOX and improve its efficacy, different drug delivery systems have been developed [21–30]. Among lipid-based systems, Doxil® and Myocet® are liposomal commercial formulations, which improved the safety profile of DOX in comparison with free DOX. However, mucositis remains one of the main recurring adverse effects [31,32]. Therefore, a formulation that will spare intestinal mucosa during chemotherapy is still a pressing necessity for cancer patients.

As liposomes, solid lipid nanoparticles (SLN) and NLC can improve bioavailability and control drug release [27,28,33], but they present advantages, as production without organic solvents and using simple and easily scale-up techniques, which turns the process simpler, safer and cheaper [34,35]. Different from SLN, NLCs are drug delivery systems composed of a mixture of solid and liquid lipids, thus forming a solid lipid matrix containing imperfections in which the APIs can be loaded [36,37]. Müller et al. [38] first described the NLCs in 2002 and after that, many studies have been carried out with different APIs, including that used in chemotherapy [39,40]. However, due to the hydrophilic characteristic of the DOX hydrochloride salt, its encapsulation in lipid nanocarriers is low [41,42] and the ion pair strategy has been used to enhance DOX incorporation in the lipid matrix. Through this strategy, DOX forms an ion pair with a lipophilic anion, improving its lipophilicity and the affinity for the lipid matrix. This strategy has improved the efficacy of DOX, as well as reduced its toxicity in different lipid-based systems [33,41,43–56].

Although there is an increasing interest in the use of NLC in cancer treatment, the use of NLCs to mitigate or prevent mucositis is poorly investigated, especially using DOX. Therefore, the aim of this study was to design and to characterize an NLC loaded with DOX (NLC–DOX), using the ion pair strategy, and compare its safety to free DOX in a mouse model of DOX-induced mucositis, which is an established model to assess the DOX-induced mucositis [19]. We found that NLC–DOX were less toxic to the animals' intestines. This study was the first to assess the impact of DOX encapsulation in NLC as a strategy to reduce the development of mucositis.

2. Materials and Methods

2.1. Materials

Doxorubicin hydrochloride (DOX) was kindly provided by ACIC Chemicals (Ontario, Canada). Oleic acid was purchased from Sigma-Aldrich (St. Louis, MO, USA). Triethanolamine (TEA) was obtained from Merck (Darmstadt, Germany). Lipoid MCT was purchased from Lipoid GmbH (Ludiwigshafen, Germany). Monooleate of sorbitan (Span 80 ®) and monooleate of sorbitan ethoxylated (Super Refined Polysorbate 80 ®) was provided by Croda Inc. (Edison, NJ, USA). Glyceryl behenate (Compritol 888 ATO ®) was provided by Gattefossé (Saint Priest, France). All other chemicals were of analytical grade.

2.2. Preparation of NLC–DOX and Free DOX Solution

NLCs were prepared by the hot melting homogenization method, as previously described [27]. During the development of the NLC–DOX we evaluated different proportions of liquid (MCT) and solid lipids (Compritol 888 ATO ®), as well as the surfactants Tween 80 ® and Span 80 ®. The better formulation was obtained by using 60:40 of solid:liquid lipids and a mixture 80:20 of Tween 80 ®:Span 80 ®. Briefly, batches (10 mL) were prepared containing an oil and aqueous phases. The oil phase (OP) was composed of 120 mg of Compritol 888 ATO ®, 80 mg of MCT, 200 mg of Tween 80 ®, 50 mg of Span 80 ®, 15 mg of DOX, 12 mg of TEA and 30 mg of oleic acid. The aqueous phase (AP) was composed of distilled water. The OP and AP were heated separately to 80 °C and then gently mixed under constant agitation, at 8000 rpm, with an Ultra Turrax T-25 homogenizer (Ika Labortechnik, Staufen, Germany) at 80 °C. The emulsion formed was homogenized for 10 min on ultrasound with high power probe (21% amplitude, Ultra-cell 750 W, Sonics Materials Inc., USA). The pH of the NLC–DOX was adjusted to 6.5 with a solution of 0.1 M HCl and the formulations were stored at 4 °C, protected from light in a nitrogen atmosphere. The non-encapsulated DOX solution (free DOX), in the same concentration of NLC–DOX (1.5 mg/mL), was prepared diluting DOX in distilled water.

2.3. Particle Size Analysis and Zeta Potential

The hydrodynamic diameter of the NLC–DOX was determined by unimodal analysis through dynamic light scattering (DLS), and the data reported were Z-average, evaluated as the intensity. The hydrodynamic diameter, polydispersity index (PDI) and Zeta potential of the NLC–DOX were determined by dynamic scattering of light and electrophoretic mobility, using a Zetasizer Nano-ZS90 (Malvern Instruments; England) at a fixed angle of 90° and temperature of 25 °C. For DLS, the NLC-DOX was diluted (1:100) in ultrapure water previously filtered through cellulose ester membrane with 0.45 µm pore diameter (HAWP04700, Merck Millipore, Burlington, MA, USA). All measurements were performed in triplicate.

2.4. Nanoparticle Tracking Analysis (NTA)

NTA experiments were performed by using the NanoSight NS300 (Malvern Instruments; Salisbury, England). After appropriate dilution of the NLC-DOX in ultrapure water, the sample was introduced into the NanoSight sample chamber with a disposable syringe. The samples were measured at room temperature for 60 s with automatic detection. The software used for capturing and analyzing the data was the NanoSight NS300 (Malvern Instruments, Salisbury, England).

2.5. Drug Encapsulation Efficiency (EE) and Drug Loading (DL)

The encapsulation efficiency (EE) and drug loading (DL) of DOX in NLC were determined by an ultrafiltration method, using centrifugal devices (Amicon® Ultra−0.5 mL 100 k; Millipore, USA). To eliminate the binding of DOX to the devices, a pretreating of the filters was performed as previously described [45]. The devices were soaked in a passivating solution (Tween 20 ®, 5% w/v), maintained overnight at room temperature and washed with distilled water prior to use. The EE and DL were calculated by using the following Equations (1) and (2), respectively:

$$EE\% = [(CT - CAP)/CT] \times 100 \qquad (1)$$

$$DL\ (mg/g) = WDL/WNP \qquad (2)$$

where CT = total DOX concentration in NLC; CAP = DOX concentration in aqueous phase (non-encapsulated drug); WDL = mg of drug loaded in NLC and WNP = g of lipids.

The CT, CAP and WDL were evaluated as described by Mussi et al. [27]. The CT was analyzed by dissolving an aliquot of the NLC dispersion in a mixture of tetrahydrofuran (THF)/methanol (MeOH) 40:60 v/v, followed by centrifugation (10 min at 2400 g) and analysis of the supernatant by UV-vis spectrophotometry at 480 nm (UV-Vis Evolution 201; ThermoFisher, Shanghai, China). The CAP was evaluated from an aliquot of the aqueous phase separated from the NLC dispersion by ultrafiltration (10 min at 2400 g), dilution with THF/MeOH and analysis by UV-vis. The WDL was derived by using the calculated EE × total (mg) of DOX added. The method for DOX quantification was previously validated. The five-point linear regression analysis resulted in the following linear equation: y = 0.01930X–0.00615 (R^2 = 0.9915).

2.6. Differential Scanning Calorimetry

Differential scanning calorimetry (DSC) analysis of formulation components (DOX and Compritol 888 ATO) and NLC-DOX were performed by using a DSC 2910 differential scanning calorimeter (TA Instruments, New Castle, DE, USA). For DSC measurements, a scan rate of 10 °C/min was used at a temperature range of 0–400 °C, under a nitrogen purge. NLC-DOX was lyophilized prior to analysis with the use of a freeze-drier (Modulyod-115, ThermoFisher, Asheville, NC, USA; Pump Edwards E2M18, West Sussex, UK). After freeze-drying, the NLCs sample, DOX and Compritol were placed directly in aluminum pans for analysis (approximately 7 mg of lipid).

2.7. ATR–FTIR Analysis

Attenuated total reflection–Fourier transform infrared (ATR–FTIR) spectra of NLC-DOX and raw materials (DOX and Compritol) were recorded within films on a Perkin Elmer FTIR spectrometer (Model Spectrum One).

2.8. Transmission Electron Microscopy (TEM) and Cryogenic TEM (Cryo-TEM)

The morphology of the NLC-DOX was evaluated by TEM. Negatively stained samples were prepared by spreading 3 µL of the NLC-DOX dispersion (diluted 1:25) onto a copper grid coated with a Lacey carbon film. After 1 min of adsorption, excess liquid was blotted off with filter paper and the grids were placed on a droplet of 2% (w/v) aqueous uranyl acetate and drained off after 1 min. The dried specimens were examined by using a 120 kV electron microscope (Tecnai-G2-Spirit-FEI/Quanta microscope; Philips, Eindhoven, Netherlands). The analyses involving TEM were conducted at the Microscopy Center of UFMG (http://www.microscopia.ufmg.br accessed on 26 August 2020).

Cryo-TEM micrographs of NLC-DOX were obtained by using a TEM (Tecnai Spirit G2-12 Biotwin-FEI, Brno, Czech Republic) operated at 120 kV. Images were recorded on the CCD Eagle (FEI), using the Serial EM software. Prior to use, the 300 mesh lacey carbon coated copper grids (EMS) were subjected to the glow discharging process with argon gas at a current of 9.2 mA for 25 s. Cryo-TEM samples were prepared by plunge freezing (Leica EM GP2). For each sample, a drop of 3 µL was placed on the carbon side of the grid, blotted for 5 s and immediately frozen in liquid ethane, and then kept in liquid nitrogen until cryo-TEM. The samples were mounted on Fischione cryo holder (Model 2550) and analyzed in the TEM at −175 °C. Pictures were processed by using ImageJ software (National Institutes of Health, Betesda, MD, USA). The analyses involving cryo-TEM were conducted at the Microscopy Center of UFMG (http://www.microscopia.ufmg.br accessed on 16 December 2020).

All the acquired images were uploaded to accessible imaging software (Image J, US National Institutes of Health, Bethesda, MD, USA). The particles were measured from images obtained from three independent NLC-DOX formulations. Before measuring the size, each photo was precisely dimensioned, using a calibrated ruler. The normal distribution of the size was analyzed by using the Shapiro–Wilk test, assuming a 95% confidence level.

2.9. In Vitro DOX Release

The release of DOX from NLC-DOX was performed by using the dialysis method. Dialysis bags with a cutoff size of 14,000 Da and diameter of 21 mm (cellulose ester membrane; Sigma-Aldrich, St. Louis, MO, USA) were filled with 2 mL of NLC-DOX, sealed and incubated with 50 mL of phosphate-buffered saline (PBS) pH 7.4, for 72 h at 37 °C, using shaking stirring (IKA® KS 4000 i control; Werke, Germany) at 120 rpm. An aqueous solution of non-encapsulated DOX (free DOX) at the same concentration (1.5 mg/mL) was used as a control. At different predetermined time intervals (1, 2, 4, 8, 24, 48 and 72 h), 2 mL of release media were taken out and replenished with an equal volume of fresh PBS. The amount of released DOX was measured by UV-vis spectrophotometry as described above. The values were plotted as a cumulative percentage of DOX release. Released DOX (%) = RF/CD × 100. Where RF = released fraction of DOX to the external medium, and CD = initial concentration of DOX inside the dialysis bag.

The regression analysis of the cumulative release of DOX from NLC-DOX and free DOX was evaluated. Different kinetic models were evaluated: zero order ($Q_t = Q_0 + K_0 t$), first order ($\ln Q_t = \ln Q_0 + K_1 t$), Higuchi ($Q_t = K_h t^{1/2}$), Hixson–Crowell ($Q_0^{1/3} - Q_t^{1/3} = K_s t$) and Korsmeyer–Peppas ($Q_t/Q_\infty = K_k t^n$); where Q_t is the amount of drug released at time t; Q_0 is the amount of the drug in the solution at time zero and K is constant of release kinetics. Determination coefficient (R^2) was used as a criterion to define the best release kinetics model [57,58]. All experiments were conducted in triplicate.

2.10. Animals and Experimental Groups

All procedures were approved by the Ethics Committee for Animal Experimentation at the Federal University of Minas Gerais (UFMG) (Protocol n° 331/2012, 22/11/2012). C57BL/6 female mice, free of specific pathogens, 6–8 weeks old, were obtained at the Central Vivarium of UFMG, weighed and randomly divided into three experimental groups. The animals were kept in collective cages with a maximum of five individuals per cage, with water and diet offered freely. The environmental conditions were controlled, using a 12-h light/dark cycle and temperature around 28 °C. The animals in the control group (Saline) received 100 µL of saline solution by intraperitoneal administration (i.p.), while the groups free DOX and NLC-DOX received DOX at 10 mg/kg by i.p. After three days, at the peak of intestinal inflammation, the animals were anesthetized with i.p. injection of ketamine (100 mg/kg) and xylazine (5 mg/kg) and blood was collected followed by cervical dislocation. The small intestine of animals was collected and divided into parts (duodenum, distal jejunum, proximal jejunum and ileum). The distal ileum portion (approximately 1 cm) was frozen at −80 °C for evaluation of cytokines. The rest of the ileum was used for histological and morphometric analysis.

2.11. Histological Analysis

Samples of the ileum of the C57BL/6 mice were fixed in formaldehyde (10%) and processed for histological analysis. The cuts obtained were stained with hematoxylin and eosin for morphological evaluation. The morphometry of villus height and crypt depth was obtained from photos of histological slides, which were analyzed by using the ImageJ software (National Institutes of Health, Betesda, MD, USA). Ten random fields per animal were computed, with tissue integrity as a limiting factor.

2.12. Analysis of Gene Expression

To evaluate the expression of cytokines in the small intestine, 1 cm of the distal ileum was extracted, using Trizol (TRI reagent, Sigma-Aldrich) following acid–alcohol affinity and kept at −80 °C until use. One microgram of total RNA was reverse-transcribed by using M-MLV RT (Promega). Gene expression was performed on n aABI PRISM 7900 sequence detection system (Applied Biosystems), using HOT FIREPol Eva Green qPCR Supermix (Solis BioDyne) according to manufacturer's instructions. Briefly, samples were exposed to 95 °C for 12 min and then subjected to 40 cycles of 95 °C for 15 s and 60 °C for 30 s. At the end of the cycling, a melting curve was performed to evaluate primer specificity. Expression of the target genes (Table 1) were normalized with GAPDH (glyceraldehyde 3- phosphate dehydrogenase), using 2-ΔΔCt. All primers were obtained at Harvard Primer Bank.

Table 1. Nucleotide sequence of the primers used.

Gene	Primer Forward	Primer Reverse
ZO-1	CCAGCTTATGAAAGGGTTGTTC	TCCTCTCTTGCCAACTTTTCTCT
Occludin	ATGTCCGGCCGATGCTCTC	TTTGGCTGCTCTTGGGTCTGTAT
IL-33	ATTTCCCCGGCAAAGTTCAG	AACGGAGTCTCATGCAGTAGA
TSLP	ACGGATGGGGCTAACTTACAA	AGTCCTCGATTTGCTCGAACT
IL-4	GGTCTCAACCCCCAGCTAGT	GCCGATGATCTCTCTCAAGTGAT
IL-13	CCTGGCTCTTGCTTGCCTT	GGTCTTGTGTGATGTTGCTCA
IL-22	ATGAGTTTTTCCCTTATGGGGAC	GCTGGAAGTTGGACACCTCAA
IL-23	ATGCTGGATTGCAGAGCAGTA	ACGGGGCACATTATTTTTAGTCT
IL-5	CTCTGTTGACAAGCAATGAGACG	TCTTCAGTATGTCTAGCCCCTG
IL-25	ACAGGACTTGAATCGGGTC	TGGTAAAGTGGGACGACGGAGTTG
GAPDH	AGGTCGGTGTGAACGGATTTG	TGTAGACCATGTAGTTGAGGTCA

2.13. Assessment of Intestinal Permeability

Intestinal permeability was determined by measuring the radioactivity diffused in the blood after administration of diethylenetriamine-pentacetic acid (DTPA) with technetium 99 m (99 mTc) [59]. Three days after administration of saline, free DOX and NLC-DOX, all mice received, by gavage, 0.1 mL of DTPA solution conjugated to 18.5 mebequerel (MBq) of 99 mTc. Four hours later, all animals were anesthetized to collect 300μL of blood in EDTA (ethylenediamine tetraacetic acid), which was placed in appropriate tubes to determine radioactivity. The data were obtained in % of dose, using the following equation: % Dose = (cpm of blood/cpm of administered dose) × 100, where cpm represents counts per minute.

2.14. Statistical Analysis

Statistical analyses were performed by using GraphPad Prism™ (version 8.2). Data were expressed as mean ± standard deviation (SD). Data normality was assessed by using the Shapiro–Wilk test. To analyze the difference in the DOX release profile and in the body weight variation of mice, two-way analysis of variance (ANOVA) was used, followed by Tukey's post-test. To compare the morphological alterations among groups, the cytokine expression by real time, intestinal permeability, occludin and ZO1, one-way ANOVA was used, followed by the Tukey's post-test. For all analyses, a significance level of 0.05 was used.

3. Results

3.1. Characterization of the Developed NLC-DOX

NLC-DOX was found to be a clear and homogeneous red suspension (Figure 1A) and could efficiently incorporate DOX. The total DOX content in the developed NLC-DOX was 99.8 ± 1.5%, with high encapsulation efficiency (84.8 ± 4.6%). The Zeta potential was −18.3 ± 5.1 mV (Figure 1B) and the average size and PDI obtained by DLS were, respectively, 69.7 ± 6.6 nm (Figure 2C) and 0.29 ± 0.07. The average size determined by NTA (Figure 1D) was slightly smaller (66.0 ± 18 nm). The size and the morphology of NLC-DOX was also evaluated by Cryo-TEM and TEM (Figure 1E,F, respectively). The TEM

(76.7 ± 30 nm) and Cryo-TEM (78.8 ± 28 nm) images showed particles homogeneous with spherical shape and normal distribution (Shapiro–Wilk test) at a confidence level of 95%.

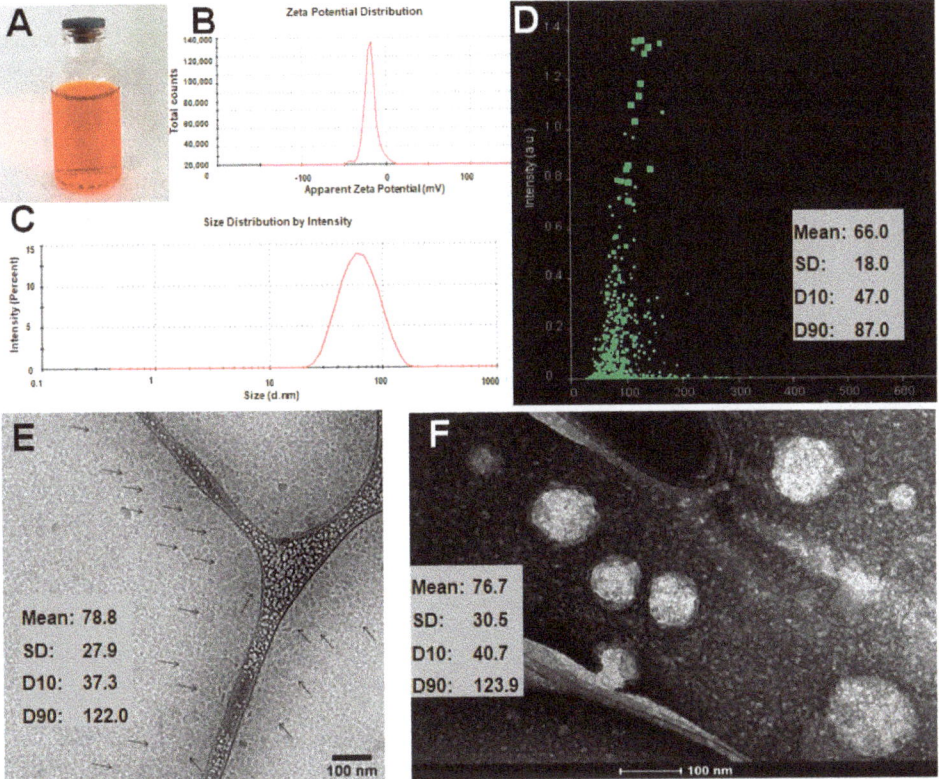

Figure 1. Characteristics of NLC-DOX. Image of NLC-DOX formulation (**A**); Zeta potential distribution determined by dynamic scattering of light and electrophoretic mobility (**B**); particle size distribution determined by DLS (**C**); particle size distribution determined by NTA (**D**); cryo-TEM image (**E**); and TEM image of NLC-DOX (**F**). Abbreviations: DOX, doxorubicin; NLC, nanostructured lipid carrier; DLS, dynamic light scattering; NTA, nanoparticle tracking analysis; TEM, transmission electronic microscopy; SD, standard deviation; D10, the size point below which 10% of NLC-DOX is contained; D90, the size point below which 90% of NLC-DOX is contained.

The thermal behavior of the NLC-DOX and its main components (DOX and the solid lipid Compritol 888 ATO) was evaluated by DSC (Figure 2A). The thermogram of pure DOX showed three endothermic peaks at temperatures between 210 and 240 °C, while the thermogram of pure Compritol 888 ATO showed only one narrow, symmetrical endotherm peak with the melt temperature of 69.79 °C. The NLC-DOX also showed only one endothermic peak at 63.85 °C, corresponding to its solid lipid matrix (Compritol 888 ATO). However, a slight decrease in the melting point (69.79 °C for pure lipid versus 63.85 °C for NLC-DOX), as well as a broadening of this peak was observed. Moreover, the presence of the endothermal melting peak of DOX was not observed in the thermogram of NLC-DOX, suggesting a high affinity of the DOX to the lipid matrix.

The FTIR spectra of DOX, NLC-DOX and Compritol 888 ATO ®, the lipid matrix of the NLC-DOX, are presented in Figure 2B–D. FTIR analysis is usually used to determine the interaction between drugs and excipients, observing the spectrum of functional groups [60]. The spectrum of the DOX (Figure 2B) shows the characteristic bands of the drug: 3525 and 3315 cm^{-1} bands, which are attributed to the O-H and a N-H group stretching vibration;

and a band at 1730 cm^{-1}, due to stretching of C=O, which are in accordance of those described in the literature [60,61]. The FTIR spectra of Compritol 888 ATO ® showed characteristic peaks in 2915 cm^{-1} (stretching of C-H), 1737 cm^{-1} (stretching of C=O) and 1465 cm^{-1} (bending of C-H). Similar results were found by [62,63]. In the spectrum of NLC-DOX, it is also possible to observe the band from N-H group at 3315 cm^{-1}, that can be attributed to DOX's molecule; and two broad bands at 2915 and 2849 cm^{-1}, that can be attributed to the stretching vibration of C-H and C-H$_2$ groups from Compritol 888 ATO ®.

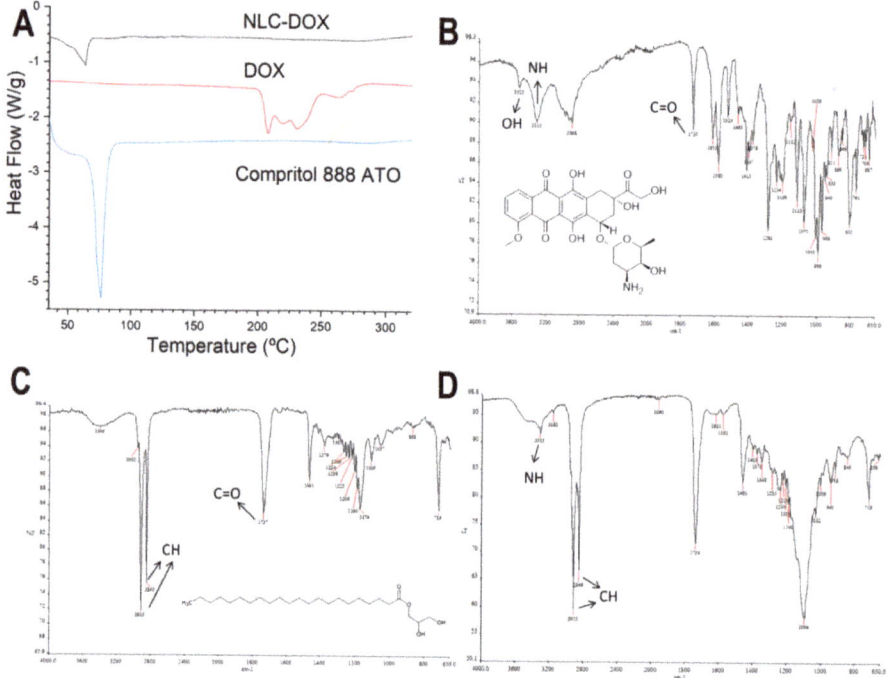

Figure 2. Characterization of the NLC-DOX formulation and its main components by differential scanning calorimetry (DSC) and attenuated total reflection–Fourier transform infrared (ATR-FTIR). DSC curves of NLC-DOX, pure DOX and Compritol 888 ATO ® (**A**); ATR-FTIT spectra of DOX (**B**), Compritol 888 ATO ® (**C**) and NLC-DOX (**D**). The arrows indicate the main absorption regions of the functional groups. Abbreviations: DOX, doxorubicin; NLC, nanostructured lipid carrier.

3.2. In Vitro DOX Release

The in vitro DOX release from NLC-DOX and free DOX was investigated by using dialysis bags in PBS buffer pH 7.4 (37 °C ± 0.5). As can be seen in Figure 3A, free DOX exhibited a rapid release of 80% of drug within 4 h, whereas the release profile of NLC-DOX indicated a sustained pattern without a burst release. The mechanism of release was evaluated by using four different kinetic models (zero-order, first-order, Higuchi and Korsmeyer–Peppas) and the regression coefficient value (R^2) was used to choose the model that best fit the data. The zero-order model presented the higher R^2 (Figure 3B), suggesting a process of constant drug release from the NLC system, independent of the DOX's concentration. This is ideal behavior for a dosage form and leads to minimum fluctuations in drug plasma levels [64].

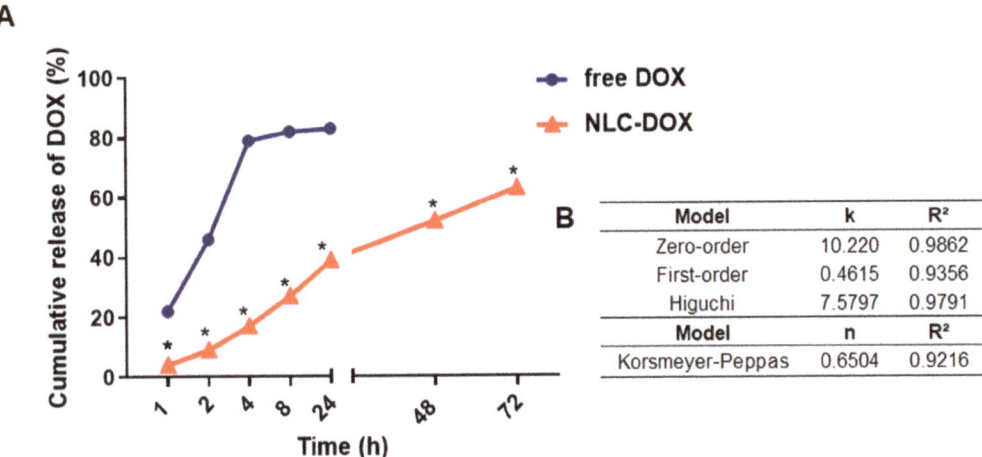

Figure 3. In vitro drug release profile of DOX from NLC-DOX and free DOX (**A**). Kinetic models applied to the release of DOX from NLC-DOX (**B**). * $p < 0.0001$. Data were presented as mean ± SD (n = 3). Abbreviations: DOX, doxorubicin; NLC, nanostructured lipid carrier; k, kinetic constant; n, diffusion exponent.

3.3. NLC-DOX Treatment Prevents Weight Loss in C57BL/6 Mice

To compare the evolution of mucositis between free DOX and NLC-DOX, we used a DOX-induced mouse model of mucositis [19]. C57BL/6 female mice (6–8 weeks) were randomly divided into three groups (Figure 4A) and inoculated i.p. with free DOX (10 mg/kg), NLC-DOX (10 mg/kg) or saline solution for the Saline group (Figure 4B). Animals treated with both DOX formulations presented weight loss in the first days of mucositis induction, which was attenuated by DOX encapsulation (NLC-DOX group) (Figure 4C). However, blood in the stool or diarrhea, common features of intestinal inflammation, were not observed in either group.

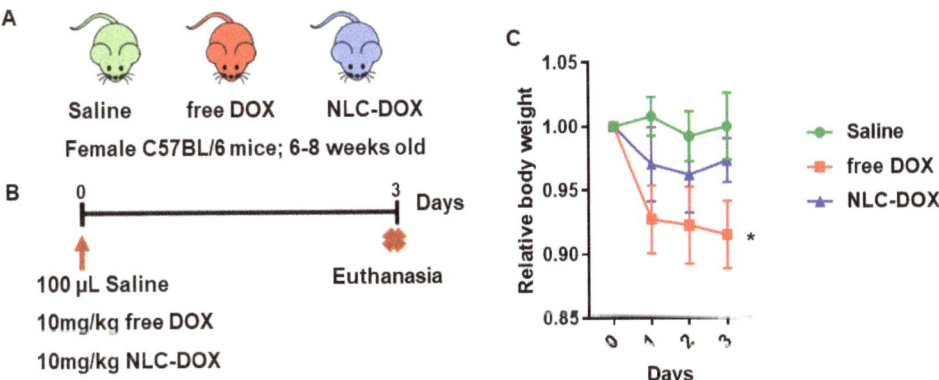

Figure 4. NLC-DOX prevents DOX-induced weight loss. (**A**) C57BL/6 mice were randomly allocated to 3 groups, Saline, free DOX and NLC-DOX (n = 5 animals/group). (**B**) Animals were injected with free DOX, NLC-DOX or saline and followed for 3 days. (**C**) Weight variation of the animals during the 3-day follow-up. The animals were weighed daily, the first weighing was performed on day zero of the protocol and the average weight per group analyzed was considered for analysis. Statistical analysis was performed by using the ANOVA test, followed by the Tukey test. * $p < 0.05$. N = 20 animals per group. Data are a pool from 4 experiments performed. Abbreviations: DOX, doxorubicin; NLC, nanostructured lipid carrier.

3.4. NLC-DOX Preserves Bowel Architecture, Prevents Mucositis-Compatible Ulcerations and Improves Intestinal Permeability

The treatment with free DOX induced changes in intestinal architecture typical of mucositis. Free DOX treated animals displayed multifocal inflammatory areas in jejune and ileum with important infiltration of mononuclear cells associated with reduced villus height, reduced crypt depth and thinning of the muscular layer (Figure 5). Ileum showed more prominent pathological changes. All of these features were improved, or even prevented, in animals treated with NLC-DOX.

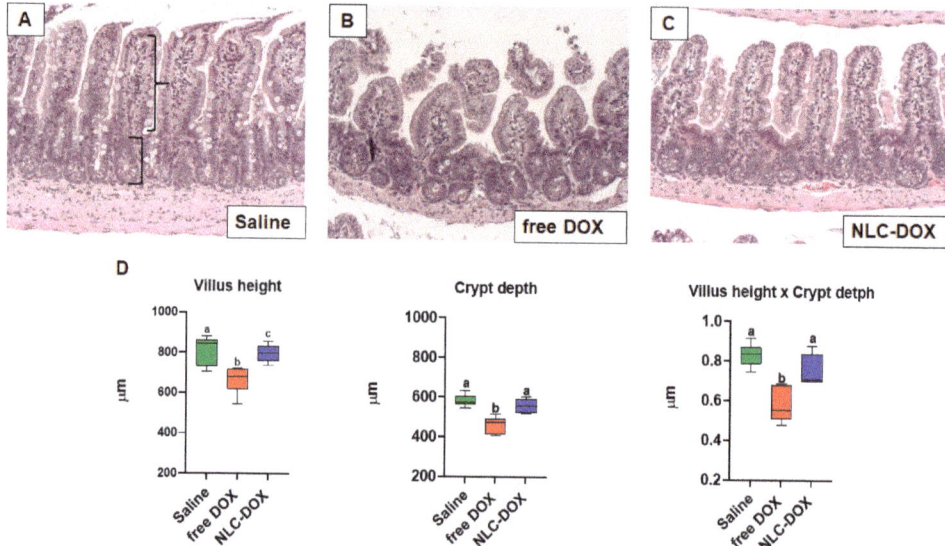

Figure 5. NLC-DOX prevented DOX-induced mucositis-associated intestinal morphological alterations. (A–C). Representative histological slides of ileum of Saline, free DOX and NLC-DOX treated animals (20× magnification). (D) Histomorphological analysis of jejune and ileum was used to quantify the height of the villus (represented by curly bracket), depth of the crypts (represented by square bracket). Statistical analysis was performed by using the ANOVA test, followed by the Tukey test. Different letters represent $p < 0.05$. N = 10 animals per group. Data are a pool from 2 experiments performed. Abbreviations: DOX, doxorubicin; NLC, nanostructured lipid carrier.

Mucositis is often associated with compromised intestinal function allowing bacteria translocation due to increased permeability. We found that associated with the inflammation and changes in intestinal architecture induced by free DOX, intestinal permeability was also increased in free DOX treated animals (Figure 6A), but totally preserved in animals treated with NLC-DOX and Saline. In addition, the maintenance of intestinal permeability in NLC-DOX was associated with increased expression of mRNA for tight junction proteins such as Occludin (Figure 6B) and ZO1 (Figure 6C) when compared to Saline or free DOX.

3.5. NLC-DOX Formulation Maintains Cytokine Expression

To gain insight about the quality of the inflammatory response triggered by DOX treatment, we evaluated signature cytokines associated with mucositis. As can be observed in Figure 7, the expression of cytokines was usually decreased in free DOX group when compared to saline group (IL-4, IL-13, TSLP and IL-9, $p < 0.05$), possibly associated to the reduced tissue viability associated to the drug cytotoxicity. However, in the group treated with NLC-DOX, the expression of cytokines was similar to the saline group, except for IL-25, a cytokine associated with intestinal protection [65], which was increased.

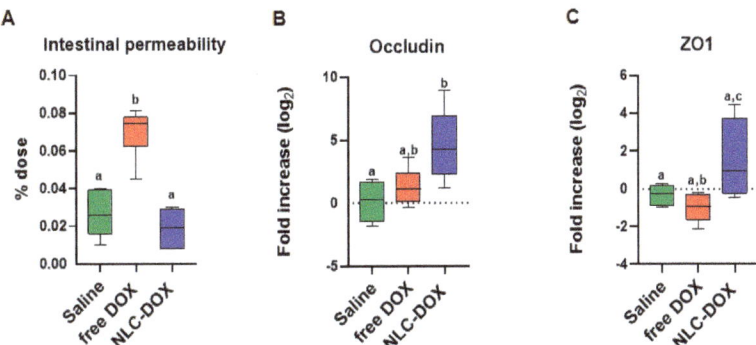

Figure 6. Intestinal permeability was preserved in NLC-DOX treatment. (**A**) Intestinal permeability by DTPA-Tc99m and mRNA expression of (**B**) Occludin and (**C**) ZO1 by real time RT-PCR in the ileum were evaluated 3 days after injection of saline, free DOX or NLC-DOX. Statistical analysis was performed by using the ANOVA test, followed by the Tukey test. Different letters represent $p < 0.05$. N = 10 animals per group. Data are a pool from 2 experiments performed. Abbreviations: DOX, doxorubicin; NLC, nanostructured lipid carrier.

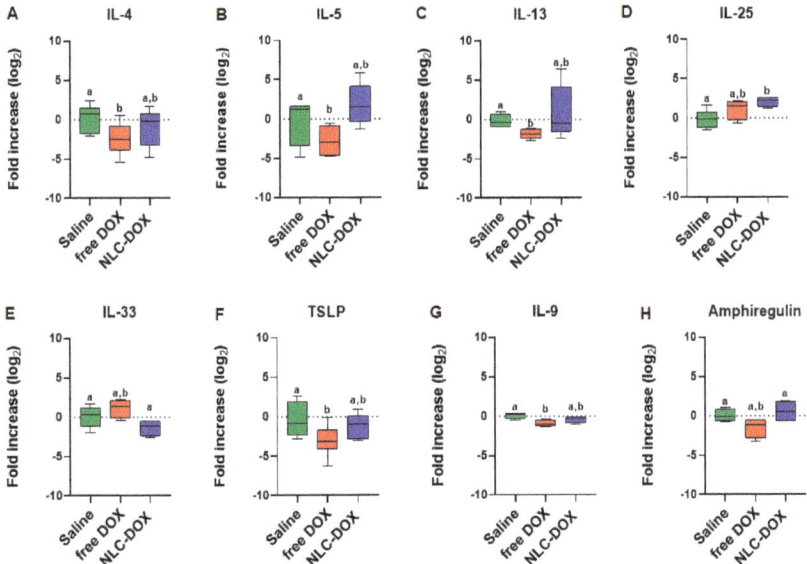

Figure 7. Cytokine expression by real time RT-PCR of (**A**) IL-4, (**B**) IL-5, (**C**) IL-13, (**D**) IL-25, (**E**) IL-33, (**F**) TSLP, (**G**) IL-9 and (**H**) Amphiregulin. Statistical analysis was performed by using the ANOVA test, followed by the Tukey test. Different letters represent $p < 0.05$. N = 15 animals per group. Data are a pool from 3 experiments performed. Abbreviations: DOX, doxorubicin; NLC, nanostructured lipid carriers.

4. Discussion

DOX is a chemotherapy drug of the anthracycline class widely used in clinical practice [66,67]. Although DOX has a relevant role in cancer therapy, its adverse effects, such as mucositis, have an important impact in the treatment and quality of life of patients [18,19]. To overcome the intense mucositis induced by DOX treatment, we proposed the loading of DOX in NLCs. This study was the first that evaluated the impact of DOX encapsulation in the lipid matrix of NLCs as a strategy to reduce mucositis.

To be used in the clinic, DOX is formulated as a hydrochloride salt, which is freely soluble in water. Therefore, its encapsulation in lipid nanocarriers is not an easy issue, being usually low [41,42]. To enhance its encapsulation in the lipid nanocarriers, the ion-pair strategy was used. Through this strategy, DOX forms an ion pair with a lipophilic anion, improving its lipophilicity and the affinity for the lipid matrix. This strategy is well described in the literature and has been used in several studies that utilized different counter ions to improve the DOX lipophilicity and its affinity for different lipid-based systems [33,41,43–56]. In the present study, OA was used as the counter ion. During the NLC production, the OA reacts with the positive electrostatic charge localized at the protonated amino nitrogen of the doxorubicin base (pKa = 9.53), forming an ion pair and improving the DOX affinity for the lipid matrix. The formation of the ion pair between OA and DOX is well described in the literature [28,51].

The developed NLC-DOX presented high encapsulation efficiency (84.8 ± 4.6%) and drug loading (55.2 ± 3.4 mg/g), minimizing the amount of soluble DOX in the external phase of the nanoparticles suspension. The obtained encapsulation efficiency (84.8 ± 4.6% EE) is in accordance with the results described by other authors (99.15–74.18% EE). However, our data concerning the drug loading (55.2 ± 3.4 mg/g) were much higher than those previously published (31 to 10.1 mg/g) [27,68–70]. Other parameters, such as morphology (spherical shape), size (66–78.8 nm), PDI (0.29 ± 0.07) and Zeta potential (−18.3 ± 5.1 mV), obtained for the developed NLC-DOX are in accordance with the literature data for parenteral formulations [27,67,68]. The negative Zeta potential can be explained by the presence of OA and non-ionic surfactants (Polysorbate 80 and Span 80) used in NLC-DOX [71,72]. The average size obtained from NTA analysis was slightly smaller (66 ± 18 nm), but very close to the average size provided for the DLS method (69.7 ± 6.6 nm). The smaller average size found for the NTA method is in accordance with the literature and corroborated the monodisperse distribution (low PDI values) measured by DLS [73,74]. Regarding the error bars of the size distribution, they are smaller with DLS, which is a consequence of the large amount of statistical data collected by this method when compared to NTA. In the NTA method, the size distributions are practically the same, but the software sometimes detects slightly more or slightly less particles between each measurement of the same sample [74].

In contrast to DLS and NTA techniques, electron microscopy—especially cryo-TEM—allows direct observation of individual NLC-DOX particles. The values obtained from TEM (76.7 ± 30 nm) and cryo-TEM (78.8 ± 28 nm) images are in a reasonable agreement with DLS and NTA analysis. Precise measurements of NLC-DOX particles from TEM and cryo-TEM images, accompanied by data provided by DLS and NTA, allowed us to obtain a more real particle size average of the developed NLC-DOX, which is a very important feature for parenteral drug delivery systems [75].

The high encapsulation efficiency and drug loading of DOX in the lipid matrix of NLCs should be the result of the intense interactions between the formulation components. In the DSC analysis, the DOX thermogram showed three endothermic melting peaks (206.8, 218.4 and 237.3 °C), which are in accordance with those described in the literature [76,77]. However, any peak of DOX was observed in the NLC-DOX thermogram, suggesting a high interaction of DOX with the lipid matrix of NLCs. This high affinity for the lipid matrix of NLCs can be the result of the ion pair formation between DOX and oleic acid (OA). The formation of an ion pair between DOX and OA has been evaluated by different authors as a strategy to improve the encapsulation efficiency of DOX in lipid nanoparticles without limiting its efficacy [27,45,78].

Another important result to note in the DSC thermogram of NLC-DOX is the characteristic endothermic peak of Compritol 888 ATO ®, the main component of the lipid matrix of the NLC-DOX. The endothermic peak of Compritol 888 ATO ® remains present in the DSC thermogram of NLC-DOX, providing evidence that the lipid matrix of NLC-DOX remains solid at room temperature. Nevertheless, this endothermic peak is broader and has a lower melting temperature (63.85 °C) when compared to the pure Compritol 888 ATO ®

(69.79 °C). The broader peak and reduction of melting temperature of the solid lipid matrix is evidence of the interactions of formulations components and liquid lipids, resulting in a less ordered lattice arrangement of solid matrix [79,80]. The reduced melting point observed for the solid lipid matrix might also be due to the nanometric size of NLC-DOX, resulting in a high surface area [81,82]. The FTIR results corroborate the data obtained in the DSC analyzes. The NLC-DOX spectrum showed bands characteristic of Compritol 888 ATO ® and some bands of DOX, but to a lesser extent. There are small differences in the absorption regions, suggesting a greater affinity between DOX and lipid matrix.

An important observation is that the developed NLC-DOX presented a controlled and sustained release of DOX during the 72 h of the study. While the free DOX released approximately 80% of DOX in the first 4 h, at the same period of time, the NLC-DOX released less than 20%. The in vitro release kinetics evaluation of NLC-DOX followed the zero-order kinetic model ($R^2 = 0.9862$). A zero-order kinetic model was also described for other authors who used NLCs to load different drug models [83,84]. However, none of them described the development of an NLC-DOX with a controlled and sustained release obeying a zero-order model. The zero-order model describes a constant release of payloads, which is ideal to achieve the desired pharmacological action with reduced side effects [64]. These controlled-release data also reflect the high encapsulation efficiency, drug loading and affinity observed in the characterization studies, suggesting that DOX is distributed throughout the solid lipid matrix of NLC. Then, the solid-lipid matrix of NLC serves as a physical barrier to the aqueous environment and the DOX it is not available to be immediately released in the receptor fluid, being released in a controlled way.

It is interesting to note that, although the encapsulation of DOX in NLC using the ion pair strategy can allow a controlled drug release at pH 7.4, it can be different in the tumor microenvironment. In other studies of our group different formulations of NLC-DOX, produced with different counter ions, showed that NLC-DOX is more efficient in reaching toxic levels of DOX in tumor cells, when compared to free DOX [33,56]. This occurs because, in the acid environment of the tumor area [85], there is an increase in the protonation of the COOH group of OA and a consequent decrease in the ion pair interaction, facilitating the release of DOX in the tumor microenvironment [71].

Considering that mucositis is one of the most serious and limiting complications of chemotherapy treatments, we aimed to evaluate if the encapsulation of DOX in an NLC matrix could provide a reduction of the mucositis process. In contrast to free DOX, NLC-DOX caused mild weight loss, one important sign of less severe mucositis [86], suggesting a more tolerable drug presentation. This can be associated with the different pattern of drug release observed for free DOX in comparison to the NLC-DOX. Since NLC-DOX provided controlled release of DOX, the impact of the drug toxicity possibly was less pronounced, allowing intestinal adjustment time.

Mucositis is characterized by villus atrophy, enterocyte damage and inflammatory cell infiltration in intestinal mucosa [6,87], which were observed in the free DOX treated group. The NLC-DOX group, on the other hand, showed preserved villus integrity and less inflammatory infiltrate compared to the free DOX group. The loss of the intestinal integrity induced by chemo and radiotherapy can increase intestinal permeability, allowing bacterial translocation and causing severe infection on the patients [88–92]. We observed that NLC-DOX treated animals showed preserved intestinal permeability. Importantly, tissue cohesion is driven by the tight junctions, proteins that promote strong cell–cell adhesion, which are important players in preserving intestinal epithelial monolayer integrity [93,94]. The NLC-DOX displayed increased expression of the two major tight junctions in the small intestine, Occludin and ZO1. We speculate that the controlled release of the drug allowed for better adjustment of the intestine to the DOX toxic mechanisms.

The expression of cytokines (inflammatory and homeostatic) associated with mucositis in the ileum of mice were also evaluated. We analyzed cytokines associated with the type 2 proinflammatory response (IL-4, IL-5, IL-13, IL-25, IL-33 and TSLP) and the cytokines involved in tissue regeneration and intestine homeostasis (IL-9 and Amphiregulin) [95,96].

Surprisingly, in the animals treated with the free DOX, an inhibition of expression of IL-4, IL-13, TSLP and IL-9 was observed in comparison to the saline group ($p < 0.05$). These results are probably associated with the intense degree of local tissue damage during the peak of tissue lesions [97]. In the animals treated with the NLC-DOX was observed the same pattern of cytokine expression in comparison to saline group ($p > 0.5$), except for IL-25 ($p < 0.05$), where a higher expression was detected. This result is in accordance with the morphology results. Since the treatment with NLC-DOX limited the mucositis process, the pattern of cytokines expression was maintained. Finally, although no difference was observed between free DOX group and NLC-DOX group for IL-9 ($p > 0.5$), a higher expression of Amphiregulin was observed for NLC-DOX group ($p < 0.05$), showing a higher ability to improve the tissue regeneration, even with a lower tissue damage. In the intestinal epithelium, cytokines such as IL-9 and Amphiregulin are involved with tissue regeneration [98–101]. Therefore, the encapsulation of DOX in NLC cannot only be able to improve the efficacy, as shown in different studies [27,67], but can also reduce the mucositis, which is an important adverse effect of DOX treatment.

5. Conclusions

The developed NLC-DOX showed spherical particles with size, PDI and Zeta potential adequate for parenteral administration, as well as high levels of DOX encapsulation and drug loading. The DSC and FTIR analyses showed a high interaction of DOX with the lipid matrix of NLC, which are in accordance with the high encapsulation and drug loading observed, resulting in a controlled drug release and, finally, preventing mucositis in the murine model. These results suggest that the developed NLC-DOX can enhance the safety of the treatment and, consequently, the quality of life of the patient.

Author Contributions: C.M.P., L.S.H., A.P.S., B.A.C. and E.B.L. conducted the experiments, analyzed the data and wrote the manuscript. G.A.C.G., H.C.S., A.A.G.F., L.A.M.F. and E.F. analyzed data and wrote the paper. All authors have read and agreed to the published version of the manuscript.

Funding: This study was financially supported by FAPEMIG (grant # APQ-00085-13), CAPES and CNPq.

Institutional Review Board Statement: The study was conducted according to the guidelines of the Declaration of Helsinki, and approved by the Ethics Committee for Animal Experimentation at the Federal University of Minas Gerais (UFMG) (Protocol n° 331/2012).

Informed Consent Statement: Not applicable.

Data Availability Statement: Data are contained within the article.

Acknowledgments: The authors would like to acknowledge the Center of Microscopy at UFMG (http://www.microscopia.ufmg.br 16/12/2020) for providing the equipment and technical support for experiments involving TEM and Cryo-TEM.

Conflicts of Interest: The authors declare no conflict of interest.

References

1. *WHO Report on Cancer: Setting Priorities, Investing Wisely and Providing Care for All*; World Health Organization: Geneva, Switzerland, 2020.
2. Liu, D.; Liu, Z.; Wang, L.; Zhang, C.; Zhang, N. Nanostructured lipid carriers as novel carrier for parenteral delivery of docetaxel. *Colloids Surf. B Biointerfaces Sci.* **2011**, *85*, 262–269. [CrossRef]
3. Fernandes, E.; Ferreira, D.; Peixoto, A.; Freitas, R.; Relvas-Santos, M.; Palmeira, C.; Martins, G.; Barros, A.; Santos, L.L.; Sarmento, B.; et al. Glycoengineered nanoparticles enhance the delivery of 5-fluoroucil and paclitaxel to gastric cancer cells of high metastatic potential. *Int. J. Pharm.* **2019**, *30*, 570. [CrossRef]
4. Awasthi, R.; Roseblade, A.; Hansbro, P.M.; Rathbone, M.J.; Dua, K.; Bebawy, M. Nanoparticles in Cancer Treatment: Opportunities and Obstacles. *Curr. Drug Targets* **2018**, *19*, 1696–1709. [CrossRef]
5. Elting, L.S.; Cooksley, C.; Chambers, M.; Cantor, S.B.; Manzullo, E.; Rubenstein, E.B. The burdens of cancer therapy. Clinical and economic outcomes of chemotherapy-induced mucositis. *Cancer* **2003**, *98*, 1531–1539. [CrossRef] [PubMed]

6. Sonis, S.T.; Elting, L.S.; Keefe, D.; Peterson, D.E.; Schubert, M.; Hauer-Jensen, M.; Bekele, B.N.; Raber-Durlacher, J.; Donnelly, J.P.; Rubenstein, E.B. Perspectives on cancer therapy-induced mucosal injury: Pathogenesis, measurement, epidemiology, and consequences for patients. *Cancer* **2004**, *100*, 1995–2025. [CrossRef] [PubMed]
7. Pulito, C.; Cristaudo, A.; La Porta, C.; Zapperi, S.; Blandino, G.; Morrone, A.; Strano, S. Oral mucositis: The hidden side of cancer therapy. *J. Exp. Clin. Cancer Res.* **2020**, *210*. [CrossRef]
8. Lai, H.C.; Yeh, Y.C.; Ting, C.T.; Lee, W.L.; Lee, H.W.; Wang, L.C.; Wang, K.Y.; Lai, H.C.; Wu, A.; Liu, T.J. Doxycycline suppresses doxorubicin-induced oxidative stress and cellular apoptosis in mouse hearts. *Eur. J. Pharmacol.* **2010**, *644*, 176–187. [CrossRef]
9. Ma, P.; Mumper, R.J. Anthracycline Nano-Delivery Systems to Overcome Multiple Drug Resistance: A Comprehensive Review. *Nano Today* **2013**, *8*, 313–331. [CrossRef] [PubMed]
10. Chaikomon, K.; Chattong, S.; Chaiya, T.; Tiwawech, D.; Sritana-Anant, Y.; Sereemaspun, A.; Manotham, K. Doxorubicin-conjugated dexamethasone induced MCF-7 apoptosis without entering the nucleus and able to overcome MDR-1-induced resistance. *Drug Des. Dev. Ther.* **2018**, *12*, 2361–2369. [CrossRef]
11. Tacar, O.; Sriamornsak, P.; Dass, C.R. Doxorubicin: An update on anticancer molecular action, toxicity and novel drug delivery systems. *J. Pharm. Pharmacol.* **2013**, *65*, 157–170. [CrossRef]
12. Goto, S.; Ihara, Y.; Urata, Y.; Izumi, S.; Abe, K.; Koji, T.; Kondo, T. Doxorubicin-induced DNA intercalation and scavenging by nuclear glutathione S-transferase π. *FASEB J.* **2001**, *15*, 2702–2714. [CrossRef] [PubMed]
13. Bodley, A.; Liu, L.F.; Israel, M.; Seshadri, R.; Koseki, Y.; Giuliani, F.C.; Kirschenbaum, S.; Silber, R.; Potmesil, M. DNA Topoisomerase II-mediated Interaction of Doxorubicin and Daunorubicin Congeners with DNA. *Cancer Res.* **1989**, *49*, 5969–5978.
14. Asensio-López, M.C.; Soler, F.; Sánchez-Más, J.; Pascual-Figal, D.; Fernández-Belda, F.; Lax, A. Early oxidative damage induced by doxorubicin: Source of production, protection by GKT137831 and effect on Ca2+ transporters in HL-1 cardiomyocytes. *Arch. Biochem. Biophys.* **2016**, *594*, 26–36. [CrossRef]
15. McCullough, R.W. US oncology-wide incidence, duration, costs and deaths from chemoradiation mucositis and antimucositis therapy benefits. *Future Oncol.* **2017**, *13*, 2823–2852. [CrossRef]
16. Lipshultz, S.E.; Cochran, T.R.; Franco, V.I.; Miller, T.L. Treatment-related cardiotoxicity in survivors of childhood cancer. *Nat. Rev. Clin. Oncol.* **2013**, *10*, 697–710. [CrossRef] [PubMed]
17. Shi, Y.; Moon, M.; Dawood, S.; McManus, B.; Liu, P.P. Mechanisms and management of doxorubicin cardiotoxicity. *Herz* **2011**, *36*, 296–305. [CrossRef] [PubMed]
18. Raber-Durlacher, J.E.; Weijl, N.I.; Abu Saris, M.; de Koning, B.; Zwinderman, A.H.; Osanto, S. Oral mucositis in patients treated with chemotherapy for solid tumors: A retrospective analysis of 150 cases. *Support Care Cancer* **2000**, *8*, 366–371. [CrossRef]
19. Kaczmarek, A.; Brinkman, B.M.; Heyndrickx, L.; Vandenabeele, P.; Krysko, D.V. Severity of doxorubicin-induced small intestinal mucositis is regulated by the TLR-2 and TLR-9 pathways. *J. Pathol.* **2012**, *226*, 598–608. [CrossRef]
20. Elad, S.; Cheng, K.K.F.; Lalla, R.V.; Yarom, N.; Hong, C.; Logan, R.M.; Bowen, J.; Gibson, R.; Saunders, D.P.; Zadik, Y.; et al. MASCC/ISOO clinical practice guidelines for the management of mucositis secondary to cancer therapy. *Cancer* **2020**. [CrossRef]
21. Kucharczyk, K.; Florczak, A.; Deptuch, T.; Penderecka, K.; Jastrzebska, K.; Mackiewicz, A.; Dams-Kozlowska, H. Drug affinity and targeted delivery: Double functionalization of silk spheres for controlled doxorubicin delivery into Her2-positive cancer cells. *J. Nanobiotechnol.* **2020**, *18*, 56. [CrossRef] [PubMed]
22. Li, J.; Li, X.; Liu, P. Doxorubicin-doxorubicin conjugate prodrug as drug self-delivery system for intracellular pH-riggered slow release. *Colloids Surf. B Biointerfaces* **2020**, *1*, 185. [CrossRef]
23. Oladipo, A.O.; Nkambule, T.T.I.; Mamba, B.B.; Msagati, T.A.M. The stimuli-responsive properties of doxorubicin adsorbed onto bimetallic Au@Pd nanodendrites and its potential application as drug delivery platform. *Mater. Sci. Eng. C* **2020**, *110*, 110696. [CrossRef]
24. Wang, C.; Qi, P.; Lu, Y.; Liu, L.; Zhang, Y.; Sheng, Q.; Wang, T.; Zhang, M.; Wang, R.; Song, S. Bicomponent polymeric micelles for pH-controlled delivery of doxorubicin. *Drug Deliv.* **2020**, *27*, 344–357. [CrossRef]
25. Sedlacek, O.; Driessche, A.V.; Uvyn, A.; Geest, B.G.D.; Hoogenboom, R. Poly(2-methyl-2-oxazoline) conjugates with doxorubicin: From synthesis of high drug loading water-soluble constructs to in vitro anti-cancer properties. *J. Control. Release* **2020**, *326*, 53–62. [CrossRef]
26. Fraix, A.; Conte, C.; Gazzano, E.; Riganti, C.; Quaglia, F.; Sortino, S. Overcoming Doxorubicin Resistance with Lipid-Polymer Hybrid Nanoparticles Photoreleasing Nitric Oxide. *Mol. Pharm.* **2020**, *17*, 2135–2144. [CrossRef] [PubMed]
27. Mussi, S.V.; Sawant, R.; Perche, F.; Oliveira, M.C.; Azevedo, R.B.; Ferreira, L.A.M.; Torchilin, V.P. Novel Nanostructured Lipid Carrier Co-Loaded with Doxorubicin and Docosahexaenoic Acid Demonstrates Enhanced in Vitro Activity and Overcomes Drug Resistance in MCF-7/Adr Cells. *Pharm. Res.* **2014**, *31*, 1882–1892. [CrossRef] [PubMed]
28. Zhao, S.; Minh, L.V.; Li, N.; Garamus, V.M.; Handge, U.A.; Liu, J.; Zou, A. Doxorubicin hydrochloride-oleic acid conjugate loaded nanostructured lipid carriers for tumor specific drug release. *Colloids Surf. B Biointerfaces* **2016**, *145*, 95–103. [CrossRef] [PubMed]
29. Popilski, H.; Feinshtein, V.; Kleiman, S.; Mattarei, A.; Garofalo, M.; Salmaso, S.; Stepensky, D. Doxorubicin liposomes cell penetration enhancement and its potential drawbacks for the tumor targeting efficiency. *Int. J. Pharm.* **2021**, *592*, 120012. [CrossRef] [PubMed]
30. Makwana, V.; Karanjia, J.; Haselhorst, T.; Anoopkumar-Dukie, S.; Rudrawar, S. Liposomal doxorubicin as targeted delivery platform: Current trends in surface functionalization. *Int. J. Pharm.* **2021**, *593*, 120117. [CrossRef]

31. Perez, A.T.; Domenech, G.H.; Frankel, C.; Vogel, C.L. Pegylated liposomal doxorubicin (Doxil) for metastatic breast cancer: The Cancer Research Network, Inc., experience. *Cancer Investig.* **2002**, *20*, 22–29. [CrossRef]
32. Leonard, R.C.F.; Williams, S.; Tulpule, A.; Levine, A.M.; Oliveros, S. Improving the therapeutic index of anthracycline chemotherapy: Focus on liposomal doxorubicin (Myocet™). *Breast* **2009**, *18*, 218–224. [CrossRef]
33. Lages, E.B.; Fernandes, R.S.; Silva, J.O.; de Souza, Â.M.; Cassali, G.D.; de Barros, A.L.B.; Ferreira, L.A.M. Co-delivery of doxorubicin, docosahexaenoic acid, and α-tocopherol succinate by nanostructured lipid carriers has a synergistic effect to enhance antitumor activity and reduce toxicity. *Biomed. Pharmacother.* **2020**, *132*, 110876. [CrossRef] [PubMed]
34. Dingler, A.; Gohla, S. Production of solid lipid nanoparticles (SLN): Scaling up feasibilities. *J. Microencapsul.* **2002**, *19*, 11–16. [CrossRef] [PubMed]
35. Mu, H.; Holm, R. Solid lipid nanocarriers in drug delivery: Characterization and design. *Expert Opin Drug Deliv.* **2018**, *15*, 771–785. [CrossRef]
36. Haider, M.; Abdin, S.M.; Kamal, L.; Orive, G. Nanostructured Lipid Carriers for Delivery of Chemotherapeutics: A Review. *Pharmaceutics* **2020**, *12*, 288. [CrossRef] [PubMed]
37. Shidhaye, S.S.; Vaidya, R.; Sutar, S.; Patwardhan, A.; Kadam, V.J. Solid lipid nanoparticles and nanostructured lipid carriers–innovative generations of solid lipid carriers. *Curr. Drug Deliv.* **2008**, *5*, 324–331. [CrossRef] [PubMed]
38. Müller, R.H.; Radtke, M.; Wissing, S.A. Solid lipid nanoparticles (SLN) and nanostructured lipid carriers (NLC) in cosmetic and dermatological preparations. *Adv. Drug Deliv. Rev.* **2002**, 131–155. [CrossRef]
39. Wu, M.; Fan, Y.; Lv, S.; Xiao, B.; Ye, M.; Zhu, X. Vincristine and temozolomide combined chemotherapy for the treatment of glioma: A comparison of solid lipid nanoparticles and nanostructured lipid carriers for dual drugs delivery. *Drug Deliv.* **2016**, *23*, 2720–2725. [CrossRef]
40. Zhang, J.; Xiao, X.; Zhu, J.; Gao, Z. Lactoferrin- and RGD-comodified, temozolomide and vincristine-coloaded nanostructured lipid carriers for gliomatosis cerebri combination therapy. *Int. J. Nanomed.* **2018**, *13*, 303. [CrossRef]
41. Mussi, S.V.; Silva, R.C.; Oliveira, M.C.; Lucci, C.M.; Azevedo, R.B.; Ferreira, L.A. New approach to improve encapsulation and antitumor activity of doxorubicin loaded in solid lipid nanoparticles. *Eur. J. Pharm. Sci.* **2013**, *23*, 282–290. [CrossRef]
42. Fulop, Z.; Gref, R.; Loftsson, T. A permeation method for detection of self-aggregation of doxorubicin in aqueous environment. *Int. J. Pharm.* **2013**, *15*, 559–561. [CrossRef] [PubMed]
43. Battaglia, L.; Gallarate, M.; Peira, E.; Chirio, D.; Muntoni, E.; Biasibetti, E.; Capucchio, M.T.; Valazza, A.; Panciani, P.P.; Lanotte, M.; et al. Solid lipid nanoparticles for potential doxorubicin delivery in glioblastoma treatment: Preliminary in vitro studies. *J. Pharm. Sci.* **2014**, *103*, 2157–2165. [CrossRef] [PubMed]
44. Ma, P.; Dong, X.; Swadley, C.L.; Gupte, A.; Leggas, M.; Ledebur, H.C.; Mumper, R.J. Development of idarubicin and doxorubicin solid lipid nanoparticles to overcome Pgp-mediated multiple drug resistance in leukemia. *J. Biomed. Nanotechnol.* **2009**, *5*, 151–161. [CrossRef]
45. Oliveira, M.S.; Mussi, S.V.; Gomes, D.A.; Yoshida, M.I.; Frezard, F.; Carregal, V.M.; Ferreira, L.A.M. α-Tocopherol Succinate Improves Encapsulation and Anticancer Activity of Doxorubicin Loaded in Solid Lipid Nanoparticles. *Colloids Surf. B Biointerfaces Sci.* **2016**, *140*, 246–253. [CrossRef]
46. Subedi, R.K.; Kang, K.W.; Choi, H.K. Preparation and characterization of solid lipid nanoparticles loaded with doxorubicin. *Eur. J. Pharm. Sci.* **2009**, *37*, 508–513. [CrossRef]
47. Miglietta, A.; Cavalli, R.; Bocca, C.; Ludovica, G.; Gasco, M.R. Cellular uptake and cytotoxicity of solid lipid nanospheres (SLN) incorporating doxorubicin or paclitaxel. *Int. J. Pharm.* **2000**, *210*, 61–67. [CrossRef]
48. Zara, G.P.; Cavalli, R.; Bargoni, A.; Fundarò, A.; Vightto, D.; Gasco, M.R. Intravenous administration to rabbits of non-stealth and stealth doxorubicin-loaded solid lipid nanoparticles at increasing concentrations of stealth agent: Pharmacokinetics and distribution of doxorubicin in brain and other tissues. *J. Drug Target* **2002**, *10*, 327–335. [CrossRef]
49. Steiniger, S.C.; Kreuter, J.; Khalansky, A.S.; Sckidan, I.N.; Bobruskin, A.I.; Smirnova, Z.S.; Severin, S.E.; UHL, R.; Kock, M.; Geiger, K.D.; et al. Chemotherapy of glioblastoma in rats using doxorubicin-loaded nanoparticles. *Int. J. Cancer* **2004**, *109*, 759–767. [CrossRef]
50. Wong, H.L.; Rauth, A.M.; Bendayan, R.; Manias, J.L.; Ramaswamy, M.; Liu, Z.; Erhan, S.Z.; Wu, X.Y. A new polymer-lipid hybrid nanoparticle system increases cytotoxicity of doxorubicin against multidrug-resistant human breast cancer cells. *Pharm. Res.* **2006**, *23*, 1574–1585. [CrossRef]
51. Zhang, X.; Sun, X.; Li, J.; Zhang, X.; Gong, T.; Zhang, Z. Lipid nanoemulsions loaded with doxorubicin-oleic acid ionic complex: Characterization, in vitro and in vivo studies. *Pharmazie* **2011**, *66*, 496–505. [PubMed]
52. Siddiqui, A.; Gupta, V.; Liu, Y.Y.; Nazzal, S. Doxorubicin and MBO-asGCS oligonucleotide loaded lipid nanoparticles overcome multidrug resistance in adriamycin resistant ovarian cancer cells (NCI/ADR-RES). *Int. J. Pharm.* **2012**, *431*, 222–229. [CrossRef] [PubMed]
53. Chen, H.H.; Huang, W.C.; Chiang, W.H.; Liu, T.I.; Shen, M.Y.; Hsu, Y.H.; Lin, S.C.; Chiu, H.C. pH-Responsive therapeutic solid lipid nanoparticles for reducing P-glycoprotein-mediated drug efflux of multidrug resistant cancer cells. *Int. J. Nanomed.* **2015**, *10*, 5035–5048. [CrossRef]
54. Colas, S.; Maheo, K.; Denis, F.; Goupille, C.; Hoinard, C.; Champeroux, P.; Tranquart, F.; Bougnoux, P. Sensitization by dietary docosahexaenoic acid of rat mammary carcinoma to anthracycline: A role for tumor vascularization. *Clin. Cancer Res.* **2006**, *19*, 5879–5886. [CrossRef] [PubMed]

55. Fundaro, A.; Cavalli, R.; Bargoni, A.; Vighetto, D.; Zara, G.P.; Gasco, M.R. Non-stealth and stealth solid lipid nanoparticles (SLN) carrying doxorubicin: Pharmacokinetics and tissue distribution after i.v. administration to rats. *Pharmacol. Res.* **2000**, *42*, 337–343. [CrossRef]
56. Borges, G.S.M.; Silva, J.O.; Fernandes, R.S.; de Souza, Â.M.; Cassali, G.D.; Yoshida, M.I.; Leite, E.A.; de Barros, A.L.B.; Ferreira, L.A.M. Sclareol is a potent enhancer of doxorubicin: Evaluation of the free combination and co-loaded nanostructured lipid carriers against breast cancer. *Life Sci.* **2019**, *232*, 116678. [CrossRef]
57. Dash, S.; Murthy, P.N.; Nath, L.; Chowdhury, P. Kinetic modeling on drug release from controlled drug delivery systems. *Acta Pol. Pharm.* **2010**, *67*, 217–223. [PubMed]
58. Lu, T.; Ten Hagen, T.L.M. Inhomogeneous crystal grain formation in DPPC-DSPC based thermosensitive liposomes determines content release kinetics. *J. Control. Release* **2017**, *247*, 64–72. [CrossRef]
59. Santos, R.G.C.; Viana, M.L.; Generoso, S.V.; Arantes, R.E.; Correia, M.I.T.D.; Cardoso, V.N. Glutamine supplementation decreases intestinal permeability and preserves gut mucosa integrity in an experimental mouse model. *J. Parenter. Enter. Nutr.* **2010**, *34*, 408–413. [CrossRef]
60. Rudra, A.; Deepa, R.M.; Ghosh, M.K.; Ghosh, S.; Mukherjee, B. Doxorubicin-loaded phosphatidylethanolamine-conjugated nanoliposomes: In Vitro characterization and their accumulation in liver, kidneys, and lungs in rats. *Int. J. Nanomed.* **2010**, *5*, 811–823. [CrossRef]
61. Li, S.; Ma, Y.; Yue, X.; Cao, Z.; Dai, Z. One-pot construction of doxorubicin conjugated magnetic silica nanoparticles. *New J. Chem.* **2009**, *33*, 2414. [CrossRef]
62. Shah, B.M.; Khunt, D.; Bhatt, H.; Misra, M.; Padh, H. Intranasal delivery of venlafaxine loaded nanostructured lipid carrier: Risk assessment and QbD based optimization. *J. Drug Deliv. Sci. Technol.* **2016**, *33*, 37–50. [CrossRef]
63. Kallakunta, V.R.; Tiwari, R.; Sarabu, S.; Bandari, S.; Repka, M.A. Effect of formulation and process variables on lipid based sustained release tablets via continuous twin screw granulation: A comparative study. *Eur. J. Pharm. Sci. Off. J. Eur. Fed. Pharm. Sci.* **2018**, *121*, 126–138. [CrossRef] [PubMed]
64. Costa, P.; Sousa Lobo, J.M. Modeling and comparison of dissolution profiles. *Eur. J. Pharm. Sci.* **2001**, *13*, 123–133. [CrossRef]
65. Von Moltke, J.; Ji, M.; Liang, H.E.; Locksley, R.M. Tuft-cell-derived IL-25 regulates an intestinal ILC2-epithelial response circuit. *Nature* **2016**, *529*, 221–225. [CrossRef]
66. Pallerla, S.; Gauthier, T.; Sable, R.; Jois, S.D. Design of a doxorubicin-peptidomimetic conjugate that targets HER2-positive cancer cells. *Eur. J. Med. Chem.* **2017**, *125*, 914–924. [CrossRef] [PubMed]
67. Fernandes, R.S.; Silva, J.O.; Mussi, S.V.; Lopes, S.C.A.; Leite, E.A.; Cassali, G.D.; Cardoso, V.N.; Townsend, D.M.; Colletti, P.M.; Ferreira, L.A.M.; et al. Nanostructured Lipid Carrier Co-loaded with Doxorubicin and Docosahexaenoic Acid as a Theranostic Agent: Evaluation of Biodistribution and Antitumor Activity in Experimental Model. *Mol. Imaging Biol.* **2018**, *20*, 437–447. [CrossRef]
68. Ni, S.; Qiu, L.; Zhang, G.; Zhou, H.; Han, Y. Lymph cancer chemotherapy: Delivery of doxorubicin-gemcitabine prodrug and vincristine by nanostructured lipid carriers. *Int. J. Nanomed.* **2017**, *12*, 1565–1576. [CrossRef]
69. Tripathi, C.B.; Parashar, P.; Arya, M. Biotin anchored nanostructured lipid carriers for targeted delivery of doxorubicin in management of mammary gland carcinoma through regulation of apoptotic modulator. *J. Liposome Res.* **2020**, *30*, 21–36. [CrossRef]
70. Wang, Y.; Zhang, H.; Hao, J.; Li, B.; Li, M.; Xiuwen, W. Lung cancer combination therapy: Co-delivery of paclitaxel and doxorubicin by nanostructured lipid carriers for synergistic effect. *Drug Deliv.* **2016**, *23*, 1398–1403. [CrossRef]
71. Oliveira, M.S.; Lima, B.H.S.; Goulart, G.A.C.; Mussi, S.V.; Borges, G.S.M.; Oréfice, R.L.; Ferreira, L.A.M. Improved Cytotoxic Effect of Doxorubicin by Its Combination with Sclareol in Solid Lipid Nanoparticle Suspension. *J. Nanosci. Nanotechnol.* **2018**, *18*, 5609–5616. [CrossRef]
72. Singh, S.; Lohani, A.; Mishra, A.K.; Verma, A. Formulation and evaluation of carrot seed oil-based cosmetic emulsions. *J. Cosmet. Laser Ther.* **2018**, 1–9. [CrossRef]
73. Guilherme, V.A.; Ribeiro, L.N.M.; Alcântara, A.C.S.; Castro, S.R.; da Silva, G.H.R.; da Silva, C.G.; Breitkreitz, M.C.; Clemente-Napimoga, J.; Macedo, C.G.; Abdalla, H.B.; et al. Improved efficacy of naproxen-loaded NLC for temporomandibular joint administration. *Sci. Rep.* **2019**, *9*, 11160. [CrossRef]
74. Filipe, V.; Hawe, A.; Jiskoot, W. Critical evaluation of Nanoparticle Tracking Analysis (NTA) by NanoSight for the measurement of nanoparticles and protein aggregates. *Pharm. Res.* **2010**, *27*, 796–810. [CrossRef]
75. Danaei, M.; Dehghankhold, M.; Ataei, S.; Hasanzadeh Davarani, F.; Javanmard, R.; Dokhani, A.; Khorasani, S.; Mozafar, M.R. Impact of Particle Size and Polydispersity Index on the Clinical Applications of Lipidic Nanocarrier Systems. *Pharmaceutics* **2018**, *10*, 57. [CrossRef]
76. Gao, L.; Li, Q.; Zhang, J.; Huang, Y.; Deng, L.; Li, C.; Tai, G.; Ruan, B. Local penetration of doxorubicin via intrahepatic implantation of PLGA based doxorubicin-loaded implants. *Drug Deliv.* **2019**, *26*, 1049–1057. [CrossRef] [PubMed]
77. Tahir, N.; Madni, A.; Correia, A.; Rehman, M.; Balasubramanian, V.; Khan, M.M.; Santos, H.A. Lipid-polymer hybrid nanoparticles for controlled delivery of hydrophilic and lipophilic doxorubicin for breast cancer therapy. *Int. J. Nanomed.* **2019**, 4961–4974. [CrossRef] [PubMed]
78. Li, X.; Jia, X.; Niu, H. Nanostructured lipid carriers co-delivering lapachone and doxorubicin for overcoming multidrug resistance in breast cancer therapy. *Int. J. Nanomed.* **2018**, *13*, 4107–4119. [CrossRef] [PubMed]

79. Jenning, V.; Mäder, K.; Gohla, S.H. Solid lipid nanoparticles (SLN) based on binary mixtures of liquid and solid lipids: A (1)H-NMR study. *Int. J. Pharm.* **2000**, *205*, 15–21. [CrossRef]
80. Castelli, F.; Puglia, C.; Sarpietro, M.G.; Rizza, L.; Bonina, F. Characterization of indomethacin-loaded lipid nanoparticles by differential scanning calorimetry. *Int. J. Pharm.* **2005**, *304*, 231–238. [CrossRef] [PubMed]
81. Sakai, H. Surface-induced melting of small particles. *Surf. Sci.* **1996**, *351*, 285–291. [CrossRef]
82. Antoniammal, P.; Arivuoli, D. Size and Shape Dependence on Melting Temperature of Gallium Nitride Nanoparticles. *J. Nanomater.* **2012**, *2012*, 11. [CrossRef]
83. Rahman, H.S.; Rasedee, A.; How, C.W.; Abdul, A.B.; Zeenathul, N.A.; Hemn, H.O.; Saeed, M.I.; Yeap, S.K. Zerumbone-loaded nanostructured lipid carriers: Preparation, characterization, and antileukemic effect. *Int. J. Nanomed.* **2013**, *8*, 2769–2781. [CrossRef]
84. Shah, N.V.; Seth, A.K.; Balaraman, R.; Aundhia, C.J.; Maheshwari, R.A.; Parmar, G.R. Nanostructured lipid carriers for oral bioavailability enhancement of raloxifene: Design and in vivo study. *J. Adv. Res.* **2016**, *7*, 423–434. [CrossRef]
85. Trédan, O.; Galmarini, C.M.; Patel, K.; Tannock, I.F. Drug resistance and the solid tumor microenvironment. *J. Natl. Cancer Inst.* **2007**, *99*, 1441–1454. [CrossRef]
86. Meirovitz, A.; Kuten, M.; Billan, S.; Abdah-Bortnyak, R.; Sharon, A.; Peretz, T.; Sela, M.; Schaffer, M.; Barak, V. Cytokines levels, Severity of acute mucositis and the need of PEG tube installation during chemo-radiation for head and neck cancer—A prospective pilot study. *Radiat. Oncol.* **2010**, *16*. [CrossRef]
87. Lee, C.S.; Ryan, E.J.; Doherty, G.A. Gastro-intestinal toxicity of chemotherapeutics in colorectal cancer: The role of inflammation. *World J. Gastroenterol.* **2014**, *20*, 3751–3761. [CrossRef]
88. Thomsen, M.; Vitetta, L. Adjunctive Treatments for the Prevention of Chemotherapy- and Radiotherapy-Induced Mucositis. *Integrative Cancer Therapies* **2018**, *17*, 1027–1047. [CrossRef] [PubMed]
89. Segers, C.; Mysara, M.; Claesen, J.; Baatout, S.; Leys, N.; Lebeer, S.; Verslegers, M.; Mastroleo, F. Intestinal mucositis precedes dysbiosis in a mouse model for pelvic irradiation. *ISME Commun.* **2021**, *1*, 24. [CrossRef]
90. de Barros, P.A.V.; Andrade, M.E.R.; Generoso, S.d.V.; Miranda, S.E.M.; dos Reis, D.C.; Leocádio, P.C.L.; de Sales E Souza, E.L.; Martins, F.d.S.; da Gama, M.A.S.; Cassali, G.D.; et al. Conjugated linoleic acid prevents damage caused by intestinal mucositis induced by 5-fluorouracil in an experimental model. *Biomed. Pharmacother.* **2018**, *103*, 1567–1576. [CrossRef] [PubMed]
91. van Vliet, M.J.; Harmsen, H.J.M.; de Bont, E.S.J.M.; Tissing, W.J.E. The Role of Intestinal Microbiota in the Development and Severity of Chemotherapy-Induced Mucositis. *PLoS Pathog.* **2010**, *6*, 5. [CrossRef] [PubMed]
92. Tulkens, J.; Vergauwen, G.; Van Deun, J.; Geeurickx, E.; Dhondt, B.; Lippens, L.; Scheerder, M.A.; Miinalainen, I.; Rappu, P.; Geest, B.G.; et al. Increased levels of systemic LPS-positive bacterial extracellular vesicles in patients with intestinal barrier dysfunction. *Gut* **2018**, *69*, 191–193. [CrossRef]
93. Groschwitz, K.R.; Hogan, S.P. Intestinal barrier function: Molecular regulation and disease pathogenesis, *J. Allergy Clin. Immunol.* **2009**, *124*, 3–20. [CrossRef]
94. Wu, T.K.; Lim, P.S.; Jin, J.S.; Wu, M.Y.; Chen, C.H. Impaired Gut Epithelial Tight Junction Expression in Hemodialysis Patients Complicated with Intradialytic Hypotension. *BioMed Res. Int.* **2018**, *2018*, 2670312. [CrossRef]
95. Licona-Limón, P.; Henao-Mejia, J.; Temann, A.U.; Gagliani, N.; Licona-Limón, I.; Ishigame, H.; Hao, L.; Herbert, D.B.R.; Flavell, R.A. Th9 Cells Drive Host Immunity against Gastrointestinal Worm Infection. *Immunity* **2013**, *39*, 744–757. [CrossRef]
96. Wynn, T. Type 2 cytokines: Mechanisms and therapeutic strategies. *Nat. Rev. Immunol.* **2015**, *15*, 271–282. [CrossRef]
97. Sonis, S.T. Pathobiology of mucositis. *Semin. Oncol. Nurs.* **2004**, *20*, 11–15. [CrossRef]
98. Zaiss, D.M.W.; Gause, W.C.; Osborne, L.C.; Artis, D. Emerging Functions of Amphiregulin in Orchestrating Immunity, Inflammation, and Tissue Repair. *Immunity* **2015**, *42*, 216–226. [CrossRef] [PubMed]
99. Turner, J.E.; Morrison, P.J.; Wilhelm, C.; Wilson, M.; Ahlfors, H.; Renauld, J.C.; Panzer, U.; Helmby, H.; Stockinger, B. IL-9-mediated survival of type 2 innate lymphoid cells promotes damage control in helminth-induced lung inflammation. *J. Exp. Med.* **2013**, *210*, 2951–2965. [CrossRef] [PubMed]
100. Chen, F.; Liu, Z.; Wu, W.; Rozo, C.; Bowdridge, S.; Millman, A.; Rooijen, N.V.; Urban, J.F., Jr.; Wynn, T.A.; Gause, W.C. An essential role for TH2-type responses in limiting acute tissue damage during experimental helminth infection. *Nat. Med.* **2012**, *18*, 260–266. [CrossRef] [PubMed]
101. Monticelli, L.A.; Osborne, L.C.; Noti, M.; Tran, S.V.; Zaiss, D.M.W.; Artis, D. IL-33 promotes an innate immune pathway of intestinal tissue protection dependent on amphiregulin–EGFR interactions. *Proc. Natl. Acad. Sci. USA* **2015**, *112*, 10762–10767. [CrossRef]

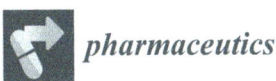

Article

Oligoarginine Peptide Conjugated to BSA Improves Cell Penetration of Gold Nanorods and Nanoprisms for Biomedical Applications

Karen Bolaños [1,2,3,*], Macarena Sánchez-Navarro [4], Andreas Tapia-Arellano [1,3], Ernest Giralt [4,5], Marcelo J. Kogan [1,3,*] and Eyleen Araya [3,6,*]

1. Departamento de Química Farmacológica y Toxicológica, Facultad de Ciencias Químicas y Farmacéuticas, Universidad de Chile, Santiago 8380494, Chile; atare_28@ciq.uchile.cl
2. Laboratorio de Comunicaciones Celulares, Centro de Estudios en Ejercicio, Metabolismo y Cancer (CEMC), Santiago 8380453, Chile
3. Advanced Center of Chronic Diseases (ACCDis), Santiago 8380494, Chile
4. Institute for Research in Biomedicine (IRB Barcelona), The Barcelona Institute of Science and Technology, Baldiri Reixac 10, 08028 Barcelona, Spain; macarena.sanchez@ipb.csic.es (M.S.-N.); ernest.giralt@irbbarcelona.org (E.G.)
5. Department of Inorganic and Organic Chemistry, University of Barcelona, Martí i Franquè s 1–11, 08028 Barcelona, Spain
6. Departamento de Ciencias Quimicas, Facultad de Ciencias Exactas, Universidad Andres Bello, Santiago 8370146, Chile
* Correspondence: k.bolaosjimenez@uandresbello.edu (K.B.); mkogan@ciq.uchile.cl (M.J.K.); eyleen.araya@unab.cl (E.A.)

Abstract: Gold nanoparticles (AuNPs) have been shown to be outstanding tools for drug delivery and biomedical applications, mainly owing to their colloidal stability, surface chemistry, and photothermal properties. The biocompatibility and stability of nanoparticles can be improved by capping the nanoparticles with endogenous proteins, such as albumin. Notably, protein coating of nanoparticles can interfere with and decrease their cell penetration. Therefore, in the present study, we functionalized albumin with the r_8 peptide (All-D, octaarginine) and used it for coating NIR-plasmonic anisotropic gold nanoparticles. Gold nanoprisms (AuNPrs) and gold nanorods (AuNRs) were coated with bovine serum albumin (BSA) previously functionalized using a cell penetrating peptide (CPP) with the r_8 sequence (BSA-r_8). The effect of the coated and r_8-functionalized AuNPs on HeLa cell viability was assessed by the MTS assay, showing a low effect on cell viability after BSA coating. Moreover, the internalization of the nanostructures into HeLa cells was assessed by confocal microscopy and transmission electron microscopy (TEM). As a result, both nanoconstructs showed an improved internalization level after being capped with BSA-r_8, in contrast to the BSA-functionalized control, suggesting the predominant role of CPP functionalization in cell internalization. Thus, our results validate both novel nanoconstructs as potential candidates to be coated by endogenous proteins and functionalized with a CPP to optimize cell internalization. In a further approach, coating AuNPs with CPP-functionalized BSA can broaden the possibilities for biomedical applications by combining their optical properties, biocompatibility, and cell-penetration abilities.

Keywords: cell internalization; albumin; BSA; CPP; gold nanorods; gold nanoprisms; arginine-rich peptide

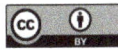

1. Introduction

Research on nanomaterials has expanded in recent years for their use in drug delivery, imaging, therapy, diagnosis, and combined therapy, among other fields [1–5]. Organic, inorganic, biological-type, or hybrids between different structures have been proposed for diverse medical/biomedical applications [6–14]. Among the prospective materials for future applications, gold nanoparticles stand out, owing to their wide-ranging potential.

AuNPs have characteristic optical properties that are derived from their localized surface plasmon resonance (LSPR), allowing them to interact with light in a different way than bulk materials do [10,15,16]. The plasmon excitation has two main decay mechanisms: radiative and non-radiative, resulting in light scattering and absorption, respectively [17]. Light scattering of AuNPs has been extensively used to design diagnostic tools, contrast agents, and Raman enhancement probes [18–20]. Conversely, absorption of light involves relaxation via electron-electron collisions or electron-lattice-phonon couplings, yielding light-to-heat conversion, [21] referred to as the photothermal effect, which can be used for drug release and photodynamic and photothermal therapy [22].

Both LSPR and the optical properties of AuNPs are highly shape- and size-dependent. In this regard, AuNRs and AuNPrs are two interesting AuNP geometries because their light absorption can be synthetically modulated. Therefore, their maximum absorption can be tuned to the biological window (the region that exhibits minimum light absorption of the biological tissues) [23–26], with a strong optical extinction and for photothermal applications [17,27].

Given the wide range of applications for AuNPs as biomedical platforms, it is essential to consider the biocompatibility of this material. AuNPrs (synthesized by sodium thiosulfate reduction) have been shown to be non-cytotoxic [28,29]. In contrast, AuNRs are commonly synthesized using the CTAB surfactant, which has shown some cytotoxic effects [30–32].

In order to avoid possible cytotoxic effects from our nanocarriers, we incorporated a protein coating on both AuNPs to increase their biocompatibility and stability [6,29,33–36]. BSA shares 76% sequence identity with human serum albumin (HSA) [37] and is well tolerated by humans [38]. This protein has been extensively used for the development of nanomaterials for biomedical applications in drug delivery, therapy (photothermal or combined), diagnosis, and theranostics [39–45].

Even though the presence of proteins as a coating on the nanoparticle's surface improves their biocompatibility and stability properties, it may also limit their internalization capacity due to alterations of the protein corona composition and, consequently, the interaction with receptors and membranes [46–48]. In this regard, the possible biomedical applications of AuNPs can be expanded as their cell internalization ability is increased. Accordingly, arginine-rich CPPs, (minimum amount of six Arg) are well known for their ability to cross biological barriers [49,50]. Although other studies have reported the conjugation of nanoparticles with internalization peptides in a direct way [51–54], it is also well known that the presence of BSA improves the circulation time of nanoparticles and controls the composition of the protein corona in physiological media, hence the importance of the inclusion of albumin in nanoparticles [37,55,56]. Therefore, we functionalized the BSA protein with r_8 to facilitate cell penetration of the AuNPs. Previous studies have shown that the use of arginine-rich CPPs increases cell penetration of the nanocarriers, opening the possibility for the improved cell internalization of AuNPs [51,57–59]. In particular, r_8 has been covalently linked to several molecules and nanosystems, such as insulin [60] liposomes, [61] quantum dots, [62] and gold nanorods, [49,58] improving their uptake and cell penetration in target sites. Nevertheless, coating AuNRs and AuNPrs (with absorption in the first biological window) with BSA, functionalized with r_8 for cell internalization, has not been reported yet. In this study, we proposed that BSA-r_8 enhances the cell internalization of AuNPs, taking as examples two promissory anisotropic AuNPs with different surface and charge: AuNRs and AuNPrs, with absorption on the first biological window (650–950 nm) [63] for possible applications in biomedical nanoplatforms.

2. Materials and Methods

2.1. Materials

HAuCl$_4$ (Gold (III) chloride hydrate), Na$_2$S$_2$O$_3$ (sodium thiosulfate), hexadecyltrimethylammonium bromide (CTAB), NaBH$_4$, and AgNO$_3$ were acquired from Sigma-Aldrich (St. Louis, MO, USA). Polyethylene Glycol 5 kDa (HS-PEG-COOH, 5 kDa) was from JenKem

Technology (Beijing, China). Milli-Q water was obtained from the purification of distilled water with the Simplicity SIMS 00001 equipment (Millipore, Molsheim, France). Cell culture plates and flasks were from Corning Costar (Corning, NY, USA). Penicillin/streptomycin and chemicals for cell culture were from Gibco (Gibco-BRL, Paisley, UK), fetal bovine serum (FBS, Biological Industries, Cromwell, CT, USA). MTS/PMS [3-(4,5-dimethylthiazol-2-yl)-5-(3-carboxymethoxyphenyl)-2-(4-sulfophenyl)-2H-tetrazolium, inner salt, MTS/phenazine methosulfate, PMS], and CellTiter 96 kit were from Promega (Promega, Madison, WI, USA). Atto-565 NHS ester (A565) was from Sigma (Sigma-Aldric Chemie, Buch, Switzerland). Other reagents were from Sigma-Aldrich.

2.2. Experimental

2.2.1. AuNRs Synthesis

AuNRs were synthesized using a previously reported seed-mediated procedure [64]. Briefly, 5 mL of a 0.3 mM $HAuCl_4$ solution in CTAB 0.1 M was reduced by ice-cold $NaBH_4$ 10 mM (300 µL), resulting in a brownish-yellow seed solution. Then, 10 mL of a 0.5 mM $HAuCl_4$ solution (in CTAB 0.1 M) was reduced by ascorbic acid in the presence of $AgNO_3$, until it reached a colorless growth solution. Finally, 120 µL of the seed solution was added to the growth solution and allowed to rest for 30 min in a thermostatic bath at 27 °C. The obtained AuNRs were centrifuged at 7030 g for 30 min, and the pellet was resuspended in Milli-Q water.

2.2.2. AuNPrs Synthesis

AuNPrs were obtained by $Na_2S_2O_3$ reduction of $HAuCl_4$, as previously reported [28,36]. A 2 mM $HAuCl_4$ solution was first reduced by 0.6 mM $Na_2S_2O_3$ and allowed to rest for 9 min. Then, a second addition of 0.6 mM $Na_2S_2O_3$ was performed, and the solution was left undisturbed for 30 min. The purple solution containing the AuNPs was centrifuged and resuspended in Milli-Q water. PEG functionalization was achieved at pH = 12 by adding 15 µL of a 2.7 mM HS-PEG5000-COOH solution and allowing conjugation under a magnetic stirrer for 3 h. Finally, AuNPrs were separated from smaller undesired AuNPs using a successive differential centrifugation procedure, as reported [36].

2.2.3. Characterization of the Nanoparticles

AuNRs and AuNPrs were characterized before and after BSA-r_8 coating by UV-Vis-NIR absorption spectra, using a Lambda 25 spectrophotometer (Perkin Elmer, Waltham, MA, USA). Dynamic light scattering (DLS) and Z potential measurements were acquired in PBS pH = 7, at 25 °C, using a Zetasizer 3000 (Malvern Instruments, Malvern, UK), as triplicates in aqueous solution at 25 °C.

TEM images of AuNRs were acquired with a JEOL JEM-1010 microscope (JEOL USA, Peabody, MA, USA), using Formvar carbon-coated copper microgrids (200 mesh; Ted Pella, Redding, CA, USA). For AuNPrs, TEM images were obtained using a Philips CM 120 transmission electron microscope with an accelerating voltage of 120 kV and a 300 mesh Formvar/Carbon-Coated Copper grid. For both AuNPs, liquid suspensions were deposited on the microgrid and allowed to stand overnight before TEM image acquisition.

2.3. Peptide Synthesis

We synthesized the all-D peptide derived from D-amino acids for this study due to their enhanced enzymatic stability [65]. Arginine-rich peptide (r_8) was synthesized by solid phase peptide synthesis (SPPS), using an H-Rink Amide Protide resin (loading: 0.56 mmol/g) in a Liberty Blue™ Automated Microwave Peptide Synthesizer. Linear D-OctoArginine was synthesized on a 0.5 mmol scale using a 5 excess of Fmoc-amino acid (0.2 M), relative to the resin. The Bromo acetic acid was coupled using 2 cycles of 30 min of 4 equivalents of OxymaPure, followed by 4 equivalents of N,N'-Diisopropylcarbodiimide, and then 4 equivalents of bromo acetic acid. Fmoc deprotection was carried out using 10% (w/v) piperazine and 0.1 M OxymaPure in a 9:1 mixture of NMP and EtOH. The resin was cleaved using TFA/H$_2$O/TIS (95%/2.5%/2.5%) for 6 h; the TFA was evaporated, dissolved in a 50/50 H$_2$O/ACN solution, and lyophilized. The peptide was purified by semi-preparative HPLC on a Waters 2700 sample manager, equipped with a Waters 2487 dual-wavelength absorbance detector, a Waters 600 controller, a Waters fraction collector and Masslynx software by using a Sunfire C18 column (150 × 10 mm × 3.5 µm, 100 Å, Waters), flow rate 6.6 mL/min; solvent A = 0.1% TFA in water and solvent B = 0.1% TFA in acetonitrile. Purity and identity were assessed by UPCL (Waters Acquity equipped with Acquity photodiode array detector, flux rate 0.610 mL/min, Acquity UPLC BEH C18 Column, 130 Å, 1.7 µm, 2.1 mm × 100 mm; solvents A = 0.045% TFA in water, and B = 0.036% TFA in acetonitrile) and UPLC-MS (Waters Acquity UPLC System equipped with ESI-SQ Detector2, flux rate 0.610 mL/min, Acquity UPLC BEH C18 Column, 130 Å, 1.7 µm, 2.1 mm × 100 mm; solvents A = 0.1% formic acid in water and B = 0.1% formic acid in acetonitrile).

The crude compound was purified by RP-HPLC at a semi-preparative scale and characterized by UPLC and UPLC-MS spectrometry (Supplementary Section 1, Figures S1 and S2) to confirm the identity of the synthesized compound, obtaining high purity (>95%). Amino acid content was analyzed by amino acid analysis; results are presented in Supplementary Section 2, Table S1.

2.4. BSA Functionalization

BSA was functionalized with r$_8$, as represented in Scheme 1, to improve the internalization properties of the nanoconstructs, and Atto-565-NHS-ester was used as a fluorescent probe for detection by fluorescence and confocal microscopy.

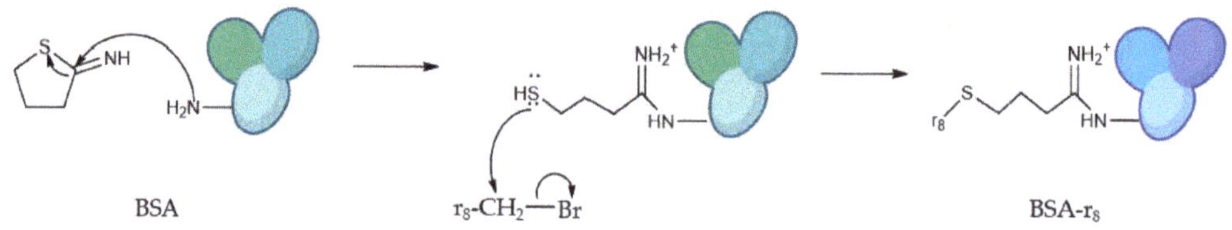

Scheme 1. Synthetic approach for BSA functionalization by r$_8$ peptide. First, 2-iminothiolane reacts with BSA amine groups in the surface of the protein, giving rise to available SH free groups, followed by r$_8$-Br reaction with the free SH groups.

BSA Labeling with r$_8$ and Atto 565

- First step: 2-Iminothiolane functionalization

A 100 mg/mL 2-Iminothiolane solution (15 µL) was added to a 10 mg/mL BSA solution (50 mg of BSA in 5 mL of PBS), in 4 intervals every 10 min (molar ratio 10:1 2-iminothiolane: BSA), and the reaction was performed for 1 h at 4 °C. The non-reacted 2-iminothiolane was removed using a P10 G25 desalting column from Sigma-Aldrich.

- Second step: r$_8$ peptide functionalization

To the previously prepared protein, 52 µL of a 100 mg/mL Br-CH$_2$-r$_8$ solution was added in 4 intervals every 10 min, and the reaction was left overnight at 4 °C (ratio 5:1 r$_8$-Br:BSA). The product was purified with a P10 G25 desalting column and analyzed by UV-Vis-NIR spectroscopy and amino acid analysis to determine the amount of r$_8$ per BSA molecule.

- Third step: amino acid analysis of BSA-r$_8$

Amino acid analysis was performed following an acid hydrolysis procedure, adding 12 N HCl and a known concentration standard (Υ-aminobutyric acid, 0.1 mM), and allowed to react at 110 °C for 72 h. Amino acid quantification was carried out in an HPLC-PDA AccQ-Tag (C18; 4 µm; 3.9 × 15 mm). The amino acid content on the functionalized BSA resulted in a 2.4 r$_8$/BSA ratio, as shown in Supplementary Section 2, Table S1.

- BSA-r₈ fluorescent labeling

Fluorescent labeling of BSA was conducted as represented in Scheme 2. To 10 mg of BSA-r₈ of the previous step, 10.7 µL of a 10 mg/mL solution of Atto 565 NHS ester was added and allowed to react for 1 h. The final product (BSA-r₈-A565) was purified with a P10 G25 desalting column and characterized by UV-Vis spectroscopy.

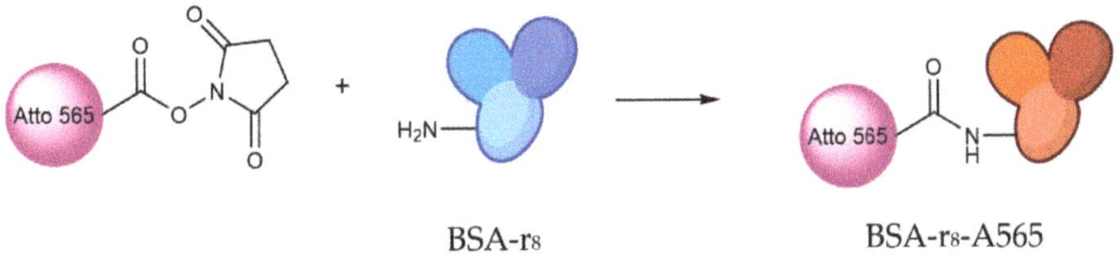

Scheme 2. Synthetic approach for BSA-r₈ functionalization by Atto565-NHS ester in the NH₂ free groups of BSA.

According to UV-Vis spectroscopy measurements, the degree of labeling (DOL) was calculated as follows:

$$DOL = \frac{Absorbance\ 565 \times \varepsilon_{Atto\ 565}}{Absorbance\ 280\ (Absorbance\ 565 \times CF_{Atto\ 565}) \times \varepsilon_{BSA}}$$

where:

$\varepsilon_{Atto\ 565} = 1.2 \times 10^5$ M^{-1} cm^{-1}, $\varepsilon_{BSA} = 4.6 \times 10^5$ M^{-1} cm^{-1}, and correction factor Atto 565 ($CF_{Atto\ 565}$) = 0.16

As a result, the DOL of BSA-r₈ A565 was 0.66 mol Atto/mol BSA.

2.5. Circular Dichroism

The BSA and BSA-r₈ 1.5×10^{-5} M samples were prepared in PBS 0.1× in the same conditions. The spectra were acquired at 20 °C, recorded from 200 to 250 nm in triplicate and condensed into a single spectrum to reduce noise at a 1 nm/s rate in a JASCO J-815 instrument (JASCO, Easton, MA, USA), using a 1 mm pathlength quartz-cuvette. The secondary structure content was calculated using the CDPro CONTIN 2DP (AUG 1982) (2DP-SW PACK) version from JASCO.

The molar ellipticity at wavelength λ ([θ$_{mrw}$]) was calculated as follows:

$$[\theta_{mrw}] = \frac{MRW \times \theta_\lambda}{10 \times d \times c}$$

where θ_λ is the observed ellipticity (degrees) at wavelength λ, d is the pathlength (cm), and c is the protein concentration (g/mL) [66].

2.6. Capping of AuNPs with BSA or BSA-r₈

BSA-r₈ or BSA capping of the AuNPs was achieved by incubation, as previously reported [36]. Briefly, to 1 mL of AuNRs or AuNPrs at a 1 nM concentration, a solution of BSA or BSA-r₈ was added (final concentration of BSA = 1 mg/mL in 0.1× PBS), incubating for 2 h at 4 °C in low-binding 1.5 mL centrifuge tubes (Eppendorf®, Hamburg, Germany), and the samples were centrifuged at 10,000 rpm for 10 min. The pellet containing the BSA or BSA-r₈ coated AuNPs was resuspended in 0.1× PBS. The protein content was quantified on the supernatants using a Micro BCA™ Protein Assay Kit from Thermo Scientific™ (Pierce, Rockford, IL, USA), according to the manufacturer's specifications, in triplicate.

2.7. Cell Culture

HeLa cells were cultured in complete DMEM, containing 1% penicillin/streptomycin, 10% FBS and 5% glutamine. The culture was maintained at 37 °C and 5% CO_2.

2.7.1. Cell Viability MTS Assays

HeLa cells (1×10^4 cells/well) were seeded in TC pretreated 96-well plates and allowed to attach at 37 °C for 24 h. The treatments were added and allowed to incubate for 24 h. The medium was then replaced by a phenol red-free medium containing the MTS/PMS containing reagent, following the manufacturer's recommendations. The absorbance of the culture medium after incubation for 1 h was recorded at 490 nm using a microplate reader. Cell viability was calculated with respect to a non-treatment control (live control). Each treatment and control were made in quintuplicate, minimum $n = 3$. Statistical analysis was performed using GraphPad Prism V5.01.

2.7.2. Confocal Microscopy

HeLa cells (3×10^5 cells/plate) were seeded on collagen pre-coated MatTek glass-bottom culture dishes (MatTek Corporation, Ashland, MA, USA) and attached for 48 h at standard culture conditions. The medium was then replaced with fresh medium, and the treatments were added considering 1 nM of each AuNP and incubated (1 or 24 h of treatment). The cells were subsequently washed 3 times with PBS, and phenol red-free medium containing the LIVE/DEAD® Cell Imaging Kit from ThermoFisher was added (Molecular Probes Inc., Eugene, OR, USA). Fluorescence was detected on a Zeiss LSM 880 laser scanning microscope (Zeiss, Berlin, Germany) with Airyscan, equipped with a CO_2 and temperature-controlled environmental chamber. Hoechst was excited with an Ar laser at 405 nm, and emission was recorded at 458 nm; Atto-565 was excited by a laser at 405 nm, and emission was recorded at 458 nm. Images were processed using Image J 1.52 p software.

2.7.3. Internalization Evaluated by Transmission Electron Microscopy

In a Petri dish (90×15 mm), 1×10^6 HeLa cells were seeded and incubated at 37 °C until a minimum confluence of 80%. The cells were then washed, the medium was replaced with a treatment containing-medium (1 nM of BSA or BSA-r_8 coated AuNPs), and the cells were incubated for 24 h. Afterwards, the cells were washed and fixed with glutaraldehyde 2.5% in PBS 0.1×. The cells were scraped and centrifuged, and the obtained pellet was fixed with OsO_4 1% in PBS for 90 min and embedded in Epon resin. The resin was sliced into slices of 80 nm thickness, and the slices were placed in a Cu grid and stained with Reynold's reagent and uranyLess staining kit, before visualization. TEM images were acquired in a JEOL JEM-1010 microscope (JEOL Ltd., Tokyo, Japan).

3. Results and Discussion

3.1. Preparation of AuNRs-BSA-r_8 and AuNPr-BSA-r_8

The r_8 peptide was synthesized and characterized by UPLC-MS, showing the characteristic $[M+2H]^{2+} = 695.02$ m/z (Figure S1). Then, BSA was functionalized with r_8 (2.4 r_8/BSA) as described in the experimental section. The degree of BSA functionalization was determined by amino acid analysis, resulting in 2.4 r_8/BSA. To determine if the functionalization of the protein led to a change in BSA secondary structure, circular dichroism spectra were obtained. Figure 1 shows the CD spectrum of BSA and BSA-r_8, indicating that they shared a similar profile, with a non-significant change from 39% and 36% alpha helix content before and after r_8 functionalization, respectively.

BSA-r_8 was functionalized with a fluorescent probe, namely A565, a known and commonly used red fluorescent probe, obtaining a 0.66 A565/BSA-r_8 degree of labeling, which resulted in BSA-A565-r_8. In this study, we tested whether AuNPrs were a suitable alternative to more-traditional AuNRs; in this sense, AuNPrs were synthesized by simply reducing Au^{3+} with $Na_2S_2O_3$, thus avoiding the involvement of cytotoxic agents [28]. AuNRs and AuNPrs were synthesized with a characteristic morphology, as TEM images show in Supplementary Section 3 (Figures S3 and S4), with a predominant aspect ratio of 3.5 for AuNRs and a 60 nm edge-length for AuNPrs.

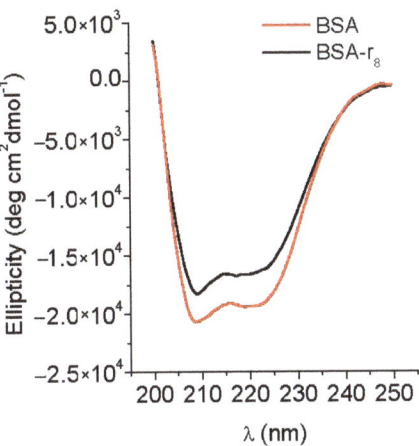

Figure 1. Circular dichroism spectrum of BSA before and after r_8 functionalization. DOL: 2.4 r_8/BSA. BSA and BSA-r_8 1.5×10^{-5} M samples were prepared in PBS.

It has been demonstrated by several spectroscopic techniques that BSA is spontaneously adsorbed in the surface of AuNPs via S-Au bonds between the free SH groups of BSA and the gold atoms in the AuNP surface [42,67–71]. Therefore, both AuNRs and AuNPrs were coated with BSA and the functionalized BSA-A565-r_8 by incubation, as summarized in Table 1 and Figures 2 and 3. Figures 2 and 3 show the UV-Vis-NIR spectra, size, and Z potential of the BSA and BSA-A565-r_8 functionalized AuNPs in PBS (pH = 7). For AuNRs, a shoulder around 558 nm appeared after BSA-A565-r_8 protein coating (Figure 2a), as well as an increment in the intensity of the first plasmon in AuNPrs (Figure 3a), confirming the presence of A565 and therefore, the functionalization of BSA on the AuNPs surface. In addition, the second plasmon of both AuNPs was shifted after the BSA and BSA-r_8-A565 coating, attributed to the modification in the dielectric constant of the AuNPs [72] (Table 1 and Figures 2a and 3a), due to the presence of the protein on the AuNPs surface, as reported in previous studies [36,73–75].

For both nanoparticles, the protein coating on the surface increased the hydrodynamic diameter in similar proportions using either the BSA or BSA-A565-r_8, as expected for the presence of the protein (Table 1 and Figures 2b and 3b). For AuNRs, hydrodynamic diameter increased from $2 \pm 1, 59 \pm 3$ nm to $3 \pm 1, 68 \pm 3$ nm and $6 \pm 1, 79 \pm 3$ nm after the BSA and BSA-A565-r_8 coating, respectively. Meanwhile, for AuNPrs, the hydrodynamic diameter shifted from $4 \pm 1, 68 \pm 4$ nm to $10 \pm 2, 142 \pm 5$ nm and $12 \pm 2, 142 \pm 5$ nm due to the BSA and BSA-A565-r_8 coating, respectively.

Regarding the Z potential, a similar trend was observed, and both nanoparticles showed similar Z potentials after the BSA or BSA-A565-r_8 coating. AuNRs showed an initial Z potential of $+45 \pm 3$ mV, due to the presence of the cationic surfactant CTAB [76,77]; in contrast, AuNPrs had an initial Z potential of -31 ± 3 mV, due to the stabilizing agent HS-PEG-COOH on the surface [36]. Then, the Z potential exhibited a shift to negative values; -21 ± 1 and -17 ± 1 for AuNR-BSA and AuNR-BSA-A565-r_8 and -14 ± 1 and -18 ± 1 mV for AuNPr-BSA and AuNPr-BSA-A565-r_8, respectively (Table 1 and Figures 2c and 3c), due to the negative charge of BSA (pI$_{BSA}$: 4.5–5.0) [78] on the surface of both AuNPs. Notably, AuNPs exhibited similar negative Z potentials, with adequate values to interact with cell membranes for internalization [60–62]. Stability of AuNR-BSA-r_8 and AuNPr-BSA-r_8 was assessed 30 days after storage at 4 °C; DLS and Z potential did not show significant differences over that time (Supplementary Section 4, Figure S5).

Table 1. Physicochemical parameters of the synthesized nanoparticles and nanoconstructs.

Samples	Long. λ_{max} (nm)	Hydrodynamic Diameter (nm)		PDI	Z Potential (mV)
		Transversal	Longitudinal		
AuNR	775	2 ± 1	59 ± 3	0.5	45 ± 3
AuNR-BSA	757	3 ± 1	68 ± 3	0.5	−21 ± 1
AuNR-BSA-A565-r$_8$	750	6 ± 1	79 ± 3	0.5	−17 ± 1
AuNPr	865	4 ± 1	68 ± 4	0.4	−31 ± 3
AuNPr-BSA	845	10 ± 2	142 ± 5	0.5	−14 ± 1
AuNPr-BSA-A565-r$_8$	829	12 ± 2	142 ± 5	0.5	−18 ± 1

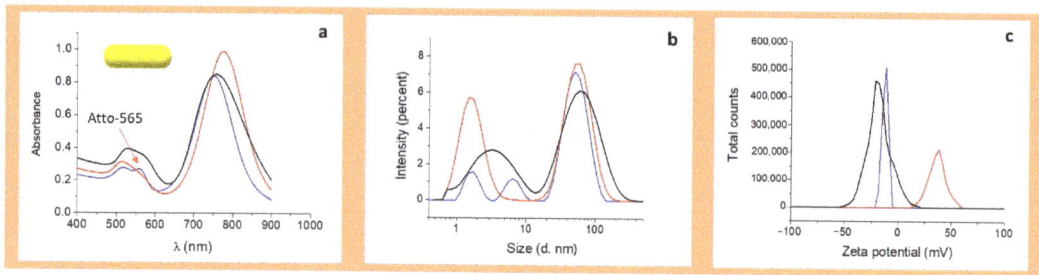

Figure 2. Characterization of BSA-A565-r$_8$ capped AuNRs: red line, AuNRs, black line AuNR-BSA, blue line AuNR-BSA-A565-r$_8$. (**a**) UV-Vis NIR spectra. The red arrow shows the presence of Atto-565. (**b**) Size distribution. (**c**) Zeta potential distribution. Acquired in PBS, pH = 7.

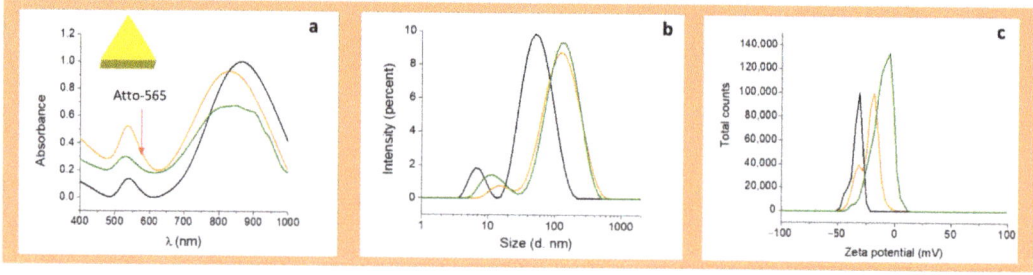

Figure 3. Characterization of BSA-A565-r$_8$ capped AuNPrs; black line AuNPrs, green line AuNPr-BSA, and orange line AuNPr-BSA-A565-r$_8$. (**a**) UV-Vis-NIR spectra. The red arrow shows the presence of Atto-565. (**b**) Size distribution. (**c**) Zeta potential distribution. Acquired in PBS, pH = 7.

3.2. Cell Viability Assays

3.2.1. Effect of AuNRs and AuNRs-BSA-A565-r$_8$ on Cell Viability

One of the main limitations of using AuNRs in biomedical applications is the cytotoxicity associated with the CTAB on the AuNP surface as the stabilizing agent in the synthesis procedure [30]. In order to overcome this issue, AuNRs can be coated with different materials, such as BSA [39,79–82] to increase their biocompatibility. In this regard, Figure 4 shows that the freshly synthesized AuNRs drastically decreased the viability of Hela cells, whereas AuNRs-A565-BSA-r$_8$ did not cause a significant effect between the 0.005–2.5 nM range at 48 h. Additionally, flow cytometry showed no effect of 1 nM AuNRs-A565-BSA-r$_8$ after 24 h of administration (Supplementary Section 5, Figure S6). Similar results were found for BSA-coated AuNPs in previous studies; the BSA coating on AuNRs improved their biocompatibility properties [83–85], highlighting the potential of coated AuNRs for bioapplications.

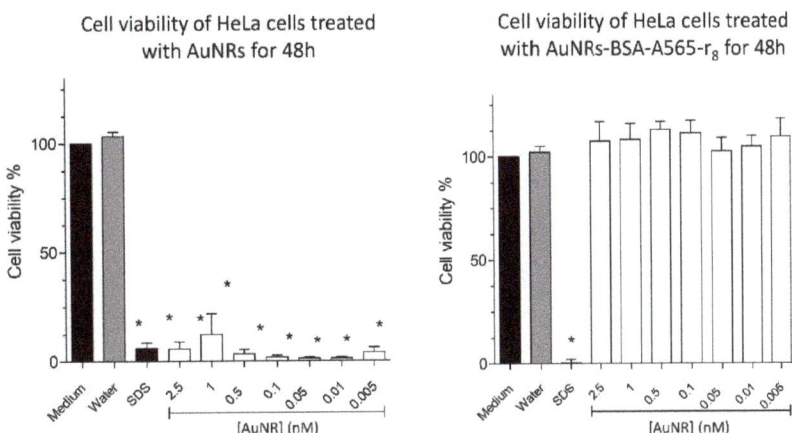

Figure 4. Effect of AuNRs and AuNR-BSA-r_8 incubated for 24 h on cell viability of HeLa cells at 48 h. The average values for n = 4 experiments are shown with error bars representing the SEM. * Significant difference according to Tukey's test $p < 0.05$ compared to medium control.

3.2.2. Effect of AuNPrs and AuNPrs-BSA-r_8 on Cell Viability

AuNPrs were functionalized with PEG-COOH to increase their colloidal stability [86] and subsequently coated with BSA-A565-r_8 (AuNPr-BSA-A565-r_8). Figure 5 shows cell viability of HeLa cells treated with AuNPrs and AuNPr-BSA-A565-r_8 at the 0.005–2.5 nM range. As expected, neither AuNPrs nor AuNPrs-BSA-r_8 showed any effect on HeLa cell viability after 48 h of treatment by MTS assay. Flow cytometry also showed non-effect of AuNPrs-BSA-r_8 1 nM in the HeLa cells after 24 h of incubation (Supplementary Section 5, Figure S6). This null effect on cell viability of AuNPrs was previously demonstrated in studies such as those of Alfranca et al. and Bao et al., using Vero cells and HT-29 cells at 72 h, respectively [29,87]

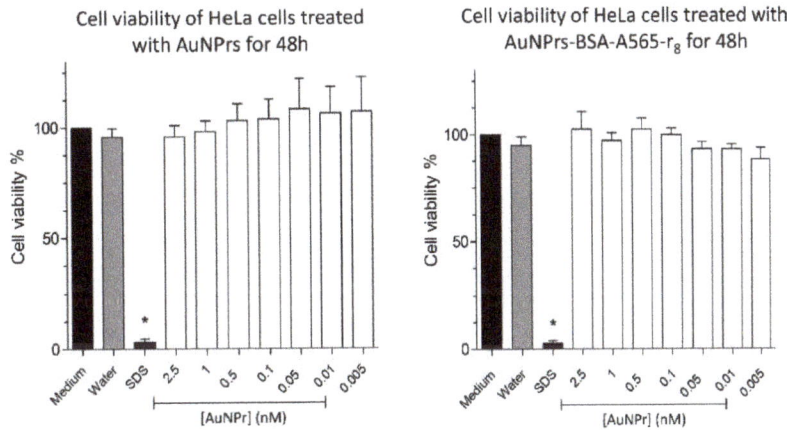

Figure 5. Effect of AuNPrs and AuNPr-BSA-r_8 incubated for 24 h on cell viability of HeLa cells at 48 h. The average values for n = 4 experiments are shown with error bars representing the SEM. * Significant difference according to Tukey's test $p < 0.05$ compared to medium control.

3.3. Cell Internalization

3.3.1. Confocal Microscopy

In a first step, we tested the internalization ability of the AuNPs capped with non-CPP functionalized BSA, as shown in Figure 6. The comparison between the BSA, AuNR-BSA, and AuNPr-BSA (labeled with A565) signals showed that BSA on the AuNP surface was not able to promote cell uptake under the studied conditions ([BSA] = 5 µM, [AuNR-BSA and AuNPr-BSA] = 1 nM, 24 h of incubation), as demonstrated by the absence of signal in the red channel.

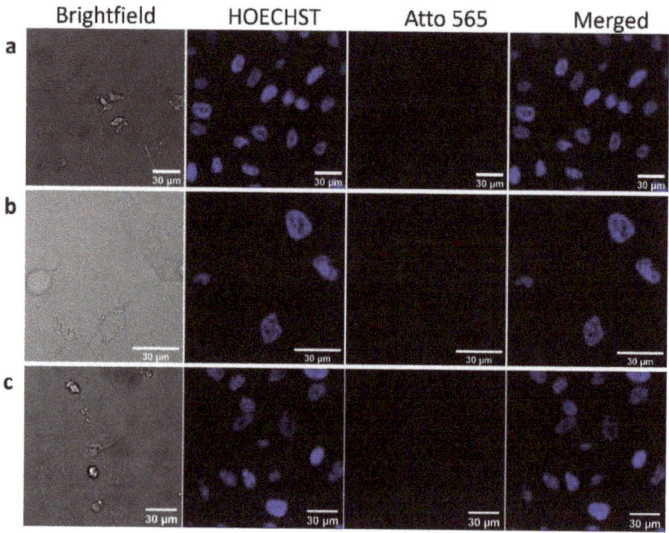

Figure 6. Confocal microscopy images of HeLa cells after treatment by: (**a**) BSA-A565, (**b**) AuNR-BSA-A565, (**c**) AuNPr-BSA-A565 incubated for 24 h. Scale 30 µm. [BSA] = 5 µM, [AuNR-BSA, AuNPr-BSA] = 1 nM. Channels: bright blue (HOECHST), red (Atto-565), blue and red (merged).

Internalization of BSA-r_8 and the AuNPs capped with BSA-r_8 (labeled with A565) was subsequently assessed by confocal microscopy. As Figure 7 shows, functionalization with r_8 increased the uptake of the protein, as well as that of the protein-coated AuNRs and AuNPrs in the red channel, using the same established conditions as in Figure 7 ([BSA] = 5 µM, [AuNR-BSA-A565-r_8] and [AuNPr-A565-r_8] = 1 nM), suggesting the prevalent role of the r_8 for cell internalization in both nanoconstructs, regardless of their surface charge.

Although discussing the exact mechanism of internalization of the proposed nanoconstructs was not the objective of our study, previous reports have indicated that nanoconstructs conjugated with CPPs are internalized in vesicles inside cells via endocytic uptake [29,51,59,88], while arginine-rich CPPs can electrostatically bind with the cell membranes, promoting translocation into the cells [29,51,59,88].

To confirm that the internalization observed through confocal microscopy corresponded to the functionalized AuNPs, and to elucidate the intracellular location of the nanoconstructs in Hela cells, we performed a TEM study, as indicated in the next section.

3.3.2. TEM for Cell Internalization

The internalization of the BSA-A565-r_8-coated AuNPs was assessed after 1 h and 24 h of incubation. Supplementary Section 6 (Figures S7 and S8) shows internalization at 1 h, indicating that the nanoconstructs started interacting with the cell membranes at this time, to become ready for the internalization process. At 24 h, in contrast, internalization of both AuNRs-BSA-A565-r_8 and AuNPr-BSA-A565-r_8 was considerable and observed under the studied conditions, as shown in Figures 8 and 9.

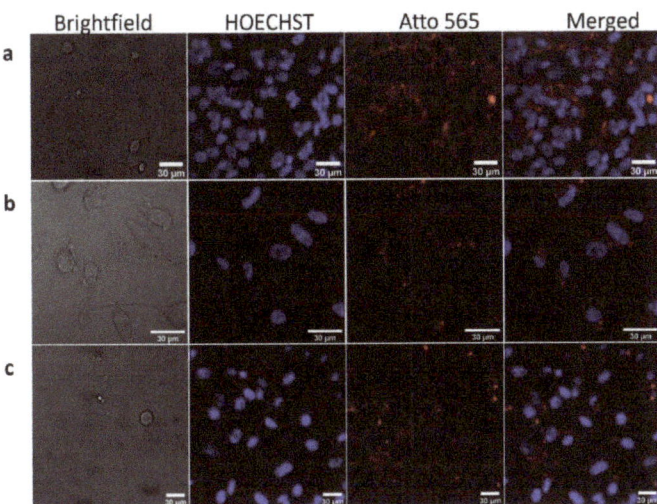

Figure 7. Confocal microscopy images of HeLa cells after treatment with: (**a**) BSA-r$_8$-A565, (**b**) AuNR-BSA-r$_8$-A565, (**c**) AuNPr-BSA-r$_8$-A565 incubated for 24 h. Scale 30 μm. [BSA-r$_8$] = 5 μM, [AuNR-BSA-A565-r$_8$ and AuNPr-A565-BSA-r$_8$] = 1 nM. Channels: bright blue (HOECHST), red (Atto-565), blue and red (merged).

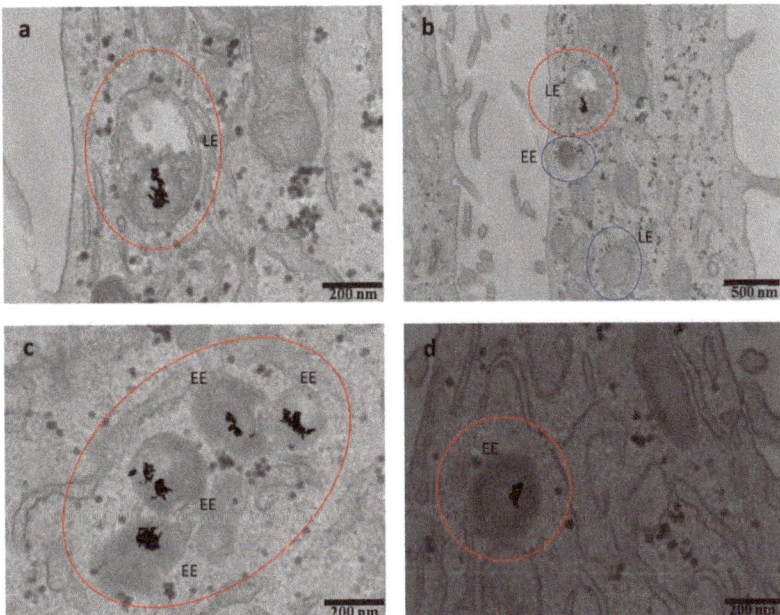

Figure 8. TEM images of HeLa cells after treatment with AuNR-BSA-r$_8$ incubated for 24 h (**a**–**d**). Red circles show the internalized AuNPs. EE: early endosomes and LE: late endosomes. Blue circles showing examples of vacant LE or EE.

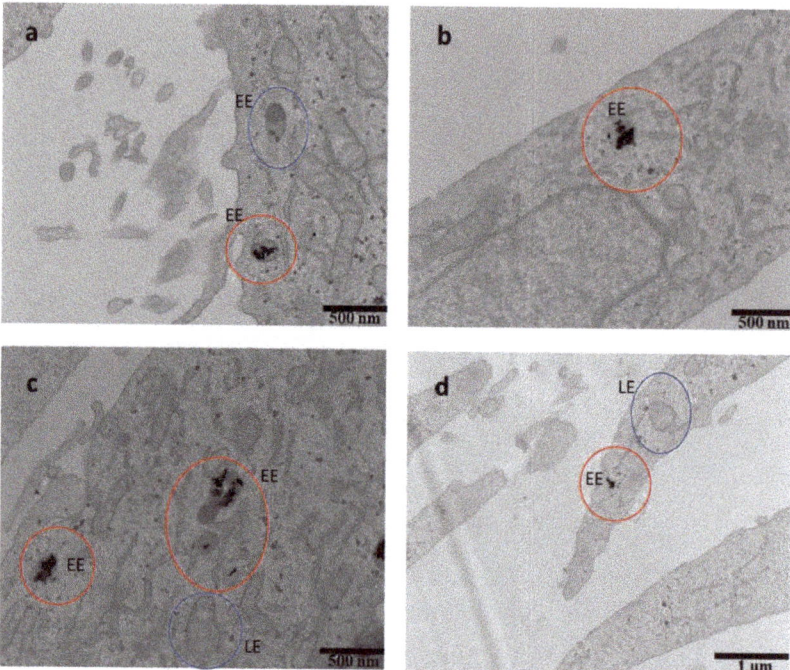

Figure 9. TEM images of HeLa cells after treatment with AuNPr-BSA-r$_8$ incubated for 24 h (**a–d**). Red circles show the internalized AuNPs. EE: early endosomes and LE: late endosomes. Blue circles showing examples of vacant LE or EE.

The TEM images allowed determination of the precise location of the AuNPs in the cells. Both AuNRs and AuNPrs-based nanocarriers seemed to be located inside the cells and accumulated into vesicles in the cytoplasm, in agreement with the proposed endocytic uptake [29,51,59,88]. According to Liu et al. [89], the vesicles were labeled considering their size as early endosomes (200 nm diameter, EE) and late endosomes (500 nm diameter, LE). In Figures 8 and 9, vacant EE and LE as well as the EE and LE where AuNPs are located were pointed out (blue and red circles, respectively). An average of 15 ± 5 AuNRs/vesicle and 18 ± 6 AuNPrs/vesicle were counted for AuNRs-BSA-A565-r$_8$ and AuNPr-BSA-A565-r$_8$, respectively (statistics of 30 vesicles from the TEM images).

4. Conclusions

In this work, we tested the internalization abilities of two novel nanoconstructs based on anisotropic AuNPs with different surface and charge, AuNRs and AuNPrs coated with BSA in the presence and absence of a CPP (r$_8$), improving AuNP internalization in the presence of r$_8$. To the best of our knowledge, this is the first report that describes the coating of AuNRs and AuNPrs (with absorption in the first biological window) with BSA functionalized with r$_8$ for improved cell internalization. These results point to the ability to improve the biocompatibility and internalization of nanoconstructs into cells by using endogenous proteins and CPPs. Nevertheless, as a further step, it would also be interesting to add targeting agents to the proposed nanoconstructs to increase their selectivity.

Supplementary Materials: The following are available online at https://www.mdpi.com/article/10.3390/pharmaceutics13081204/s1: Figure S1: Structure of the Br-CH$_2$-r$_8$ peptide, Figure S2: UPLC trace (a) and MS spectra (b) of Br-r$_8$ (BrCH2CO-r$_8$), Figure S3: Microscopy characterization of AuNRs: a, b. representative TEM images, scale 200 nm, c. Aspect ratio frequency distri-bution (length/width), statistics of at least 50 AuNRs, Figure S4: Microscopy characterization of AuNPrs: a, b. representative TEM images, scale 200 nm, c. Edge length (nm) frequency distribution (length/width), statistics of at least 50 AuNPrs, Figure S5: Characterization of BSA-r_8 capped AuNPs after 24 h, DLS and Zeta potential, Figure S6: Flow cytometry of Hela cells incubated by 24 h with: a. water, b. AuNR-BSA-r_8 1 nM in AuNRs, c. AuNPr-BSA-r_8 1 nM AuNPrs, Figure S7: TEM images of HeLa cells after treatment by AuNR-BSA-r_8 incubated by 1 h, Figure S8: TEM images of HeLa cells after treatment by AuNPr-BSA-r_8 incubated by 1 h, Table S1: Amino acid analysis of BSA-r8 after acid digestion, using Υ-aminobutiric acid as standard (aaba).

Author Contributions: Conceptualization, K.B., M.J.K. and E.A.; methodology, K.B., M.S.-N. and A.T.-A.; formal analysis, K.B., M.J.K. and E.A.; resources, E.G., M.J.K. and E.A.; writing—original draft preparation, K.B.; writing—review and editing, all authors; supervision, E.A. and M.J.K.; project administration, E.A. and M.K; funding acquisition, E.G., E.A. and M.J.K. All authors have read and agreed to the published version of the manuscript.

Funding: K.B. acknowledges ANID, Chile, Doctoral fellowship 21180258 and Advanced Center for Chronic Diseases. A.T.-A. acknowledges PhD fellowship number 21151461 and 23190312. E.A. acknowledges Fondecyt 1190623. M.J.K. acknowledges FONDECYT 1211482, FONDAP 15130011 and FONDEQUIP EQM170111. M.S.-N. and E.G. acknowledge MINECO-FEDER (BIO 2016-75327-R) and the Generalitat de Catalunya (XRB and 2017SGR-998). IRB Barcelona is the recipient of a Severo Ochoa Award of Excellence from MINECO (Government of Spain).

Institutional Review Board Statement: Not applicable.

Informed Consent Statement: Not applicable.

Data Availability Statement: Not applicable.

Acknowledgments: The authors acknowledge the support of the IRB Advanced Microscopy Core Facility, Mass Spectrometry Core Facility of IRB Barcelona, and Electronic Microscopy Facility from Centres Científics i Tecnològics Universitat de Barcelona.

Conflicts of Interest: The authors report no conflict of interest in this work.

References

1. Callaghan, C.; Peralta, D.; Liu, J.; Mandava, S.H.; Maddox, M.; Dash, S.; Tarr, M.A.; Lee, B.R. Combined Treatment of Tyrosine Kinase Inhibitor-Labeled Gold Nanorod Encapsulated Albumin with Laser Thermal Ablation in a Renal Cell Carcinoma Model. *J. Pharm. Sci.* **2016**, *105*, 284–292. [CrossRef]
2. Popp, M.K.; Oubou, I.; Shepherd, C.; Nager, Z.; Anderson, C.; Pagliaro, L. Photothermal Therapy Using Gold Nanorods and Near-Infrared Light in a Murine Melanoma Model Increases Survival and Decreases Tumor Volume. *J. Nanomater.* **2014**, *2014*, 450670. [CrossRef]
3. Song, X.; Liang, C.; Gong, H.; Chen, Q.; Wang, C.; Liu, Z. Photosensitizer-Conjugated Albumin-Polypyrrole Nanoparticles for Imaging-Guided in Vivo Photodynamic/Photothermal Therapy. *Small* **2015**, *11*, 3932–3941. [CrossRef] [PubMed]
4. Yeo, E.L.L.; Cheah, J.U.J.; Neo, D.J.H.; Goh, W.I.; Kanchanawong, P.; Soo, K.C.; Thong, P.S.P.; Kah, J.C.Y. Exploiting the protein corona around gold nanorods for low-dose combined photothermal and photodynamic therapy. *J. Mater. Chem. B* **2017**, *5*, 254–268. [CrossRef]
5. Bayda, S.; Adeel, M.; Tuccinardi, T.; Cordani, M.; Rizzolio, F. The history of nanoscience and nanotechnology: From chemical-physical applications to nanomedicine. *Molecules* **2020**, *25*, 112. [CrossRef]
6. Huang, H.; Lovell, J.F. Advanced Functional Nanomaterials for Theranostics. *Adv. Funct. Mater. Theranostics* **2017**, *27*, 1603524. [CrossRef]
7. Han, J.; Zhao, D.; Li, D.; Wang, X.; Jin, Z.; Zhao, K. Polymer-based nanomaterials and applications for vaccines and drugs. *Polymers* **2018**, *10*, 31. [CrossRef]
8. Aguilar, Z.P. Types of Nanomaterials and Corresponding Methods of Synthesis. In *Nanomaterials for Medical Applications*; Elsevier: Amsterdam, The Netherlands, 2013; pp. 33–82; ISBN 9780123850898.
9. Klebowski, B.; Depciuch, J.; Parlinska-Wojtan, M.; Baran, J. Applications of Noble Metal-Based Nanoparticles in Medicine. *Int. J. Mol. Sci.* **2018**, *19*, 4031. [CrossRef]
10. Vetterlein, C.; Vásquez, R.; Bolaños, K.; Acosta, G.A.; Guzman, F.; Albericio, F.; Celis, F.; Campos, M.; Kogan, M.J.; Araya, E. Exploring the influence of Diels–Alder linker length on photothermal molecule release from gold nanorods. *Colloids Surf. B Biointerfaces* **2018**, *166*, 323–329. [CrossRef]
11. Inostroza-Riquelme, M.; Vivanco, A.; Lara, P.; Guerrero, S.; Salas-Huenuleo, E.; Chamorro, A.; Leyton, L.; Bolaños, K.; Araya, E.; Quest, A.; et al. Encapsulation of Gold Nanostructures and Oil-in-Water Nanocarriers in Microgels with Biomedical Potential. *Molecules* **2018**, *23*, 1208. [CrossRef]

12. An, Y.H.; Lee, J.; Son, D.U.; Kang, D.H.; Park, M.J.; Cho, K.W.; Kim, S.; Kim, S.H.; Ko, J.; Jang, M.H.; et al. Facilitated Transdermal Drug Delivery Using Nanocarriers-Embedded Electroconductive Hydrogel Coupled with Reverse Electrodialysis-Driven Iontophoresis. *ACS Nano* **2020**, *14*, 4523–4535. [CrossRef] [PubMed]
13. Lin, W.; Ma, G.; Yuan, Z.; Qian, H.; Xu, L.; Sidransky, E.; Chen, S. Development of Zwitterionic Polypeptide Nanoformulation with High Doxorubicin Loading Content for Targeted Drug Delivery. *Langmuir* **2019**, *35*, 1273–1283. [CrossRef] [PubMed]
14. Esteban-Fernández de Ávila, B.; Lopez-Ramirez, M.A.; Mundaca-Uribe, R.; Wei, X.; Ramírez-Herrera, D.E.; Karshalev, E.; Nguyen, B.; Fang, R.H.; Zhang, L.; Wang, J. Multicompartment Tubular Micromotors Toward Enhanced Localized Active Delivery. *Adv. Mater.* **2020**, *32*, 1–10. [CrossRef] [PubMed]
15. Pérez-Hernández, M.; Del Pino, P.; Mitchell, S.G.; Moros, M.; Stepien, G.; Pelaz, B.; Parak, W.J.; Gálvez, E.M.; Pardo, J.; De La Fuente, J.M. Dissecting the molecular mechanism of apoptosis during photothermal therapy using gold nanoprisms. *ACS Nano* **2015**, *9*, 52–61. [CrossRef]
16. Fazio, B.; D'Andrea, C.; Foti, A.; Messina, E.; Irrera, A.; Donato, M.G.; Villari, V.; Micali, N.; Maragò, O.M.; Gucciardi, P.G. SERS detection of Biomolecules at Physiological pH via aggregation of Gold Nanorods mediated by Optical Forces and Plasmonic Heating. *Sci. Rep.* **2016**, *6*, 1–13. [CrossRef]
17. Kelly, K.L.; Coronado, E.; Zhao, L.L.; Schatz, G.C. The Optical Properties of Metal Nanoparticles: The Influence of Size, Shape, and Dielectric Environment. *J. Phys. Chem. B* **2003**, *107*, 668–677. [CrossRef]
18. Mezni, A.; Dammak, T.; Fkiri, A.; Mlayah, A.; Abid, Y.; Smiri, L.S. Photochemistry at the surface of gold nanoprisms from surface-enhanced raman scattering blinking. *J. Phys. Chem. C* **2014**, *118*, 17956–17967. [CrossRef]
19. Santos, N.C.; Domingues, M.M.; Felício, M.R.; Gonçalves, S.; Carvalho, P.M. Application of Light Scattering Techniques to Nanoparticle Characterization and Development. *Front. Chem.* **2018**, *6*, 1–17. [CrossRef]
20. Liu, H.; Pierre-Pierre, N.; Huo, Q. Dynamic light scattering for gold nanorod size characterization and study of nanorod-protein interactions. *Gold Bull.* **2012**, *45*, 187–195. [CrossRef]
21. Sasidharan, S.; Bahadur, D.; Srivastava, R. Albumin stabilized gold nanostars: A biocompatible nanoplatform for SERS, CT imaging and photothermal therapy of cancer. *RSC Adv.* **2016**, *6*, 84025–84034. [CrossRef]
22. Bai, X.; Wang, Y.; Song, Z.; Feng, Y.; Chen, Y.; Zhang, D.; Feng, L. The basic properties of gold nanoparticles and their applications in tumor diagnosis and treatment. *Int. J. Mol. Sci.* **2020**, *21*, 2480. [CrossRef]
23. Khandelia, R.; Bhandari, S.; Pan, U.N.; Ghosh, S.S.; Chattopadhyay, A. Gold Nanocluster Embedded Albumin Nanoparticles for Two-Photon Imaging of Cancer Cells Accompanying Drug Delivery. *Small* **2015**, *11*, 4075–4081. [CrossRef]
24. Gonçalves, A.S.C.; Rodrigues, C.F.; Moreira, A.F.; Correia, I.J. Strategies to improve the photothermal capacity of gold-based nanomedicines. *Acta Biomater.* **2020**, *116*, 105–137. [CrossRef] [PubMed]
25. De Matteis, V.; Rizzello, L. Noble Metals and Soft Bio-Inspired Nanoparticles in Retinal Diseases Treatment: A Perspective. *Cells* **2020**, *9*, 679. [CrossRef]
26. Okoampah, E.; Mao, Y.; Yang, S.; Sun, S.; Zhou, C. Gold nanoparticles–biomembrane interactions: From fundamental to simulation. *Colloids Surf. B Biointerfaces* **2020**, *196*, 111312. [CrossRef]
27. Link, S.; El-sayed, M.A. Shape and size dependence of radiative, non-radiative and photothermal properties of gold nanocrystals. *Int. Rev. Phys. Chem.* **2000**, *19*, 409–453. [CrossRef]
28. Pelaz, B.; Grazu, V.; Ibarra, A.; Magen, C.; Del Pino, P.; De La Fuente, J.M. Tailoring the synthesis and heating ability of gold nanoprisms for bioapplications. *Langmuir* **2012**, *28*, 8965–8970. [CrossRef] [PubMed]
29. Alfranca, G.; Artiga, Á.; Stepien, G.; Moros, M.; Mitchell, S.G.; De La Fuente, J.M. Gold nanoprism-nanorod face off: Comparing the heating efficiency, cellular internalization and thermoablation capacity. *Nanomedicine* **2016**, *11*, 2903–2916. [CrossRef] [PubMed]
30. Wang, L.; Li, J.; Pan, J.; Jiang, X.; Ji, Y.; Li, Y.; Qu, Y.; Zhao, Y.; Wu, X.; Chen, C. Revealing the binding structure of the protein corona on gold nanorods using synchrotron radiation-based techniques: Understanding the reduced damage in cell membranes. *J. Am. Chem. Soc.* **2013**, *135*, 17359–17368. [CrossRef] [PubMed]
31. Alkilany, A.M.; Nagaria, P.K.; Hexel, C.R.; Shaw, T.J.; Murphy, C.J.; Wyatt, M.D. Cellular uptake and cytotoxicity of gold nanorods: Molecular origin of cytotoxicity and surface effects. *Small* **2009**, *5*, 701–708. [CrossRef]
32. Parab, H.J.; Chen, H.M.; Lai, T.C.; Huang, J.H.; Chen, P.H.; Liu, R.S.; Hsiao, M.; Chen, C.H.; Tsai, D.P.; Hwu, Y.K. Biosensing, cytotoxicity, and cellular uptake studies of surface-modified gold nanorods. *J. Phys. Chem. C* **2009**, *113*, 7574–7578. [CrossRef]
33. Koryakina, I.; Kuznetsova, D.S.; Zuev, D.A.; Milichko, V.A.; Timin, A.S.; Zyuzin, M.V. Optically Responsive Delivery Platforms: From the Design Considerations to Biomedical Applications. *Nanophotonics* **2020**, *9*, 39–74. [CrossRef]
34. Bhushan, B.; Khanadeev, V.; Khlebtsov, B.; Khlebtsov, N.; Gopinath, P. Impact of albumin based approaches in nanomedicine: Imaging, targeting and drug delivery. *Adv. Colloid Interface Sci.* **2017**, *246*, 13–39. [CrossRef]
35. Min, Y.; Caster, J.M.; Eblan, M.J.; Wang, A.Z. Clinical Translation of Nanomedicine. *Chem. Rev.* **2015**, *115*, 11147–11190. [CrossRef]
36. Bolaños, K.; Celis, F.; Garrido, C.; Campos, M.; Guzmán, F.; Kogan, M.J.; Araya, E. Adsorption of bovine serum albumin on gold nanoprisms: Interaction and effect of NIR irradiation on protein corona. *J. Mater. Chem. B* **2020**, *8*, 8644–8657. [CrossRef] [PubMed]
37. Loureiro, A.; Azoia, N.G.; Gomes, A.C.; Cavaco-Paulo, A. Albumin-Based Nanodevices as Drug Carriers. *Curr. Pharm. Des.* **2016**, *22*, 1371–1390. [CrossRef]

38. Lee, E.S.; Youn, Y.S. Albumin-based potential drugs: Focus on half-life extension and nanoparticle preparation. *J. Pharm. Investig.* **2016**, *46*, 305–315. [CrossRef]
39. Bolaños, K.; Kogan, M.J.; Araya, E. Capping gold nanoparticles with albumin to improve their biomedical properties. *Int. J. Nanomed.* **2019**, *14*, 6387–6406. [CrossRef]
40. Ding, C.; Xu, Y.; Zhao, Y.; Zhong, H.; Luo, X. Fabrication of BSA@AuNC-Based Nanostructures for Cell Fluoresce Imaging and Target Drug Delivery. *ACS Appl. Mater. Interfaces* **2018**, *10*, 8947–8954. [CrossRef] [PubMed]
41. Zu, L.; Liu, L.; Qin, Y.; Liu, H.; Yang, H. Multifunctional BSA-Au nanostars for photoacoustic imaging and X-ray computed tomography. *Nanomed. Nanotechnol. Biol. Med.* **2016**, *12*, 1805–1813. [CrossRef] [PubMed]
42. Rahdar, S.; Rahdar, A.; Ahmadi, S.; Trant, J.F. Adsorption of bovine serum albumin (BSA) by bare magnetite nanoparticles with surface oxidative impurities that prevent aggregation. *Can. J. Chem.* **2019**, *97*, 577–583. [CrossRef]
43. Shanwar, S.; Liang, L.; Nechaev, A.V.; Basheva, D.K.; Balalaeva, I.V.; Vodeneev, V.A.; Roy, I.; Zvyagin, A.V.; Guryev, E.L. Controlled Formation of a Protein Corona Composed of Denatured BSA on Upconversion Nanoparticles Improves Their Colloidal Stability. *Pharmceutics* **2021**, *14*, 1657.
44. Lillo, C.R.; Calienni, M.N.; Rivas, B.; Prieto, M.J.; Rodriguez, D.; Tuninetti, J.; Toledo, P.; Alonso, V.; Moya, S.; Gonzalez, M.C.; et al. BSA-capped gold nanoclusters as potential theragnostic for skin diseases: Photoactivation, skin penetration, in vitro and in vivo toxicity. *Mater. Sci. Eng. C* **2020**, *112*, 110891. [CrossRef]
45. Sabbarwal, S.; Dubey, A.K.; Pandey, M.; Kumar, M. Synthesis of Biocompatible, BSA capped Fluorescent CaCO3 Pre-Nucleation Nanoclusters for Cell Imaging Applications. *J. Mater. Chem. B* **2020**, *8*, 5729–5744. [CrossRef] [PubMed]
46. Bros, M.; Nuhn, L.; Simon, J.; Moll, L.; Mailänder, V.; Landfester, K.; Grabbe, S. The protein corona as a confounding variable of nanoparticle-mediated targeted vaccine delivery. *Front. Immunol.* **2018**, *9*, 1–10. [CrossRef]
47. Falahati, M.; Attar, F.; Sharifi, M.; Haertlé, T.; Berret, J.; Khan, R.H.; Saboury, A.A. A health concern regarding the protein corona, aggregation and disaggregation. *Biochim. Biophys. Acta-Gen. Subj.* **2019**, *1863*, 971–991. [CrossRef] [PubMed]
48. Francia, V.; Yang, K.; Deville, S.; Reker-Smit, C.; Nelissen, I.; Salvati, A. Corona Composition Can Affect the Mechanisms Cells Use to Internalize Nanoparticles. *ACS Nano* **2019**, *13*, 11107–11121. [CrossRef] [PubMed]
49. Bode, S.A.; Timmermans, S.B.P.E.; Eising, S.; Van Gemert, S.P.W.; Bonger, K.M.; Löwik, D.W.P.M. Click to enter: Activation of oligo-arginine cell-penetrating peptides by bioorthogonal tetrazine ligations. *Chem. Sci.* **2019**, *10*, 701–705. [CrossRef]
50. Åmand, H.L.; Rydberg, H.A.; Fornander, L.H.; Lincoln, P.; Nordén, B.; Esbjörner, E.K. Cell surface binding and uptake of arginine- and lysine-rich penetratin peptides in absence and presence of proteoglycans. *Biochim. Biophys. Acta-Biomembr.* **2012**, *1818*, 2669–2678. [CrossRef]
51. Allolio, C.; Magarkar, A.; Jurkiewicz, P.; Baxová, K.; Javanainen, M.; Mason, P.E.; Šachl, R.; Cebecauer, M.; Hof, M.; Horinek, D.; et al. Arginine-rich cell-penetrating peptides induce membrane multilamellarity and subsequently enter via formation of a fusion pore. *Proc. Natl. Acad. Sci. USA* **2018**, *115*, 11923–11928. [CrossRef] [PubMed]
52. Zhao, P.; Li, F.; Huang, Y. *Nanotechnology-Based Targeted Drug Delivery Systems and Drug Resistance in Colorectal Cancer*; Elsevier Inc.: Amsterdam, The Netherlands, 2020; ISBN 9780128199374.
53. Pan, Z.; Kang, X.; Zeng, Y.; Zhang, W.; Peng, H.; Wang, J.; Huang, W.; Wang, H.; Shen, Y.; Huang, Y. A mannosylated PEI-CPP hybrid for TRAIL gene targeting delivery for colorectal cancer therapy. *Polym. Chem.* **2017**, *8*, 5275–5285. [CrossRef]
54. Garcia, J.; Fernández-Blanco, Á.; Teixidó, M.; Sánchez-Navarro, M.; Giralt, E. d-Polyarginine Lipopeptides as Intestinal Permeation Enhancers. *ChemMedChem* **2018**, *13*, 2045–2052. [CrossRef] [PubMed]
55. An, F.F.; Zhang, X.H. Strategies for preparing albumin-based nanoparticles for multifunctional bioimaging and drug delivery. *Theranostics* **2017**, *7*, 3667–3689. [CrossRef]
56. Palanikumar, L.; Al-Hosani, S.; Kalmouni, M.; Nguyen, V.P.; Ali, L.; Pasricha, R.; Barrera, F.N.; Magzoub, M. pH-responsive high stability polymeric nanoparticles for targeted delivery of anticancer therapeutics. *Commun. Biol.* **2020**, *3*, 1–17. [CrossRef] [PubMed]
57. Riveros, A.L.; Eggeling, C.; Riquelme, S.; Adura, C.; López-Iglesias, C.; Guzmán, F.; Araya, E.; Almada, M.; Juárez, J.; Valdez, M.A.; et al. Improving cell penetration of gold nanorods by using an amphipathic arginine rich peptide. *Int. J. Nanomed.* **2020**, *15*, 1837–1851. [CrossRef]
58. Garcia, J.; Fernández-Pradas, J.M.; Lladó, A.; Serra, P.; Zalvidea, D.; Kogan, M.; Giralt, E.; Sánchez-Navarro, M. The combined use of gold nanoparticles and infrared radiation enables cytosolic protein delivery. *Chem. A Eur. J.* **2020**. [CrossRef]
59. Nakase, I.; Noguchi, K.; Aoki, A.; Takatani-Nakase, T.; Fujii, I.; Futaki, S. Arginine-rich cell-penetrating peptide-modified extracellular vesicles for active macropinocytosis induction and efficient intracellular delivery. *Sci. Rep.* **2017**, *7*, 1–12. [CrossRef] [PubMed]
60. Kamei, N.; Morishita, M.; Takayama, K. Importance of intermolecular interaction on the improvement of intestinal therapeutic peptide/protein absorption using cell-penetrating peptides. *J. Control. Release* **2009**, *136*, 179–186. [CrossRef]
61. Jiang, Y.; Zhang, Z.; Zhang, Y.; Lv, H.; Zhou, J.; Li, C.; Hou, L.; Zhang, Q. Dual-functional liposomes based on pH-responsive cell-penetrating peptide and hyaluronic acid for tumor-targeted anticancer drug delivery. *Biomaterials* **2012**, *33*, 9246–9258. [CrossRef] [PubMed]
62. Ishikawa, M.; Biju, V. *Luminescent Quantum Dots, Making Invisibles Visible in Bioimaging*, 1st ed.; Elsevier Inc.: Amsterdam, The Netherlands, 2011; Volume 104, ISBN 9780124160200.

63. Cassano, S.D.; Voliani, V. Photothermal effect by NIR-responsive excretable ultrasmall-in-nano architectures. *Mater. Horiz.* **2019**, *6*, 531–537. [CrossRef]
64. Scarabelli, L.; Sánchez-Iglesias, A.; Pérez-Juste, J.; Liz-Marzán, L.M. A "Tips and Tricks" Practical Guide to the Synthesis of Gold Nanorods. *J. Phys. Chem. Lett.* **2015**, *6*, 4270–4279. [CrossRef]
65. Melchionna, M.; Styan, K.; Marchesan, S. The unexpected advantages of using D-amino acids for peptide self-assembly into nanostructured hydrogels for medicine. *Curr. Top. Med. Chem.* **2016**, *16*, 2009–2018. [CrossRef]
66. Kelly, S.M.; Jess, T.J.; Price, N.C. How to study proteins by circular dichroism. *Biochim. Biophys. Acta Proteins Proteom.* **2005**, *1751*, 119–139. [CrossRef]
67. Grönbeck, H.; Curioni, A.; Andreoni, W. Thiols and disulfides on the Au(111) surface: The headgroup-gold interaction. *J. Am. Chem. Soc.* **2000**, *122*, 3839–3842. [CrossRef]
68. Maleki, M.S.; Moradi, O.; Tahmasebi, S. Adsorption of albumin by gold nanoparticles: Equilibrium and thermodynamics studies. *Arab. J. Chem.* **2017**, *10*, 491–502. [CrossRef]
69. de Oliveira Noman, L.; Sant'Ana, A.C. The control of the adsorption of bovine serum albumin on mercaptan-modified gold thin films investigated by SERS spectroscopy. *Spectrochim. Acta Part. A Mol. Biomol. Spectrosc.* **2018**, *204*, 119–124. [CrossRef]
70. Pramanik, S.; Banerjee, P.; Sarkar, A.; Bhattacharya, S.C. Size-dependent interaction of gold nanoparticles with transport protein: A spectroscopic study. *J. Lumin.* **2008**, *128*, 1969–1974. [CrossRef]
71. Treuel, L.; Malissek, M.; Gebauer, J.S.; Zellner, R. The influence of surface composition of nanoparticles on their interactions with serum albumin. *ChemPhysChem* **2010**, *11*, 3093–3099. [CrossRef] [PubMed]
72. del Caño, R.; Mateus, L.; Sánchez-Obrero, G.; Sevilla, J.M.; Madueño, R.; Blázquez, M.; Pineda, T. Hemoglobin bioconjugates with surface-protected gold nanoparticles in aqueous media: The stability depends on solution pH and protein properties. *J. Colloid Interface Sci.* **2017**, *505*, 1165–1171. [CrossRef] [PubMed]
73. Leopold, L.F.; Tódor, I.S.; Diaconeasa, Z.; Rugină, D.; Ștefancu, A.; Leopold, N.; Coman, C. Assessment of PEG and BSA-PEG gold nanoparticles cellular interaction. *Colloids Surf. A Physicochem. Eng. Asp.* **2017**, *532*, 70–76. [CrossRef]
74. Binaymotlagh, R.; Hadadzadeh, H.; Farrokhpour, H.; Haghighi, F.H.; Abyar, F.; Mirahmadi-Zare, S.Z. In situ generation of the gold nanoparticles–bovine serum albumin (AuNPs–BSA) bioconjugated system using pulsed-laser ablation (PLA). *Mater. Chem. Phys.* **2016**, *177*, 360–370. [CrossRef]
75. Alsamamra, H.; Hawwarin, I.; Sharkh, S.A.; Abuteir, M. Study the Interaction between Gold Nanoparticles and Bovine Serum Albumin: Spectroscopic Approach. *J. Bioanal. Biomed.* **2018**, *10*, 43–49. [CrossRef]
76. Vio, V.; Riveros, A.L.; Tapia-Bustos, A.; Lespay-Rebolledo, C.; Perez-Lobos, R.; Muñoz, L.; Pismante, P.; Morales, P.; Araya, E.; Hassan, N.; et al. Gold nanorods/siRNA complex administration for knockdown of PARP-1: A potential treatment for perinatal asphyxia. *Int. J. Nanomed.* **2018**, *13*, 6839–6854. [CrossRef] [PubMed]
77. Li, D.; Zhang, M.; Xu, F.; Chen, Y.; Chen, B.; Chang, Y.; Zhong, H.; Jin, H.; Huang, Y. Biomimetic albumin-modified gold nanorods for photothermo-chemotherapy and macrophage polarization modulation. *Acta Pharm. Sin. B* **2018**, *8*, 74–84. [CrossRef] [PubMed]
78. Kun, R.; Szekeres, M.; Dékány, I. Isothermal titration calorimetric studies of the pH induced conformational changes of bovine serum albumin. *J. Therm. Anal. Calorim.* **2009**, *96*, 1009–1017. [CrossRef]
79. Zhao, J.; Stenzel, M.H. Entry of nanoparticles into cells: The importance of nanoparticle properties. *Polym. Chem.* **2018**, *9*, 259–272. [CrossRef]
80. Wu, B.; Deng, S.; Zhang, S.; Jiang, J.; Han, B.; Li, Y. PH sensitive mesoporous nanohybrids with charge-reversal properties for anticancer drug delivery. *RSC Adv.* **2017**, *7*, 46045–46050. [CrossRef]
81. Jurašin, D.D.; Ćurlin, M.; Capjak, I.; Crnković, T.; Lovrić, M.; Babič, M.; Horák, D.; Vrček, I.V.; Gajović, S. Surface coating affects behavior of metallic nanoparticles in a biological environment. *Beilstein J. Nanotechnol.* **2016**, *7*, 246–262. [CrossRef] [PubMed]
82. Zhang, L.; Xia, K.; Bai, Y.Y.; Lu, Z.; Tang, Y.; Deng, Y.; Chen, J.; Qian, W.; Shen, H.; Zhang, Z.; et al. Synthesis of gold nanorods and their functionalization with bovine serum albumin for optical hyperthermia. *J. Biomed. Nanotechnol.* **2014**, *10*, 1440–1449. [CrossRef]
83. Wang, X.; Li, J.; Kawazoe, N.; Chen, G. Photothermal Ablation of Cancer Cells by Albumin-Modified Gold Nanorods and Activation of Dendritic Cells. *Materials* **2018**, *12*, 31. [CrossRef]
84. Zhou, B.; Song, J.; Wang, M.; Wang, X.; Howard, E.W.; Zhou, F.; Qu, J.; Chen, W.R. BSA-bioinspired gold nanorods loaded with immunoadjuvant for the treatment of melanoma by combined photothermal therapy and immunotherapy. *Nanoscale* **2018**, *10*, 21640–21647. [CrossRef] [PubMed]
85. Adura, C.; Guerrero, S.; Salas, E.; Medel, L.; Riveros, A.; Mena, J.; Arbiol, J.; Albericio, F.; Giralt, E.; Kogan, M.J. Stable conjugates of peptides with gold nanorods for biomedical applications with reduced effects on cell viability. *ACS Appl. Mater. Interfaces* **2013**, *5*, 4076–4085. [CrossRef]
86. Charbgoo, F.; Nejabat, M.; Abnous, K.; Soltani, F.; Taghdisi, S.M.; Alibolandi, M.; Thomas Shier, W.; Steele, T.W.J.; Ramezani, M. Gold nanoparticle should understand protein corona for being a clinical nanomaterial. *J. Control. Release* **2018**, *272*, 39–53. [CrossRef]
87. Bao, C.; Beziere, N.; Del Pino, P.; Pelaz, B.; Estrada, G.; Tian, F.; Ntziachristos, V.; De La Fuente, J.M.; Cui, D. Gold nanoprisms as optoacoustic signal nanoamplifiers for in vivo bioimaging of gastrointestinal cancers. *Small* **2013**, *9*, 68–74. [CrossRef] [PubMed]
88. Ambrosone, A.; Del Pino, P.; Marchesano, V.; Parak, W.J.; De La Fuente, J.M.; Tortiglione, C. Gold nanoprisms for photothermal cell ablation in vivo. *Nanomedicine* **2014**, *9*, 1913–1922. [CrossRef] [PubMed]
89. Liu, M.; Li, Q.; Liang, L.; Li, J.; Wang, K.; Li, J.; Lv, M.; Chen, N.; Song, H.; Lee, J.; et al. Real-Time visualization of clustering and intracellular transport of gold nanoparticles by correlative imaging. *Nat. Commun.* **2017**, *8*, 1–10. [CrossRef] [PubMed]

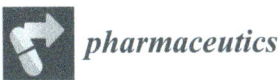

Article

Modification of Proliferation and Apoptosis in Breast Cancer Cells by Exposure of Antioxidant Nanoparticles Due to Modulation of the Cellular Redox State Induced by Doxorubicin Exposure

Laura Denise López-Barrera [1], Roberto Díaz-Torres [2], Joselo Ramón Martínez-Rosas [1], Ana María Salazar [3], Carlos Rosales [4] and Patricia Ramírez-Noguera [1,*]

1. Departamento de Ciencias Biológicas, Facultad de Estudios Superiores Cuautitlán, Universidad Nacional Autónoma de México (UNAM), Ciudad Universitaria, 4510, 4513, Mexico City CP 54714, Mexico; laura.lobar@cuautitlan.unam.mx (L.D.L.-B.); mvzjoselomartinez@gmail.com (J.R.M.-R.)
2. Departamento de Ingeniería y Tecnología, Facultad de Estudios Superiores Cuautitlán, Universidad Nacional Autónoma de México (UNAM), Ciudad Universitaria, 4510, 4513, Mexico City CP 54714, Mexico; diaztorres_r@hotmail.com
3. Departamento de Medicina Genómica y Toxicología Ambiental, Instituto de Investigaciones Biomédicas, Universidad Nacional Autónoma de México (UNAM), Ciudad Universitaria, 4510, 4513, Mexico City CP 54714, Mexico; anamsm@biomedicas.unam.mx
4. Departamento de Inmunología, Instituto de Investigaciones Biomédicas, Universidad Nacional Autónoma de México (UNAM), Ciudad Universitaria, 4510, 4513, Mexico City CP 54714, Mexico; carosal@biomedicas.unam.mx
* Correspondence: ramireznoguera@unam.mx; Tel.: +52-5623-19-99 (ext. 3-9429)

Abstract: In this report, we investigated whether the use of chitosan-carrying-glutathione nanoparticles (CH-GSH NPs) can modify proliferation and apoptosis, and reduce cell damage induced by doxorubicin on breast cancer cells. Doxorubicin is a widely used antineoplasic agent for the treatment of various types of cancer. However, it is also a highly toxic drug because it induces oxidative stress. Thus, the use of antioxidant molecules has been considered to reduce the toxicity of doxorubicin. CH-GSH NPs were characterized in size, zeta potential, concentration, and shape. When breast cancer cells were treated with CH-GSH nanoparticles, they were localized in the cellular cytoplasm. Combined doxorubicin exposure with nanoparticles increased intracellular GSH levels. At the same time, decreasing levels of reactive oxygen species and malondialdehyde were observed and modified antioxidant enzyme activity. Levels of the Ki67 protein were evaluated as a marker of cell proliferation and the activity of the Casp-3 protein related to cell apoptosis was measured. Our data suggests that CH-GSH NPs can modify cell proliferation by decreasing Ki67 levels, induce apoptosis by increasing caspase-3 activity, and reduce the oxidative stress induced by doxorubicin in breast cancer cells by modulating molecules associated with the cellular redox state. CH-GSH NPs could be used to reduce the toxic effects of this antineoplastic. Considering these results, CH-GSH NPs represent a novel delivery system offering new opportunities in pharmacy, material science, and biomedicine.

Keywords: glutathione; nanoparticles; oxidative stress; doxorubicin; breast cancer

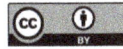

1. Introduction

Breast cancer is one of the leading health problems worldwide. Its incidence is estimated at 11.6%, placing it among the first three types of cancer diagnosed in both men and women [1]. Approximately half of the people diagnosed with breast cancer usually present recurrences even after treatment and about one-third of these patients die from the disease [2]. About 80% of breast carcinomas are positive for hormonal (progesterone and estrogen) receptors. These tumors are treated with drugs such as tamoxifen that blocks estrogen-induced cell growth. Other breast tumors (about 15%) express the human epidermal growth factor receptor (HER2). These tumors are treated with a monoclonal antibody such as trastuzumab, which is specific against HER2. The third group of breast tumors does not express hormonal receptors or HER2 and is known as triple-negative.

These tumors tend to be more aggressive, and their treatment is based on the general inhibition of cell replication on all dividing cells [2].

Doxorubicin (Dox) is a potent broad-spectrum antineoplastic agent belonging to the anthracycline family and is used to treat various cancer types including breast cancer. Its action mechanism is associated with inhibiting cell replication by binding to the enzyme topoisomerase II, causing DNA alterations, and favoring the aging of cells [3]. Unfortunately, it also induces oxidative stress that can affect both dividing and non-dividing cells. Consequently, doxorubicin can trigger undesirable side effects due to general cell toxicity. Dox stimulates the formation of free radicals (O_2^-, H_2O_2, and $^\bullet OH$) and reactive oxygen species (ROS) through Fenton chemistry reactions during the metabolic transformation of doxorubicin to doxorubicinol. Besides, this antineoplastic can activate the NADPH oxidase and modify calcium metabolism [4]. Exposure to doxorubicin has also been reported to decrease the Ki67 protein levels associated with cell proliferation and to increase the number of apoptotic cells in a dose-dependent manner [5].

There is a growing interest in finding ways of reducing oxidative stress in tissues during doxorubicin treatment. A promising approach is the use of antioxidant molecules [6,7]. Glutathione (GSH) is one of the primary endogenous antioxidants at the cellular level and is associated with various events such as proliferation, apoptosis, and redox state regulation. It is synthesized exclusively in the cell cytoplasm and once used and in its oxidized state, it cannot be incorporated into the cell, thus it must be synthesized to maintain the levels in an optimal state [8]. Moreover, GSH is recognized as a fundamental antioxidant molecule for cellular protection from toxins, both endogenous and environmental, including several anti-cancer cytotoxic drugs [9].

Transporting GSH and other agents into cells to reduce the toxic effects of anti-cancer drugs requires the use of innovative delivery systems [10]. Nanotechnology in cancer treatment represents a novel alternative to deliver agents to cells due to the physicochemical properties of many different nanoparticles. Chitosan (CH), a natural polymer, has been used to create nanoparticles (NPs) that are ideal delivery systems. They are easy to produce, have a shallow immunogenic profile, diffuse quickly into cells, and are biodegradable and biocompatible. In addition, CH NPs can easily interact with many other molecules due to their chemical structure [11]. CH NPs have already been reported to deliver molecules that can regulate inflammation events and sensitize cancer cells to X-ray radiation [12,13]. This report explored the use of CH-GSH NPs to modify proliferation, apoptosis, and the cellular redox state through the modulation of oxidative stress induced by doxorubicin in two breast cancer cell lines.

2. Materials and Methods

2.1. Preparation and Characterization of Nanoparticles

Chitosan-carrying-glutathione nanoparticles (CH-GSH NPs) were prepared by the ionic gelation technique as previously described [14]. CH-GSH NPs were also coupled to rhodamine-123 at a concentration of 0.5 mg/mL in methanol for confocal microscopy analysis. Rhodamine-123 was added to the already formed CH-GSH NPs at 1: 4 ratio overnight. Nanoparticles were ultracentrifuged with glycerol at 27,000 rpm for 1 h and the ring formed containing the nanoparticles was resuspended in 1% acetic acid. Next, nanoparticles were characterized in concentration with a hydrodynamic diameter and zeta potential using the equipment Nanosight and Zetasizer from Malvern Panalytical, Malvern, UK Quantification of the encapsulated GSH was determined indirectly by the DTNB technique at a wavelength of 425 nm as described [15]. Finally, were observed the shape of CH-GSH NPs through transmission electron microscopy.

2.2. Cell Lines

The breast cancer cell lines MCF-7 (ATCC HTB-22) and MDA MB-231 (ATCC HTB-26) were used. MCF-7 cells are positive for functional estrogen receptors and MDA MB-231 cells are negative for estrogen receptors, progesterone receptors, and the E-cadherin. Cells were cultured in a DMEM medium supplemented with 12% fetal bovine serum (FSB), antibiotic 1% (penicillin/streptomycin) at 37 °C in a 5% CO_2 incubator. Cells were cultured in either 24-well or 6-well tissue culture plates until they were confluent before performing the various assays described next.

2.3. Confocal Microscopy Analysis

NPs coupled to rhodamine-123 were added to MCF-7 and MDA MB-231 cells, and two concentrations of NPs were used, namely 1.8×10^8 nanoparticles/mL (equivalent to 0.08 mM GSH) and 1.4×10^9 nanoparticles/mL (equivalent to 0.64 mM GSH), for 2 h. Then, cells were washed with PBS, fixed with 3% paraformaldehyde, and stained with DAPI (0.1 µg/mL). Finally, cells were observed with the confocal microscopy Zeiss LSM800. The images were taken at a 63× magnification at an λ ext 360/em 460 (DAPI) and λ ext 507/em 529 nm (Rhodamine 123).

2.4. Cytotoxicity

To evaluate the cytotoxic effect, cells were exposed to 5 µM of Dox for 12 h, then washed once with PBS, and were exposed for 2 h to CH NPs and CH-GSH NPs at a concentration of 1.8×10^8 or 1.4×10^9 NP/mL. We used the resazurin technique. This assay evaluates cells' ability to reduce resazurin to resorufin and can be read at a wavelength of 570/600 nm [16]. The cells were placed in 24-well plates; treatments were added; cells were washed with PBS; resazurin was added at a concentration of 0.01% and was left to incubate for 30 min at 37 °C; and lastly, the lectures were made. To know the differences between the treatments with NPs, Dox, and the untreated cells, the following calculation was performed:

$$\frac{(A\ 1) - (A\ 2)\ treated\ cells}{(A\ 1) - (A\ 2)\ Untreated\ cells} \times 100 = \%\ Cell\ viability$$

where:
   A1 = absorbance at 570 nm and
   A2 = absorbance at 600 nm.

2.5. Biomarkers of Oxidative Stress

2.5.1. Intracellular and Extracellular GSH Concentrations

Confluent cells cultured in 6-well plates were exposed to 5 µM Dox for 12 h. After time, the medium was removed, and cells were washed with PBS. Then, CH NPs or CH-GSH NPs were added for 2 h at a concentration of 1.8×10^8 or 1.4×10^9 NPs/ mL. At the end of the exposure time, the culture medium was removed and washed with PBS twice, placed in 100 µL of lysis buffer (0.1% Triton, 5 mM EDTA, 1 mM PMSF), and scraped on ice. The cell suspension was centrifuged at 13,000 rpm for 10 min at 4 °C and the supernatant (cell lysate) was transferred to a clean tube. The amount of total protein in the cell lysates was determined according to the Bradford method [17]. The extracellular concentration of GSH was indirectly measured using the culture medium of the cells treated with nanoparticles. The concentration of intracellular and extracellular GSH was determined with the 2,2-dithiobisnitrobenzoic acid (DTNB) assay [15]. This assay is based on the reaction of GSH with DTNB, forming a yellow adduct product (GS-TNB) that can be read spectrophotometrically at a wavelength of 425 nm.

2.5.2. Malondialdehyde Concentration

Malondialdehyde (MDA) concentration was determined with the thiobarbituric acid reactive species assay (TBARS) [18] with some modifications. This assay is based on the reaction of MDA with thiobarbituric acid to form a pink adduct product. The product can be read spectrophotometrically at a wavelength of 540 nm. Cells were treated with 5 µM Dox for 12 h, after which the medium was removed, and cells were washed twice with PBS. Then, CH NPs or CH-GSH NPs were added for 2 h at a concentration of 1.8×10^8 or 1.4×10^9 NPs/mL. At the end of the incubation time, the medium was removed, and two washes were carried out with PBS; 100 µL of lysis buffer was added; and the cells were scraped on ice. The cell suspension obtained is centrifuged at 13,000 rpm for 10 min and the supernatant obtained is separated. The cell lysate was mixed at a 1:1 ratio with 0.67% (m/v) thiobarbituric acid and incubated at 90 °C for 30 min. Finally, samples were read spectrophotometrically at a wavelength of 540 nm.

2.5.3. Measurement of ROS

The detection of reactive oxygen species was performed with the dichlorofluorescein diacetate (DCFDA) assay [19] with some modifications. Cells were treated for 12 h with 5 µM Dox, underwent two washes carried out with PBS, and CH NPs and CH-GSH NPs were added at a concentration of 1.8×10^8 or 1.4×10^9. At the end of the exposure time, the culture medium was removed, and the cells were washed twice with PBS. The fluorogenic dye 2′,7′-DCFDA was added to the cells at 5 µM and were incubated for 15 min at 37 °C. In the presence of the reactive oxygen species and other peroxides, DCFDA is oxidized to 2′,7′-dichlorofluorescein (DCF), a fluorescent product that can be detected with a fluorometer at excitation light λ_{ex} = 488 nm and emission light λ_{em} = 525 nm.

2.5.4. Antioxidant Enzymes' Activity

To estimate the activity of antioxidant enzymes, the cells were treated with Dox at a concentration of 5 µM for 12 h. After that time, two washes with PBS were carried out and CH NPs and CH-GSH NPs were added to the cells for 2 h at a concentration of 1.8×10^8 and 1.4×10^9 NPs/mL. Confluent cells were scraped and placed in 100 µL lysis buffer (0.1% Triton, 5 mM EDTA, 1 mM PMSF). Cells were centrifuged at 13,000 rpm for 10 min at 4 °C and cell lysate was transferred to a clean tube.

Catalase activity was estimated as previously reported [20]. Regarding the cell lysate, 100 µL was taken and 100 µL of the reaction medium containing ×100 (1%) was added, after which the cells were incubated at 37 °C for 15 min. Then, 100 µL of a 30% H_2O_2 solution was added. The enzyme-generated oxygen bubbles trapped by triton X-100 were visualized as foam. The height of the foam layer corresponds to the catalase activity and it is compared to a calibration curve made with known concentrations of catalase.

The activity of glutathione peroxidase GPx was estimated as previously reported [21]. The technique is based on measuring the decrease in NADPH absorbance at 340 nm absorption by a coupled reaction with glutathione reductase (GPx). The GPx uses GSH to convert H_2O_2 to H_2O. As a result, the GSSG produced is regenerated by GRx with the conversion of NADPH to $NADP^+$.

The activity of GRx was estimated as previously reported [21]. The cells were processed in the same way as glutathione peroxidase. Glutathione reductase activity reduces the oxidized form of glutathione, disulfide glutathione (GSSG), to reduced glutathione. Considering this reaction is coupled to NADPH's oxidation and NADPH absorbs light at 340 nm, a decrease in absorbance reflects its oxidation.

2.6. Caspase-3 Activity

To evaluate the effect on apoptosis, the cells were treated with Dox at a concentration of 5 µM for 12 h; subsequently, two washes with PBS were carried out and CH NPs and CH-GSH NPs were added for 2 h at a concentration of 1.8×10^8 and 1.4×10^9 NPs/mL. At the end of the exposure time, the cells were washed with PBS and 100 µL of lysis buffer was added. Cells were scraped on ice. The suspension obtained was centrifuged at 13,000 rpm for 10 min. The supernatant (cell lysate) was collected to evaluate caspase-3 activity. Caspase-3 activity was measured in the cell lysate using the CaspACE assay System colorimetric kit, which consists of a colorimetric assay based on the spectrophotometric detection of p-nitroanilide chromophore at a wavelength of 405 nm [22].

2.7. Quantification of Ki67

To determine the effect on proliferation, the amount of antigen was measured by an ELISA test in which a color change from blue to yellow in the plate containing the antibody coupled to a chromogen is proportional to the Ki67 in the sample, which can be read at a wavelength of 450 nm [23]. The cells are treated with Dox at a concentration of 5 µM for 12 h; subsequently, two washes with PBS were carried out and CH NPs and CH-GSH NPs were added for 2 h at a concentration of 1.8×10^8 and 1.4×10^9 NPs/mL. At the end of the exposure time, the cells were washed with PBS, 100 µL of lysis buffer was added, the cells were scraped on ice, and the suspension obtained was centrifuged at 13,000 rpm for 10 min. The supernatant obtained is added to the microplate to determine the presence of the antigen.

2.8. Statistical Analysis

Three independent biological experiments were carried out in triplicates for each experiment. The results obtained were analyzed using a one-way analysis of variance (ANOVA), followed by multiple comparisons of means according to Tukey's statistical test, considering a significant difference at $p < 0.05$. OriginLab graphing and data analysis software was used.

3. Results and Discussion

3.1. Characterization of Nanoparticles

The CH-GSH NPs were prepared according to the ionic gelation method described in the experimental section. NPs were characterized by measuring their hydrodynamic diameter, polydispersion index (PDI), zeta potential, concentration, and GSH encapsulation percentage (Table 1). CH-GSH NPs labeled with rhodamine 123 had a hydrodynamic diameter between 100 and 150 nm. The particle size is an important parameter because it is assumed that most nanoparticles can be transported into the cells by endocytosis [24]. The polydispersion index indicated that both preparations of nanoparticles were homogeneous suspensions. This argument was further supported by the zeta potential which suggested that the nanoparticles remained in suspension without precipitation [25]. The percentage of GSH encapsulation was 99.23%, indicating that enough GSH was captured in the NPs. Considering GSH is very hydrophilic, it cannot enter cells unless it is trapped inside a nanocarrier. In addition, analysis of the nanoparticles' characterization by transmission electron microscopy showed that most particles were spherical (Figure 1).

Table 1. Characterization results.

Nanoparticles	Hydrodynamic Diameter (nm) ± SD	Polydispersion Index (PDI)	Z Potential (mV) ± SD	Amount of NP (NPs/mL)	Encapsulation of GSH (%)
CH-GSH NPs	147.1 ± 75.40	0.246	15.2 ± 3.10	3.718×10^{10}	99.23
CH NPs	126.7 ± 57.57	0.276	18.7 ± 2.04	3.718×10^{10}	-
CH-GSH NPs R-123	129.8 ± 55.01	0.264	23.2 ± 1.12	5.343×10^{10}	99.23

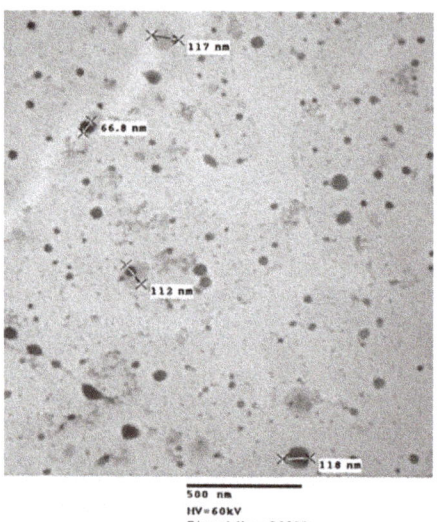

Figure 1. Image of transmission electron microscopy of CH-GSH NPs.

3.2. Chitosan-Carrying-Glutathione Nanoparticles (CH-GSH NPs) Are Localized into the Cells

Cells were exposed to two different concentrations of CH-GSH NPs labeled with rhodamine-123 for 2 h and then subsequently stained with DAPI to differentiate the nucleus. Two different breast cancer cell lines readily internalized the NPs, accumulated in the cytoplasm near the nucleus' periphery. As shown in Figure 2, CH-GSH NPs are in the cytoplasm in both cell lines. We used two different NPs concentrations; however, no significant differences were observed in the images obtained. Qualitative observations suggest a greater sensitivity in the distribution of CH-GSH NP in the cytoplasm of MDA MB-231 cells even at the lowest exposure dose compared to the MCF-7 cell line. In this case, the higher doses tested showed a minor inclusion in MCF-7 cells. These results suggest sharp differences to the nanoparticles studied.

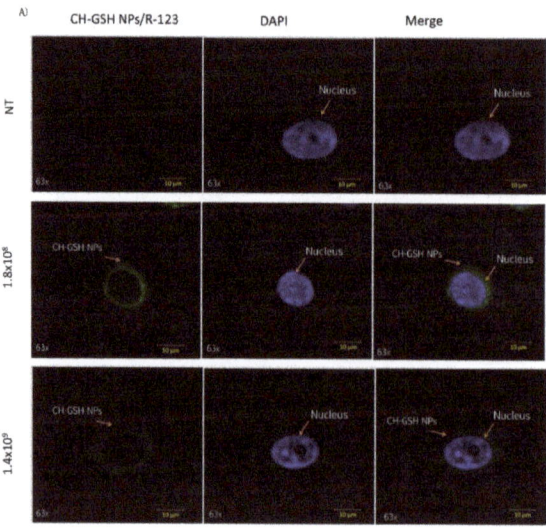

Figure 2. *Cont.*

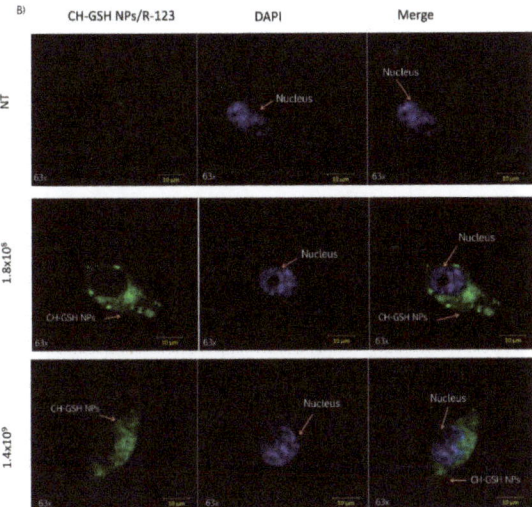

Figure 2. Confocal microscopy images of cells exposed to a concentration of 1.8×10^8 NPs/mL and 1.4×10^9 NPs/mL at the time of 2 h. Untreated cells (NT), (**A**) MCF-7 and (**B**) MDA MB-231 cells.

3.3. Nanoparticles Do Not Reduce the Cell Viability and Do Not Alter Cytotoxicity Induced by Doxorubicin

To demonstrate that exposure to NPs did not compromise cell viability, a resazurin assay was performed [16]. As shown in Figure 3, the exposure to 5 µM of doxorubicin and its combination with nanoparticles in the two concentrations did not show significant differences between them, suggesting that the presence of NPs does not alter the cytotoxic capacity of doxorubicin.

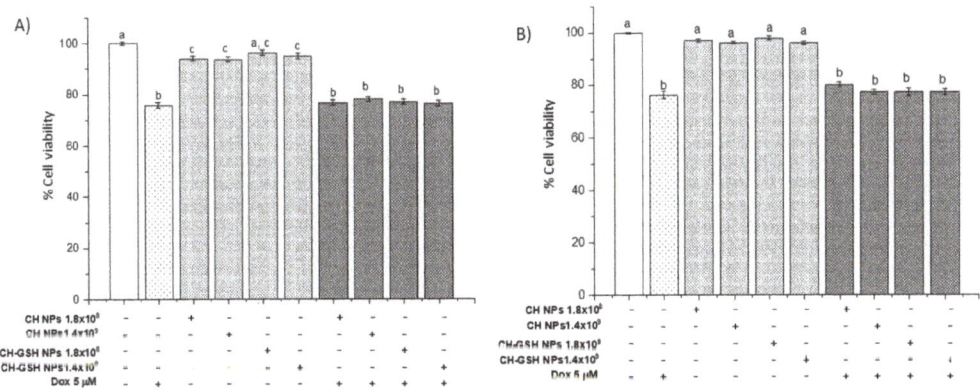

Figure 3. Viability of cells exposed to doxorubicin for 12 h and then 2 h with NPs. (**A**) MCF-7 and (**B**) MDA MB-231 cells. Bars with equal letters indicate no significant differences between the means (Tukey's test, $p < 0.05$).

3.4. Doxorubicin Exposure with a Nanoparticle Increase the Intracellular GSH Levels

Total intracellular and extracellular GSH concentrations were determined in cells exposed to the NPs. Intracellular GSH concentration increased significantly compared with the untreated cells when the cells were exposed to CH-GSH NPs and CH-NPs with the highest concentration tested. The MDA MB-231 cells were the exception (Figure 4A,C). For

MDA MB-231 cells, the NPs treatment did not change the intracellular concentration of GSH (Figure 4C). These results suggest differences in the susceptibility of exposed cells by having available GSH content in the NPs. The exposure only to nanoparticles in the cells does not modify the intracellular GSH and statistically GSH levels are like those obtained in the untreated cells. In combined treatments, levels may increase due to previous exposure to the stress-inducing agent doxorubicin.

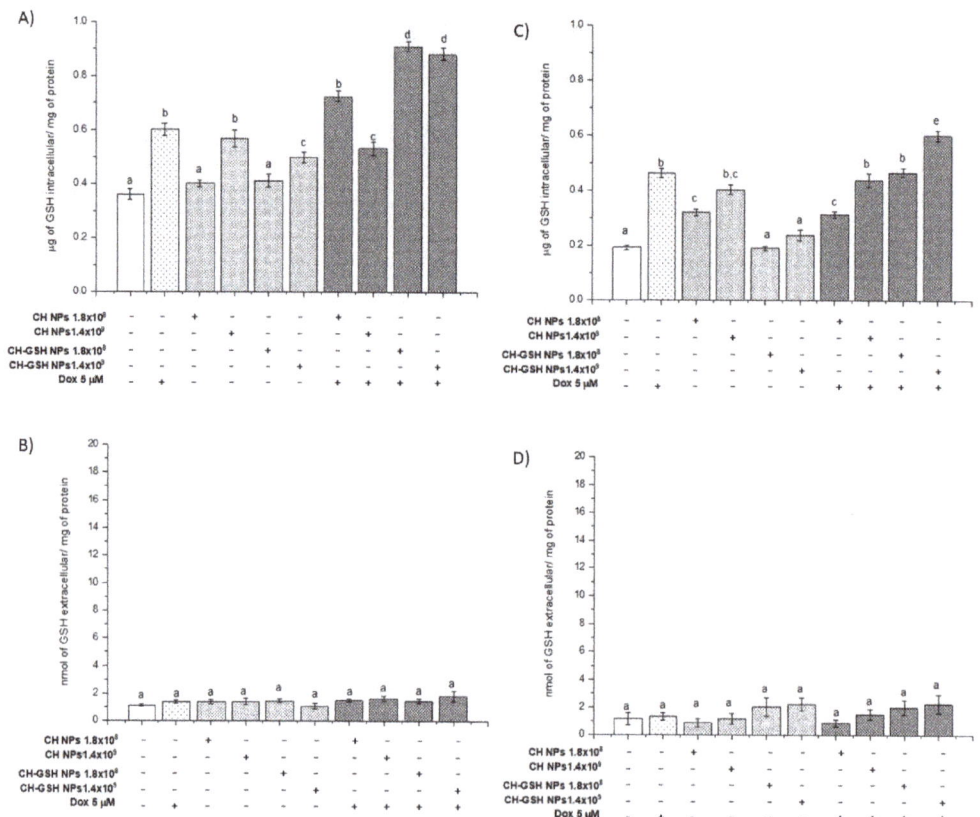

Figure 4. GSH intra (**A,C**) and extracellular (**B,D**) levels of cells exposed to doxorubicin for 12 h and then 2 h with CH-GSH NPs or CH-NPs. MCF-7 (**A,B**) and MDA MB-231 (**C,D**) cells. Bars with equal letters indicate no significant differences between the means (Tukey's test, $p < 0.05$).

Exposing cells to doxorubicin (Dox) significantly increased the intracellular GSH concentration and this concentration was higher in the combined exposure to Dox and CH-GSH NPs. This increase was more evident in MCF7 cells than in MDA MB-231 cells (Figure 4A,C). We quantified the extracellular GSH levels in the culture medium used in cells exposed to Dox. CH-GSH NPs and CH-NPs in Figure 4B,D showed no significant differences between extracellular GSH levels in any culture media for the treatments and any cell lines. This finding indicates that the NPs do not leak the GSH. The contrast between intracellular and extracellular GSH values suggests nanoparticles' inclusion, correlates with confocal microscopy images, and suggests the bioavailability of thiol in NPs.

Interestingly, the results show an increase in the GSH concentration dose-response when MDA MB-231 cells were exposed to CH-NP. This effect was not present in the same way in the MCF-7 cells; it was only significant in the maximum concentration studied and this amount was higher than that induced when the cells were exposed to

CH-GSH NPs. There is documented evidence that demonstrates the ability of CH-NP to modulate various cellular signals associated with exogenous stimuli such as radiosensitization, antioxidation, and changes in cell unions, among many others. In addition to this, the physicochemical nature of the nanoparticles can generate cellular responses that significantly promote changes in the concentration of GSH; in turn, this promotes different effects related to enzymatic or non-enzymatic events, which finally control its cellular concentration [8,9]. NPs, as a xenobiotic agent, could exert this type of phenomenon that should be further studied.

3.5. Lipoperoxidation Levels Are Reduced by the Combination of Doxorubicin and NPs

Malondialdehyde (MDA) is the final product of lipid oxidation. Thus, it is an indicator of cellular damage due to oxidative stress. The treatment of MCF-7 cells with Dox resulted in a marked increase in MDA concentration (Figure 5A). A similar result was observed in MDA MB-231 cells (Figure 5B). Exposure of cells to the CH-GSH NPs did not change the basal concentration of MDA in MCF7, indicating that the NPs alone did not induce oxidative stress on the cells. This effect differed in MDA MB-231 cells (Figure 5B), suggesting differential sensibility to induce MDA. The physicochemical properties of CH-NPs promote increasing levels of MDA. Combined exposure to Dox and subsequently to CH-GSH NPs resulted in a substantial reduction of MDA concentration (Figure 5). This result suggests that CH-GSH NPs have a protective antioxidant effect. Even cells exposed to CH-GSH NPs maintained MDA levels like untreated cells, while exposure to Dox significantly increased MDA levels in both cell lines (Figure 5). Therefore, these data suggest that the GSH into NPs could interact directly with ROS and free radicals or be used by antioxidant enzymes to reduce oxidative stress produced by the exposure to Dox [8].

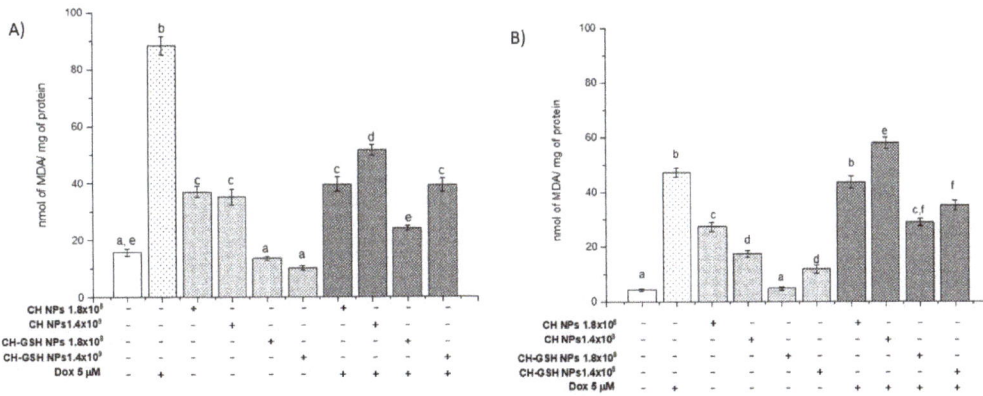

Figure 5. MDA levels of cells exposed to Dox for 12 h and then 2 h with CH-GSH NPs or CH-NPs. (**A**) MCF-7 and (**B**) MDA MB-231 cells. Bars with equal letters indicate no significant differences between the means (Tukey's test, $p < 0.05$).

3.6. Exposure to the Combination of Doxorubicin and CH-GSH NPs Reduces ROS Levels

Considering the NPs could modify the amount of intracellular GSH and the lipid peroxidation by reactive species decreased significantly in the combined exposures compared to Dox alone, we decided to estimate ROS using 2, 7 dichlorofluorescein diacetate (DCFDA). Figure 6A,B shows normalized results considering the untreated cells as baseline ROS levels. Cells exposed to CH-GSH NPs did not change the basal levels of ROS. As anticipated, cells exposed to Dox had a higher amount of ROS. In contrast, the combined exposure to Dox and CH-GSH NPs resulted in a marked reduction of ROS levels. This implies that the modulating effects modify the amount of ROS at the cellular level due to CH-GSH NPs indeed inducing a protective antioxidant effect in cells exposed to Dox.

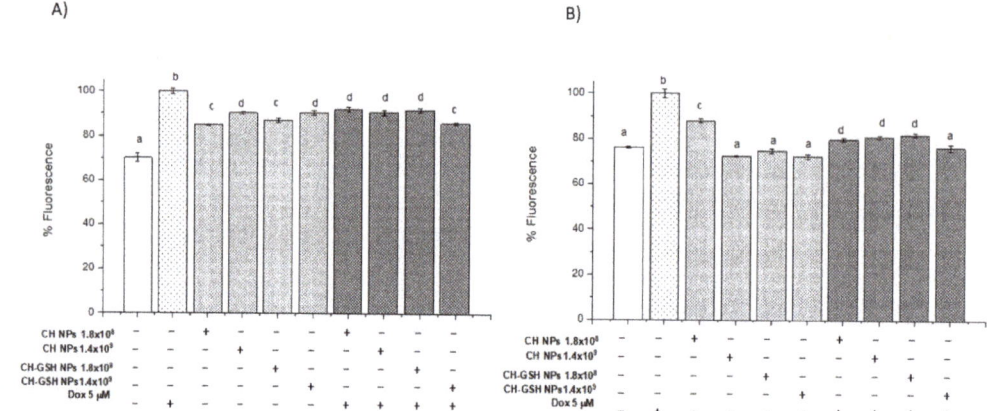

Figure 6. Combined exposure to Dox and CH-GSH NPs or CH-NPs reduced ROS levels. The cells were exposed to Dox for 12 h and then 2 h with CH-GSH NPs. (**A**) MCF-7 and (**B**) MDA MB-231 cells. Bars with equal letters indicate no significant differences between the means (Tukey's test, $p < 0.05$).

Cell responses to CH-GSH NPs and CH-NP previously exposed to doxorubicin promoted a significant decrease in ROS generation compared to the amount of ROS in cells exposed to doxorubicin in both exposed cell lines. There is evidence reported concerning the CH-NP inducing antioxidant effects due to its ability to provide chelating ligands in the amino and hydroxyl groups in positions C-3 and C-2 in monomers, and effectively chelate heavy metals as Fe^{2+}.

It has also been reported that these reactive groups may be responsible for the capture of some free radicals [26–28].

Notably, ROS levels also decreased in cells treated with doxorubicin and CH-NPs in MCF-7 cells compared with cells exposed to Dox. These effects may be related to their antioxidant capacity previously reported to CH-NPs and the cellular effects on inducing gene expression and biochemical regulation related to the modulation of the intracellular redox status.

3.7. Doxorubicin Decreases the Activity of Antioxidant Enzymes Induced by CH-GSH NPs but It Depends on the Cell Type

We quantified the specific activity of catalase. In Figure 7, CH-GSH NPs only modified MDA MB-231 cells' activity, while in MCF-7 cells, there is no difference concerning the untreated cells. However, when cells are exposed to Dox and CH-GSH NPs, the activity is diminished compared to the Dox-induced. As previously observed, the GSH from NPs modified ROS levels, decreasing catalase activity for this reason. Catalase is the enzyme responsible for the degradation of H_2O_2 to H_2O. Thus, it has a protective antioxidant effect on the cell. The catalase activity in MCF-7 cells did not change after exposing the cells to CH-GSH NPs (Figure 7A).

In contrast, the catalase activity in MDA MB-231 cells was increased by exposing the cells to NPs (Figure 7B). This variation in response reflects important metabolic differences in both cell lines. Despite this, both cell lines presented a marked increase in catalase activity after the treatment with Dox, inhibited by NPs presence.

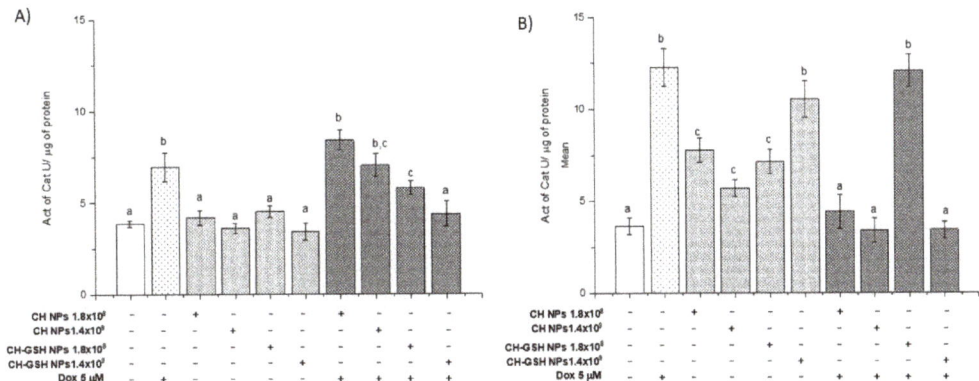

Figure 7. The activity of catalase. The cells were exposed to Dox for 12 h and then 2 h with CH-GSH NPs or CH-NPs. (**A**) MCF-7 and (**B**) MDA MB-231 cells. Bars with equal letters indicate no significant differences between the means (Tukey's test, $p < 0.05$).

The activity of glutathione peroxidase (GPx) (Figure 8) shows that the enzyme activity only modified MDA MB-231 cells in a concentration of 1.8×10^8. When cells are exposed to Dox combined with CH-GSH NPs, the activity increases in levels like Dox-induced in the MCF-7 cells and the activity decreased in the MDA MB-231 cells. The enzyme GPx is part of the intrinsic antioxidant mechanisms by reducing peroxides with the aid of GSH as a reducing agent at the cellular level. The basal activity of GPx in MCF-7 cells did not change after exposing them to CH-GSH NPs (Figure 8A). In contrast, GPx activity in MDA MB-231 cells was increased after exposing the cells to a concentration of 1.8×10^8 NPs (Figure 8B). Again, this variation in response seems to reflect important metabolic differences in both cell lines. Both cell lines presented a marked increase in GPx activity after the treatment with Dox (Figure 8), which was not inhibited by the NPs presence in MCF-7 cells (Figure 8A). In contrast, the NPs induced a significant decrease in GPx activity in MDA MB-231 cells after the treatment with Dox (Figure 8B).

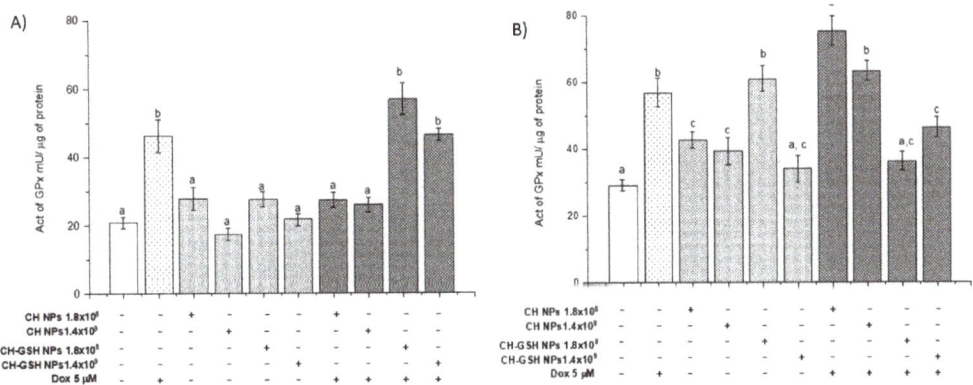

Figure 8. The activity of GPx. The cells were exposed to Dox for 12 h and then 2 h with CH-GSH NPs or CH-NPs. (**A**) MCF-7 and (**B**) MDA MB-231 cells. Bars with equal letters indicate significant differences between the means (Tukey's test, $p < 0.05$).

Glutathione (GSH) functions as a reducing agent during the elimination of peroxides by being oxidized and converted into disulfide glutathione (GSSG). Later, the enzyme glutathione reductase (GRx) uses GSSG as a substrate to regenerate GSH [21]. GRx is induced under oxidative stress. Thus, its activity is also indicative of the antioxidant state of a cell. The basal activity of GRx in MCF-7 cells and MDA MB-231 cells did not change after exposing them to CH-GSH NPs (Figure 9). Both cell lines presented a marked increase in GRx activity after the treatment with Dox, wholly blocked in the NPs presence. The result suggested that NPs induced a decrease in the ROS amount in the cell and consequently the cell did not require the activation of GRx.

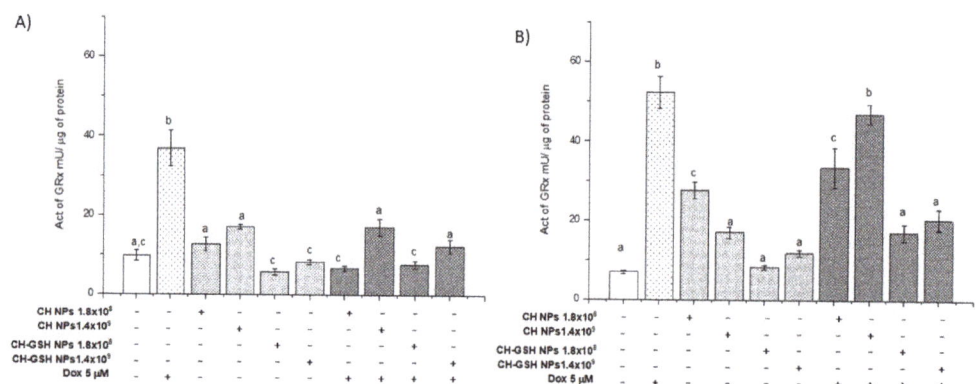

Figure 9. The activity of GRx. The cells were exposed to Dox for 12 h and then 2 h with CH-GSH NPs or CH-NPs. (**A**) MCF-7 and (**B**) MDA MB-231 cells. Bars with equal letters indicate no significant differences between the means (Tukey's test, $p < 0.05$).

3.8. CH-GSH NPs Induce Apoptosis by Increasing Caspase-3 Activity

In addition to the treatments mentioned, Z-VAD-FMK, an inhibitor of caspase-3 activity, was added to demonstrate that activity is decreased when exposed to doxorubicin. In Figure 10, exposure to CH-GSH NPs increases caspase-3 activity, more evident in MDA-MB-231 cells than in MCF-7 cells. When exposure to doxorubicin followed by CH-GSH NPs occurs, it can be observed that in MCF-7 cells, the activity seems to decrease (Figure 10A). In contrast, in MDA-MB-231 cells, the activity increases concerning that induction by doxorubicin (Figure 10B). Wójcik et al., 2015, and Daga et al., 2016, suggested that the combined exposure of GSH and doxorubicin induced cell-signaling, related to the increase of apoptosis effects [29,30].

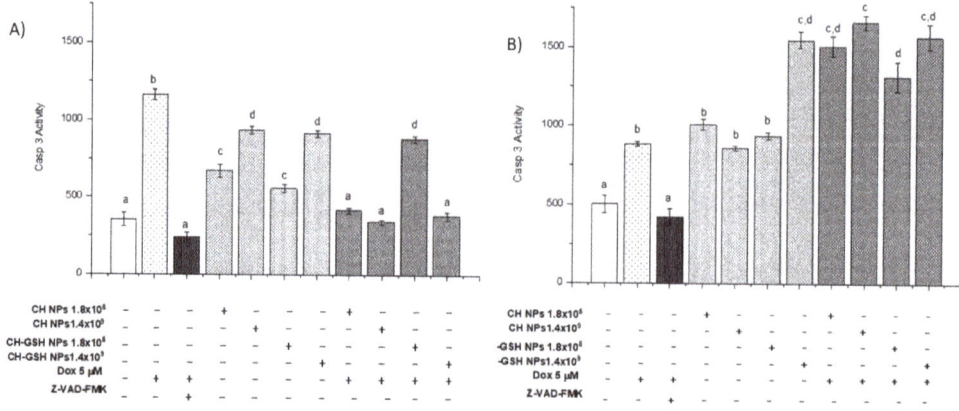

Figure 10. The activity of caspase-3. The cells were exposed to Dox for 12 h and then 2 h with CH-GSH NPs or CH-NPs. (**A**) MCF-7 and (**B**) MDA MB-231 cells. Bars with equal letters indicate no significant differences between the means (Tukey's test, $p < 0.05$).

In this work, the effects associated with apoptosis were not exclusive to the chemotherapeutic agent and glutathione; some authors report events in which chitosan has an essential role in apoptosis. In studies carried out on bladder tumor cells, Hasegawa et al. showed that chitosan could induce apoptosis through the activation of caspase-3. However, the mechanism of action through which it carries out this activation is unknown [31]. Lee et al., 2011, showed that a derivative of chitosan, diethylaminoethyl chitosan, could induce apoptosis in Hela cells through the regulation of enzymes (caspase-3, -8, and -9); p53 and BAX expression. Modifying the expression of BCL2 proteins. This would generate a disruption of the mitochondrial membrane and an oxidation–reduction imbalance [32].

Wimardhani et al., 2014, reported that the exposure of Ca9-22 cells with chitosan derivatives induced the appearance of early apoptotic cells, increased caspase-3 activity, and the arrest of G1/S of the cell cycle, suggesting that chitosan could be used as a natural anti-cancer agent [33]. Therefore, the caspase-3 activity increase could be due to the exposure to doxorubicin, GSH of NPs, and chitosan.

3.9. CH-GSH NPs Impair Cell Proliferation by Decreasing Ki67 Levels

Ki67 levels were measured as a molecular marker of cell proliferation. The Ki67 antigen has a specific expression in the M phase of the cell cycle; it is commonly visualized with the MIB1 antibody [34]. Our data showed that the CH-GSH NPs in both concentrations significantly decreased the percentage of Ki-67 concerning the NT cells in both cell lines (Figure 11). It has been reported that GSH levels can regulate the activity of genes associated with proliferation, differentiation, and apoptosis, and a high level of GSH is essential for normal cellular functions, signal translation, and protection against certain carcinogens [35]. When cells are exposed to both doxorubicin and CH-GSH NPs, the levels remain like those obtained with cells exposed only to doxorubicin. The above suggests that NPs could not affect doxorubicin-induced proliferation but could modify the redox state as observed when ROS levels were estimated.

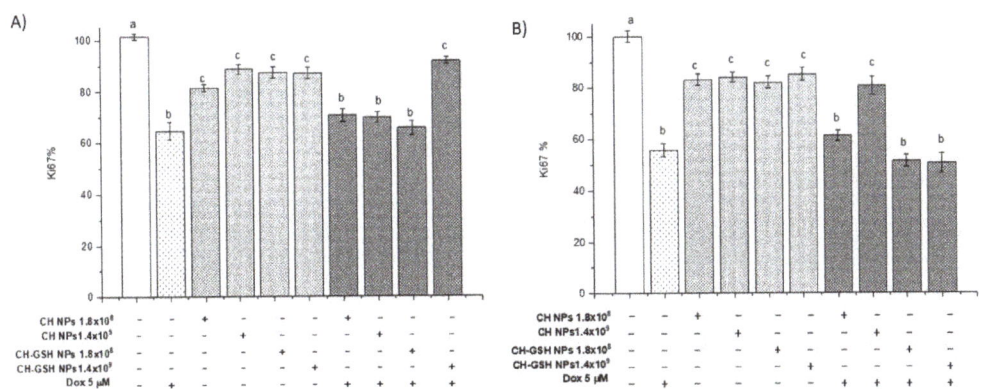

Figure 11. Ki67 levels. The cells were exposed to Dox for 12 h and then 2 h with CH-GSH NPs. (**A**) MCF-7 and (**B**) MDA MB-231 cells. Bars with equal letters indicate no significant differences between the means (Tukey's test, $p < 0.05$).

Furthermore, there is evidence that the decrease in Ki67 levels is related to some chitosan derivatives, which modify various cell-signaling pathways directly or indirectly related to cell proliferation and apoptosis. Chitosan can inhibit pro-inflammatory molecules such as TNF-α, blocking the activation of NFkB and reducing the expression of genes that protect and induce cell proliferation [36]. In addition, it can activate the transcription factor Nrf2 through the PI3/Akt pathway. Rojo de la Vega et al. reported that a decrease in the expression of Nrf2 promotes the activation of CDk2 and CDk4 inhibitor p21 [37]. Another study suggests that some cells treated with chitosan derivatives can increase the expression of TGF-β that activates an intracellular-signaling cascade associated with Smad proteins and thus favors the transcription of genes associated with cell cycle inhibition [38]. MCF-7 cells showed increased sensitivity to NPs' exposure compared to MDA MB-231 cells in the various tests performed. This finding may be due to its metabolism. It has been reported that Dox modifies the metabolism of both cell lines by affecting more the metabolic profile of MDA-MB-231 cells than of MCF-7 cells, showing changes in ketonic bodies, glycolysis, and energetic and lipid metabolism [16,39]. MDA MB-231 cells have a higher consumption of glucose and upregulated redox pathways than MCF-7 [40].

Conversely, the observed effect may be due to, as some authors mentioned, the fact that combined exposure of NPs with various agents enhances cell sensibilization. Zalbielca et al., 2017, and Willmann et al., 2015, showed that combined exposure of NPs of Dox/GSH has higher cytotoxic effects than free Dox in feline fibrosarcoma cell lines. In a study in MCF-7 cells with metallic NPs and radiation, there was a higher effect on the combination exposure, wherein NPs act as nano-sensitizers [6,41]. Uma et al., 2016, suggested that gold NPs act as sensitizing agents in MDA-MB-231 and MCF-7 cells, modifying cell-cycle effects, viability, and DNA damage [42]. Alvandifar et al. used a combined exposition of PLGA and verapamil NPs to improve this chemotherapeutic effectiveness and decrease the dose to have a higher effect [43]. These results suggest that the combined exposure of nanoparticles and doxorubicin may decrease the resistance of MDA MB-231 cells to these types of drugs.

4. Conclusions

The results obtained in this research suggest that CH-GSH NPs modify Ki67 levels and alter the apoptosis by increasing caspase-3 activity and the cellular redox state, reducing the oxidative stress generated by doxorubicin exposure. It has been documented that GSH may play a dual role in tumor progression or cancer cell death concerning cancer. The above is probably due to the fine biochemical regulation in its synthesis and the relationship of its oxidation–reduction modulating effects, as well as other enzymatic and non-enzymatic mechanisms. The effects of doxorubicin are variable and include the ability to induce resistance to chemotherapy; modify the initiation and progression of cancer; activate cell-signaling pathways related to stressful microenvironments; promote apoptosis in tumor cells; and have the radio-sensitization be induced by this antioxidant. We observed higher sensitivity of MCF-7 cells to CH-GSH NPs than MDA MB-231 cells; this may be due to each cells' genotypic characteristics.

As a GSH delivery entity, CH-NPs attract attention. The results of this work show their capacity to diffuse quickly into cells and exert significant effects to modulate the oxidative stress induced by doxorubicin in breast cancer cells. Considering this, CH-GSH NPs must be studied as a potential designed delivery system that offers a new biomaterial with biomedical opportunities to study the molecular, biochemical, and biological mechanisms related to the cellular redox status. This information will be useful to design better therapies based on antioxidant nanoparticles.

Author Contributions: Conceptualization, L.D.L.-B. and P.R.-N.; data curation, L.D.L.-B., R.D.-T. and P.R.-N.; formal analysis, L.D.L.-B., R.D.-T., A.M.S., C.R. and P.R.-N.; funding acquisition, R.D.-T. and P.R.-N.; investigation, L.D.L.-B. and J.R.M.-R.; methodology, L.D.L.-B., J.R.M.-R. and P.R.-N.; project administration, R.D.-T. and P.R.-N.; resources, P.R.-N.; supervision, R.D.-T., A.M.S., C.R. and P.R.-N.; validation, L.D.L.-B. and R.D.-T.; visualization, L.D.L.-B., R.D.-T., A.M.S., C.R. and P.R.-N.; writing—original draft preparation, L.D.L.-B., R.D.-T., J.R.M.-R., A.M.S., C.R. and P.R.-N. All authors have read and agreed to the published version of the manuscript.

Funding: This research was funded by PAPIIT IN214321 from Dirección General de Asuntos del Personal Académico, Universidad Nacional Autónoma de México.

Institutional Review Board Statement: Not applicable.

Informed Consent Statement: Not applicable.

Data Availability Statement: The data presented in this study are available on request for the corresponding author.

Acknowledgments: The authors acknowledge the invaluable support of M en C Elizabeth Soria Castro in the TEM analysis. L. D. López-Barrera received a scholarship number 639023 from CONACYT as a doctorate student.

Conflicts of Interest: The authors declare no conflict of interest.

References

1. Bray, F.; Ferlay, J.; Soerjomataram, I.; Siegel, R.L.; Torre, L.A.; Jemal, A. Global Cancer Statistics 2018: GLOBOCAN Estimates of Incidence and Mortality Worldwide for 36 Cancers in 185 Countries. *CA Cancer J. Clin.* **2018**, *68*, 394–424. [CrossRef] [PubMed]
2. Pardee, J.D. *Understanding Breast Cancer. Cell Biology and Therapy—A Visual Approach*; Morgan & Claypool Life Sciences: San Rafael, CA, USA, 2008.
3. Renu, K.; Abilash, V.G.; Tirupathi Pichiah, P.B.; Arunachalam, S. Molecular Mechanism of Doxorubicin-Induced Cardiomyopathy–An Update. *Eur. J. Pharmacol.* **2018**, *818*, 241–253. [CrossRef]
4. Chegaev, K.; Riganti, C.; Rolando, B.; Lazzarato, L.; Gazzano, E.; Guglielmo, S.; Ghigo, D.; Fruttero, R.; Gasco, A. Doxorubicin-Antioxidant Co-Drugs. *Bioorg. Med. Chem. Lett.* **2013**, *23*, 5307–5310. [CrossRef]
5. Czeczuga-Semeniuk, E.; Anchim, T. The Effect of Doxorubicin and Retinoids on Proliferation, Necrosis and Apoptosis in MCF-7 Breast Cancer Cells. *Folia Histochem. Cytobiol.* **2004**, *42*, 7.
6. Zabielska-Koczywąs, K.; Dolka, I.; Król, M.; Żbikowski, A.; Lewandowski, W.; Mieczkowski, J.; Wójcik, M.; Lechowski, R. Doxorubicin Conjugated to Glutathione Stabilized Gold Nanoparticles (Au-GSH-Dox) as an Effective Therapeutic Agent for Feline Injection-Site Sarcomas—Chick Embryo Chorioallantoic Membrane Study. *Molecules* **2017**, *22*, 253. [CrossRef] [PubMed]
7. Songbo, M.; Lang, H.; Xinyong, C.; Bin, X.; Ping, Z.; Liang, S. Oxidative Stress Injury in Doxorubicin-Induced Cardiotoxicity. *Toxicol. Lett.* **2019**, *307*, 41–48. [CrossRef]
8. Kalinina, E.V.; Chernov, N.N.; Novichkova, M.D. Role of Glutathione, Glutathione Transferase, and Glutaredoxin in Regulation of Redox-Dependent Processes. *Biochem. Mosc.* **2014**, *79*, 1562–1583. [CrossRef]
9. Hui Wu, J.H.; Batist, G. Glutathione and Glutathione Analogues; Therapeutic Potentials. *Biochim. Biophys. Acta BBA-Gen. Subj.* **2013**, *1830*, 3350–3353. [CrossRef] [PubMed]
10. Raj, S.; Khurana, S.; Choudhari, R.; Kesari, K.K.; Kamal, M.A.; Garg, N.; Ruokolainen, J.; Das, B.C.; Kumar, D. Specific Targeting Cancer Cells with Nanoparticles and Drug Delivery in Cancer Therapy. *Semin. Cancer Biol.* **2019**, S1044579X19302160. [CrossRef] [PubMed]
11. Rahmani, S.; Hakimi, S.; Esmaeily, A.; Samadi, F.Y.; Mortazavian, E.; Nazari, M.; Mohammadi, Z.; Tehrani, N.R.; Tehrani, M.R. Novel Chitosan Based Nanoparticles as Gene Delivery Systems to Cancerous and Noncancerous Cells. *Int. J. Pharm.* **2019**, *560*, 306–314. [CrossRef]
12. Ma, L.; Shen, C.; Gao, L.; Li, D.; Shang, Y.; Yin, K.; Zhao, D.; Cheng, W.; Quan, D. Anti-Inflammatory Activity of Chitosan Nanoparticles Carrying NF-KB/P65 Antisense Oligonucleotide in RAW264.7 Macrophage Stimulated by Lipopolysaccharide. *Colloids Surf. B Biointerfaces* **2016**, *142*, 297–306. [CrossRef]
13. Piña Olmos, S.; Díaz Torres, R.; Elbakrawy, E.; Hughes, L.; Mckenna, J.; Hill, M.A.; Kadhim, M.; Ramírez Noguera, P.; Bolanos-Garcia, V.M. Combinatorial Use of Chitosan Nanoparticles, Reversine, and Ionising Radiation on Breast Cancer Cells Associated with Mitosis Deregulation. *Biomolecules* **2019**, *9*, 186. [CrossRef] [PubMed]
14. López-Barrera, L.D.; Díaz-Torres, R.; López-Macay, A.; López-Reyes, A.G.; Pina Olmos, S.; Ramírez-Noguera, P. Oxidative Stress Modulation Induced by Chitosan-Glutathione Nanoparticles in Chondrocytes. *Pharmazie* **2019**, *74*, 406–411. [CrossRef] [PubMed]
15. Hu, M.L. Measurement of Protein Thiol Groups and Glutathione in Plasma. *Methods Enzymol.* **1994**, *233*, 380–385. [CrossRef]
16. Präbst, K.; Engelhardt, H.; Ringgeler, S. Basic Colorimetric Proliferation Assays: MTT, WST, and Resazurin. Colorimetric Proliferation Assays Methods. *Mol. Biol.* **2017**, *1601*, 1–17. [CrossRef]
17. Bradford, M.M. A Rapid and Sensitive Method for the Quantitation of Microgram Quantities of Protein Utilizing the Principle of Protein-Dye Binding. *Anal. Biochem.* **1976**, *72*, 248–254. [CrossRef]
18. Ohkawa, H.; Ohishi, N.; Yagi, K. Assay for Lipid Peroxides in Animal Tissues by Thiobarbituric Acid Reaction. *Anal. Biochem.* **1979**, *95*, 351–358. [CrossRef]
19. Wang, H.; Joseph, J.A. Quantifying cellular oxidative stress by dichlorofluorescein assay using microplate reader. *Free Radic. Biol. Med.* **1999**, *27*, 612–616. [CrossRef]
20. Iwase, T.; Tajima, A.; Sugimoto, S.; Okuda, K.; Hironaka, I.; Kamata, Y.; Takada, K.; Mizunoe, Y. A Simple Assay for Measuring Catalase Activity: A Visual Approach. *Sci. Rep.* **2013**, *3*, 3081. [CrossRef]
21. Esworthy, R.S.; Chu, F.F.; Doroshow, J.H. Analysis of Glutathione-Related Enzymes. *Curr. Protoc. Toxicol.* **1999**, 7.1.1–7.1.32. [CrossRef]
22. Promega. *CaspACE TM Assay System, CaspACE TM Assay System, Colorimetric*; Promega: Madison, WI, USA, 2018.
23. CUSABIO. Human Antigen KI-67 (Ki-67). *ELISA Kit* **2018**, *67*, 1–14.
24. Monopoli, M.P.; Pitek, A.S.; Lynch, L.; Dawson, D.A. Formation and Characterization of the Nanoparticle–Protein Corona. *Nanomater. Interfaces Biol. Methods Protoc.* **2013**, *1025*, 137–155. [CrossRef]

25. Hans, M.L.; Lowman, A.M. Biodegradable Nanoparticles for Drug Delivery and Targeting. *Curr. Opin. Solid State Mater. Sci.* **2002**, *6*, 319–321. [CrossRef]
26. Chang, S.H.; Wu, W.C.H.; Tsai, G.J. Effects of chitosan molecular weight on its antioxidant and antimutagenic properties. *Carbohydr. Polym.* **2018**, *181*, 1026–1032. [CrossRef]
27. Choi, H.; Nam, J.-P.; Nah, J.-W. Application of chitosan and chitosan derivatives as biomaterials. *J. Ind. Eng. Chem.* **2016**, *33*, 1–10. [CrossRef]
28. Kim, K.W.; Thomas, R.L. Antioxidative activity of chitosans with varying molecular weights. *Food Chem.* **2006**, *101*, 308–313. [CrossRef]
29. Wójcik, M.; Lewandowski, W.; Król, M.; Pawłowski, K.; Mieczkowski, J.; Lechowski, R.; Zabielska, K. Enhancing antitumor efficacy of doxorubicin by non-covalent conjugation to gold nanoparticles-In vitro studies on Feline fibrosarcoma cell lines. *PLoS ONE* **2015**. [CrossRef]
30. Daga, M.; Ulllio, C.; Argenziano, M.; Dianzani, C.; Cavalli, R.; Trotta, F.; Barrera, G. GSH-targeted nanosponges increase doxorubicin-induced toxicity "in vitro" and "in vivo" in cancer cells with high antioxidant defenses. *Free. Radic. Biol. Med.* **2016**, *97*, 24–37. [CrossRef]
31. Hasegawa, M.; Yagi, K.; Iwakawa, S.; Hirai, M. Chitosan induces apoptosis via caspase-3 activation in bladder tumor cells. *Jpn. J. Cancer Res. Gann* **2001**, *92*, 459–466. [CrossRef]
32. Lee, S.; Ryu, B.; Je, J.; Kim, S. Diethylaminoethyl chitosan induces apoptosis in HeLa cells via activation of caspase-3 and p53 expression. *Carbohydr. Polym.* **2011**, *84*, 571–578. [CrossRef]
33. Wimardhani, Y.S.; Suniarti, D.F.; Freisleben, H.J.; Wanandi, S.I.; Siregar, N.C.; Ikeda, M.A. Chitosan exerts anti-cancer activity through induction of apoptosis and cell cycle arrest in oral cancer cells. *J. Oral Sci.* **2014**, *56*, 119–126. [CrossRef] [PubMed]
34. Mohamed, H.; Samy, N.; Afify, M.; Abd, N.; Maksoud, E. Ki-67 as a potential biomarker in patients with breast cancer. *J. Genet. Eng. Biotechnol.* **2008**, *16*, 479–484. [CrossRef]
35. Abdalla, M.Y. Glutathione as Potential Target for Cancer Therapy; More or Less is Good? *Jordan J. Biol. Sci.* **2011**, *4*, 119–124.
36. Kadry, M.O.; Abdel-Megeed, R.M.; El-Meliegy, E.; Abdel-Hamid, A.H.Z. Crosstalk between GSK-3, c-Fos, NFκB and TNF-α signaling pathways play an ambitious role in Chitosan Nanoparticles Cancer Therapy. *Toxicol. Rep.* **2018**, *5*, 723–727. [CrossRef] [PubMed]
37. Rojo de la Vega, M.; Chapman, E.; Zhang, D.D. NRF2 and the Hallmarks of Cancer. *Cancer Cell* **2018**, *2*, 1–23. [CrossRef]
38. Farhadihosseinabadi, B.; Zarebkohan, A.; Eftekhary, M.; Heiat, M.; Moosazadeh Moghaddam, M.; Gholipourmalekabadi, M. Crosstalk between chitosan and cell signaling pathways. *Cell. Mol. LifeSci.* **2019**. [CrossRef]
39. Maria, R.M.; Altei, W.F.; Selistre-de-Araujo, H.S.; Colnago, L.A. Effects of Doxorubicin, Cisplatin, and Tamoxifen on the Metabolic Profile of Human Breast Cancer MCF-7 Cells As Determined by 1 H High-Resolution Magic Angle Spinning Nuclear Magnetic Resonance. *Biochemistry* **2017**, *56*, 2219–2224. [CrossRef]
40. Maria, R.M.; Altei, W.F.; Selistre-de-Araujo, H.S.; Colnago, L.A. Impact of chemotherapy on metabolic reprogramming: Characterization of the metabolic profile of breast cancer MDA-MB-231 cells using 1 H HR-MAS NMR spectroscopy. *J. Pharm. Biomed. Anal.* **2017**, *146*, 324–328. [CrossRef]
41. Willmann, L.; Schlimpert, M.; Halbach, S.; Erbes, T.; Stickeler, E.; Kammerer, B. Metabolic profiling of breast cancer: Differences in central metabolism between subtypes of breast cancer cell lines. *Chromatogr. B* **2015**, *1000*, 95–104. [CrossRef]
42. Uma, S.; Govindaraju, K.; Ganesh, K.; Prabhu, D.; Arulvasu, C.; Karthick, V.; Changmai, N. Anti-proliferative effect of biogenic gold nanoparticles against breast cancer cell lines (MDA-MB-231 & MCF-7). *Appl. Surf. Sci.* **2016**, *371*, 415–424. [CrossRef]
43. Alvandifar, F.; Ghaffari, B.; Goodarzi, N.; Ravari, N.S.; Karami, F.; Amini, M.; Souri, E.; Khoshayand, M.R.; Esfandyari-Manesh, M.; Jafari, R.M.; et al. Dual Drug Delivery System of PLGA Nanoparticles to Reverse Drug Resistance by Altering BAX/Bcl-2. *J. Drug Deliv. Sci. Technol.* **2018**, *47*, 291–298. [CrossRef]

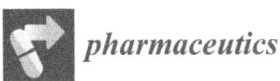

Article

Targeting Tumor Cells with Nanoparticles for Enhanced Co-Drug Delivery in Cancer Treatment

Wen-Ying Huang [1],[†], Chih-Ho Lai [2],[†], Shin-Lei Peng [3], Che-Yu Hsu [4], Po-Hung Hsu [5], Pei-Yi Chu [4], Chun-Lung Feng [6] and Yu-Hsin Lin [4],[7],[8],*

[1] Department of Applied Cosmetology, Hung-Kuang University, Taichung 433304, Taiwan; beca690420@sunrise.hk.edu.tw
[2] Molecular Infectious Disease Research Center, Department of Microbiology and Immunology, Chang Gung University and Chang Gung Memorial Hospital, Taoyuan 333323, Taiwan; chlai@mail.cgu.edu.tw
[3] Department of Biomedical Imaging and Radiological Science, China Medical University, Taichung 404, Taiwan; speng@mail.cmu.edu.tw
[4] Department of Pharmacy, National Yang Ming Chiao Tung University, Taipei 112304, Taiwan; claire5588tv@gmail.com (C.-Y.H.); ositachu3@gmail.com (P.-Y.C.)
[5] Center for Advanced Molecular Imaging and Translation, Chang Gung Memorial Hospital, Taoyuan 333, Taiwan; bloodbull@gmail.com
[6] Division of Hepatogastroenterology, Department of Internal Medicine, China Medical University Hospital, Taichung 404332, Taiwan; fjld6604@yahoo.com.tw
[7] Center for Advanced Pharmaceutics and Drug Delivery Research, Department and Institute of Pharmacology, Institute of Biopharmaceutical Sciences, Faculty of Pharmacy, National Yang Ming Chiao Tung University, Taipei 11221, Taiwan
[8] Department of Medical Research, China Medical University Hospital, China Medical University, Taichung 404333, Taiwan
* Correspondence: ylhsin@ym.edu.tw or ylhsin@nycu.edu.tw; Tel.: +886-2-28267000 (ext. 7932)
† The first two authors (Wen-Ying Huang and Chih-Ho Lai) contributed equally to this work.

Abstract: Gastric cancer (GC) is a fatal malignant tumor, and effective therapies to attenuate its progression are lacking. Nanoparticle (NP)-based solutions may enable the design of novel treatments to eliminate GC. Refined, receptor-targetable NPs can selectively target cancer cells and improve the cellular uptake of drugs. To overcome the current limitations and enhance the therapeutic effects, epigallocatechin-3-gallate (EGCG) and low-concentration doxorubicin (DX) were encapsulated in fucoidan and D-alpha-tocopherylpoly (ethylene glycol) succinate-conjugated hyaluronic acid-based NPs for targeting P-selectin-and cluster of differentiation (CD)44-expressing gastric tumors. The EGCG/DX-loaded NPs bound to GC cells and released bioactive combination drugs, demonstrating better anti-cancer effects than the EGCG/DX combination solution. In vivo assays in an orthotopic gastric tumor mouse model showed that the EGCG/DX-loaded NPs significantly increased the activity of gastric tumors without inducing organ injury. Overall, our EGCG/DX-NP system exerted a beneficial effect on GC treatment and may facilitate the development of nanomedicine-based combination chemotherapy against GC in the future.

Keywords: gastric cancer; nanoparticle; fucoidan; D-alpha-tocopherylpoly (ethylene glycol) succinate; combination chemotherapy

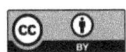

1. Introduction

The stomach is located in the upper abdomen between the esophagus and small intestine. Its primary function is to store and partially digest food after ingestion [1,2]. Abnormal growth and multiplication of gastric cells can lead to gastric cancer (GC). Most GCs are adenocarcinomas that arise from the mucosal tissue lining inside the stomach. Abnormal cells may penetrate deeper into the stomach wall or spread to nearby organs or tissues [3]. Cell adhesion molecules are the major elements of the metastasis process [4]. In particular, P-selectin is an adhesion molecule that mediates the interaction of platelets and endothelial cells with monocytes, neutrophils, and tumor cells [5]. P-selectin also binds to several human cancers, such as GC, colon cancer, and breast cancer [6,7]. Cluster of differentiation (CD)44-positive GC cells show self-renewal properties and the ability to produce differentiated offspring, consistent with the cancer stem cell phenotype [8]. CD44-positive GC cells are reported to contribute to increased resistance to radiation- or chemotherapy-induced cancer cell death [9].

Cancer nanotechnology is being vigorously developed for applications in cancer imaging, molecular diagnosis, and targeted therapy [10–12]. Compared with their single- or dual-ligand-targeting nanoparticle (NP) counterparts, non-targeted NPs significantly increase metastasis deposition. Multiligand NPs are obtained by modulating the surfaces of NPs with more than one type of targeting ligand. These facilitate high-precision targeting of different metastatic subpopulations that express different targetable receptors otherwise missed by single-ligand NPs [13,14]. Fucoidan (FD) is the active ingredient of seaweed that induces cell apoptosis, inhibits the proliferation of cancer cells, and is reported to have a strong affinity for P-selectin, which interacts with sulfated oligosaccharides [15–17]. Hyaluronic acid (HA) is a natural linear polysaccharide, composed of repeating disaccharide units of $\beta(1,3)$-N-acetylglucosamine (GlcNAc) and $\beta(1,4)$-glucuronic acid (GlcUA), which forms van der Waals bonds and hydrogen bonds with migrating cells via the CD44 ligand receptors [18,19]. D-alpha-tocopheryl poly(ethylene glycol) (PEG) succinate (TPGS) is a water-soluble derivative of natural vitamin E and prevents P-glycoprotein (P-gp) adenosine triphosphatase (ATPase) from hydrolyzing ATP by blocking the ATP-binding sites, thus inhibiting ATPase activity [20]. Herein, we prepared a TPGS-conjugated HA (TH) copolymer that can simultaneously interact with membrane-bound CD44 and reduce P-gp expression in GC cells.

Doxorubicin (DX), an anthracycline antibiotic, is currently the most effective chemotherapeutic drug used to treat GC, ovarian cancer, and breast cancer. DX acts as a DNA intercalator and topoisomerase II inhibitor. However, it exhibits strong cardiotoxicity [19,21]. The standard dose of 20 mg/m^2 is widely used for GC, but an overall response to DX monotherapy is observed in only 17% of GC patients [22–24]. Epigallocatechin-3-gallate (EGCG), a bioactive polyphenol compound in green tea, has antioxidant and anti-inflammatory properties and can be utilized in disease management [25]. EGCG can sensitize the efficacy of DX, enhancing its therapeutic effect in hepatocellular or prostate cancer [26,27]. Combination chemotherapy is a promising method for improving cancer treatment. However, clinical combination therapy is limited by the unique pharmacokinetics of the combined drugs, resulting in uneven drug distribution [28,29]. We established tumor-targeting NPs, combining FD binding to P-selectin-expressing tumors and TH targeting CD44-expressing tumors to reduce P-gp expression. Gelatin is a natural polymer containing residues of glycine, proline, hydroxyproline, and alanine, which are common amino acids. Gelatin-polyphenol interactions primarily occur through hydrogen bonds between hydrophobic amino acids (mainly proline residues) and the phenol ring of polyphenols [30,31]. Thus, in this study, we used PEG-gelatin (PG) to load the anticancer agents EGCG and DX to enhance their loading efficiency and sustained release, thereby attempting to maximize their combined therapeutic effect and minimize systemic toxicity (Figure 1a).

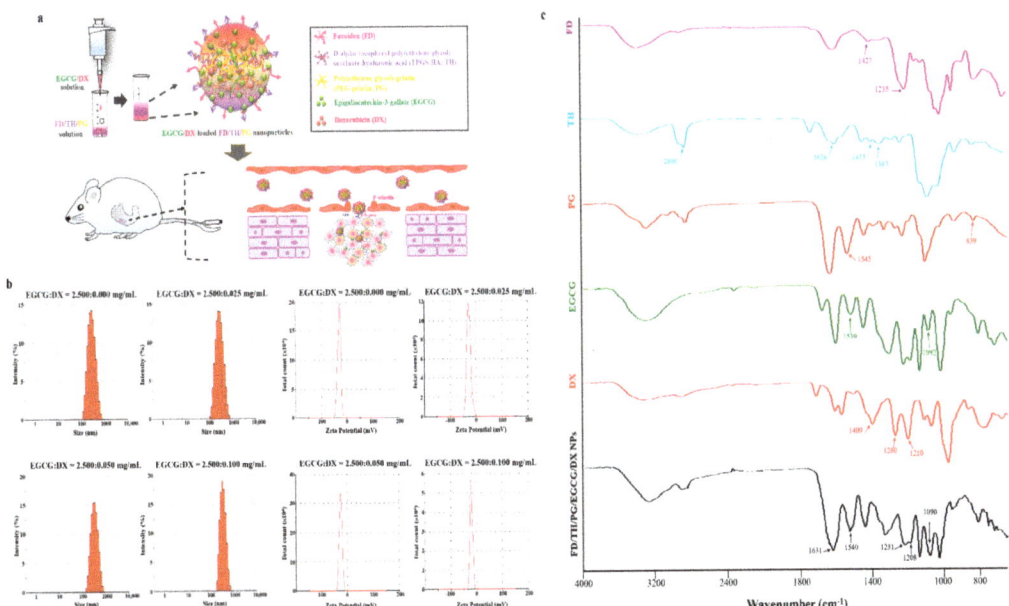

Figure 1. (**a**) NPs were prepared by adding EGCG/DX solution into FD/TH/PG solution under gentle stirring at 37 °C; the schematic representation of the strategy for using EGCG/DX-loaded FD/TH/PG NPs on carcinoma cells is shown; (**b**) Particle size distributions and zeta potential values of EGCG/DX-loaded FD/TH/PG NPs made with different DX concentrations; (**c**) Fourier transform infrared analyses of FD, TH, PG, EGCG, DX, and FD/TH/PG/EGCG/DX NPs.

2. Materials and Methods

2.1. Preparation and Characterization of EGCG/DX-Loaded FD/TH/PG NPs

TH and PG were synthesized according to the protocols suggested by Chen et al. [32]. For TH copolymer preparation, 0.2 mmol dicyclohexylcarbodiimide and 0.2 mmol 4-dimethylaminopyridine were dissolved in 5.0 mL of acetonitrile and added to an aqueous HA solution in deionized (DI) water (20.0 mg/mL in 10.0 mL). The solution was then stirred for 1.0 h to activate the carboxylic groups of HA. Subsequently, 0.1 g of TPGS was dissolved in 2.0 mL of DI water, then slowly added to the above mixed solution and stirred for 24.0 h under a nitrogen atmosphere. The PG copolymer was prepared by dissolving the 2.0 g of gelatin into 20.0 mL of dimethyl sulfoxide (DMSO). The resultant mixture was serviced as solvent for 0.6 g of methoxypolyethylene glycol succinimidyl ester (mPEG-NHS), and then stirred for 4 h. The unconjugated reagents were removed by dialyzing in 5.0 L of DI water, which was replaced five times per day. After the resultant TH and PG were lyophilized in a freeze dryer, Fourier transform infrared (FTIR) spectroscopy was used to detect the presence of purified compound in the sample.

NPs composed of the FD-TH complex with PG containing encapsulated EGCG and DX were prepared as follows. First, the EGCG-loaded FD/TH/PG NPs were formulated by optimizing the relative concentration of FD:TH. A series of FD:TH aqueous solutions (0.00:0.00, 1.20:1.20, 2.40:2.40 and 3.60:3.60 mg/mL in 0.50 mL) were added to aqueous PG solution (15.00 mg/mL in 0.50 mL) and then slowly shaken for 0.5 h at 37 °C. Next, EGCG aqueous solution (5.00 mg/mL in 1.00 mL) was added to 1.0 mL of aqueous FD/TH/PG solutions. The reaction mixture was stirred for 30 min. Then, NPs with different FD:TH:PG:EGCG compositions (0.00:0.00:3.75:2.50, 0.30:0.30:3.75:2.50, 0.60:0.60:3.75:2.50, and 0.90:0.90:3.75:2.50 mg/mL) were completed. After encapsulating DX in these NPs, DX was dissolved in DI water (0.00, 0.10, 0.20, and 0.40 mg/mL in 0.50 mL) and then poured into the EGCG aqueous solution (10.00 mg/mL in 0.50 mL) to form EGCG/DX aqueous solutions (5.00:0.00, 5.00:0.05, 5.00:0.10, and 5.00:0.20 mg/mL in 1.00 mL). The mixture of EGCG/DX solutions (1.00 mL) and FD/TH/PG solution in DI water (1.00 mL) was stirred at 37 °C for 30 min. When the centrifugation was completed, the particle size distributions and zeta potentials of the obtained NPs were analyzed by a Zetasizer Nano apparatus (Malvern Instruments Ltd., Worcestershire, England, UK). The residual EGCG or DX content in the supernatant was assessed. The drug-loading efficiency of the NPs was determined using a reversed-phase high-performance liquid chromatography (HPLC) equipped with a C18 column and UV detector (230 nm).

2.2. Assessing pH Sensitivity and Evaluating Drug Release Profiles in EGCG/DX-Loaded FD/TH/PG NPs

The size distributions and morphological changes of NPs at pH 7.4, 6.5, and 5.0 were assessed using a Zetasizer instrument and transmission electron microscopy (TEM, JEOL Ltd., Tokyo, Japan) to evaluate the stability of the NPs. Buffers with pH 7.4, 6.5, and 5.0 were used to simulate the circulatory system, tumor tissue, and endosomal compartment environment, respectively [33]. The pH sensitivity of NPs was determined by using an HPLC system to measure the release of EGCG and DX under different pH environments. Briefly, 2.0 mg/mL of NP solution was immersed in a dialysis bag and dialyzed against different pH values of 5.0 (10.0 mM acetic acid/sodium acetate), 6.5, and 7.4 (10.0 mM phosphate-buffered saline (PBS)), respectively. The released solution was sampled at specific time intervals and replaced with an equal volume of fresh buffer. The amount of drug release under different pH environments was evaluated with a standard calibration curve and the experiment was repeated five times under each condition.

2.3. GC Cell Culture and the Anticancer Function

Stable luciferase-expressing human GC cells (Luc MKN45) were supplied by the Japanese Collection of Research Bioresources Cell Bank (JCRB No. JCRB1379). Luc MKN45 cells can be easily detected in animals using an in vivo imaging system (IVIS, PerkinElmer Inc., Waltham, MA, USA). The culture was started in a Petri dish at a seeding density of 3×10^5 viable cells/mL in Roswell Park Memorial Institute (RPMI) 1640 medium supplemented with 10% fetal bovine serum (FBS) and 4 µg/mL of puromycin to maintain luciferase expression in a humidified atmosphere of 5% CO_2/95% air at 37 °C. The cells were harvested for subculture every three days with 0.25% trypsin plus 0.05% ethylenediaminetetraacetic acid (EDTA) solution and used for the cytotoxicity experiments. In the cell cytotoxicity experiment, Luc MKN45 cells were seeded in 96-well plates at a cell density of 1.0×10^4 cells/well. After overnight incubation, the growth medium was replaced by PBS with 5% FBS containing distinct concentrations of EGCG solution (0–450 mg/L), DX solution (0–9 mg/L), EGCG/DX solution, or EGCG/DX-loaded NPs (EGCG concentration 0–450 mg/L; DX concentration 0–9 mg/L) for 2.0 h. The examined samples were extracted, and the cells were washed with PBS twice. After culturing in the growth medium for another 22.0 h, cells were incubated in growth medium with 1 mg/mL of 3-(4,5-dimethylthiazol-2-yl)-2,5-diphenyltetrazolium bromide (MTT) to evaluate the cell viability. The additive effect of the EGCG/DX combination on cancer cell viability was determined according to the Chou–Talalay method. The combination index (CI) was calculated using the following equation:

$$CI = D_E/D_{xE} + D_D/D_{xD}, \qquad (1)$$

where D_E and D_D are the concentrations of EGCG and DX, respectively, used to achieve x% drug effect in the combined therapy. D_{xE} and D_{xD} are the concentrations of EGCG and DX, respectively, used alone to achieve x% drug effect. A CI value lower than 1.0 indicates a synergistic effect, a value equal to 1.0, an additive effect, and a value higher than 1.0, an antagonistic effect of the combined drug action [34–36]. The association between drug concentration and inhibitory concentration (IC) for cell viability reduction was calculated and an isobologram and a combination index (CI)—fraction affected (Fa) plot were created.

2.4. In Vitro Drug Cellular Uptake and Cell Distribution of NPs

Luc MKN45 cells carrying fluorescent-dye-conjugated EGCG and DX in NPs were assessed by flow cytometry for the quantification analysis of cellular uptake ratio of EGCG and DX. The cellular uptakes of DX and EGCG were determined by detecting the fluorescence of DX itself (EX470/EM585) and cyanine5 hydrazide (Cy5)-conjugated EGCG (Cy5-EGCG), respectively. The synthesis of fluorescent Cy5-EGCG was prepared by pouring Cy5 solution (1.0 mg/0.1 mL in DMSO) into EGCG aqueous solution (0.2 g/20.0 mL). After continuous stirring for 12.0 h, the fluorescence sample was freeze-dried. The 20.0 mL of DI water was added to the lyophilized Cy5-EGCG sample to precipitate and remove unreacted fluorescent dye. The suspension was centrifuged for several times for separating the precipitated Cy5 dye until no more fluorescent dye precipitation. The prepared Cy5-EGCG solutions were lyophilized with a freeze dryer. Fluorescent Cy5-EGCG/DX-loaded FD/TH/PG NPs were prepared as described before. In brief, Luc MKN45 cells were treated with Cy5-EGCG/DX solution and Cy5-EGCG/DX-loaded NPs for 2.0 h. The medium was washed with PBS and suspended and collected in 0.5 mL of PBS. A Becton Dickinson FACSCalibur flow cytometer (Becton Dickinson, Franklin Lakes, NJ, USA) was used to assess the Cy5-EGCG and DX content in 1.0×10^4 cells, and the Cell Quest software WinMDI (Verity Software House, Inc., Topsham, ME, USA) was used for analysis.

The cellular distribution of fluorescent NPs was further observed by confocal laser scanning microscopy (CLSM, Zeiss LSM 880, Jena, Germany). Fluorescent rhodamine 6G-conjugated EGCG (Rh6G-EGCG) was prepared by the procedure of Cy5-EGCG. In addition, fluorescent polymer Cy5 hydrazide-labeled FD (Cy5-FD), Alexa594 hydrazide-labeled TH (Alexa594-TH), and Atto425 N-hydroxysuccinimide ester-labeled PG (Atto425-PG) were synthesized. These fluorescent solutions (Cy5, Alexa594, and Atto425; 1.0 mg/0.1 mL in DMSO) were gently poured into aqueous FD solutions, TH and PG (0.2 g/20.0 mL) in DI water, respectively. The reaction mixtures were stirred for 12.0 h and dialyzed against DI water in the dark for detaching the unconjugated fluorescent dye. The residue of Cy5-FD, Alexa594-TH, and Atto425-PG solutions were lyophilized in a freeze dryer to prepare distinct fluorescence samples. In brief, Luc MKN45 cells at a density of 3×10^5 cells/cm^2 were seeded on glass coverslips. After preculture for 24.0 h and incubation of fluorescent Rh6G-EGCG/DX solutions and Rh6G-EGCG/DX-loaded Cy5-FD/Alexa594-TH/Atto425-PG NPs for 2.0 h, the medium was washed with PBS. The cells were fixed with 3.7% paraformaldehyde (PFA), and the nuclei were stained with 4,6-diamidino-2-phenylindole (DAPI) and observed by CLSM.

2.5. Evaluation of NP Binding to P-Selectin and CD44s

To determine the capability of FD and TH in NPs in terms of the binding specificity of P-selectin and CD44, human recombinant P-selectin or CD44 (0.5 µg/50 µL) was added to high-hydrophobicity 96-well ELISA plates and incubated overnight at 4 °C. After being washed with PBS, the wells were blocked with 0.1 mL bovine serum albumin (BSA) for 1.0 h. After washing with PBS again, the wells were incubated with different concentrations of fluorescent Rh6G-FD/fluoresceinamine (FA)-TH/PG solution or Rh6G-FD/FA-TH/PG/EGCG NPs for 30 min and gently washed thrice with PBS. Fluorescence images were taken with an EnSpire™ (PerkinElmer Inc., Waltham, MA, USA) Multilabel Plate Reader by averaging 16 reads per well (excitation 525 nm/emission 548 nm for Rh6G-FD; excitation 480 nm/emission 520 nm for FA–TH). Test fluorescent sample solutions (400 µg/mL) and anti-P-selectin or anti-CD44 antibody (2.0 µg/mL) were added to the wells of the previously coated P-selectin or CD44 for the comparisons of binding specificity. The total volume of the resultant mixture in each well was 50 µL. After incubating for 0.5 h, fluorescence measurements were executed. The effect of the prepared NPs on cell surface protein expression was evaluated by culturing 3 mL of Luc MKN45 cells at a density of 3×10^5/mL on glass coverslips for 24.0 h at 37 °C.

The fluorescent Rh6G-FD/FA-TH/PG/EGCG NPs were treated to the cells for 2.0 h. Then, NPs were fixed in 1.0% PFA and stained for P-selectin or CD44 for immunofluorescence experiments. The fixed cells were blocked in PBS with 1.0% BSA and Tween 20 for

1 h, and a mixture solution of primary antibodies (rabbit anti-P-selectin antibody or mouse anti-CD44 antibody) was used for treatment overnight at 4 °C. After washing with PBS, the incubation of cells in a mixture of anti-rabbit Cy5® secondary antibody or anti-mouse Alexa Fluor® 594 secondary antibody was performed for 1.0 h in the dark. Subsequently, the cells were uniformly mounted on slides and examined using CLSM.

2.6. Flow Cytometric Analysis of Cell Cycle and Western Blotting Investigation of Apoptosis-Related Proteins

The incubation of Luc MKN45 cells in the tested EGCG/DX-loaded NPs (EGCG concentration 0–200 mg/L; DX concentration 0–4 mg/L) for 2.0 h was used to evaluate the efficiency of EGCG/DX-loaded NPs on the cell cycle. Then, the cells were washed with PBS and incubated in cell cultured medium for 22.0 h. The cells were again washed with ice-cold PBS and fixed in ice-cold 70% ethanol. After the cells were washed with PBS for the third time, hypotonic buffer was utilized for suspending cells. Subsequently, cells were incubated for 1.0 h at 37 °C. The propidium iodide (PI; 1.00 mg/mL, 0.01 mL) was applied to the buffer, and the cells were again incubated for 0.5 h at 4 °C in the dark. The stages of the cell cycle were evaluated by PI and a Becton Dickinson FACSCalibur flow cytometer. After treating Luc MKN45 cells with EGCG/DX-loaded NPs with different drug concentrations, Western blotting analysis was utilized to assess the expression of apoptotic proteins. Cell lysis was performed by using freeze-thaw cycles, and the cell lysates were centrifuged at $6000 \times g$ at 4 °C. Cell protein lysates were separated into the same amounts with electrophoresis using sodium dodecyl sulfate-polyacrylamide gel electrophoresis, and the isolated proteins were resettled to polyvinylidene difluoride (PVDF) membranes. The PVDF membranes were put in 5% (w/v) nonfat dry milk buffer for 1.0 h and then probed with the following primary antibodies at 4 °C overnight: rabbit polyclonal anti-caspase-9 and anti-poly(ADP-ribose) polymerase (PARP), mouse monoclonal anti-caspase-3, and anti-α-tubulin. Finally, the PVDF membranes were incubated with horseradish peroxidase-conjugated secondary antibodies for 1.0 h, and the immune complexes were evaluated using enhanced chemiluminescence.

2.7. Estimation of Anti-Tumor Activity of Bioluminescent Imaging and IVIS Spectrum Detection on Nanoparticles in Tumors

Animal use and care in this study complied with the 1996 revision of the Guide for the Care and Use of Laboratory Animals prepared by the Institute of Laboratory Animal Resources, National Research Council and published by the National Academy Press. Male six-week-old mice with severe combined immunodeficiency (SCID) and weighing 25 g, purchased from the National Laboratory Animal Center, were placed in the Laboratory Animal Center at Yang Ming Chiao Tung University, Taiwan. The animal care guidelines and all experimental protocols were approved by the Institutional Animal Care and Use Committee (IACUC 1070307). The mice were kept under standard conditions (lights on from 6 AM to 6 PM) and allowed to adapt to local conditions for one week. To establish an orthotopic gastric tumor mouse model, the Luc MKN45 cells were inoculated via the orthotopic implantation method. In brief, after sterilizing the shaved abdominal skin, an incision was made to expose the stomach and the injection of Luc MKN45 cells ($1 \times 10^7/100$ μL) mixed in matrix gel (Becton Dickinson, Franklin Lakes, NJ, USA) suspension into the gastric wall was performed sub-serosally. Once the stomach was returned to the peritoneal cavity, the abdominal wall and skin were sutured closed.

After the stable detection of an orthotopic gastric tumor was achieved, drug treatment was initialized. The tumor growth was monitored using IVIS spectrum detection by capturing bioluminescence signals from Luc MKN45 cells. The mice were divided into three groups randomly with six mice each, with the injection of FD/TH/PG solution (control group), 20.0 mg/kg of EGCG/0.4 mg/kg DX in EGCG/DX solution, or EGCG/DX-loaded FD/TH/PG NPs via tail vein, respectively. Luciferin was injected intraperitoneally into the mice and waited for 10 min for bioluminescence expression and images were taken by IVIS. The quantification of the bioluminescence signals was used to monitor the tumor growth. The animals were sacrificed after the final observation and organs were taken for histological examination by hematoxylin and eosin (H&E) or immunohistochemical (IHC) staining. The efficiency of EGCG/DX-loaded NPs on tumor status was assessed by IHC staining of M30 (apoptosis marker) and Ki-67 (proliferation marker). After dewaxing the paraffin, the tissue sections were immersed in a series of concentrations of ethanol and xylene for rehydration. The sections were stained with primary antibodies of M30 CytoDeath (Peviva, Bromma, Stockholm, Sweden) and Ki67 (Thermo Fisher Scientific, Grand Island, NY, USA) after blocking with BSA. Then, secondary peroxidase antibodies were used for the probe. Finally, the distribution expression of M30 and Ki67 and tissue inflammation at different magnifications were observed under a light microscope. Meanwhile, in the in vivo NP distribution study, fluorescent-labeled Rh6G-EGCG/DX-loaded Cy5-FD/Alexa594-TH/VioTag750-PG NPs were injected via tail vein to evaluate their distribution during the treatment. After euthanizing the mice at 24 h, fluorescence images of organs and tissues were obtained in the IVIS. Moreover, the mice also received fluorescent Rh6G-FD/FA-TH/PG/EGCG NPs via 24.0 h intravenous injection. Subsequently, the gastric tumor slides were assessed using immunofluorescence staining with rabbit anti-P-selectin antibody or mouse anti-CD44 primary antibodies, probed with secondary antibodies (anti-rabbit Cy5® or anti-mouse Alexa Fluor® 594), then examined using CLSM.

2.8. Statistical Analysis

One-way analysis of variance was used to analyze differences in the measured characteristics of the treatment groups. The confidence intervals were determined using Statistical Analysis System, version 6.08 (SAS Institute, Cary, NC, USA). The mean ± standard deviation (SD) was used to represent all data and $p < 0.05$ was considered statistically significant.

3. Results

3.1. Preparation and Characterization of EGCG/DX-Loaded FD/TH/PG NPs

To create NPs that can be combined with EGCG and DX, first, the optimal material FD:TH ratio should be determined when preparing EGCG-loaded NPs and then the concentration of DX should be adjusted to create EGCG/DX-loaded NPs. As shown in Table 1, as the amount of FD/TH incorporated in FD/TH/PG/EGCG NPs increased, the mean particle size of the NPs was 214.68 ± 18.78 to 741.79 ± 198.79 nm and their polydispersity index (PDI) was 0.25 ± 0.08 to 0.95 ± 0.26. When the FD:TH:PG ratio was 0.60:0.60:3.75 mg/mL, the NPs formed a dissoluble opalescent suspension after centrifugation. The particle size was 224.68 ± 18.78 nm and the zeta potential -26.14 ± 1.75 mV, with a significantly narrow distribution (0.25 ± 0.08) (Table 1). However, when the FD:TH:PG ratio increased to 0.90:0.90:3.75 mg/mL, the average particle size of the NPs increased, as did their PDI (to 0.4), indicating high heterogeneity. To further load DX into NPs, NPs containing different concentrations of EGCG and DX were prepared using a gelation technique in which the EGCG/DX solution was added to the FD/TH/PG aqueous solution. The HPLC analysis method showed that, at an EGCG:DX ratio of 2.50:0.05 mg/mL, the loading efficiency of EGCG and DX in the NPs was $59.07\% \pm 7.06\%$ and $63.46\% \pm 4.59\%$, respectively. The subsequent experiment required a narrower distribution (PDI = 0.21 ± 0.05) (Table 2 and Figure 1b).

Table 1. Effect of different FD/TH proportions on particle sizes, polydispersity indices, zeta potential values, and drug loading efficiency of the prepared EGCG-loaded FD/TH/PG NPs ($n = 5$). ■ Precipitation of aggregates after centrifugation was observed.

	PG at 3.75 mg/mL; EGCG at 2.50 mg/mL			
FD:TH (mg/mL)	Mean Particle Size (nm)	Polydispersity Indices	Zeta Potential Value (mV)	Loading Efficiency (%)
0.00:0.00	■	■	■	■
0.30:0.30	741.79 ± 198.79	0.95 ± 0.26	−17.72 ± 5.67	59.86 ± 9.87
0.60:0.60	214.68 ± 18.78	0.25 ± 0.08	−26.14 ± 1.75	63.48 ± 7.39
0.90:0.90	315.27 ± 47.84	0.41 ± 0.13	−29.76 ± 4.65	69.87 ± 3.14

Table 2. Effect of varying DX concentration on EGCG/DX-loaded FD/THA/PG particle sizes, polydispersity indices, zeta potential values, and drug loading efficiency ($n = 5$).

	FD at 0.60 mg/mL; TH at 0.60 mg/mL; PG at 3.75 mg/mL				
EGCG:DX (mg/mL)	Mean Particle Size (nm)	Polydispersity Indices	Zeta Potential Value (mV)	Loading Efficiency (%)	
				EGCG	DX
2.500:0.000	214.68 ± 18.78	0.25 ± 0.08	−26.14 ± 1.75	63.48 ± 7.39	ND
2.500:0.025	205.43 ± 11.95	0.28 ± 0.06	−25.84 ± 3.23	61.74 ± 3.49	59.43 ± 9.34
2.500:0.050	221.26 ± 13.26	0.21 ± 0.05	−23.30 ± 2.13	59.07 ± 7.06	63.46 ± 4.59
2.500:0.100	254.84 ± 18.75	0.38 ± 0.10	−22.87 ± 3.58	57.39 ± 8.74	67.78 ± 9.62

In FTIR investigates of EGCG/DX-loaded FD/TH/PG NPs, the representative peaks at 1235 and 1427 cm^{-1} ascribed to FD were dispensed to sulfate esters (O=S=O) and CH$_2$ (galactose, xylose) scissoring vibrations or CH$_3$ (fucose, O-acetyls) asymmetric bending vibrations. The synthesized TH copolymer was analyzed with FTIR and showed representative peaks at 1363 and 2880 cm^{-1}, conforming to the −CH$_2$ group on PEG and the −CH stretching band of TPGS, and peaks at 1413 and 1626 cm^{-1}, reflecting the contribution of C−O stretches symmetrically and C=O stretches asymmetrically, corresponding to the carboxyl group on HA. In the PEG-conjugated gelatin (PG) spectrum, characteristic peaks at 839 and 1545 cm^{-1} were observed, corresponding to bending C−C and −NH stretching vibrations on PEG and gelatin. Finally, EGCG/DX-loaded FD/TH/PG complex spectra showed characteristic peaks at 1090 and 1208 cm^{-1}, corresponding to the C−OH deformation of EGCG and DX, respectively. Moreover, the NH bending peak on PG shifted from 1545 cm^{-1} to 1540 cm^{-1}; the S=O or C=O stretching peaks on FD or TH shifted from 1235 cm^{-1} or 1626 cm^{-1} to 1231 cm^{-1} or 1631 cm^{-1}, respectively. This indicates that the H atoms of EGCG or DX interacted via hydrogen bonds with the N atoms of PG (C−OH···N−C) or the O atoms of FD or TH (C−OH···O=S or O=C) (Figure 1c).

3.2. Characterization of the Morphology and Drug Release Profile of EGCG/DX-Loaded FD/TH/PG NPs

We evaluated the pH sensitivity of the NPs and the distinct drug release profile of EGCG/DX-loaded NPs using TEM and HPLC, respectively (Figure 2). At pH 7.4 and 6.5 (simulating the physiological fluids and tumor tissues), the NPs shown as stable spheres with a matrix structure with particle sizes of 200–230 nm, because EGCG and DX form hydrogen bonds with PG or TH. The drug release percentage from NPs over 3.0 h incubation was 6.21% ± 0.87% (EGCG) and 9.54% ± 0.15% (DX) at pH 7.4 and 7.94% ± 0.69% (EGCG) and 9.87% ± 1.35% (DX) at pH 6.5. At pH 5.0 (simulating an acidic environment in endosomal of cancer cells), some of the −COO− groups were moderately protonated in TH, affecting the negative electrostatic repulsion of NPs, which become unstable and partially collapse but with increased particle size (418.31 ± 69.75 nm) (Figure 2a). Under those conditions, the EGCG release was 24.58% ± 1.64% and the DX release was 28.17% ± 3.68% within 3.0 h. In addition, the hydrogen bonding between the N or O atom in PG or TH, and the H atom in the hydroxyl group of EGCG or DX caused slower drug release from EGCG/DX-loaded NPs, reaching 59.74% ± 3.31% and 75.74% ± 2.08% for EGCG and DX, respectively, over 24.0 h (Figure 2b).

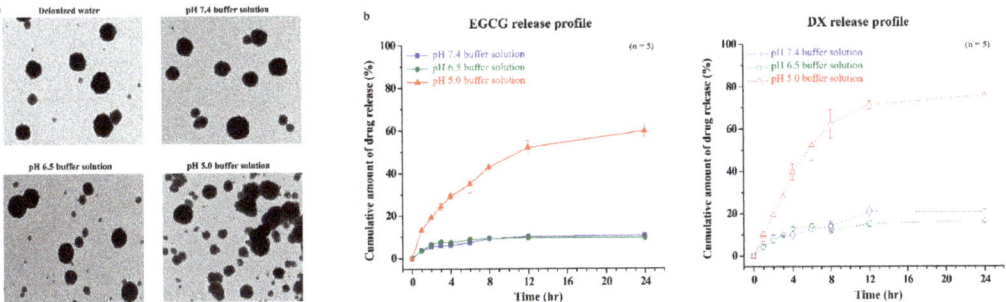

Figure 2. (**a**) Transmission electron micrographs of nanoparticles in buffer solution with different pH values; (**b**) The release profile of EGCG and DX in varying pH environments at 37 °C. Data is expressed as mean ± SD (n = 5).

3.3. Effects of FD/TH Solutions and EGCG/DX-Loaded FD/TH/PG Nanoparticles on Binding of P-Selectin and CD44

To study the targeting of P-selectin and CD44 by Rh6G-FD/FA-TH/PG solution or Rh6G-FD/FA-TH/PG/EGCG NPs with different FD or TH molecule concentrations (100, 200 and 400 μg/mL), their fluorescence intensity was quantified by spectrofluorometry. The evident fluorescence intensities at Rh6G-FD or FA-TH concentrations of 100 μg/mL to 400 μg/mL were 207.19 ± 24.09 to 659.21 ± 85.31 or 173.39 ± 35.19 to 480.11 ± 51.26 (only FD/TH/PG solutions), respectively and 373.91 ± 59.08 to 911.21 ± 52.61 or 231.39 ± 40.09 to 662.31 ± 60.76 (EGCG/DX-loaded FD/TH/PG NPs), respectively. Additionally, Rh6G-FD or FA-TH fluorescence analysis indicated that the contact degree of EGCG/DX-loaded NPs with P-selectin or CD44 was greater than that of FD/TH/PG solutions. The addition of P-selectin or CD44 reduced the adhesion of targeting proteins to FD or TH by approximately 50% due to blockage by the competing anti-targeting P-selectin or CD44 protein antibodies (Figure 3a). Therefore, we evaluated the benefits of the relative composition of FD and TH in P-selectin- and CD44-targeted NPs. The prepared NPs interact with protein expression on GC cell surface was observed by CLSM. After 2.0 h of incubation with fluorescent Rh6G-FD/FA-HA/PG/EGCG NPs, fluorescence signals (Rh6G-FD (red dot) and FA-TH (orange dot)) of the NPs were observed in the cell cytoplasm and intercellular spaces, and then the NPs could exhibit co-localize and interact with P-selectin (purple dots) and CD44 (green dots) in gastric cancer cells (blue or red arrows indicate superimposed red/purple or orange/green dots) (Figure 3b).

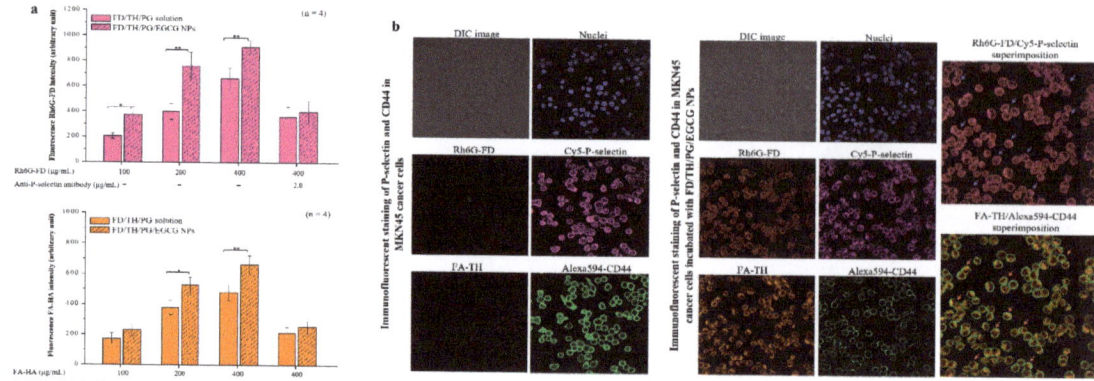

Figure 3. (**a**) Binding assays of fluorescence Rh6G-FD and FA-TH to immobilized recombinant P-selectin and CD44 protein. Data is expressed as mean ± SD (n = 4). Asterisk symbols * and ** represent statistically significant differences with p value < 0.05 and < 0.01, respectively; (**b**) Immunofluorescence staining of P-selectin and CD44 proteins in MKN45 cancer cells incubated with Rh6G-FD/FA-TH/PG/EGCG NPs.

3.4. Evaluating the Anticancer Effect of EGCG/DX-Loaded FD/TH/PG NPs and the Combination Index Determination

To evaluate the potential inhibitory effect of EGCG or DX alone and the synergy of the EGCG/DX solution, the effects of EGCG/DX-loaded NP treatment on GC cell viability was analyzed. Both EGCG and DX significantly affected cell growth at high concentrations of 450 and 9 mg/L, respectively, and the cell viability decreased to 50.59% ± 3.46% and 50.81% ± 5.11%, respectively (Figure 4). We also compared the efficacy of EGCG/DX solution and EGCG/DX-loaded NP on inhibiting GC growth. The cell survival after EGCG/DX-loaded NP treatment was obviously lower than that after EGCG/DX solution treatment. The anti-cancer activity of EGCG/DX-loaded FD/TH/PG NPs (EGCG concentration, 150–450 mg/L; DX concentration, 3–9 mg/L) on Luc MKN45 cells was significantly higher than that of the EGCG/DX combined solution (p < 0.05; Figure 4c). The therapeutic IC50 of EGCG/DX-loaded NPs was 200/4 mg/L, which was half that of the EGCG/DX combined solution (400/8 mg/L).

In addition, the CI-Fa plot and isobologram are described in Figure 4d. EGCG/DX combination treatment had a slightly synergistic effect on the cell viability, with CI of IC_{10} and IC_{20} being 0.86 and 0.94, respectively. EGCG/DX-loaded NP treatment showed a better synergistic antiproliferation effect, with CIs of IC_{10}, IC_{20}, IC_{30}, IC_{40}, and IC_{50} being 0.56, 0.48, 0.70, 0.80, and 0.89, respectively, compared with EGCG/DX combination solution. This result showed that GCG/DX-loaded FD/TH/PG NP targeting cancer therapy has better benefits than EGCG/DX combined drug therapy.

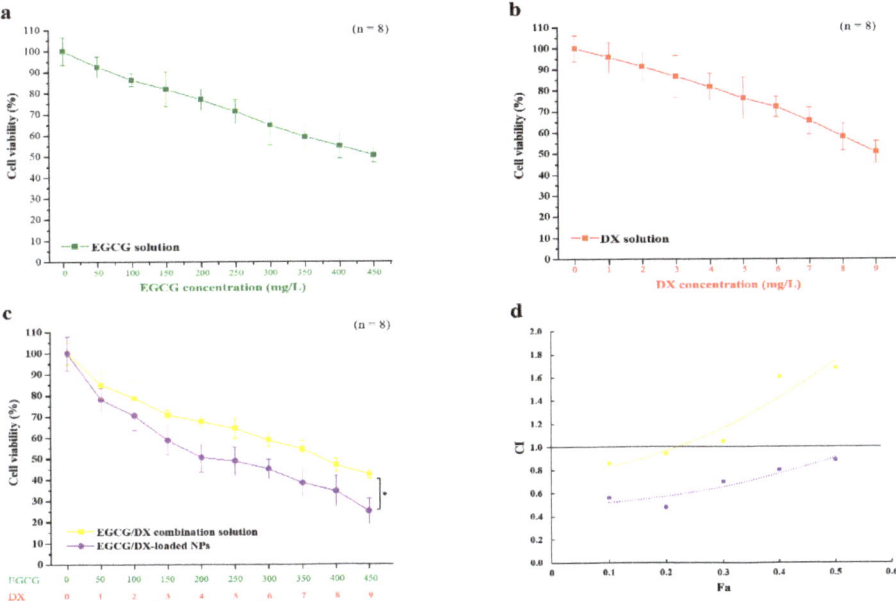

Figure 4. The effects of EGCG, DX, EGCG/DX combination solution, and EGCG/DX-loaded NPs on Luc MKN45 cell viability: (**a**) A 2.0 h dose response treatment with EGCG; (**b**) A 2.0 h dose response treatment with DX; (**c**) A 2.0 h dose response treatment with EGCG/DX solution and EGCG/DX-loaded NPs; cell viability was assessed at 24.0 h for a–c; data are expressed as mean ± SD (n = 8). Asterisk * represents statistically significant difference with p value < 0.05. (**d**) Combination index–fraction affected (CI-Fa) plot; CI < 1.0 indicates synergistic effects, CI = 1.0 indicates additive effects and CI > 1.0 indicates antagonistic effects of the combined drug action. Dots below the slanted line indicate synergistic effects.

3.5. Internalization of EGCG and DX and Cellular Uptake of Complexes Contained within Fluorescent Nanoparticles

To confirm the cellular uptake ability, fluorescence-activated cell sorting analysis was made after the cells were treated with both the drug combination and NPs containing Cy5-EGCG and DX. Flow cytometry examination was performed with Luc MKN45 cells after treatment with FD/TH/PG NPs loaded with EGCG/DX. The cellular uptake and fluorescence intensity of Cy5-EGCG were 86.53% ± 3.25% and 27,639.98 ± 254.91, respectively, while those of DX reached 60.42% ± 1.56% and 13,493.23 ± 143.87, respectively, after exposure for 2.0 h. In contrast, after treatment with only EGCG/DX solution, the cellular uptake and total fluorescence intensity of Cy5-EGCG were 56.29% ± 1.32% and 18,783.54 ± 198.40, respectively and those of DX were 28.62% ± 0.97% and 6275.41 ± 60.43, respectively (Figure 5a). This difference in drug absorption capacity is closely related to the presence of EGCG/DX in NPs, which successfully identified the specific targets, namely P-selectin and CD44, on the cell surface.

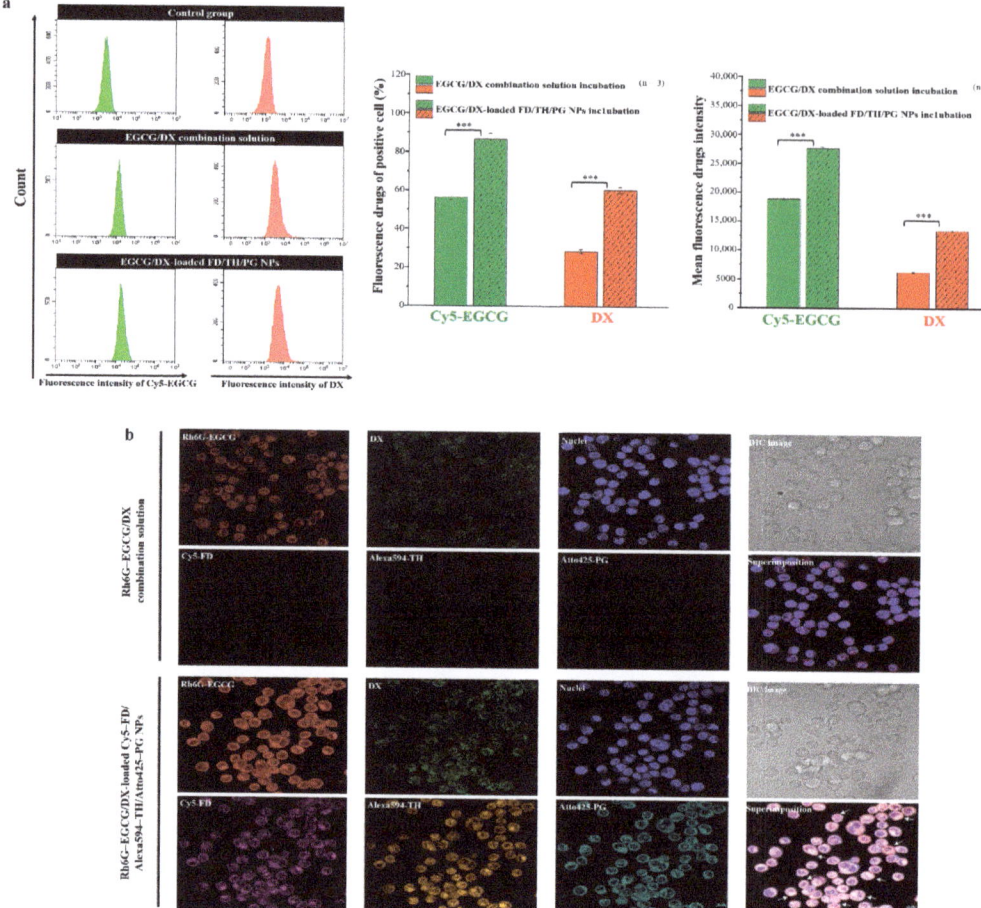

Figure 5. (**a**) In vitro cellular uptake of Cy5-GCG and DX was assessed using flow cytometry after treatment with EGCG/DX combination solution and EGCG/DX-loaded NPs; (**b**) Confocal images of gastric cancer cells viewing cellular distribution of the Rh6G-EGCG/DX combination solution and Rh6G-EGCG/DX-loaded Cy5-FD/Alexa594-TH/Atto425-PG NPs, *** represent statistically significant differences with p value < 0.001.

CLSM was used to compare and evaluate the delivery efficiency of EGCG/DX solution and EGCG/DX-loaded FD/TH/PG NPs after 2.0 h treatment, and DAPI with fluorescence expression was used to stain cell nuclei. Cy5-FD, Alexa594-TH, and Atto425-PG were co-localized in the cells. The internalization of EGCG and DX was evaluated by observing Rh6G-EGCG and DX fluorescence performance signals. Drug content (Rh6G-EGCG and DX) was higher in GC cells treated with the EGCG/DX-loaded NPs than in those treated with the EGCG/DX solution, indicating that the NP system infiltrated cancer cells and improved the delivery of EGCG and DX (Figure 5b).

3.6. Cell Cycle Arrest and Apoptosis Effects of NPs Loaded with EGCG/DX

To investigate whether the decrease in the growth rate of cells treated with test samples is associated with cell cycle arrest, we analyzed PI-stained Luc MKN45 cells treated with EGCG/DX-loaded NPs containing different EGCG and DX concentrations within 24.0 h by flow cytometry. As shown in Figure 6a, after EGCG/DX-loaded NP treatment, the cells displayed significant accumulation in the G2/M phase compared to the control group.

In particular, EGCG/DX-loaded NPs significantly reduced the G0/G1 population (from 57.28% ± 2.35% to 18.66% ± 4.51%), the number of cells undergoing the S phase slightly decreased (from 16.48% ± 0.87% to 12.11% ± 5.03%), and the accumulation of G2/M in cells (from 25.11% ± 1.73% to 67.86% ± 3.95%) increased in an EGCG/DX dose-dependent manner, indicating that EGCG/DX-loaded NPs affect cell cycle arrest at the G2/M phase in GC cells. To determine whether the EGCG/DX-loaded NPs can induce cell apoptosis, we performed Western blotting and evaluated the ratios of cleaved caspase-9, caspase-3, and poly(ADP-ribose) polymerase (PARP) levels to their total protein expression (cleaved form plus proform). α-Tubulin was used as an internal control. Twenty-four hours after the samples were treated with different drug concentrations, EGCG/DX (200/4 mg/mL) was found to increase the cleaved protein to total protein expression ratios of caspase-9, caspase-3, and PARP by approximately 18%, 45%, and 69%, respectively, compared with that in the untreated group (Figure 6b).

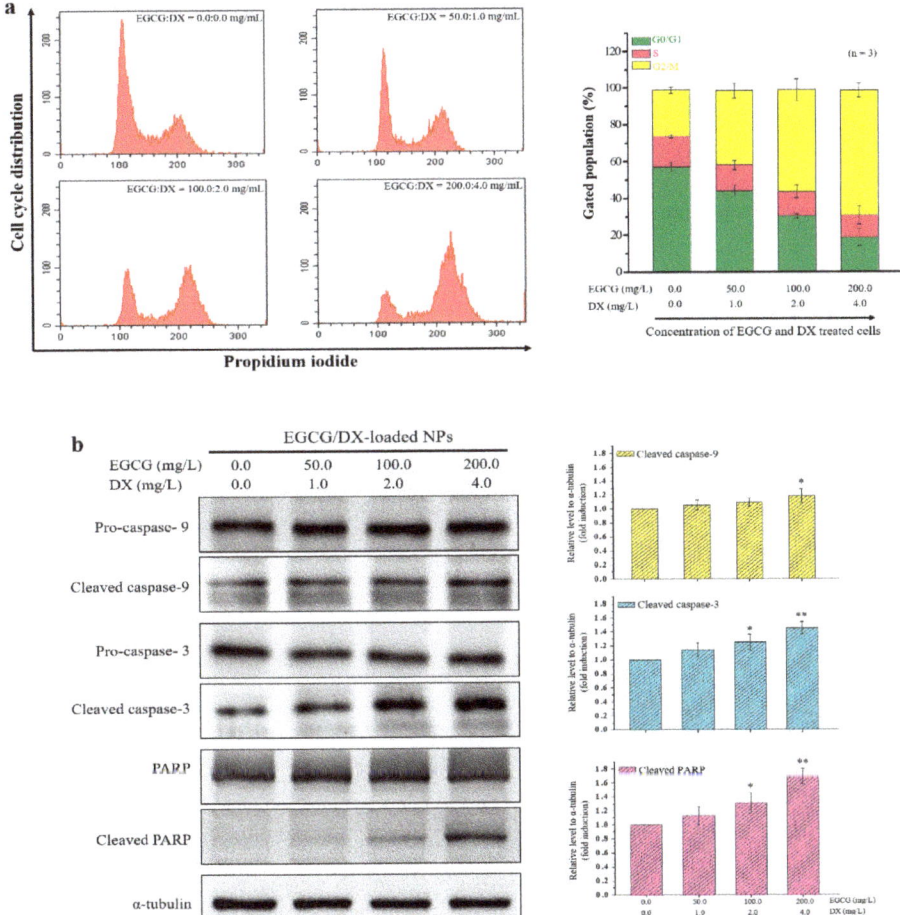

Figure 6. (**a**) The proportions of cells in the G0/G1, S, and G2/M phases, after treatment with EGCG/DX-loaded FD/TH/PG NPs are indicated. The cells were stained with propidium iodide and the cell cycle distribution was analyzed using flow cytometry. (**b**) Western blotting analysis of apoptosis-related caspase-9, caspase-3, and PARP in MKN45 cells after incubation with EGCG/DX-loaded FD/TH/PG NPs and α-tubulin was used as an internal control. * Statistically significant difference of $p < 0.05$ and ** $p < 0.01$, respectively as compared with the without sample treatment group.

3.7. Bioluminescent Imaging to Evaluate Anticancer Activity in an Orthotopic Gastric Tumor Mouse Model

We examined tumor-specific effects of EGCG/DX-loaded NPs in the gastric tumor mouse model of a luciferase-expressing gastric tumor. Male SCID mice were inoculated with EGCG/DX combination solution (20 mg/kg EGCG/0.4 mg/kg DX) and EGCG-loaded FD/TH/PG NPs or FD/TH/PG solution as a control by using intravenous tail injection every three days for a total of five injections. The bioluminescence signals of gastric tumor pointedly increased by 3.87-fold ± 0.39-fold (FD/THA/PG solution) and 3.10-fold ± 0.29-fold (EGCG/DX solution) at day 18. Furthermore, EGCG/DX-loaded FD/THA/PG NPs (2.16 ± 0.35 units) better inhibited tumor growth, with a lower relative photon flux compared with mice in other treatment groups (Figure 7a). There was no difference in body weight loss in our EGCG/DX-loaded NPs group and it was also superior to that in the FD/TH/PG control solution, indicating significant antitumor activity (Figure 7a). We also used IVIS to further evaluate the local accumulation of NPs. After fluorescent Rh6G-EGCG/DX-loaded Cy5–FD/Alexa594-TH/VioTag750-PG NPs were used for tail vein injection, fluorescent signals were detected on different tissues by IVIS technology. The gastric tumor was visualized by detecting bioluminescent signals formed by stable luciferase-expressing Luc MKN45 cells. The intensity of the fluorescent signals (Rh6G-EGCG and DX) at the tumor site significantly increased locally within 24.0 h, indicating continuous and sustained drug delivery by NPs targeting P-selectin and CD44 in the tumor. After 24.0 h, the mice were sacrificed to determine the total fluorescent counts in tumor and normal tissues and an increase in the NP distribution in the tumor led to a decrease in their distribution in other organs. Therefore, the tumor-targeting ability of EGCG/DX-loaded FD/TH/PG NPs was effective in the orthotopic gastric tumor mouse model (Figure 7b).

3.8. Histological and Immunohistochemical Analyses of Cancer Biomarkers

After the experimental mice were sacrificed, H&E staining was used for histological examination of gastric tumors and other organ biopsies (Figure 8). Compared with the EGCG/DX-loaded NP groups, tumor sections from the EGCG/DX combination group had more granular eosinophil infiltration (black arrow). The EGCG/DX-loaded NP group showed increased tumor necrosis, characterized as grade 2 tissue necrosis (necrosis of tumor cells or disappearance of more than 2/3 cells; the right side of the red line) compared with the EGCG/DX combination group (Figure 8a). Additionally, immunohistochemical analysis presented that after EGCG/DX-loaded FD/TH/PG NP treatment, M30 expression in tumors increased, while Ki67 expression diminished (i.e., coffee dots; green arrows, Figure 8a). These findings showed that targeted NPs induce GC cells apoptosis, resulting in a significant increase in anticancer activity with tumor necrosis. In the EGCG/DX combination group, the lung tissue showed inflammatory cell exudation, red blood cells scattered in multiple alveolar cavities, and thickened interstitial pulmonary edema (i.e., black arrows, Figure 8b). In contrast, the pathological damage was evidently minor in the EGCG/DX-loaded NP group, in which the alveolar structures were clear, and signs of inflammation decreased (i.e., black arrows, Figure 8b). Moreover, the hepatocyte swelling density and neutrophil infiltration situation of liver tissue biopsies in the EGCG/DX-loaded NP group was less than those in the EGCG/DX combined group (i.e., red arrows, Figure 8b). Therefore, targeting NPs can not only significantly improve the antitumor ability of drugs against GC, but also reduce the inflammatory response in the body.

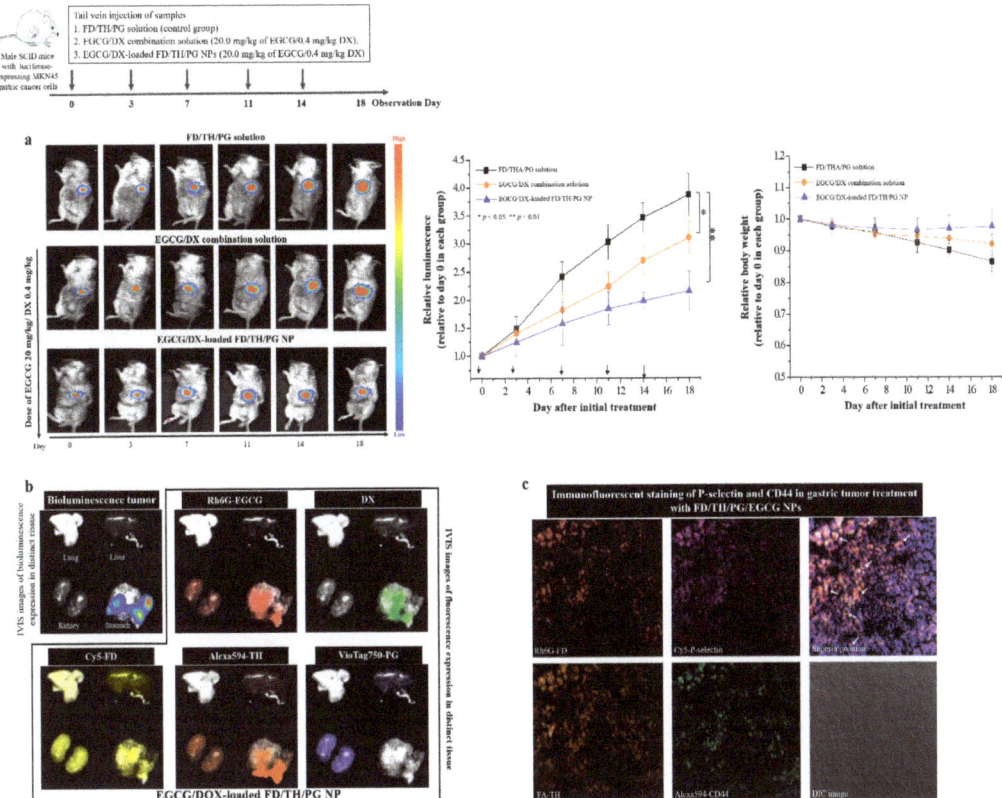

Figure 7. (a) The antitumor effects of different samples in orthotopic Luc MKN45 xenograft mice model. Mice were divided into three groups of six mice each and treated with FD/TH/PG solution (■), EGCG/DX combination solution (●), or EGCG/DX-loaded FD/TH/PG NPs (▲). * Statistically significant difference of $p < 0.05$ and ** $p < 0.01$. (b) Distributions of fluorescent Rh6G-EGCG/DX-loaded Cy5-FD/Alexa594–TH/VivoTag750-PG in tumor and organs after treatment. Gastric tumors were detected with a bioluminescent in vivo imaging system. (c) Immunofluorescence staining of P-selectin and CD44 proteins in gastric tumor slides treated with Rh6G–FD/FA-TH/PG/EGCG NPs.

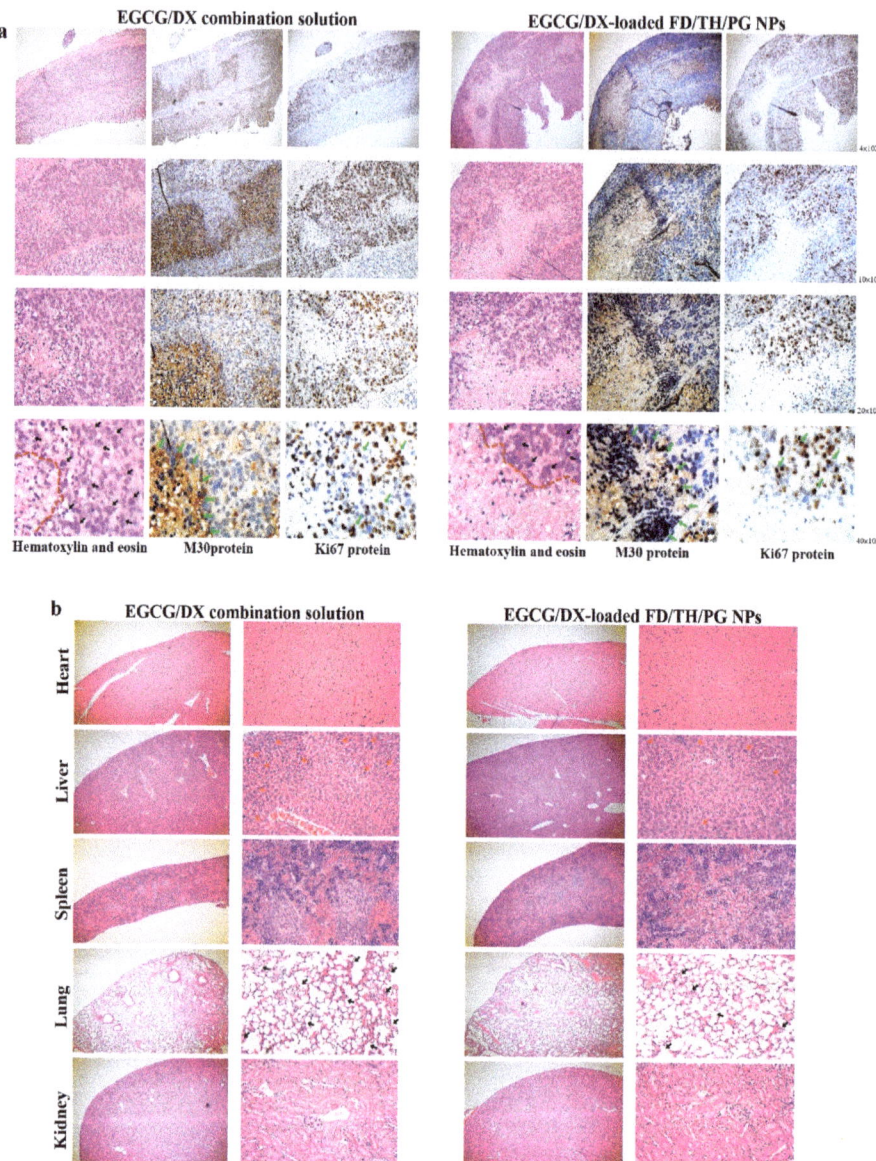

Figure 8. (a) Histological analysis and immunohistochemical analysis of Ki67 (proliferation marker) or M30 (apoptosis marker) of gastric tumor biopsy after treatment with EGCG/DX combination solution or EGCG/DX-loaded FD/TH/PG NPs; (b) Histological analysis of different organs in mice bearing gastric tumor after treatment with EGCG/DX combination solution or EGCG/DX-loaded FD/TH/PG NPs.

4. Discussion

Cell adhesion is the process by which cells interact and attach to neighboring cells through specialized molecules, regulating cell motility and migration [37,38]. Adhesion molecules of the selectin family (E-, L-, and P-selectin) are a class of membrane-bound protein that participate in the initial adhesion of leukocytes to the site of infection or inflammation [37]. P-selectin expression increases in the vasculature of human cancers and facilitates metastasis by promoting the adhesion of circulating cancer cells to activated platelets and endothelial cells in distant organs [39,40]. P-selectin can also bind with high affinity to some sulfatides and sulfated polysaccharides, such as heparin, dextran sulfate, and FD [41,42]. Park et al. used FD extracted from *Fucus vesiculosus* to cause autophagic cell death of human GC cells and show antiproliferation activity via Beclin1 upregulation and the conversion of microtubule-associated protein (MAP) light chain 3-I (LC3-I) to LC3-II [43]. P-selectin binds to CD44 and promotes the capture of vascular endothelial cells and cancer cells by leukocytes [44]. HA, a major extracellular matrix component, is a physiological ligand that is overexpressed in CD44 on the surface of malignant tumor cells and can be used to selectively activate multiple oncogenic signaling pathways that lead to tumor cell-specific phenotypes [45]. CLSM showed that the fluorescence signals (Rh6G-FD (red dot) and FA-TH (orange dot)) of the prepared NPs were co-localized and interacted with P-selectin (purple dot) and CD44 (green dot) in gastric tumor tissue (white arrows)(Figure 7c). Rh6G-EGCG and DX fluorescence signals emanated by Rh6G-EGCG/DX-loaded Cy5-FD/Alexa594-TH/Atto425-PG NPs were attached to Luc MKN45 cells, and more drugs (EGCG and DX) were released into the cell cytoplasm compared with EGCG/DX combination treatment (Figure 5). Furthermore, the carrier EGCG/DX induced cell cycle arrest in the G2/M phase, inhibited GC proliferation, and enhanced the expression of apoptosis-related proteins (Figure 6).

Tumor cell growth generates a complex physiological environment that is distinct from regions surrounding healthy tissues. Both the extracellular and intracellular pH values of tumor cells are considered to be acidic and lower than those of normal cells [46,47]. Physiological pH is generally believed to be in the range of 7.2–7.4 for normal tissues and the circulatory system [48]. However, the pH value of tumor cells is weakly acidic, between 6.5 and 7.0, and the pH value of endosomes and lysosomes is between 5.0 and 6.0 [49]. Therefore, the pH of the tumor microenvironment and tumor cells plays an important role in the development and treatment of cancer. The NP system adopts a pH-sensitive adjustment strategy to prevent the untimely release of drugs. In the present study, NPs containing EGCG/DX were designed with a matrix structure that minimizes drug release into normal physiological environments, such as nontarget tissues and blood, and promotes the release of EGCG and DX into lysosomes and late endosomes of the tumor cells. The cumulative release of EGCG and DX at pH 5.0 amounted to 59.74% ± 3.31% and 75.74% ± 2.08%, respectively (Figure 2). Specifically, in vivo experiments confirmed that the lower bioluminescence intensity after intravenous injection of EGCG/DX-loaded NP (20 mg/kg EGCG/0.4 mg/kg DX) treatment significantly inhibited tumor growth (Figure 7). Histological analyses showed that the delivery of EGCG/DX to tumors through NPs can induce GC cell apoptosis, as indicated by increased levels of caspase-cleaved cytokeratin 18 (M30, ccK18) as an apoptotic cell death pharmacodynamic biomarker, accompanied by a reduction in inflammatory pulmonary lesions (Figure 8).

5. Conclusions

In summary, we applied an FD-based and TH-based NP system for the active, targeted co-delivery of EGCG and DX through P-selectin and CD44 ligand recognition to GC cells. Drug release was regulated by the NP system using a pH-sensitive adjustment strategy. In addition, the NPs prepared for the co-drug delivery system significantly improved the synergistic anti-cancer effect of EGCG and DX compared with that of the EGCG/DX combination solution. Targeting enhanced NP distribution in GC cells and decreasing it in major organs in the orthotopic gastric tumor could lead to the development of novel cancer therapies and facilitate their clinical trials.

Author Contributions: W.-Y.H. and C.-H.L. contributed equally to this work and should be considered co-first authors. W.-Y.H. and C.-H.L. conceived and designed this work. S.-L.P., C.-Y.H., and P.-H.H. performed the experimental study. P.-Y.C. and C.-L.F. analyzed the data and discussed the results. Y.-H.L. supervised the research and obtained funding. All authors have read and agreed to the published version of the manuscript.

Funding: This work is particularly supported by Ministry of Science and Technology, grant number MOST 107-2221-E-010-004-MY3 and Yin Yen-Liang Foundation Development and Construction Plan of the School of Medicine, National Yang-Ming University. The funders had no role in study design, data collection and analysis, decision to publish or preparation of the manuscript.

Institutional Review Board Statement: The study was conducted according to the guidelines of the Declaration of Helsinki, and approved by the Institutional Animal Care and Use Committee of Laboratory Animal Center at Yang Ming Chiao Tung University (IACUC 1070307 and 1 January 2019 of approval).

Acknowledgments: We thank the Laboratory of the Leiss LSM 880 confocal Spectral microscopy experiment and BD FACSCalibur flow cytometer provided by core facility of National Yang Ming Chiao Tung University. The authors would like to thank Enago (www.enago.tw) for the English language review.

Conflicts of Interest: The authors declare no conflict of interest.

References

1. Scheuble, N.; Schaffner, J.; Schumacher, M.; Windhab, E.J.; Liu, D.; Parker, H.; Steingoetter, A.; Fischer, P. Tailoring Emulsions for Controlled Lipid Release: Establishing in vitro–in Vivo Correlation for Digestion of Lipids. *ACS Appl. Mater. Interfaces* **2018**, *10*, 17571–17581. [CrossRef]
2. Sensoy, I. A review on the food digestion in the digestive tract and the used in vitro models. *Curr. Res. Food Sci.* **2021**, *4*, 308–319. [CrossRef]
3. Shang, A.P.J. Multidisciplinary approach to understand the pathogenesis of gastric cancer. *World J. Gastroenterol.* **2005**, *11*, 4131–4139. [CrossRef] [PubMed]
4. Zetter, B.R. Adhesion molecules in tumor metastasis. *Semin. Cancer Biol.* **1993**, *4*, 219–229. [PubMed]
5. Chen, J.-L.; Chen, W.-X.; Zhu, J.-S.; Chen, N.-W.; Zhou, T.; Yao, M.; Zhang, D.-Q.; Wu, Y.-L. Effect of P-selectin monoclonal antibody on metastasis of gastric cancer and immune function. *World J. Gastroenterol.* **2003**, *9*, 1607–1610. [CrossRef] [PubMed]
6. Stone, J.P.; Wagner, D.D. P-selectin mediates adhesion of platelets to neuroblastoma and small cell lung cancer. *J. Clin. Investig.* **1993**, *92*, 804–813. [CrossRef] [PubMed]
7. Li, L.; Short, H.J.; Qian, K.-X.; Elhammer, A.P.; Geng, J.-G.. Characterization of Glycoprotein Ligands for P-Selectin on a Human Small Cell Lung Cancer Cell Line NCI-H345. *Biochem. Biophys. Res. Commun.* **2001**, *288*, 637–644. [CrossRef] [PubMed]
8. Takaishi, S.; Okumura, T.; Tu, S.; Wang, S.S.; Shibata, W.; Vigneshwaran, R.; Gordon, S.A.; Shimada, Y.; Wang, T.C. Identification of Gastric Cancer Stem Cells Using the Cell Surface Marker CD44. *STEM CELLS* **2009**, *27*, 1006–1020. [CrossRef] [PubMed]
9. Zavros, Y. Initiation and Maintenance of Gastric Cancer: A Focus on CD44 Variant Isoforms and Cancer Stem Cells. *Cell. Mol. Gastroenterol. Hepatol.* **2017**, *4*, 55–63. [CrossRef]
10. Guagliardo, R.; Merckx, P.; Zamborlin, A.; De Backer, L.; Echaide, M.; Pérez-Gil, J.; De Smedt, S.C.; Raemdonck, K. Nanocarrier Lipid Composition Modulates the Impact of Pulmonary Surfactant Protein B (SP-B) on Cellular Delivery of siRNA. *Pharmaceutics* **2019**, *11*, 431. [CrossRef]
11. Wang, M.D.; Shin, D.M.; Simons, J.W.; Nie, S. Nanotechnology for targeted cancer therapy. *Expert Rev. Anticancer. Ther.* **2007**, *7*, 833–837. [CrossRef]
12. Santos-Rebelo, A.; Garcia, C.; Eleutério, C.; Bastos, A.; Coelho, S.C.; Coelho, M.A.N.; Molpeceres, J.; Viana, A.S.; Ascensão, L.; Pinto, J.F.; et al. Development of Parvifloron D-Loaded Smart Nanoparticles to Target Pancreatic Cancer. *Pharmaceutics* **2018**, *10*, 216. [CrossRef]
13. Covarrubias, G.; He, F.; Raghunathan, S.; Turan, O.; Peiris, P.M.; Schiemann, W.P.; Karathanasis, E. Effective treatment of cancer metastasis using a dual-ligand nanoparticle. *PLoS ONE* **2019**, *14*, e0220474. [CrossRef]
14. Abyaneh, H.S.; Soleimani, A.H.; Vakili, M.R.; Soudy, R.; Kaur, K.; Cuda, F.; Tavassoli, A.; Lavasanifar, A. Modulation of Hypoxia-Induced Chemoresistance to Polymeric Micellar Cisplatin: The Effect of Ligand Modification of Micellar Carrier Versus Inhibition of the Mediators of Drug Resistance. *Pharmaceutics* **2018**, *10*, 196. [CrossRef]
15. Manivasagan, P.; Bharathiraja, S.; Moorthy, M.S.; Oh, Y.-O.; Song, K.; Seo, H.; Oh, J. Anti-EGFR Antibody Conjugation of Fucoidan-Coated Gold Nanorods as Novel Photothermal Ablation Agents for Cancer Therapy. *ACS Appl. Mater. Interfaces* **2017**, *9*, 14633–14646. [CrossRef]
16. Yamasaki-Miyamoto, Y.; Yamasaki, M.; Tachibana, H.; Yamada, K. Fucoidan Induces Apoptosis through Activation of Caspase-8 on Human Breast Cancer MCF-7 Cells. *J. Agric. Food Chem.* **2009**, *57*, 8677–8682. [CrossRef] [PubMed]
17. Jafari, M.; Sriram, V.; Xu, Z.; Harris, G.M.; Lee, J.-Y. Fucoidan-Doxorubicin Nanoparticles Targeting P-Selectin for Effective Breast Cancer Therapy. *Carbohydr. Polym.* **2020**, *249*, 116837. [CrossRef] [PubMed]
18. Boeriu, C.G.; Springer, J.; Kooy, F.K.; Broek, L.A.M.V.D.; Eggink, G. Production Methods for Hyaluronan. *Int. J. Carbohydr. Chem.* **2013**, *2013*, 1–14. [CrossRef]

19. Mi, F.-L.; Wang, L.-F.; Chu, P.-Y.; Peng, S.-L.; Feng, C.-L.; Lai, Y.-J.; Li, J.-N.; Lin, Y.-H. Active Tumor-Targeted co-Delivery of Epigallocatechin Gallate and Doxorubicin in Nanoparticles for Combination Gastric Cancer Therapy. *ACS Biomater. Sci. Eng.* **2018**, *4*, 2847–2859. [CrossRef] [PubMed]
20. Yang, C.; Wu, T.; Qi, Y.; Zhang, Z. Recent Advances in the Application of Vitamin E TPGS for Drug Delivery. *Theranostics* **2018**, *8*, 464–485. [CrossRef] [PubMed]
21. Ghanem, A.A.; Emara, H.A.; Muawia, S.; El Maksoud, A.I.A.; Al-Karmalawy, A.A.; Elshal, M.F. Tanshinone IIA synergistically enhances the antitumor activity of doxorubicin by interfering with the PI3K/AKT/mTOR pathway and inhibition of topoisomerase II: In vitro and molecular docking studies. *New J. Chem.* **2020**, *44*, 17374–17381. [CrossRef]
22. Kulig, J.; Kolodziejczyk, P.; Sierzega, M.; Bobrzynski, L.; Jedrys, J.; Popiela, T.; Dadan, J.; Drews, M.; Jeziorski, A.; Krawczyk, M.; et al. Adjuvant Chemotherapy with Etoposide, Adriamycin and Cisplatin Compared with Surgery Alone in the Treatment of Gastric Cancer: A Phase III Randomized, Multicenter, Clinical Trial. *Oncology* **2010**, *78*, 54–61. [CrossRef]
23. Moertel, C.G.; Lavin, P.T. Phase II–III chemotherapy studies in advanced gastric cancer. Eastern Cooperative Oncology Group. *Cancer Treat. Rep.* **1979**, *63*, 1863–1869. [PubMed]
24. Wöhrer, S.S.; Raderer, M.; Hejna, M. Palliative chemotherapy for advanced gastric gancer. *Ann. Oncol.* **2004**, *15*, 1585–1595. [CrossRef] [PubMed]
25. Almatroodi, S.A.; Almatroudi, A.; Khan, A.A.; Alhumaydhi, F.A.; Alsahli, M.A.; Rahmani, A.H. Potential Therapeutic Targets of Epigallocatechin Gallate (EGCG), the Most Abundant Catechin in Green Tea, and its Role in the Therapy of Various Types of Cancer. *Molecules* **2020**, *25*, 3146. [CrossRef]
26. Liang, G.; Tang, A.; Lin, X.; Li, L.; Zhang, S.; Huang, Z.; Tang, H.; Li, Q.Q. Green tea catechins augment the antitumor activity of doxorubicin in an in vivo mouse model for chemoresistant liver cancer. *Int. J. Oncol.* **2010**, *37*, 111–123. [CrossRef]
27. Stearns, M.E.; Amatangelo, M.D.; Varma, D.; Sell, C.; Goodyear, S.M. Combination Therapy with Epigallocatechin-3-Gallate and Doxorubicin in Human Prostate Tumor Modeling Studies: Inhibition of Metastatic Tumor Growth in Severe Combined Immunodeficiency Mice. *Am. J. Pathol.* **2010**, *177*, 3169–3179. [CrossRef] [PubMed]
28. Omabe, K.; Paris, C.; Lannes, F.; Taïeb, D.; Rocchi, P. Nanovectorization of Prostate Cancer Treatment Strategies: A New Approach to Improved Outcomes. *Pharmaceutics* **2021**, *13*, 591. [CrossRef]
29. Liu, Y.; Fang, J.; Kim, Y.-J.; Wong, M.K.; Wang, P. Codelivery of Doxorubicin and Paclitaxel by Cross-Linked Multilamellar Liposome Enables Synergistic Antitumor Activity. *Mol. Pharm.* **2014**, *11*, 1651–1661. [CrossRef]
30. Bello, A.B.; Kim, D.; Kim, D.; Park, H.; Lee, S.-H. Engineering and Functionalization of Gelatin Biomaterials: From Cell Culture to Medical Applications. *Tissue Eng. Part B Rev.* **2020**, *26*, 164–180. [CrossRef]
31. Shutava, T.G.; Balkundi, S.S.; Vangala, P.; Steffan, J.J.; Bigelow, R.L.; Cardelli, J.A.; O'Neal, D.P.; Lvov, Y.M. Layer-by-Layer-Coated Gelatin Nanoparticles as a Vehicle for Delivery of Natural Polyphenols. *ACS Nano* **2009**, *3*, 1877–1885. [CrossRef]
32. Chen, M.-L.; Lai, C.-J.; Lin, Y.-N.; Huang, C.-M.; Lin, Y.-H. Multifunctional nanoparticles for targeting the tumor microenvironment to improve synergistic drug combinations and cancer treatment effects. *J. Mater. Chem. B* **2020**, *8*, 10416–10427. [CrossRef]
33. Chu, P.-Y.; Tsai, S.-C.; Ko, H.-Y.; Wu, C.-C.; Lin, Y.-H. Co-Delivery of Natural Compounds with a Dual-Targeted Nanoparticle Delivery System for Improving Synergistic Therapy in an Orthotopic Tumor Model. *ACS Appl. Mater. Interfaces* **2019**, *11*, 23880–23892. [CrossRef] [PubMed]
34. Xin, X.; Lin, F.; Wang, Q.; Yin, L.; Mahato, R.I. ROS-Responsive Polymeric Micelles for Triggered Simultaneous Delivery of PLK1 Inhibitor/miR-34a and Effective Synergistic Therapy in Pancreatic Cancer. *ACS Appl. Mater. Interfaces* **2019**, *11*, 14647–14659. [CrossRef] [PubMed]
35. Chou, T.-C. Drug Combination Studies and Their Synergy Quantification Using the Chou-Talalay Method. *Cancer Res.* **2010**, *70*, 440–446. [CrossRef] [PubMed]
36. Zhou, D.-H.; Wang, X.; Yang, M.; Shi, X.; Huang, W.; Feng, Q. Combination of Low Concentration of (−)-Epigallocatechin Gallate (EGCG) and Curcumin Strongly Suppresses the Growth of Non-Small Cell Lung Cancer in Vitro and in Vivo through Causing Cell Cycle Arrest. *Int. J. Mol. Sci.* **2013**, *14*, 12023–12036. [CrossRef] [PubMed]
37. Hanley, W.D.; Napier, S.L.; Burdick, M.; Schnaar, R.; Sackstein, R.; Konstantopoulos, K. Variant isoforms of CD44 are P- and L-selectin ligands on colon carcinoma cells. *FASEB J.* **2005**, *20*, 337–339. [CrossRef] [PubMed]
38. Hanurry, E.Y.; Mekonnen, T.W.; Andrgie, A.T.; Darge, H.F.; Birhan, Y.S.; Hou, W.-H.; Chou, H.-Y.; Cheng, C.-C.; Lai, J.-Y.; Tsai, H.-C. Biotin-Decorated PAMAM G4.5 Dendrimer Nanoparticles to Enhance the Delivery, Anti-Proliferative, and Apoptotic Effects of Chemotherapeutic Drug in Cancer Cells. *Pharmauceutics* **2020**, *12*, 443. [CrossRef] [PubMed]
39. Shamay, Y.; Elkabets, M.; Li, H.; Shah, J.; Brook, S.; Wang, F.; Adler, K.; Baut, E.; Scaltriti, M.; Jena, P.; et al. P-selectin is a nanotherapeutic delivery target in the tumor microenvironment. *Sci. Transl. Med.* **2016**, *8*, 345ra87. [CrossRef]
40. Läubli, H.; Borsig, L. Selectins promote tumor metastasis. *Semin. Cancer Biol.* **2010**, *20*, 169–177. [CrossRef] [PubMed]
41. Preobrazhenskaya, M.E.; Berman, A.E.; Mikhailov, V.I.; Ushakova, N.A.; Mazurov, A.V.; Semenov, A.V.; Usov, A.I.; Ni-fant'ev, N.E.; Bovin, N.V. Fucoidan inhibits leukocyte recruitment in a model peritoneal inflammation in rat and blocks interaction of P-selectin with its carbohydrate ligand. *Biochem. Mol. Biol. Int.* **1997**, *43*, 443–451. [CrossRef]
42. Mulligan, M.S.; Iizuka, M.; Miyasaka, M.; Suzuki, M.; Kawashima, H.; Hasegawa, A.; Kiso, M.; Warner, R.L.; Ward, P.A. Anti-inflammatory effects of sulfatides in selectin-dependent acute lung injury. *Int. Immunol.* **1995**, *7*, 1107–1113. [CrossRef] [PubMed]

43. Park, H.S.; Kim, G.-Y.; Nam, T.-J.; Kim, N.D.; Choi, Y.H. Antiproliferative Activity of Fucoidan Was Associated with the Induction of Apoptosis and Autophagy in AGS Human Gastric Cancer Cells. *J. Food Sci.* **2011**, *76*, T77–T83. [CrossRef]
44. Chen, C.; Zhang, Q.; Liu, S.; Parajuli, K.R.; Qu, Y.; Mei, J.; Chen, Z.; Zhang, H.; Khismatullin, D.B.; You, Z. IL-17 and insulin/IGF1 enhance adhesion of prostate cancer cells to vascular endothelial cells through CD44-VCAM-1 interaction. *Prostate* **2015**, *75*, 883–895. [CrossRef]
45. Bourguignon, L.Y.W. Matrix Hyaluronan-CD44 Interaction Activates MicroRNA and LncRNA Signaling Associated With Chemoresistance, Invasion, and Tumor Progression. *Front. Oncol.* **2019**, *9*, 492. [CrossRef] [PubMed]
46. Saghaeidehkordi, A.; Chen, S.; Yang, S.; Kaur, K. Evaluation of a Keratin 1 Targeting Peptide-Doxorubicin Conjugate in a Mouse Model of Triple-Negative Breast Cancer. *Pharmaceutics* **2021**, *13*, 661. [CrossRef] [PubMed]
47. Hao, G.; Xu, Z.P.; Li, L. Manipulating extracellular tumour pH: An effective target for cancer therapy. *RSC Adv.* **2018**, *8*, 22182–22192. [CrossRef]
48. E Gerweck, L.; Seetharaman, K. Cellular pH gradient in tumor versus normal tissue: Potential exploitation for the treatment of cancer. *Cancer Res.* **1996**, *56*, 1194–1198.
49. Abazari, R.; Ataei, F.; Morsali, A.; Slawin, A.M.Z.; Carpenter-Warren, C.L. A luminescent amine-functionalized metal-organic framework conjugated with folic acid as a targeted biocompatible pH-responsive nanocarrier for apoptosis induction in breast cancer cells. *ACS Appl. Mater. Interfaces* **2019**, *1*, 45442–45454. [CrossRef]

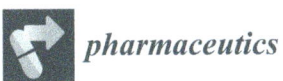 *pharmaceutics*

Article

AS1411 Aptamer Linked to DNA Nanostructures Diverts Its Traffic Inside Cancer Cells and Improves Its Therapeutic Efficacy

Giulia Vindigni [1,†], Sofia Raniolo [1,2,†], Federico Iacovelli [2], Valeria Unida [2], Carmine Stolfi [1], Alessandro Desideri [2] and Silvia Biocca [1,*]

[1] Department of Systems Medicine, University of Rome Tor Vergata, Via Montpellier 1, 00133 Rome, Italy; giulia.vindigni@uniroma2.it (G.V.); sofia.raniolo@uniroma2.it (S.R.); carmine.stolfi@uniroma2.it (C.S.)
[2] Department of Biology, University of Rome Tor Vergata, Via della Ricerca Scientifica 1, 00133 Rome, Italy; federico.iacovelli@uniroma2.it (F.I.); valeria.unida@gmail.com (V.U.); desideri@uniroma2.it (A.D.)
* Correspondence: biocca@med.uniroma2.it; Tel.: +39-06-72596418
† These authors contributed equally to this work.

Abstract: The nucleolin-binding G-quadruplex AS1411 aptamer has been widely used for cancer therapy and diagnosis and linked to nanoparticles for its selective targeting activity. We applied a computational and experimental integrated approach to study the effect of engineering AS1411 aptamer on an octahedral truncated DNA nanocage to obtain a nanostructure able to combine selective cancer-targeting and anti-tumor activity. The nanocages functionalized with one aptamer molecule (Apt-NC) displayed high stability in serum, were rapidly and selectively internalized in cancer cells through an AS1411-dependent mechanism, and showed over 200-fold increase in anti-cancer activity when compared with the free aptamer. Comparison of Apt-NCs and free AS1411 intracellular distribution showed that they traffic differently inside cells: Apt-NCs distributed through the endo-lysosomal pathway and were never found in the nuclei, while the free AS1411 was mostly found in the perinuclear region and in nucleoli. Molecular dynamics simulations indicated that the aptamer, when linked to the nanocage, sampled a limited conformational space, more confined than in the free state, which is characterized by a large number of metastable conformations. A different intracellular trafficking of Apt-NCs compared with free aptamer and the confined aptamer conformations induced by the nanocage were likely correlated with the high cytotoxic enhancement, suggesting a structure–function relationship for the AS1411 aptamer activity.

Keywords: G-quadruplex; nucleolin; DNA nanocages; intracellular localization; cancer targeting; molecular dynamics simulations

1. Introduction

Aptamers are short single-stranded DNA or RNA oligonucleotides with stable three-dimensional structures capable of binding with high affinity to a variety of molecular targets [1]. A unique class of aptamers is constituted of G-rich sequences that, under physiological conditions, spontaneously fold into non-canonical four-stranded structures named G-quadruplexes. These are characterized by the stacking of two or more successive planes of four guanine residues arranged in a square planar array via Hoogsteen hydrogen bonding (a G-quartet). G-quadruplex structures are highly polymorphic, and a single sequence can fold into several different conformations, depending on the relative orientations of strands and types of loops [2–4]. The 26-base G-rich AS1411 aptamer has been identified as an anti-cancer agent, which specifically recognizes nucleolin on the cancer cell surface with high selectivity and affinity [5,6]. As other G-quadruplex aptamers, AS1411 adopts a mixture of multiple structures in solution, and one of them has been solved through NMR spectroscopy, studying a DNA sequence named AT11, where a single guanine has been substituted by a thymine. This mutated version shows a preferential G-quadruplex conformation and exhibits an anti-proliferative activity comparable to that of AS1411 [4,7].

The AS1411 target molecule, nucleolin, is a multifunctional cyto-nucleoplasmic protein mostly localized in the nucleoli in normal cells and aberrantly overexpressed in many types of cancers, where it is also located on the cell surface [8]. In cancer cells, the surface nucleolin acts as a receptor of oncogenic ligands and shows protumorigenic function regulating the biosynthesis of specific oncomiRNAs [9]. Following its interaction with nucleolin, AS1411 inhibits cancer cells proliferation and induces cell death, with little effects on normal cells. AS1411 exhibits antiproliferative effects by upregulating p53, downregulating Bcl-2, and inhibiting cancer cell migration and invasion in an Akt1-dependent manner [10–12]. Due to its unique properties, AS1411 has been used for its anticancer therapeutic effect and, when linked to nanoparticles, as a selective tumor-targeting ligand [13,14]. Notably, AS1411 aptamer treatment was evaluated in phase II clinical trials in patients with acute myeloid leukemia and renal cell carcinoma [15], but it never reached phase III.

In the last years, we have been involved in the in silico, in vitro, and in cell characterization of a DNA-based truncated octahedral nanocage family [16–21]. These nanocages are made by 12 double helices, obtained by assembling 8 oligonucleotides whose ends are covalently linked in order to produce fully covalent structures, which ensure high stability in biological fluids and inside cells. We have characterized the receptor-mediated cell internalization of DNA nanostructures and their efficacy in selective doxorubicin delivery and miRNA silencing in cancer cells [22–24]. When functionalized with folate molecules and tailored with anti-miR21 complementary sequences, DNA nanocages induce selective miR21 sequestering and cytotoxicity to tumor cells overexpressing the α isoform of the folate receptor [25].

In this work, with the aim of increasing AS1411 stability and therapeutic efficacy, we designed octahedral DNA nanocages harboring one AS1411 molecule (Apt-NC) and studied its efficiency as targeting ligand and cytotoxic molecule against cancer cells. We studied the in vitro and intracellular stability, the time-dependent cell internalization, the targeting selectivity, and the therapeutic efficacy of the new assembled nanocages. Interestingly, the AS1411-functionalized nanocages displayed higher cytotoxic efficacy and different intracellular trafficking than the free AS1411 aptamer. Molecular dynamics simulations of two 3D models of free AS1411 in comparison with the aptamer-functionalized nanocage indicated that the free aptamer sampled a large number of metastable conformations, while the conformations were more localized and confined into a low-energy conformational basin when linked to the nanocage. These results indicate that the nanocage constrains the aptamer in a more defined conformation, likely correlated to the different intracellular localization and higher therapeutic effect.

2. Materials and Methods

2.1. Preparation of Aptamer-Functionalized DNA Nanocages

AS1411-functionalized nanocages (Apt-NC) and non-functionalized nanocages (NC) were prepared as described [21]. A biotin molecule was added on one edge of the structure for the detection of nanostructures through the streptavidin–biotin reaction. Briefly, nanocages were assembled by mixing equimolar amounts of 8 oligonucleotides in TAM buffer (40 mM Tris–acetic acid, pH 7.0, 12.6 mM magnesium acetate). The sequences of the oligonucleotides used for the assembly of NCs and the sequence of free AS1411 aptamer are reported in Supplementary Table S1. After assembly, nanocages were incubated for 2 h at 25 °C with T4 DNA ligase (New England Biolabs Inc., Ipswich, MA, USA) to covalently link the obtained structures and run on native 5% polyacrylamide gels in TAEM buffer (40 mM Tris–acetic acid, pH 7.0, 1 mM EDTA, 12.6 mM magnesium acetate). The band corresponding to the correctly assembled nanocages was cut out of the gel, eluted, and concentrated by 2-propanol precipitation.

2.2. Cell Cultures

HeLa cells, derived from human cervix cancer, and CHO, Chinese hamster ovary, cells were grown in DMEM (Dulbecco's modified Eagle medium, Euroclone, Devon, UK) and DMEM/F-12 (Dulbecco's modified Eagle medium/Nutrient Mixture F-12, Euroclone, Devon, UK), respectively, supplemented with 10% FBS (Gibco, Paisleg, UK), 1 mM L-glutamine (Sigma Aldrich, St Louis, MO, USA), 1mM sodium pyruvate (Biowest, Miami, FL, USA), and 100 U/ml penicillin–streptomycin (Euroclone, Devon, UK).

2.3. DNA Nanocages Stability

Biotinylated cages were incubated in TBS (Tris-HCl 50 mM, NaCl 150 mM, pH 7.8) or in culture medium supplemented with 10% FBS at 37 °C for different times. Each sample was then digested with proteinase K (100 µg/mL) for 1 h at 37 °C, and analyzed by DNA blot, as previously described [21]. Biotin detection was carried out using streptavidin–HRP (horseradish peroxidase) (Abcam Inc., Toronto, ON, Canada), and visualized by enhanced chemiluminescence (ECL Extend, Euroclone, Devon, UK). For image processing and densitometric analysis, photographic films were digitized by scanning and bands analyzed by ImageJ software.

2.4. Purification of DNA Nanocages and DNA Blot

Cells were plated in 48-well plates one day before treatments. After incubation with DNA nanocages for different time periods, cells were lysed, centrifuged, digested with proteinase K, and DNA blot was performed as previously described [21].

2.5. Confocal Analysis

Cells were seeded onto poly-L-lysine-coated glass cover-slides. For binding experiments, cells were incubated with biotinylated nanocages in DMEM 10% FBS for 1 h at 4 °C, washed in PBS, fixed in 4% paraformaldehyde, and incubated for 5 min with NaBH$_4$. For uptake experiments, cells were incubated with nanocages at 37 °C for different time periods, fixed with 4% paraformaldehyde, and permeabilized for 4 min with Tris/Triton (Tris HCl 0.1 M, Triton 0.1%, pH 7.7). Rabbit polyclonal anti-flotillin-1 antibody (Santa Cruz Biotechnology Inc., Dallas, TX, USA) was used to detect the flotillin-1 protein. Early endosomes were visualized with polyclonal EEA1 antibody (Abcam Inc., Toronto, ON, Canada) and lysosomes with mouse monoclonal anti-LAMP-1 antibody (Abcam Inc., Toronto, ON, Canada). Donkey anti-rabbit IgG and donkey anti-mouse IgG, both Rhodamine Red-X-conjugated AffiniPure (Jackson ImmunoResearch, Cambridgeshire, UK) were used as secondary antibodies [24]. Biotinylated cages were detected by using streptavidin–FITC (Jackson ImmunoResearch, Cambridgeshire, UK). The nuclei were stained with DAPI (Invitrogen, Carlsbad, CA, USA). Images were obtained with a laser confocal fluorescent microscope Olympus FV1000 at 60× magnification, and the fluorescence signal was evaluated with the IMARIS software. Co-localization events were evaluated as previously described [24].

2.6. Cell Viability Assay

HeLa and CHO cells were plated in 96-well plates at a density of 5×10^3 cells/well and 7×10^3 cells/well, respectively, grown for 24 h, and treated with different concentrations of Apt-NCs, NCs, or free AS1411 aptamer for 24 h at 37 °C. The MTS assay (3-(4,5-dimethylthiazol-2-yl)-5-(3-carboxymethoxyphenyl)-2-(4-sulfophenyl)-2H-tetrazolium) (Promega, WI, USA) was used for evaluating cell proliferation. Multiskan Ascent 96/384 plate reader (MTX Lab Systems, Bradenton, FL, USA) was used for measuring the absorbance at 492 nm. Cell viability was normalized to control condition (untreated cells).

2.7. Statistical Analysis

All experiments were carried out in triplicate and data analyzed using GraphPad Prism. Results were expressed as a mean ± S.E.M and statistical analyses performed using

Student's *t*-test. Differences were considered statistically significant when $p < 0.05$ (*), $p < 0.01$ (**) and $p < 0.001$ (***).

2.8. Computational Methods

Two models of the AS1411 G-quadruplex were generated. The first one (Supplementary Figure S1, AS1411) was generated starting from the PDB structure with ID:2N3M corresponding to the AT11 variant of the aptamer [4] using the fiber module of the 3DNA program [26] to generate the PDB file. The nucleotide sequence of the strand composing the G-quadruplex was modified through the 3DNA mutate_bases module [26] to fully match the AS1411 oligonucleotide sequence. The PyMol sculpting module [27] was used to generate an additional conformation, imposing guanines 11 as part of the first G-quartet of the aptamer (Supplementary Figure S1, AS1411*). The structures were minimized using the UCSF Chimera program [28] to remove any clashes and unwanted interactions introduced by the modeling procedure. The octahedral scaffold of the DNA nanocages was built through our Polygen software [16] designing eight oligonucleotide sequences (Supplementary Table S1) based on those previously used to experimentally assemble different truncated octahedral geometries [22,29]. The AS1411-NC and AS1411*-NC structures were modeled using the SYBYL 6.0 program (TRIPOS, http://www.tripos.com, accessed on 30 June 2021), manually adding one copy of the AS1411 aptamer to the octahedral scaffold, using a 7-thymidine spacer to keep the structure accessible for nucleolin targeting. The system topologies and the coordinates of AS1411, AS1411*, AS1411-NC, and AS1411*-NC models, used as input for the AMBER 16 MD package [30], were generated through the AmberTools tLeap module, parametrizing the structures through the AMBER ff19SB force field with the parmbsc1 corrections [31]. The structures were immersed in a rectangular box filled with TIP3P water molecules, imposing a minimum distance between the solute and the box of 14 Å, neutralizing the charges adding Mg^{2+} counterions to the solvated systems in favorable positions, as implemented in the tLeap program, together with 4 K^+ ions for G-quadruplex stabilization [32]. All systems were minimized using 2500 steps of the steepest descent algorithm to remove unfavorable interactions and prevent Mg^{2+} ions from binding to DNA, applying harmonic restraints of 50 kcal·mol^{-1}·Å^{-2}. The systems were then equilibrated to 300 K in the NVT ensemble for 500 ps using the Langevin thermostat, with a coupling coefficient of 1.0 ps and including cartesian restraint of 15 kcal·mol^{-1}·Å^{-2} on nucleotide atoms. After the equilibration phase, the systems were subjected to an equilibrium simulation of 500 ps removing all constraints and to relax all atoms. The systems were then simulated using the NPT ensemble for a period of 10 ns, applying periodic boundary conditions, a 2.0 fs time-step, and the PME method [33] for the long-range electrostatic interactions with a cutoff of 9.0 Å for the evaluation of short-range nonbonded interactions. The SHAKE algorithm [34] was used to constrain covalent bonds involving hydrogen atoms. The temperature was fixed at 303 K using the Langevin dynamics [35], while pressure was kept constant at 1 atm through the Langevin piston method [36]. Atomic positions were saved every 1000 steps (2.0 ps) for the analyses.

2.9. Gaussian Accelerated Molecular Dynamics Simulations

For each system, 100 ns dual-boost Gaussian accelerated molecular dynamics (GaMD) simulations [37] were performed, saving the atomic positions every 1000 steps. GaMD is an enhanced sampling method in which a harmonic boost potential is applied to smooth the potential energy surfaces and reduce the systems energy barriers [37]. Using this approach, it is possible to sample a large conformational space, which cannot be normally accessed by classical MD simulations. Moreover, by constructing a boost potential following Gaussian distribution, using cumulant expansion to the second order, GaMD simulations can be correctly reweighted to recover the original biomolecular free energy profiles [37]. GaMD simulations were entirely performed using an NVIDIA TITAN XP GPU using the default parameters suggested for the method (http://miao.compbio.ku.edu/GaMD/, last accessed 30 June 2021).

2.10. Trajectory Analysis

The GROMACS 2020.3 analysis tools [38] were used to compute the root mean square fluctuations (RMSFs) and principal component analysis (PCA) over the entire 100 ns trajectories. A clustering analysis was performed on all the saved configurations through the gmx cluster module of GROMACS using the GROMOS algorithm [39], forcing a cut-off of 0.12 nm for the geometrical clustering procedure. In order to recover the original free-energy profiles of the simulated structures, the GaMD trajectories were reweighted using PyReweighting, a toolkit of Python scripts designed to facilitate the GaMD simulation analyses [37]. The UCSF Chimera program [28] was used to generate the pictures of the representative structures.

3. Results

3.1. Design, Assembly, and In Vitro Stability of AS1411 Functionalized DNA Nanocages

AS1411 has been shown to adopt multiple conformations characterized by very similar hydrodynamic and electrophoretic properties [7]. A single G-quadruplex conformation, named AT11, can be obtained by mutating a guanine in thymine in the position 10 [4]. The AT11 structure was obtained by NMR spectroscopy, and we started from this PDB structure to build the AS1411 atomic 3D model, introducing the original AS1411 sequence through the 3DNA mutate_bases module (Supplementary Figure S1) [26]. A second 3D model of the aptamer, called AS1411*, was generated replacing guanine 10 with guanine 11 in the formation of the first G-quartet of the aptamer (Supplementary Figure S1). A 3D model with one AS1411 or AS1411* aptamer (Apt) attached to a DNA nanocage (NC) was built to form the Apt-NC structure (Figure 1A). The octahedral nanocage was obtained from 8 oligonucleotide sequences (OL1–OL8, Supplementary Table S1) to form a scaffold made up of 12 double stranded B-DNA helices forming the edges of a covalently closed octa-hedron, connected by short single-stranded five-thymidine linkers, corresponding to the square truncated faces [21,23,25]. AS1411 aptamer was connected to the nanocage scaffold through a seven-nucleotide linker made by thymidine, using a modified oligonucleotide (OL8$_{Apt}$) (Supplementary Table S1).

The assembly of AS1411-octahedral nanocages was performed as described [21], using the oligonucleotides reported in Supplementary Table S1. In electrophoresis, the assembled nanocages ran in the gel as a single well-defined product with a molecular weight of about 530 bp (Supplementary Figure S2). As depicted in Figure 1A, Apt-NCs were functionalized with a biotin molecule on one edge of the structure. The presence of biotin enabled detection of the assembled nanocages after transfer from the gel to a membrane, through the streptavidin (HRP)–biotin reaction in the DNA blot, a system with a sensitivity up to 100 times higher than the ethidium bromide staining, as we calculated in a comparative test.

Figure 1B shows the stability of biotinylated Apt-NCs incubated at 37 °C in DMEM cell culture medium supplemented with 10% FBS for different time points. After incubation, each sample was treated with proteinase K (100 µg/mL), run in 5% polyacrylamide gel, and analyzed in DNA blot using streptavidin–HRP [21]. Apt-NCs were stable and fully intact for at least 5 h of incubation with serum, then they started to be slowly degraded as a function of time and were still detectable after 48 h (Figure 1B, top panel). In detail, the half-life of Apt-NCs in DMEM–10% FBS was 25 h, calculated by the relative intensity of each band visualized through DNA blot (Figure 1B, bottom panel). Since K$^+$ ions act as stabilizing agents for G-quadruplex structures [40], we tested the in vitro stability of Apt-NCs in serum in the absence or in the presence of 5 mM KCl. DNA blot analysis showed that the presence of only K$^+$ ions increased the resistance of Apt-NCs to serum nucleases, extending their half-life from 16 to 22 h (Supplementary Figure S3). Notably, the presence of both monovalent and bivalent cations in DMEM culture medium guaranteed excellent stability to Apt-NCs (Figure 1B).

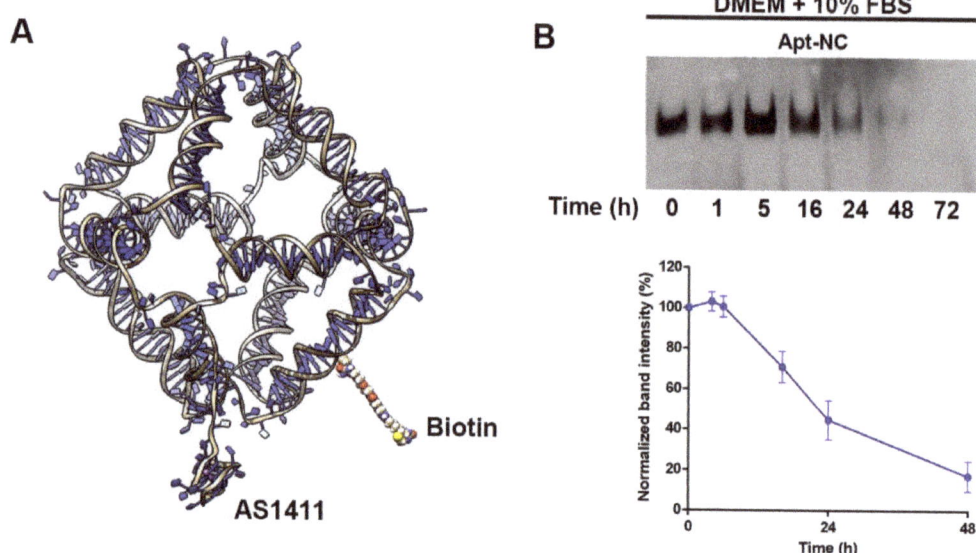

Figure 1. (**A**) Schematic representation of the Apt-NC nanostructure model. (**B**) DNA blot analysis of Apt-NCs incubated in DMEM supplemented with 10% FBS at 37 °C for different times, as indicated. Apt-NCs before incubation with serum proteins are indicated as time 0. Biotinylated Apt-NCs were detected with streptavidin–HRP. The graph shows the densitometric analysis of three different experiments, performed using the ImageJ software. The relative intensity of each band was normalized to the intensity of the band corresponding to time 0 and reported in the graph. Values are expressed as an average ± SEM.

3.2. Intracellular Stability and Targeting Efficiency

The targeting efficiency and intracellular stability of AS1411-modified NCs were studied by DNA blot in HeLa cells, a human cervical cancer cell line with high surface nucleolin expression [41]. Figure 2 shows HeLa cells incubated with 30 nM biotinylated Apt-NCs or non-functionalized NCs (NC) for 1 and 24 h at 37 °C. After incubation, nanostructures were purified from cell lysates and analyzed by DNA blot, using streptavidin–HRP [21]. Lanes 1, 4, 7, and 10 show the band corresponding to DNA nanocages before incubation with cells (time 0). After purification from cell extracts, Apt-NCs ran as one band in the gel, with a mobility comparable to the input (time 0), confirming that we were visualizing only Apt-NCs that were intact inside cells. Interestingly, a similar band intensity was detected at 1 and 24 h of incubation (compare lanes 2–3), suggesting that Apt-NCs were rapidly internalized inside cells, but they did not accumulate in a time-dependent manner. Notably, NCs without aptamer functionalization were almost non-detectable (lanes 5–6), demonstrating that efficient cell uptake occurred only through a nucleolin-mediated AS1411-dependent mechanism. As a control, non-cancer CHO cells, which express very low amount of membrane nucleolin [42], did not show any significant entry of nanocages after 1 and 24 h of incubation with either biotinylated Apt-NCs (lanes 8–9) or non-functionalized NCs (lanes 11–12).

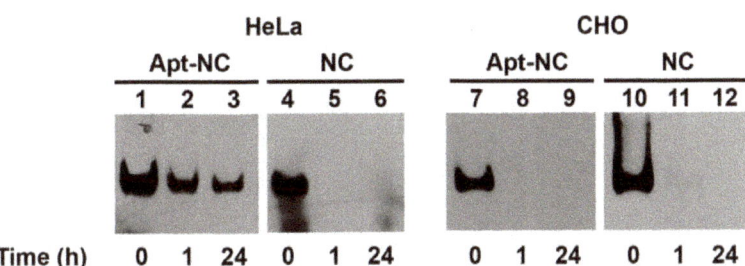

Figure 2. DNA blot of Apt-NC (lanes 2–3 and 8–9) and non-functionalized NC (lanes 5–6 and 11–12) purified from HeLa and CHO cell extracts after 1 and 24 h incubation. In lanes 1, 4, 7, and 10, 30 ng of nanocages before incubation with cells (time 0) are shown. Biotinylated nanostructures were detected with the streptavidin (HRP)–biotin reaction.

3.3. Intracellular Trafficking of Apt-NCs

The membrane binding and cellular internalization of AS1411-functionalized NCs were studied by confocal microscopy in HeLa cells. To distinguish between membrane-bound and internalized nanostructures, cells were incubated at 4 °C or at 37 °C, respectively. At 4 °C, nanostructures can only enter the cell through direct translocation, because endocytosis, an energy-dependent process, is inhibited at this temperature. Moreover, for visualizing the membrane-bound nanostructures, cells were only fixed, whilst for studying the internalized NCs, cells were incubated for different time periods, then fixed and permeabilized. Representative confocal images of biotinylated-Apt-NC binding at 4 °C and uptake at 37 °C are shown in Figure 3A. Apt-NCs efficiently bound to HeLa cells and appeared as many small green fluorescent dots on the plasma membrane (Figure 3A, panel a). At 37 °C, after 30 minutes, most of the green fluorescent dots were already visible inside cells (Figure 3A, panel b) and remain visible after 4 h of incubation (Figure 3A, panel c), showing a vesicular distribution. In line with DNA blot experiments shown in Figure 2, very low fluorescent signal is observed in HeLa cells treated with NCs (Figure 3A, panel d), confirming that nanocages are entering in cells through a AS1411-dependent mechanism.

The nucleolin-dependent internalization mechanism was clarified by performing a double fluorescence staining of Apt-NCs and Flotillin-1, a lipid raft marker protein which associates with nucleolin in membrane lipid rafts [43]. As shown in Figure 3B (panels a–e), after 30 min of incubation, the green punctate staining of Apt-NCs (panel b) significantly overlapped with the red fluorescence of flotillin-1 (panel c), as confirmed by merged images of green and red fluorescence in panel d. The correlation of the intensity values of the green and red pixels is reported in the scatter plot (panel e) used to calculate the Pearson's coefficient (PCC) [44]. The PCC was 0.47 ± 0.03, confirming that Apt-NCs were internalized through a nucleolin-mediated mechanism involving flotillin endocytosis.

The intracellular distribution was further studied by colocalization analysis of Apt-NCs with the early endosomal antigen (EEA1) after 1 h incubation or the lysosomal-associated membrane protein 1 (LAMP-1) [24] after 4 h incubation. Figure 3B shows representative images of double immunofluorescence of Apt-NCs, shown as green dots inside cells (panels g and l), and EEA1 and LAMP-1 (panels h and m) as red dots. The intracellular distribution was only partially overlapping, as visualized in merged images (panels i and n) and the corresponding scatter plots (panels j and o). The correlation of the intensity values of the green and red pixels evaluated by the Pearson's coefficient (PCC) [44], analyzing the scatter plot, is shown in panels e and j. In detail, the PCC was 0.20 ± 0.02 with the EEA1 marker after 30 min of internalization and 0.27 ± 0.01 with the LAMP-1 marker after 4 h, indicating that Apt-NCs partially trafficked through the endo-lysosomal pathway.

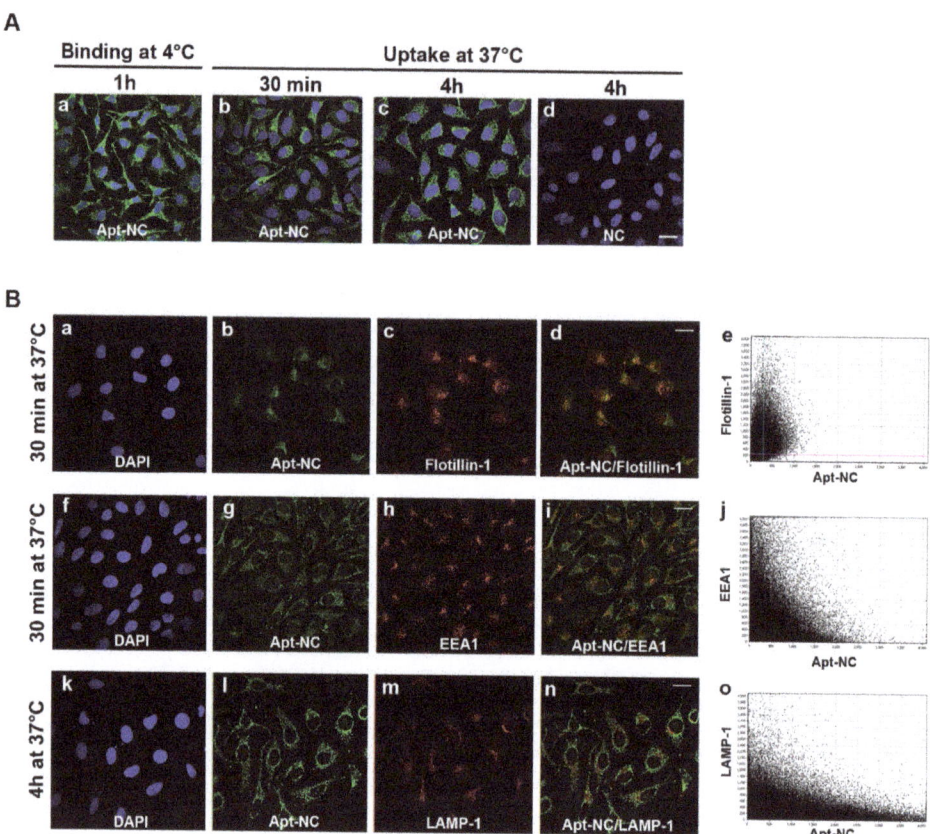

Figure 3. (**A**) Confocal analysis of membrane-binding and intracellular distribution of Apt-NCs. HeLa cells were incubated with 60 nM of biotinylated Apt-NCs (panels **a–c**) or non-functionalized NCs (panel **d**) for 1 h at 4 °C (panel **a**) or for 30 min and 4 h at 37 °C (panels **b–d**), as indicated. (**B**) Co-localization analysis of Apt-NCs (panels **b,g,l**) with flotillin-1 (panel **c**), endosomal marker EEA1 (panel **h**), and lysosomal marker LAMP-1 (panel **m**). The (**b,c**) images are merged in (panel **d,g,h**) images are merged in (panel **i**), and the (**l**) and m images are merged in (panel **n**). Cell nuclei are visualized in (panels **a,f,k**). The correlation of the intensity values of the green and red pixels was performed using the IMARIS software and scatter plots are reported in (panels **e,j,o**). Biotinylated NCs were visualized using streptavidin–FITC and nuclei were stained with DAPI. Scale bar: 20 µm.

Guided by these observations, we compared the intracellular distribution of free AS1411 and Apt-NC in HeLa cells and verified whether the presence of a large excess of free AS1411 was able to impair the uptake and the intracellular distribution of Apt-NCs. HeLa cells were incubated with Apt-NCs (Figure 4, panels a and b) or AS1411-Cy5 (Figure 4, panels c and d) for 1 h at 37 °C and analyzed by confocal microscopy. Apt-NCs appeared as green fluorescent punctate staining in the cytoplasm (Figure 4, panel b), whilst free AS1411-Cy5 appeared as red dots mostly localized in nucleoli and in the perinuclear region (Figure 4, panel d). It was evident that Apt-NCs and free AS1411 aptamer trafficked inside cells differently and that the AS1411-functionalized nanocages were never found in the nuclei.

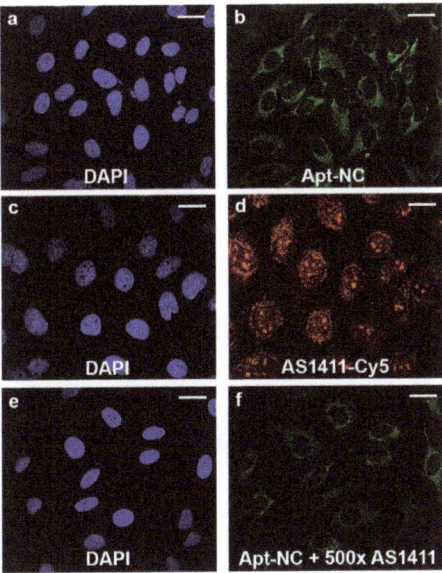

Figure 4. Comparison of intracellular distribution of Apt-NCs and Cy5-AS1411. Cells were incubated with 60 nM biotinylated Apt-NCs (panels **a**,**b**) or 3 µM free Cy5-AS1411 (panels **c**,**d**) for 1 h at 37 °C. (panels **e**,**f**) show cells incubated with Apt-NCs in the presence of 500 molar excess of free AS1411. Biotinylated Apt-NCs were visualized using streptavidin–FITC, and nuclei were stained with DAPI. Scale bar: 20 µm.

Interestingly, incubation of Apt-NCs in the presence of 500 times molar excess of free AS1411 (Figure 4, panel f) did not lead to significant reduction of the green signal (compare panels b and f), as also confirmed by green fluorescence intensity profiles of the confocal images (Supplementary Figure S4), indicating that cell uptake of Apt-NCs was not impaired by the presence of a large excess of free aptamer and demonstrating that the receptor-mediated uptake of AS1411-linked to the nanocages in HeLa cells had a higher efficiency compared with the free aptamer. All together, these results suggest that AS1411-NC functionalization may facilitate AS1411-nucleolin or other membrane proteins interactions, activating a different entry pathway.

3.4. Cytotoxic Effect of Apt-NCs

The cytotoxic activity of Apt-NCs was tested in comparison with non-functionalized NCs and free AS1411 in cancer HeLa and non-cancer CHO cells. Cells were treated for 24 h with NCs at concentrations ranging from 3.75 nM to 60 nM and with free AS1411 at concentrations ranging from 3.75 nM to 30 µM (Figure 5). Figure 5A shows that incubation of HeLa cells with free AS1411 aptamer was not cytotoxic up to micromolar concentrations. On the other hand, we observed a dose-dependent reduction of cell viability of HeLa cells when treated with Apt-NCs already in the nanomolar range, indicating more than 200-fold increase in cytotoxicity, in comparison with the free aptamer (Figure 5A). No significant reduction in cell viability was observed when treating HeLa cells with NCs not functionalized with the aptamer. As a control, we analyzed the cytotoxic effect of Apt-NCs and free AS1411 on the non-cancer cell line CHO (Figure 5B). No reduction in cell proliferation was observed in CHO cells at all tested concentrations, demonstrating that AS1411 linked to DNA nanocages is not toxic in non-cancer cells. In agreement with this result, free AS1411 induced low cytotoxicity in CHO as in other non-cancer cells [42]. Flow cytofluorimetry was performed for detecting apoptotic cells by a double staining with annexin V–FITC/propidium iodide (PI) (Supplementary Figure S5). In detail, after 24 h treatment with Apt-NCs the percentage of apoptotic cells reached 33.2 ± 1.2% at 45 nM, while in cells treated with pristine NCs at the same concentration, the percentage was 9.8 ± 1.9%, similar to that observed in untreated control cells (9.9 ± 0.3%). The analysis confirmed the MTS results, showing that Apt-NCs induced a significant dose-dependent apoptosis in HeLa cells while no effect was observed in non-cancer CHO cells.

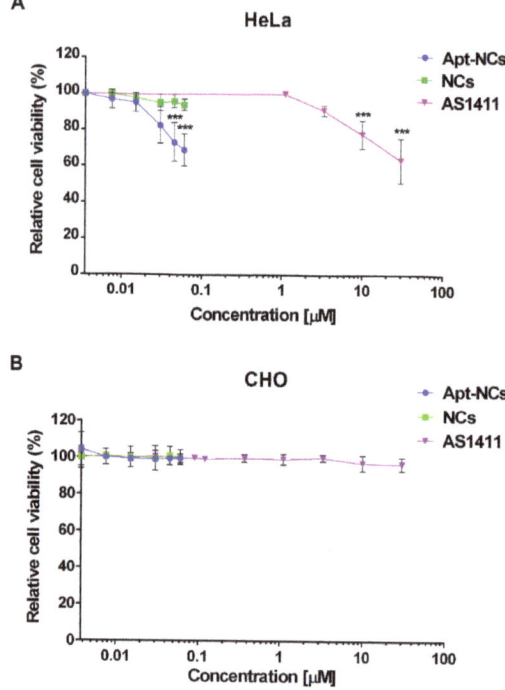

Figure 5. Cytotoxic effect of Apt-NCs in HeLa (**A**) and CHO cells (**B**). Cell proliferation after 24 h treatment with Apt-NCs, non-functionalized NCs, and free AS1411 at different concentrations was assessed by MTS. The values are the means of six replicates normalized to untreated cells. Statistical significance: (***) $p < 0.001$ (Student's t-test) compared with NCs treated cells in the case of Apt-NCs and untreated cells in the case of AS1411.

3.5. GaMD Simulations

G-quadruplex-forming sequences are remarkably polymorphic. A single sequence may reach a different 3D structure depending on the physicochemical conditions, such as different folding conditions or presence of a different counterion bound in its core. The high-resolution 3D structure of AS1411 has never been reported due to the high complexity resulting from the simultaneous presence of several conformers that has been demonstrated through multiple spectroscopic techniques [7]. We performed four 100 ns long GaMD simulations, two for each model generated for the free aptamers (AS1411 and AS1411*) and two for the models of the aptamers linked to the octahedral nanocage (AS1411-NC and AS1411*-NC), in the presence of potassium ions. Figure 6 shows that the RMSF values, describing the time-averaged deviation of C2' atom positions of the nucleotides, were higher for the free AS1411 (black line) than for the NC-linked aptamer (AS1411-NC) (red line), suggesting a lower conformational space sampling for the latter structure. A similar result was obtained comparing the RMSF of the free AS1411* and of the AS1411*-NC models (Supplementary Figure S6). A PCA analysis of the motions, coupling the projection of the first two main motions to the reweighting of the GaMD simulations, was carried out to recover the original free energy profile of the molecules (Figure 7 and Supplementary Figure S6). In this representation, the conformational space sampled by the structure is directly proportional to the number of points plotted on the graph, while the color indicates the energy of the sampled conformations, whose values increase from blue to red. The free AS1411 and AS1411* structures (Figure 7A and Supplementary Figure S7A) sampled several metastable conformations, characterized by small energy differences of about 1–2 kcal/mol. On the other hand, in the AS1411-NC and AS1411*-NC structures, the aptamer sampled a more localized conformational space, confined into low-energy basins (Figure 7B and Supplementary Figure S7B). Indeed, by clustering the different frames obtained from the four trajectories, we found two main representative clusters for the AS1411-NC and AS1411*-NC (Supplementary Figure S8, green and yellow bars), while the two free aptamer structures were characterized by more than 40 low-populated different clusters (Supplementary Figure S8, red and blue bars), confirming a much lower conformational variability for the aptamer linked to the nanocage scaffold.

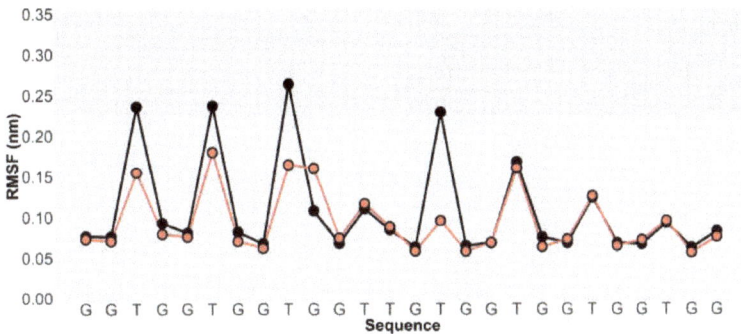

Figure 6. RMSF values calculated for the C2′ atoms of the AS1411 aptamer. Black and red filled circles indicate the values calculated for the free and cage-linked aptamers, respectively.

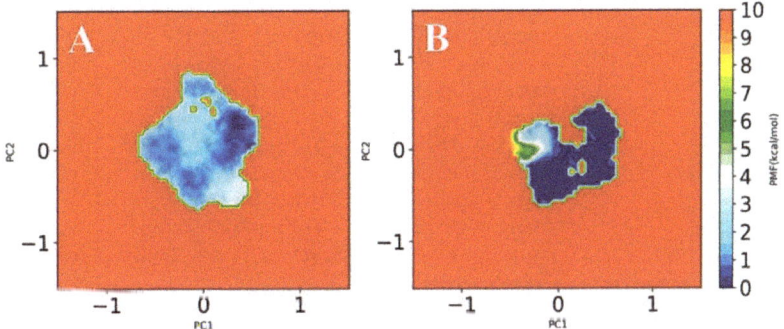

Figure 7. Free energy principal component projection of the free (**A**) and cage-linked (**B**) AS1411 aptamers.

4. Discussion

Here we report a marked enhancement of the G-quadruplex AS1411 therapeutic efficiency due to its functionalization over octahedral DNA nanocages. Aptamer-linked nanocages (i) are stable both in serum and inside cells, similarly to other previously characterized covalently linked DNA nanostructures [21,22,29], (ii) are selectively and efficiently internalized by cancer cells, and (iii) increase the cytotoxic efficacy by more than two orders of magnitude compared with a free aptamer. At least two main explanations can be conceived for the enhanced AS1411 cytotoxicity observed in cancer cells when linked to DNA nanostructures: (i) a more defined conformation adopted by the cage-linked AS1411 and (ii) a different intracellular entry pathway in cancer cells followed by the cage-linked AS1411 compared with free aptamer.

Analysis of the conformational variability of two 3D models of the free aptamers (AS1411 and AS1411*) and of the aptamers linked to the octahedral nanocage (AS1411-NC and AS1411*-NC) through GaMD simulations showed that the free AS1411 or AS1411* aptamers generated more than 40 conformational clusters, indicating that the free aptamer samples many metastable conformations, characterized by small energy differences. On the other hand, MD simulations of Apt-NC pointed out that the nanocage scaffold constrains the aptamer to adopt a more defined conformation, independently of the starting structure, mainly described by two representative clusters (Supplementary Figure S6). Consequently, the structure of the free aptamer appears to be more floating, as confirmed by the RMSF analyses. These results are likely correlated to the higher efficiency of the cage linked AS1411 in targeting nucleolin and/or other membrane proteins in cancer cells and in improving cell toxicity compared with the free aptamer. Indeed, this may represent an example of structure–function relationship, since the enhanced AS1411 cytotoxicity appears correlated to a confinement of the aptamer in a more defined conformation than that of the free aptamer.

AS1411 has been linked to various types of nanoparticles due to its selective binding to nucleolin, a protein overexpressed on the cell surface and inside cancer cells [45–49]. Notably, a marked improvement of cytotoxicity has been previously obtained by increasing the loading (more than 100 molecules) of AS1411 on the surface of gold nanostars [50]. However, the here described inhibition of cancer cell proliferation by AS1411 linked to NCs (up to two orders of magnitude greater than that by the free aptamer) is the most powerful reported so far.

We demonstrated that the aptamer AS1411 confers a selective targeting activity to Apt-NCs, when compared with pristine nanocages, showing a clear targeting preference for the nucleolin-positive HeLa cancer cells compared with the nucleolin-negative control cells. Apt-NCs are efficiently taken up by cancer cells using a flotillin-dependent endocytosis mechanism, traffic through the endo-lysosomal pathway, and never reach the nuclei, whilst AS1411 traffics both to the cytoplasm and to the nuclei, accumulating in nucleoli. By competition experiments, we also demonstrated that aptamer-linked nanocages display a higher internalization efficiency than free AS1411. The different intracellular traffic and localization may be responsible for the higher cytotoxicity, changing the mechanism of action of AS1411, although further studies are required to definitely confirm it and to identify the pathway.

The proposed AS1411-functionalized DNA nanocages are very stable and, beyond the marked increase of cytotoxicity to cancer cells, present the advantage of being a potential multifunctional scaffold. In fact, the octahedral DNA nanocages can be tailored with sequestering units for selective oncomiR inhibition [25] and/or loaded with DNA intercalating drugs, such as doxorubicin [23,25], and used as multipurpose delivery vehicles.

Supplementary Materials: The following are available online at https://www.mdpi.com/article/10.3390/pharmaceutics13101671/s1, Table S1: Sequences of the oligos for the assembly of octahedral DNA nanocages, Figure S1: Schematic representation of G-quadruplex folding topology of AS1411 and AS1411* in K$^+$ solution, Figure S2: Gel electrophoresis analysis of pristine (NCs) and AS1411-functionalized nanocages (Apt-NCs), Figure S3: Stability of Apt-NCs in the absence or presence of K$^+$ ions, Figure S4: Intensity profiles of streptavidin–FITC signal, Figure S5: Annexin V-FITC/propidium iodide assay in HeLa and CHO cells, Figure S6: RMSF values calculated for the C2′ atoms of the AS1411* structures, Figure S7: Free energy principal component projection of the isolated (A) and cage-linked (B) AS1411* aptamers, Figure S8: Bar chart representing the distribution of the clustered AS1411, AS1411-NC, AS1411*, and AS1411*-NC conformations.

Author Contributions: G.V., S.R. and V.U. designed and performed experiments, analyzed data, and helped writing the manuscript; F.I. and C.S. designed experiments and analyzed data, A.D. designed experiments and helped writing the manuscript, and S.B. designed experiments, analyzed and interpreted data, and wrote the manuscript. All authors have read and agreed to the published version of the manuscript.

Funding: This work was supported by PRIN 2017 "Progetto di Rilevante Interesse Nazionale (PRIN) grant (to S.B.) and Associazione Italiana per la Ricerca sul Cancro FIRC-AIRC fellowship for Italy (to S.R. and F.I.).

Institutional Review Board Statement: Not applicable.

Informed Consent Statement: Not applicable.

Data Availability Statement: Not applicable.

Acknowledgments: We thank E. Romano from the Centre of Advanced Microscopy "Patrizia Albertano" for the skillful assistance in confocal analysis.

Conflicts of Interest: The authors declare no conflict of interest.

References

1. Keefe, A.D.; Pai, S.; Ellington, A. Aptamers as therapeutics. *Nat. Rev. Drug Discov.* **2010**, *9*, 537–550. [CrossRef]
2. Burge, S.; Parkinson, G.N.; Hazel, P.; Todd, A.K.; Neidle, S. Quadruplex DNA: Sequence, topology and structure. *Nucleic Acids Res.* **2006**, *34*, 5402–5415. [CrossRef]
3. Patel, D.J.; Phan, A.T.; Kuryavyi, V. Human telomere, oncogenic promoter and 5′-UTR G-quadruplexes: Diverse higher order DNA and RNA targets for cancer therapeutics. *Nucleic Acids Res.* **2007**, *35*, 7429–7455. [CrossRef]
4. Do, N.Q.; Chung, W.J.; Truong, T.H.A.; Heddi, B.; Phan, A.T. G-quadruplex structure of an anti-proliferative DNA sequence. *Nucleic Acids Res.* **2017**, *45*, 7487–7493. [CrossRef]
5. Bates, P.J.; Laber, D.; Miller, D.M.; Thomas, S.D.; Trent, J.O. Discovery and development of the G-rich oligonucleotide AS1411 as a novel treatment for cancer. *Exp. Mol. Pathol.* **2009**, *86*, 151–164. [CrossRef]
6. Bates, P.J.; Reyes-Reyes, E.; Malik, M.T.; Murphy, E.M.; O'Toole, M.G.; Trent, J.O. G-quadruplex oligonucleotide AS1411 as a cancer-targeting agent: Uses and mechanisms. *Biochim. Biophys. Acta Gen. Subj.* **2017**, *1861*, 1414–1428. [CrossRef] [PubMed]
7. Dailey, M.M.; Miller, M.C.; Bates, P.J.; Lane, A.N.; Trent, J.O. Resolution and characterization of the structural polymorphism of a single quadruplex-forming sequence. *Nucleic Acids Res.* **2010**, *38*, 4877–4888. [CrossRef] [PubMed]
8. Christian, S.; Pilch, J.; Akerman, M.E.; Porkka, K.; Laakkonen, P.; Ruoslahti, E. Nucleolin expressed at the cell surface is a marker of endothelial cells in angiogenic blood vessels. *J. Cell Biol.* **2003**, *163*, 871–878. [CrossRef] [PubMed]
9. Abdelmohsen, K.; Gorospe, M. RNA-binding protein nucleolin in disease. *RNA Biol.* **2012**, *9*, 799–808. [CrossRef] [PubMed]
10. Cheng, Y.; Zhao, G.; Zhang, S.; Nigim, F.; Zhou, G.; Yu, Z.; Song, Y.; Chen, Y.; Li, Y. AS1411-Induced Growth Inhibition of Glioma Cells by Up-Regulation of p53 and Down-Regulation of Bcl-2 and Akt1 via Nucleolin. *PLoS ONE* **2016**, *11*, e0167094. [CrossRef]
11. Girvan, A.C.; Teng, Y.; Casson, L.K.; Thomas, S.D.; Jüliger, S.; Ball, M.; Klein, J.B.; Pierce, W.M.; Barve, S.S.; Bates, P.J. AGRO100 inhibits activation of nuclear factor-κB (NF-κB) by forming a complex with NF-κB essential modulator (NEMO) and nucleolin. *Mol. Cancer Ther.* **2006**, *5*, 1790–1799. [CrossRef]
12. Soundararajan, S.; Chen, W.; Spicer, E.K.; Courtenay-Luck, N.; Fernandes, D.J. The Nucleolin Targeting Aptamer AS1411 Destabilizes Bcl-2 Messenger RNA in Human Breast Cancer Cells. *Cancer Res.* **2008**, *68*, 2358–2365. [CrossRef]
13. Li, F.; Lu, J.; Liu, J.; Liang, C.; Wang, M.; Wang, L.; Li, D.; Yao, H.; Zhang, Q.; Wen, J.; et al. A water-soluble nucleolin aptamer-paclitaxel conjugate for tumor-specific targeting in ovarian cancer. *Nat. Commun.* **2017**, *8*, 1–14. [CrossRef]
14. Murphy, E.M.; Centner, C.S.; Bates, P.J.; Malik, M.T.; Kopechek, J.A. Delivery of thymoquinone to cancer cells with as1411-conjugated nanodroplets. *PLoS ONE* **2020**, *15*, e0233466. [CrossRef]
15. Rosenberg, J.E.; Bambury, R.M.; Van Allen, E.; Drabkin, H.A.; Lara, P.N.; Harzstark, A.L.; Wagle, N.; Figlin, R.A.; Smith, G.W.; Garraway, L.A.; et al. A phase II trial of AS1411 (a novel nucleolin-targeted DNA aptamer) in metastatic renal cell carcinoma. *Investig. N. Drugs* **2013**, *32*, 178–187. [CrossRef] [PubMed]
16. Alves, C.; Iacovelli, F.; Falconi, M.; Cardamone, F.; Della Rocca, B.M.; De Oliveira, C.L.P.; Desideri, A. A Simple and Fast Semiautomatic Procedure for the Atomistic Modeling of Complex DNA Polyhedra. *J. Chem. Inf. Model.* **2016**, *56*, 941–949. [CrossRef]
17. Falconi, M.; Oteri, F.; Chillemi, G.; Andersen, F.F.; Tordrup, D.; Oliveira, C.; Pedersen, J.S.; Knudsen, B.R.; Desideri, A. Deciphering the Structural Properties That Confer Stability to a DNA Nanocage. *ACS Nano* **2009**, *3*, 1813–1822. [CrossRef] [PubMed]
18. Franch, O.; Iacovelli, F.; Falconi, M.; Juul, S.; Ottaviani, A.; Benvenuti, C.; Biocca, S.; Ho, Y.-P.; Knudsen, B.R.; Desideri, A. DNA hairpins promote temperature controlled cargo encapsulation in a truncated octahedral nanocage structure family. *Nanoscale* **2016**, *8*, 13333–13341. [CrossRef] [PubMed]

19. Juul, S.; Iacovelli, F.; Falconi, M.; Kragh, S.L.; Christensen, B.; Frøhlich, R.; Franch, O.; Kristoffersen, E.L.; Stougaard, M.; Leong, K.W.; et al. Temperature-Controlled Encapsulation and Release of an Active Enzyme in the Cavity of a Self-Assembled DNA Nanocage. *ACS Nano* **2013**, *7*, 9724–9734. [CrossRef]
20. Oliveira, C.L.P.; Juul, S.; Jørgensen, H.L.; Knudsen, B.; Tordrup, D.; Oteri, F.; Falconi, M.; Koch, J.; Desideri, A.; Pedersen, J.S.; et al. Structure of Nanoscale Truncated Octahedral DNA Cages: Variation of Single-Stranded Linker Regions and Influence on Assembly Yields. *ACS Nano* **2010**, *4*, 1367–1376. [CrossRef]
21. Vindigni, G.; Raniolo, S.; Ottaviani, A.; Falconi, M.; Franch, O.; Knudsen, B.R.; Desideri, A.; Biocca, S. Receptor-Mediated Entry of Pristine Octahedral DNA Nanocages in Mammalian Cells. *ACS Nano* **2016**, *10*, 5971–5979. [CrossRef]
22. Raniolo, S.; Iacovelli, F.; Unida, V.; Desideri, A.; Biocca, S. In Silico and In Cell Analysis of Openable DNA Nanocages for miRNA Silencing. *Int. J. Mol. Sci.* **2019**, *21*, 61. [CrossRef]
23. Raniolo, S.; Vindigni, G.; Ottaviani, A.; Unida, V.; Iacovelli, F.; Manetto, A.; Figini, M.; Stella, L.; Desideri, A.; Biocca, S. Selective targeting and degradation of doxorubicin-loaded folate-functionalized DNA nanocages. *Nanomed. Nanotechnol. Biol. Med.* **2018**, *14*, 1181–1190. [CrossRef]
24. Raniolo, S.; Vindigni, G.; Unida, V.; Ottaviani, A.; Romano, E.; Desideri, A.; Biocca, S. Entry, fate and degradation of DNA nanocages in mammalian cells: A matter of receptors. *Nanoscale* **2018**, *10*, 12078–12086. [CrossRef]
25. Raniolo, S.; Unida, V.; Vindigni, G.; Stolfi, C.; Iacovelli, F.; Desideri, A.; Biocca, S. Combined and selective miR-21 silencing and doxorubicin delivery in cancer cells using tailored DNA nanostructures. *Cell Death Dis.* **2021**, *12*, 1–9. [CrossRef] [PubMed]
26. Lu, X.-J.; Olson, W.K. 3DNA: A versatile, integrated software system for the analysis, rebuilding and visualization of three-dimensional nucleic-acid structures. *Nat. Protoc.* **2008**, *3*, 1213–1227. [CrossRef] [PubMed]
27. De Lano, W.L. *The PyMOL Molecular Graphics System, Version 1.8*; Schrödinger, LLC.: San Carlos, CA, USA, 2002. [CrossRef]
28. Pettersen, E.F.; Goddard, T.D.; Huang, C.C.; Couch, G.S.; Greenblatt, D.M.; Meng, E.C.; Ferrin, T. UCSF Chimera?A visualization system for exploratory research and analysis. *J. Comput. Chem.* **2004**, *25*, 1605–1612. [CrossRef] [PubMed]
29. Raniolo, S.; Croce, S.; Thomsen, R.P.; Okholm, A.H.; Unida, V.; Iacovelli, F.; Manetto, A.; Kjems, J.; Desideri, A.; Biocca, S. Cellular uptake of covalent and non-covalent DNA nanostructures with different sizes and geometries. *Nanoscale* **2019**, *11*, 10808–10818. [CrossRef]
30. Salomon-Ferrer, R.; Case, D.A.; Walker, R.C. An overview of the Amber biomolecular simulation package. *Wiley Interdiscip. Rev. Comput. Mol. Sci.* **2012**, *3*, 198–210. [CrossRef]
31. Ivani, I.; Dans, P.D.; Noy, A.; Pérez, A.; Faustino, I.; Hospital, A.; Walther, J.; Andrio, P.; Goñi, R.; Balaceanu, A.; et al. Parmbsc1: A refined force field for DNA simulations. *Nat. Methods* **2015**, *13*, 55–58. [CrossRef]
32. Havrila, M.; Stadlbauer, P.; Islam, B.; Otyepka, M.; Sponer, J. Effect of Monovalent Ion Parameters on Molecular Dynamics Simulations of G-Quadruplexes. *J. Chem. Theory Comput.* **2017**, *13*, 3911–3926. [CrossRef]
33. Toukmaji, A.Y.; Sagui, C.; Board, J.A.; Darden, T.A. Efficient particle-mesh Ewald based approach to fixed and induced dipolar interactions. *J. Chem. Phys.* **2000**, *113*, 10913–10927. [CrossRef]
34. Ryckaert, J.-P.; Ciccotti, G.; Berendsen, H.J. Numerical integration of the cartesian equations of motion of a system with constraints: Molecular dynamics of n-alkanes. *J. Comput. Phys.* **1977**, *23*, 327–341. [CrossRef]
35. Goga, N.; Rzepiela, A.J.; de Vries, A.H.; Marrink, S.J.; Berendsen, H.J.C. Efficient Algorithms for Langevin and DPD Dynamics. *J. Chem. Theory Comput.* **2012**, *8*, 3637–3649. [CrossRef] [PubMed]
36. Feller, S.E.; Zhang, Y.; Pastor, R.W.; Brooks, B.R. Constant pressure molecular dynamics simulation: The Langevin piston method. *J. Chem. Phys.* **1995**, *103*, 4613–4621. [CrossRef]
37. Miao, Y.; Feher, V.A.; McCammon, J.A. Gaussian Accelerated Molecular Dynamics: Unconstrained Enhanced Sampling and Free Energy Calculation. *J. Chem. Theory Comput.* **2015**, *11*, 3584–3595. [CrossRef]
38. Abraham, M.J.; Murtola, T.; Schulz, R.; Páll, S.; Smith, J.; Hess, B.; Lindahl, E. GROMACS: High performance molecular simulations through multi-level parallelism from laptops to supercomputers. *SoftwareX* **2015**, *1–2*, 19–25. [CrossRef]
39. Daura, X.; Gademann, K.; Jaun, B.; Seebach, D.; Van Gunsteren, W.F.; Mark, A.E. Peptide Folding: When Simulation Meets Experiment. *Angew. Chem. Int. Ed.* **1999**, *38*, 236–240. [CrossRef]
40. Bagheri, Z.; Ranjbar, B.; Latifi, H.; Zibaii, M.I.; Moghadam, T.T.; Azizi, A. Spectral properties and thermal stability of AS1411 G-quadruplex. *Int. J. Biol. Macromol.* **2015**, *72*, 806–811. [CrossRef]
41. Jing, Y.; Cai, M.; Zhou, L.; Jiang, J.; Gao, J.; Wang, H. Aptamer AS1411 utilized for super-resolution imaging of nucleolin. *Talanta* **2020**, *217*, 121037. [CrossRef]
42. Reyes-Reyes, E.; Šalipur, F.R.; Shams, M.; Forsthoefel, M.; Bates, P.J. Mechanistic studies of anticancer aptamer AS1411 reveal a novel role for nucleolin in regulating Rac1 activation. *Mol. Oncol.* **2015**, *9*, 1392–1405. [CrossRef] [PubMed]
43. Chen, X.; Shank, S.; Davis, P.B.; Ziady, A.G. Nucleolin-Mediated Cellular Trafficking of DNA Nanoparticle Is Lipid Raft and Microtubule Dependent and Can Be Modulated by Glucocorticoid. *Mol. Ther.* **2011**, *19*, 93–102. [CrossRef] [PubMed]
44. Bolte, S.; Cordelières, F.P. A guided tour into subcellular colocalization analysis in light microscopy. *J. Microsc.* **2006**, *224*, 213–232. [CrossRef] [PubMed]
45. Charoenphol, P.; Bermudez, H. Aptamer-Targeted DNA Nanostructures for Therapeutic Delivery. *Mol. Pharm.* **2014**, *11*, 1721–1725. [CrossRef] [PubMed]
46. Yu, Z.; Li, X.; Duan, J.; Yang, X.-D. Targeted Treatment of Colon Cancer with Aptamer-Guided Albumin Nanoparticles Loaded with Docetaxel. *Int. J. Nanomed.* **2020**, *15*, 6737–6748. [CrossRef]

47. Zhang, Y.; Ma, W.; Mao, C.; Shao, X.-R.; Xie, X.; Wang, F.; Liu, X.; Li, Q.; Lin, Y. DNA-Based Nanomedicine with Targeting and Enhancement of Therapeutic Efficacy of Breast Cancer Cells. *ACS Appl. Mater. Interfaces* **2019**, *11*, 15354–15365. [CrossRef]
48. Xiao, D.; Li, Y.; Tian, T.; Zhang, T.; Shi, S.; Lu, B.; Gao, Y.; Qin, X.; Zhang, M.; Wei, W.; et al. Tetrahedral Framework Nucleic Acids Loaded with Aptamer AS1411 for siRNA Delivery and Gene Silencing in Malignant Melanoma. *ACS Appl. Mater. Interfaces* **2021**, *13*, 6109–6118. [CrossRef]
49. Zhou, Y.; Yang, Q.; Wang, F.; Zhou, Z.; Xu, J.; Cheng, S.; Cheng, Y. Self-Assembled DNA Nanostructure as a Carrier for Targeted siRNA Delivery in Glioma Cells. *Int. J. Nanomed.* **2021**, *16*, 1805–1817. [CrossRef] [PubMed]
50. Dam, D.H.M.; Culver, K.S.B.; Odom, T.W. Grafting Aptamers onto Gold Nanostars Increases in vitro Efficacy in a Wide Range of Cancer Cell Types. *Mol. Pharm.* **2014**, *11*, 580–587. [CrossRef]

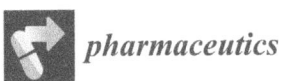

Article

Antigen-Capturing Mesoporous Silica Nanoparticles Enhance the Radiation-Induced Abscopal Effect in Murine Hepatocellular Carcinoma Hepa1-6 Models

Kyungmi Yang [1,2,†], Changhoon Choi [1,†], Hayeong Cho [3], Won-Gyun Ahn [1], Shin-Yeong Kim [1], Sung-Won Shin [1,2], Yeeun Kim [1], Taekyu Jang [3], Nohyun Lee [3,*] and Hee Chul Park [1,2,*]

[1] Department of Radiation Oncology, Samsung Medical Center, Seoul 06351, Korea; kyungmi.yang@samsung.com (K.Y.); chchoi93@gmail.com (C.C.); mementoamor@icloud.com (W.-G.A.); kkdnsy@naver.com (S.-Y.K.); camuserik@gmail.com (S.-W.S.); yeeun17.kim@sbri.co.kr (Y.K.)
[2] School of Medicine, Sungkyunkwan University, Seoul 06351, Korea
[3] School of Advanced Materials Engineering, Kookmin University, Seoul 02707, Korea; gkdud5305@naver.com (H.C.); wkdxorb55@kookmin.ac.kr (T.J.)
* Correspondence: nohyunlee@kookmin.ac.kr (N.L.); hee.ro.park@samsung.com (H.C.P.)
† These authors contributed equally to this work.

Abstract: Immunomodulation by radiotherapy (RT) is an emerging strategy for improving cancer immunotherapy. Nanomaterials have been employed as innovative tools for cancer therapy. This study aimed to investigate whether mesoporous silica nanoparticles (MSNs) enhance RT-mediated local tumor control and the abscopal effect by stimulating anti-cancer immunity. Hepa1-6 murine hepatocellular carcinoma syngeneic models and immunophenotyping with flow cytometry were used to evaluate the immune responses. When mice harboring bilateral tumors received 8 Gy of X-rays on a single tumor, the direct injection of MSNs into irradiated tumors enhanced the growth inhibition of irradiated and unirradiated contralateral tumors. MSNs enhanced RT-induced tumor infiltration of cytotoxic T cells on both sides and suppressed RT-enhanced infiltration of regulatory T cells. The administration of MSNs pre-incubated with irradiated cell-conditioned medium enhanced the anti-tumor effect of anti-PD1 compared to the as-synthesized MSNs. Intracellular uptake of MSNs activated JAWS II dendritic cells (DCs), which were consistently observed in DCs in tumor-draining lymph nodes (TDLNs). Our findings suggest that MSNs may capture tumor antigens released after RT, which is followed by DC maturation in TDLNs and infiltration of cytotoxic T cells in tumors, thereby leading to systemic tumor regression. Our results suggest that MSNs can be applied as an adjuvant for in situ cancer vaccines with RT.

Keywords: mesoporous silica nanoparticles; radiotherapy; immunotherapy; tumor microenvironment; abscopal effect

Citation: Yang, K.; Choi, C.; Cho, H.; Ahn, W.-G.; Kim, S.-Y.; Shin, S.-W.; Kim, Y.; Jang, T.; Lee, N.; Park, H.C. Antigen-Capturing Mesoporous Silica Nanoparticles Enhance the Radiation-Induced Abscopal Effect in Murine Hepatocellular Carcinoma Hepa1-6 Models. *Pharmaceutics* **2021**, *13*, 1811. https://doi.org/10.3390/pharmaceutics13111811

Academic Editors: Marina Santiago Franco and Yu Seok Youn

Received: 5 October 2021
Accepted: 26 October 2021
Published: 29 October 2021

Publisher's Note: MDPI stays neutral with regard to jurisdictional claims in published maps and institutional affiliations.

Copyright: © 2021 by the authors. Licensee MDPI, Basel, Switzerland. This article is an open access article distributed under the terms and conditions of the Creative Commons Attribution (CC BY) license (https://creativecommons.org/licenses/by/4.0/).

1. Introduction

In recent years, immunotherapy has gained interest as an option in cancer treatment. Immune checkpoint inhibitors targeting cytotoxic T lymphocyte-associated protein 4 (CTLA-4), programmed cell death protein 1 (PD1), and programmed cell death ligand 1 (PD-L1) have been approved by the United States Food and Drug Administration (FDA) and are considered promising systemic therapies based on clinical trials for various types of cancers [1]. Radiotherapy (RT) is one of the major types of cancer treatments and is known to modulate cancer immunity. Preclinical studies and some clinical cases have reported surprising results of the abscopal effect of combining immunotherapy with RT [2]. However, this has not yet become standard treatment in the clinic, and not all patients have experienced this positive outcome. Clinical trials to determine the optimal combination of RT and immunotherapy are ongoing.

Immunotherapy has been tested clinically for hepatocellular carcinoma (HCC), which is the second leading cause of cancer-related deaths worldwide [3–5]. Studies have shown positive results, with objective response rates of up to 20% [5]. Despite these encouraging results, immunotherapy does have clinical limitations, such as a relatively low response rate and acquired resistance [6]. In particular, immune checkpoint inhibitors are known to be less effective for HCC because of the lack of tumor-infiltrating lymphocytes and the immunosuppressive tumor microenvironment [7]. Thus, there is an unmet need to find innovative ways to enhance such treatment effects [8]. RT, one of the strategies to overcome this problem, has been considered as an option to boost the efficacy of immunotherapy for HCC [9]. Clinically, in a study investigating the role of RT in advanced HCC patients treated with nivolumab, patients with previous or concurrent RT showed better clinical outcomes than those without RT [10]. We previously studied a syngeneic murine HCC model and confirmed the abscopal effect and immunological mechanisms of the combination of RT and anti-PD1 antibody [11]. However, the mechanism by which RT stimulates the immune system is not yet clear, and effective immune modulation by RT itself needs to be tested to better understand the synergy between RT and immunotherapy. Researchers have suggested that RT induces immunogenic cell death and that this property could be useful for in situ vaccination [12].

Various types of engineered nanomaterials have been developed for medicinal purposes. Among them, mesoporous silica nanoparticles (MSNs) have attracted growing attention as nanocarriers for drug delivery or antigen targeting for vaccination. Owing to their large surface area and porous structure, MSNs possess the absorbing property of small biomaterials, such as proteins [13]. They effectively deliver absorbed biomaterials to target cells [14,15]. Researchers have made progress in the development of this property of MSNs for cancer treatment. In addition to chemotherapeutic drug delivery, MSNs have been studied for cancer vaccination, which could elicit an anti-cancer immune response by delivering cancer antigens to antigen-presenting cells [16].

In this study, we used a syngeneic murine HCC model to investigate anti-cancer immune stimulation by using MSNs in combination with RT. We tested the hypothesis that MSNs effectively deliver RT-releasing cancer antigens to local immune cells and investigated whether MSNs can enhance local tumor control and the abscopal effect.

2. Materials and Methods

2.1. Synthesis and Characterization of Nanoparticles

MSNs were synthesized via the sol-gel reaction of silane agents in the presence of structure-directing agents [17]. We dissolved 3 g of cetyltrimethylammonium chloride (CTAC, 25% solution, 12 mL, Sigma-Aldrich, St. Louis, MO, USA) and 60 mg of triethanolamine (Sigma-Aldrich, St. Louis, MO, USA) in 120 mL of deionized water. After heating to 95 °C, 2.25 mL of tetraethyl orthosilicate (TEOS, Acros Organics, Fair Lawn, NJ, USA) was added. After 2 h, the solution was cooled to room temperature, and the nanoparticles were collected by centrifugation at 11,000 rpm for 30 min and washed with ethanol three times. To extract residual structure-directing agents from the pores of MSNs, 1.3 mL of hydrochloric acid was added to the solution, which was refluxed for 3 h. For amine functionalization, 2.8 mL of (3-aminopropyl) triethoxysilane (APTES, 99%, Sigma-Aldrich, St. Louis, MO, USA) was added to the pore-extracted MSN solution and reacted for 3 h at 80 °C.

Fluorescently labeled MSNs were prepared by the co-addition of a fluorescence dye-conjugated silane agent with TEOS. The fluorescence dye-conjugated silane agent was synthesized by reacting 5 mg of fluorescein isothiocyanate (FITC, Sigma-Aldrich, St. Louis, MO, USA) with 44 µL of APTES in 1 mL of ethanol for 12 h in the dark. Immediately after the addition of TEOS (2.25 mL) to a solution containing CTAC (12 mL) and triethanolamine (60 mg), 250 µL of pre-conjugated FITC-APTES solution was added. After 2 h, the solution was cooled to room temperature, and the nanoparticles were collected by centrifugation at 11,000 rpm for 30 min and washed with ethanol three times. To extract residual structure-directing agents from the pores of MSNs, 1.3 mL of hydrochloric acid was added to the solution, which was refluxed for 3 h. For amine functionalization, 2.8 mL of APTES was added and reacted for 3 h at 80 °C.

The morphology of the MSNs was analyzed using a transmission electron microscope (JEM-2010, JEOL, Mitaka, Tokyo, Japan) at an accelerating voltage of 200 kV. A transmission electron microscopy (TEM) sample was prepared by dropping a diluted solution containing MSNs on a TEM grid, which was followed by air drying. TEM images were obtained without staining. The hydrodynamic sizes and zeta potentials of MSNs were measured by dynamic light scattering (Zetasizer ZS90, Malvern Instrument, Malvern, Worcestershire, UK). The Brunauer-Emmett-Teller (BET) surface area and pore volume of MSNs were measured by nitrogen (N_2) adsorption using a BELSORP-mini II (BEL, Toyonaka, Osaka, Japan).

2.2. Measurement of Antigen-Capturing Capacity

Fluorescein-conjugated ovalbumin (F-OVA, Invitrogen, Carlsbad, CA, USA) was used as a model antigen to evaluate the antigen-capturing capacity of MSNs. MSNs (1 mg) were incubated with 0.2 mg of F-OVA at 4 °C for 24 h. Next, the mixture was centrifuged at 11,000 rpm for 15 min. The F-OVA content was measured using a spectrophotometer (RF-6000, Shimadzu, Nakagyo, Kyoto, Japan). The amount of adsorbed MSNs was calculated from the change in the amount of F-OVA before and after adsorption.

2.3. Cell Culture

Murine hepatoma Hepa1-6 cells were purchased from the American Type Culture Collection (ATCC, Manassas, VA, USA). Hepa1-6 cells were cultured in Dulbecco's modified Eagle's medium (DMEM, Gibco, Carlsbad, CA, USA) containing 10% fetal bovine serum (FBS, Gibco) at 37 °C under a humidified atmosphere of 5% CO_2.

2.4. Measurement of Tumor Growth in Mice Co-Treated with MSNs and Radiation

Five-week-old male C57BL/6 mice were purchased from Orient Bio (Seongnam, Gyeonggi, Korea). All animal procedures were conducted in accordance with the appropriate regulatory standards under the study protocol (ID: 20181227001). To observe the abscopal effect, a bilateral syngeneic HCC model was established as previously described [11]. Briefly, Hepa1-6 cells (1×10^6 cells) were injected into the right hind leg of the mice, and the same number of Hepa1-6 cells was injected into the left leg of the same mice 3 days after the first injection. The mice were randomized into four groups (n = 10 per group): (i) sham treatment, (ii) radiation treatment, (iii) MSN treatment and (iv) radiation + MSNs. The right leg bearing a Hepa1-6 tumor was given with sham treatment or irradiated with 8 Gy of X-ray 14 days after cell inoculation. Irradiation was performed using a linear accelerator (Varian Medical System, Palo Alto, CA, USA), as previously described [8]. The as-synthesized MSNs (400 µg per tumor) were intratumorally injected into the irradiated tumors twice on days 14 and 15 after cell inoculation. The size of the tumors in both legs was measured every 2–3 days using calipers. The tumor volume was calculated using the formula: volume (mm^3) = ($W^2 \times L$)/2 (W, width (mm); L, length (mm)), as previously described [11,18]. The mice were sacrificed 42 days after cell inoculation.

2.5. Flow Cytometry Analysis

Tumors were harvested from both legs of the mice on days 20 and 42 after cell injection. A single-cell suspension was prepared as described previously [11]. Briefly, after the removal of red blood cells, the cells were fixed with Cytofix (BD554655, BD Biosciences, San Jose, CA, USA) for 30 min at 4 °C and resuspended in staining buffer (BD554656). The cells were permeabilized using the Fix/Perm kit (00-5523, eBioscience, San Diego, CA, USA). For T cell analysis, cells were stained with anti-Foxp3 (BD560408) and anti-IFNγ (BD557724) antibodies for 30 min at 4 °C. After washing, the cells were stained with antibodies specific for CD4 (BD552051), CD8 (BD560469), CD25 (BD551071), and CD45 (BD559864). Data were acquired using a BD FACSVerse flow cytometer (BD Biosciences) and analyzed using FlowJo software version 10.6.1 (Three Star Inc., Ashland, OR, USA).

For dendritic cell (DC) analysis, inguinal lymph nodes of the irradiated tumor side were harvested four days after irradiation, and DCs were isolated using the EasySep mouse plasmacytoid DC isolation kit (STEMCELL Technologies, Vancouver, BC, Canada). The DCs were stained with anti-CD11c (BD553801), anti-CD80 (BD560016), anti-CD86 (BD560582) and anti-MHC II (BD562363), and subjected to flow cytometry.

2.6. Pre-Incubation of MSNs with Irradiated Cell Conditioned Medium

Hepa1-6 cells were seeded in a 100 mm dish and irradiated with 100 Gy of γ-rays using an IBL437C blood irradiator (CIS Bio International, Gif-sur-Yvette, Essone, France). After 48 h of incubation without FBS, the conditioned medium (CM) was collected and centrifuged at $1500\times g$ for 10 min to remove cell debris. The MSNs were resuspended at a concentration of 2.5 mg/mL in the cell culture supernatant and incubated for 72 h at 4 °C. After centrifugation at 11,000 rpm for 15 min, CM-incubated MSNs (CM-MSNs) were collected and washed twice with PBS. CM-MSNs were resuspended in PBS at a final concentration of 8 mg/mL.

2.7. Cellular Uptake of MSNs

The immortalized immature DC line JAWS II was purchased from ATCC. JAWS II cells were seeded onto a cover slip (Paul Marienfeld GmbH & Co. KG, Lauda-Königshofen, Baden-Württemberg, Germany) and incubated with 250 µg/mL of rhodamine-preloaded MSNs for two days. Cells were fixed with 4% formaldehyde and permeabilized with 0.01% Triton X-100. Cells were stained with Alexa-Fluor488-conjugated phalloidin (Life Technologies, Eugene, OR, USA) and DAPI (Sigma-Aldrich, St. Louis, MO, USA). Fluorescence images were acquired using a Zeiss Observer D1 fluorescence microscope (Carl Zeiss, Oberkochen, Baden-Württemberg, Germany). The activation of JAWS II cells by CM-MSNs was determined by flow cytometry. JAWS II cells (5×10^6 cells) were seeded in 12-well plates and incubated with 100 or 200 µg/mL of CM-MSNs for two days. Cells were stained with anti-CD40 (BD562846), anti-CD80, anti-CD86, anti-MHC I (BD742859), anti-MHC II and anti-PD-L1 (12-5982-82, eBioscience, San Diego, CA, USA). Stained cells were analyzed by a BD FACSVerse flow cytometry.

2.8. Measurement of Tumor Growth in Mice Co-Treated with CM-MSNs and Anti-PD1

To test the immune-boosting effect of CM-MSNs, a single Hepa1-6 tumor model was established by injecting into the right hind leg of C57BL/6 mice. When the tumors were palpable, the mice were randomly divided into four groups ($n = 4$ per group): (i) MSNs + isotype IgG, (ii) MSNs + anti-PD1, (iii) CM-MSNs + isotype IgG and (iv) CM-MSNs + anti-PD1. Isotype IgG and anti-PD1 (BE0089 and BE0146; Bio X Cell, West Lebanon, NH, USA) were intraperitoneally administered at a dose of 2 mg/kg twice per week. MSNs or CM-MSNs (8 mg/kg) were subcutaneously injected into the left hind leg on the same day as the antibody injection. Tumor size was measured every 2–3 days using calipers, as described above. The mice were sacrificed 28 days after cell inoculation.

2.9. Immunohistochemistry

Formalin-fixed paraffin-embedded tumor tissue specimens were prepared as described previously [18]. For immunohistochemistry (IHC), the tumors were sliced into 4-µm-thick sections, deparaffinized in xylene, rehydrated in graded alcohol, and washed with 0.01 M PBS, pH 7.4. Heat-induced epitope retrieval was performed using citrate buffer (pH 6.0; Dako, Carpinteria, CA, USA), followed by blocking with a blocking buffer (Dako). The tissue sections were stained with anti-CD4 and CD8 antibodies, followed by incubation with horseradish peroxidase-conjugated secondary antibodies and 3,3'-diaminobenzidine substrate chromogen solution (DAB, Dako). IHC images were obtained using an Aperio

ScanScope AT slide scanner (Leica Biosystems Inc., Buffalo Grove, IL, USA) and analyzed using ImageScope software 12.4.3 (Leica Biosystems, Buffalo Grove, IL, USA).

2.10. Statistical Analysis

All quantitative data are presented as the mean ± standard deviation (SD) or standard error of the mean (SEM). Statistical analyses were performed using Prism 9.2 (GraphPad Software, San Diego, CA, USA). *p*-values were calculated using one-way analysis of variance (ANOVA), Kruskal-Wallis test, or unpaired two-tailed *t*-test. Statistical significance was set at $p < 0.05$.

3. Results

3.1. Characterization of MSNs

MSNs were synthesized via the sol–gel reaction of TEOS in the presence of CTAC as a pore-directing agent. TEM images showed that the MSNs had a spherical mesoporous structure (Figure 1A). The average size of MSNs was 100.82 ± 13.41 nm (Figure 1B). To optimize the antigen-capturing capacity, the surface of the MSNs was modified using APTES. The zeta potential of the strongly negative as-synthesized MSNs changed to a positive value after surface modification, confirming successful amine functionalization (Figure 1C). The hydrodynamic diameter of MSNs measured by dynamic light scattering was 104.22 nm (Figure 1D). The BET surface area and pore size determined via N_2 adsorption/desorption experiments were 325.31 m^2/g and 4.21 nm, respectively (Figure 1E). The antigen-capturing capacity of MSNs was estimated by the adsorption of F-OVA. Poly(lactic-*co*-glycolic acid) (PLGA) was employed as a control because its antigen-capturing capacity was recently reported [19]. After incubation of F-OVA with PLGA and MSNs, only 9% and 7% of F-OVA was adsorbed, respectively (Figure 1D). Surface modification with APTES significantly increased the affinity to F-OVA and 45% of F-OVA was captured by amine-functionalized MSNs. The interaction between MSNs and F-OVA can be attributed mainly to electrostatic interactions. After the adsorption of F-OVA, the zeta potential and hydrodynamic size of MSN were changed to −11.1 mV and 191 nm, respectively (Figure 1C,D). Owing to the enhanced capturing capacity, subsequent experiments were performed using amine-functionalized MSNs.

3.2. Effects of Intratumorally Injected MSNs on Radiation-Induced Abscopal Tumor Growth

Given that MSNs with a tumor microenvironment can capture biomaterials released after RT, we tested the effect of intratumoral injection of MSNs on radiation-induced tumor growth inhibition. To observe the abscopal effect, the bilateral Hepa1-6 tumor model was used, as in a previous study [11]. Hepa1-6 cells were injected into both legs 3 days apart. X-rays (8 Gy) were delivered to the primary tumor site in the right hind leg, and MSNs were directly injected into the same primary tumor (Figure 2A). Radiation alone significantly decreased the growth of primary tumors but not secondary tumors ($p < 0.001$; Figure 2B–E). Intratumoral administration of MSNs did not affect the growth of unirradiated primary and secondary tumors, but it significantly decreased the growth of both primary and secondary tumors when injected into irradiated primary tumors (Figure 2B–E) compared with sham treatment. The difference in tumor volume between radiation and radiation plus MSNs was not statistically significant. These data indicate that MSNs in combination with RT inhibited the growth of distal and primary tumors.

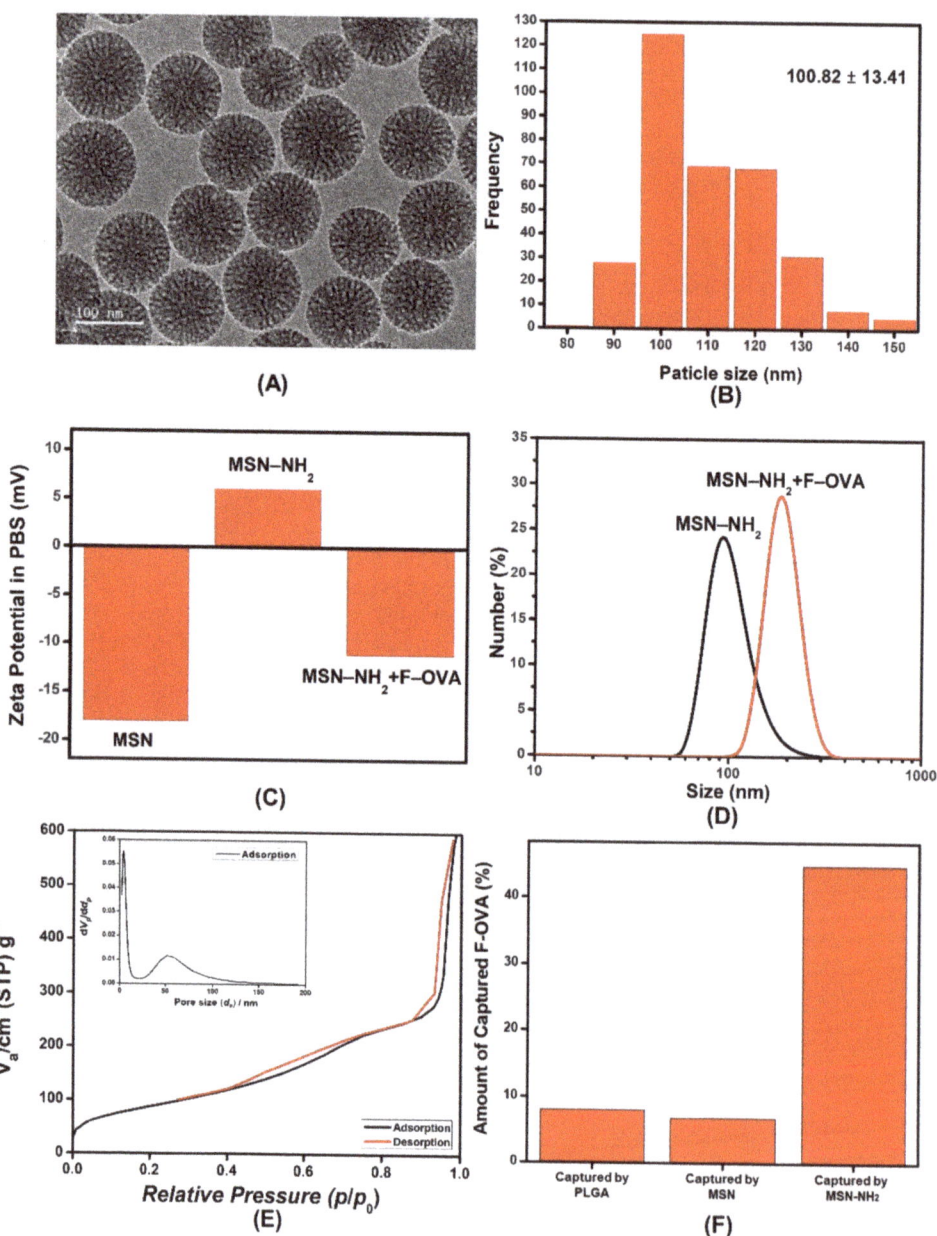

Figure 1. Synthesis of mesoporous silica nanoparticles (MSNs) with antigen-capturing capacity. (**A**) Transmission electron microscopy image of MSNs and (**B**) diagraph showing size distribution. (**C**) Zeta potentials of MSN, MSN-NH$_2$ and MSN-NH$_2$ after capturing fluorescein-conjugated ovalbumin (F-OVA). (**D**) Hydrodynamic diameter of MSN-NH$_2$ before and after capturing F-OVA. (**E**) N$_2$ absorption/desorption isotherms of MSNs. (Inset: pore size distribution from the adsorption branch). (**F**) Amount of F-OVA captured by poly-lactic-*co*-glycolic acid (PLGA), MSNs and MSN-NH$_2$.

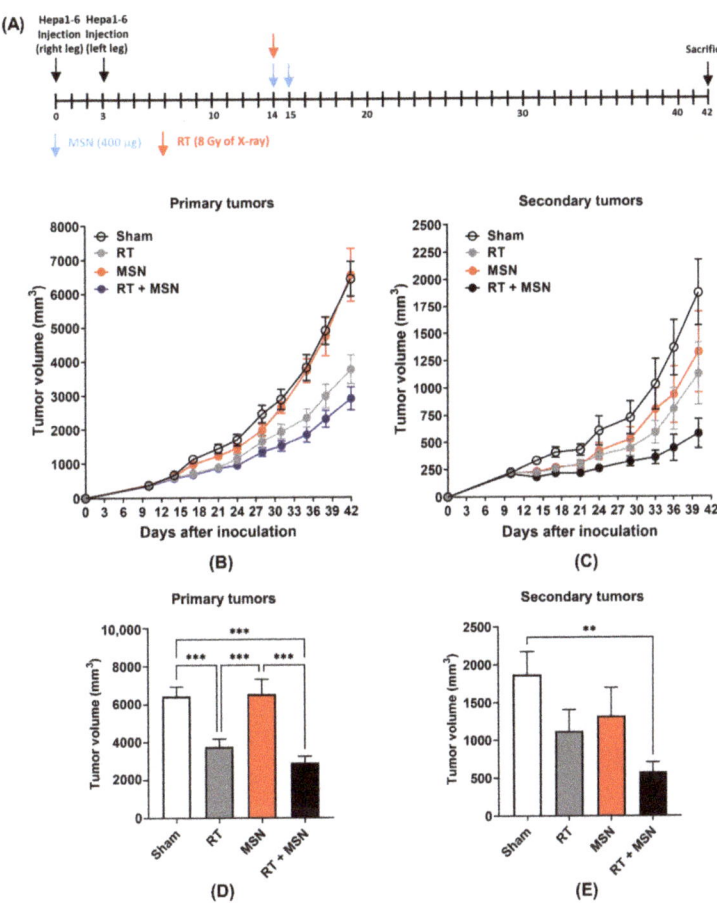

Figure 2. Intratumoral administration of MSNs enhances the radiation-induced abscopal effect in a bilateral Hepa1-6 tumor model. (**A**) Schedule of MSN or radiation treatment. (**B**) Growth curves of irradiated primary Hepa1-6 tumors implanted into C57BL/6 mice. (**C**) Growth curves of unirradiated secondary Hepa1-6 tumors in the same mice receiving RT. (**D,E**) Comparison of tumor volumes between treatment groups 42 days after tumor inoculation. ** $p < 0.01$; *** $p < 0.001$.

3.3. Effects of Intratumorally Injected MSNs on Tumor-Infiltrating Lymphocytes

To further understand how MSNs facilitate radiation-induced abscopal effects, we evaluated the immunophenotype of tumor-infiltrating T lymphocytes. Primary and secondary tumors were harvested 6 and 28 days after irradiation (Figure 3A). Flow cytometric analysis revealed that in the tumors harvested on day 6, radiation increased the percentage of CD4+IFNγ+ T cells ($p < 0.05$) and CD8+IFNγ+ T cells ($p < 0.05$) in the primary tumors but not in the secondary tumors compared to the sham treatment (Figure 3B,C). Injection of MSNs into the irradiated primary tumors, but not the unirradiated tumors, further augmented the percentage of activated T cells, although this increase did not reach statistical significance. Instead, MSNs significantly decreased the number of CD4 + CD25 + Foxp3 + regulatory T cells (Tregs) in primary tumors (Figure 3B). In the tumors harvested on day 28, the number of activated CD4 + or CD8 + T cells significantly increased in the secondary tumors as well as the primary tumors co-treated with MSNs and radiation compared to that in sham or single treatments (Figure 3D,E). This correlates with a greater reduction in tumor size (Figure 2D,E). Radiation increased the number of Tregs in the unirradiated secondary tumors, which was suppressed by co-treatment with MSNs (Figure 3C,E). These data suggest that MSNs may enhance RT-induced tumor regression at the distal site via modulation of the T cell response.

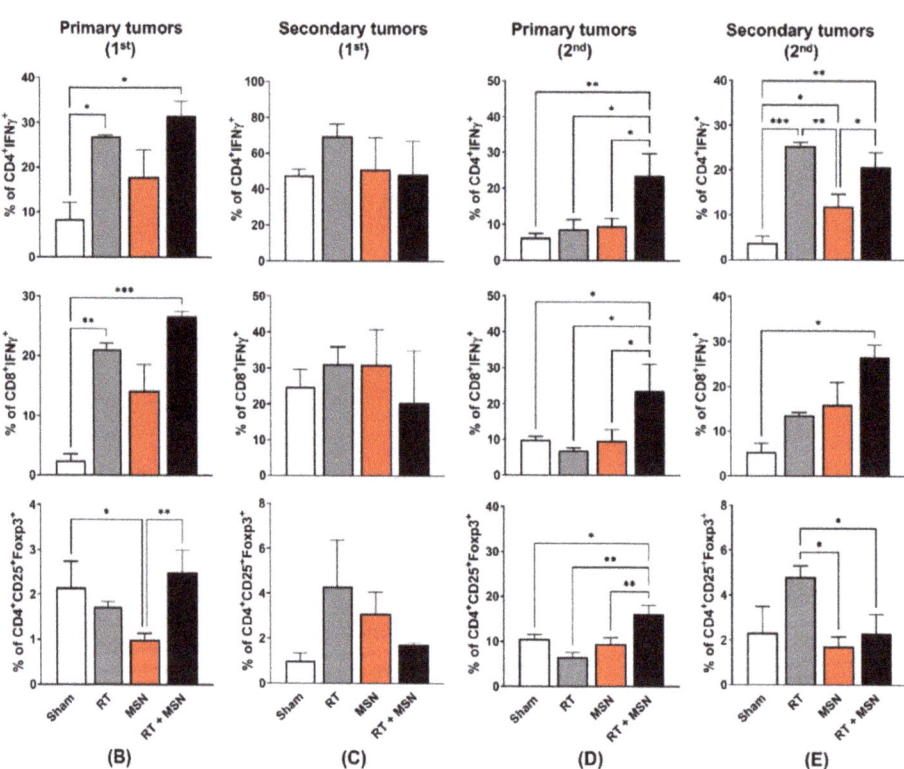

Figure 3. Direct injection of MSNs into irradiated primary tumors increases the number of cytotoxic T cells infiltrating the distal tumors. (**A**) Illustration of the treatment schedule and timing of tumor harvesting. (**B,C**) Profiling of activated T cells and Treg cells from primary (**B**) and secondary tumor tissues (**C**) harvested 20 days after tumor inoculation. (**D,E**) Profiling of activated T cells and Treg cells from primary (**D**) and secondary tumor tissues (**E**) harvested 42 days after tumor inoculation. * $p < 0.05$; ** $p < 0.01$; *** $p < 0.001$.

3.4. Effects of MSNs on Dendritic Cell Activation

It is likely that the systemic anti-tumor effect of MSNs is linked to the activation of DCs residing in lymph nodes. To verify this, we tested whether MSNs could activate DCs in vitro. To recapitulate the in vivo situation, conditioned medium (CM) was prepared from Hepa1-6 cells irradiated with 100 Gy of γ-rays and incubated with MSNs to generate CM-MSNs (Figure 4A). First, to test whether DCs can take up CM-MSNs, immortalized immature dendritic JAWS II cells were incubated with rhodamine-preloaded CM-MSNs. Fluorescence imaging showed an efficient uptake of nanoparticles into the cytoplasm of JAWS II cells without visible toxicity (Figure 4B). Flow cytometry showed that CM-MSNs increased the surface expression of DC maturation markers, including CD86, MHC I and MHC II, in a dose-dependent manner (Figure 4C). CM-MSNs also upregulated PD-L1 expression in JAWS II cells. In contrast, MSNs without preconditioning in medium did not activate JAWS II cells at 200 µg/mL (Figure 4D).

Next, we examined whether MSNs injected into irradiated tumors facilitated DC maturation in tumor-draining lymph nodes (TDLNs) collected from mice. In mice bearing bilateral Hepa1-6 tumors, the right hind legs were exposed to X-rays (8 Gy) and then injected with FITC-preloaded MSNs or PBS. TDLNs were collected 3 days after irradiation and subjected to flow cytometry (Figure 4E). DCs obtained from mice co-treated with radiation, and MSNs showed an increase in the FITC-positive cell population compared to that in mice treated with radiation alone ($p < 0.001$; Figure 4F), suggesting uptake of MSNs by DCs. Injection of MSNs into irradiated tumors increased the expression of DC maturation markers such as CD80, CD86 and MHC II in DCs from TDLNs (Figure 4F), which is consistent with the in vitro results.

3.5. Effects of CM-MSNs on Hepa1-6 Tumor Growth in a Syngeneic Mouse Model

To test the function of CM-MSNs as a cancer vaccine therapy in vivo, we inoculated Hepa1-6 cells into the right hind legs and then evaluated the combined effect of the nanomaterials and anti-PD1 on tumor growth (Figure 5A). Treatment with CM-MSNs delayed tumor growth compared to treatment with the as-synthesized MSNs (Figure 5B,C). CM-MSNs augmented anti-PD1-mediated tumor growth inhibition to a greater extent than the as-synthesized MSNs ($p < 0.05$; Figure 5B,C). Immunohistochemical analysis of CD4 and CD8 in Hepa1-6 tumor tissues showed that CM-MSNs and anti-PD1 greatly increased the infiltration of both CD4- and CD8-positive cells within the tumor tissues (Figure 5D,E). These data suggest that CM-MSNs could be applied in cancer vaccine therapies to boost cancer immunotherapy.

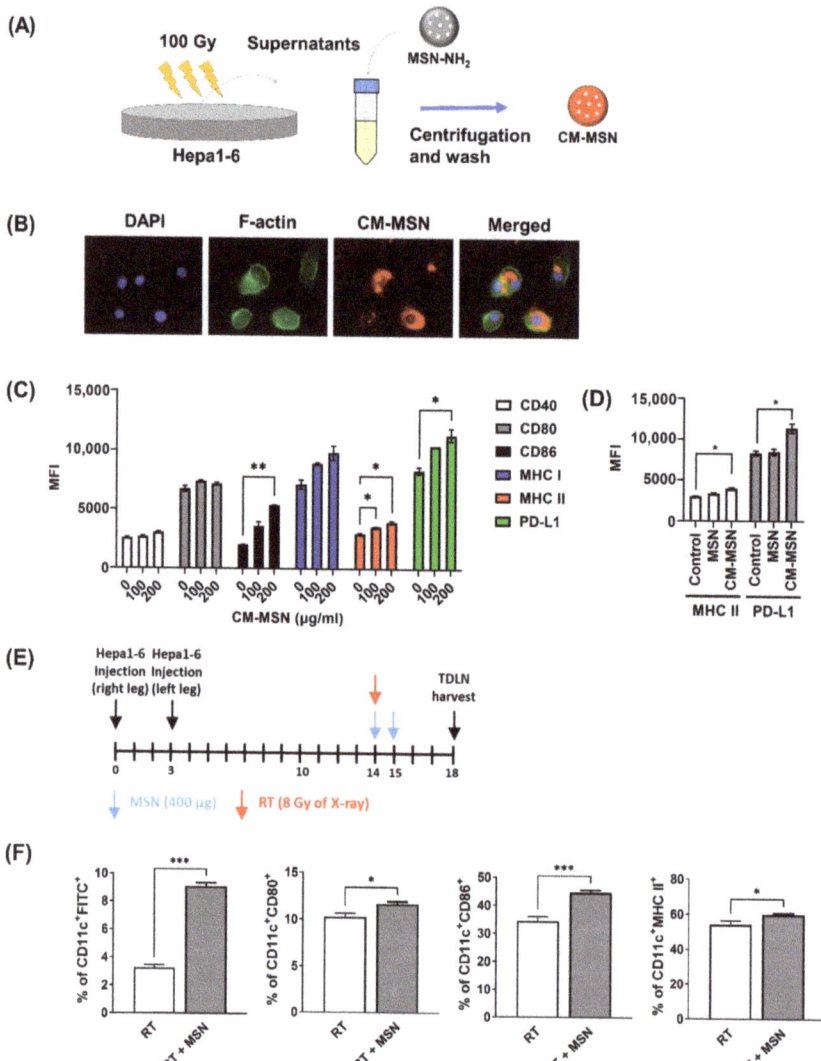

Figure 4. MSNs pre-incubated with the irradiated cell conditioned medium activates dendritic cells in vitro and in vivo. (**A**) Schematic diagram for the preparation of conditioned medium-incubated MSNs (CM-MSNs). (**B**) Uptake of CM-MSNs into JAWS II cells. Representative images of CM-MSNs labeled with rhodamine. (**C**) CM-MSNs activated JAWS II, an immortalized immature dendritic cell line. (**D**) MSNs without preconditioning did not activate JAWS II cells. (**E**) Schedule of timing of harvesting tumor-draining lymph nodes. (**F**) Flow cytometry data showing the MSN-increased population of activated DCs in TDLNs. * $p < 0.05$; ** $p < 0.01$; *** $p < 0.001$.

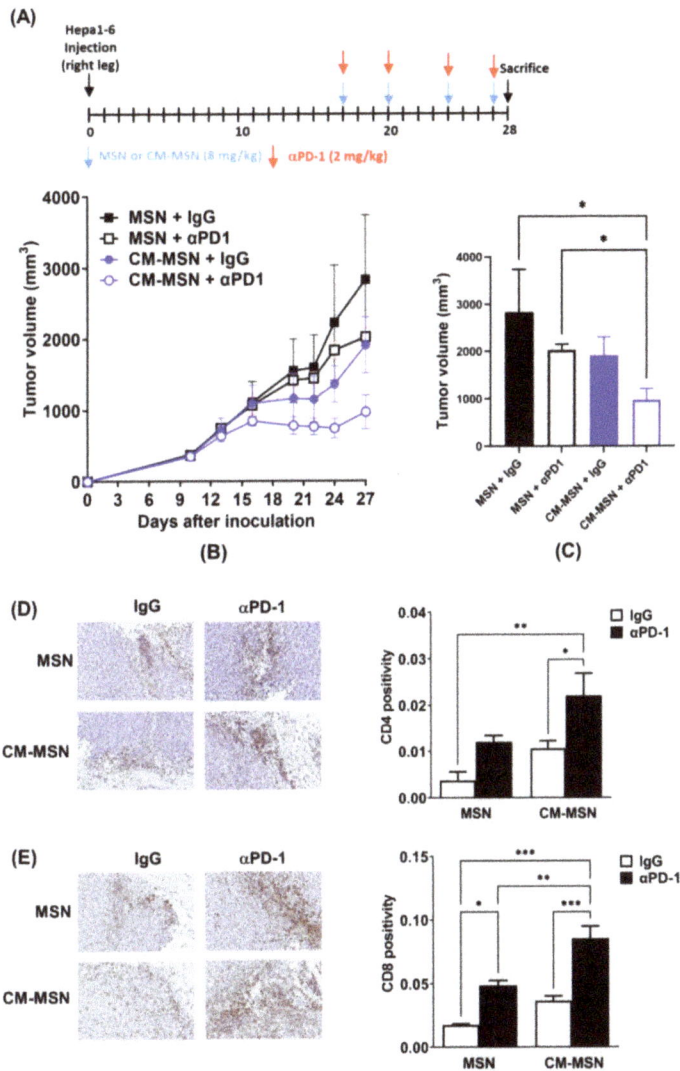

Figure 5. MSNs pre-incubated with irradiated cell conditioned medium augments the anti-tumor effect of programmed cell death protein 1 (anti-PD1) in a syngeneic hepatocellular carcinoma (HCC) model. (**A**) Schedule of MSN or anti-PD-1 treatment. (**B**) Growth curves of Hepa1-6 tumors implanted into C57BL/6 mice. (**C**) Comparison of tumor volume 27 days after tumor inoculation. (**D**) Representative immunohistochemistry (IHC) images and quantitative data of CD4 staining in Hepa1-6 tumor tissues. (**E**) Representative IHC images and quantitative data of CD8 staining in Hepa1-6 tumor tissues. * $p < 0.05$; ** $p < 0.01$; *** $p < 0.001$.

4. Discussion

MSNs have a large surface area and porous structure that aid in absorbing nano-level materials such as drugs, proteins, and DNA fragments [15]. Based on this ability, numerous studies on MSNs have been conducted for various therapeutic purposes, including drug delivery, diagnosis and imaging [13,15]. MSNs have also been explored for cancer vaccination because MSNs that absorb tumor antigens increase the anti-tumor adaptive immune response [20]. Hong et al. [21] showed that the encapsulation of ovalbumin in MSNs enhanced DC internalization, lysosomal degradation escape, and cross-presentation, resulting in tumor growth inhibition. The efficacy and clearance of MSNs depend on their physical characteristics, such as surface charge, diameter, and pore size [13]. In terms of size, MSNs with diameters of 30–200 nm are efficient for drug loading, and those less than 100 nm are sufficient for lymph node drainage [21]. Larger pore sizes have shown better antigen-presenting functions [22]. In this study, we designed MSNs that can capture antigens released after RT and tested their efficacy in combination with RT. PLGA particles have been shown to improve the abscopal effect by capturing RT-releasing antigens [19]. The measurement of antigen-capturing capacity revealed that the as-synthesized MSNs adsorbed a similar amount of F-OVA as the PLGA particles. However, the amine functionalization of MSNs increased the absorption capacity by more than 6-fold. Since the interaction between MSNs and biomolecules depends on physicochemical properties such as electrostatic interactions, hydrogen bonding, and hydrophobic interactions, we expect that the antigen-capturing capacity can be further improved using various silane agents.

Based on the finding that MSNs efficiently captured F-OVA, we speculated that MSNs directly injected into tumors could absorb biomolecules from irradiated tumor cells, thereby eliciting anti-tumor immunity. In the bilateral Hepa1-6 tumor model, MSNs plus RT showed better regression of both primary and secondary tumors. Since MSNs alone did not show any significant effect on tumor growth, it is likely that the capturing process of RT-released antigens by MSNs is necessary for boosting systemic anti-tumor effects. CM-MSNs were prepared to mimic the MSN-absorbing antigens released during RT treatment in vivo. As expected, CM-MSNs showed better tumor control and boosted the anti-cancer effect of the anti-PD1 antibody compared with the as-synthesized MSNs. The action of CM-MSNs may be related to the increase in the number of CD4+ and CD8+ T lymphocytes infiltrating the tumor tissues, which was further enhanced by co-treatment with anti-PD1. These data suggest that MSNs could work as an effective nanocarrier for RT-released antigens and exert a systemic anti-tumor effect. Finally, we expect that CM-MSNs or a combination of MSNs and RT will make the outcome of immunotherapy much stronger and more sustainable.

The key steps in anti-cancer immunity are the maturation of DCs for antigen presentation and the activation of tumor-infiltrating T lymphocytes [23]. Similar to the mechanism of general vaccination, cell-mediated immune responses proceed as follows: drainage to lymph nodes, uptake by DCs, maturation of DCs, and presentation of peptide–MHC I complexes to CD8 + T cells, which are termed as the DUMP cascade process [24]. In this study, the uptake of CM-MSNs by DCs and subsequent DC activation in TDLNs was confirmed in vitro and in vivo (Figure 4). To test the early and late responses of T lymphocytes to RT and MSNs, tumors were harvested on days 6 and 26, and the immune cell populations were profiled (Figure 3). While the infiltration of cytotoxic T cells in the primary tumors was increased by either RT or RT plus MSNs in the early phase, there was no significant increased infiltration in secondary tumors. In the late phase, the number of cytotoxic T cells increased in the group treated with RT plus MSNs in both primary and secondary tumors, suggesting that MSNs may boost the RT-induced abscopal effect in the late phase. In addition, regulatory T cell numbers increased in the secondary tumors in the group that received RT alone, but not in the group treated with RT plus MSNs, which may endow effector T cells with cytotoxic activity. It could be inferred that MSNs balance immunity toward anti-tumor responses within the tumor microenvironment through continuous antigen delivery [14]. Taken together, our data suggest that MSNs capturing RT-induced antigens may strengthen the DUMP cascade, resulting in a significant suppression of both local and abscopal tumors via systemic anti-tumor immunity [21].

High doses of RT kill tumor cells, thus releasing large amounts of various antigens, including damaged double-stranded DNA, which is a powerful stimulator of the immune system [25]. The antigens that were released by RT and captured by MSNs may be nonselective. These antigens can be mixed with neoantigens from tumors and self-antigens shared with normal tissue [26,27]. However, theoretically, there might be no immune response to the materials from normal tissues as an immune tolerance [28]. This study found that CM-MSN or MSNs as adjuvants with RT acted in similar way as in vivo vaccines [29]. Despite many efforts, numerous typical cancer vaccines have failed [29]. One of the reasons is immune resistance to vaccine therapy because most cancer vaccines have a specific antigen target [30]. In contrast, in situ vaccines have the advantage of generating multiple antigens that can act simultaneously [31]. In addition, to overcome this resistance, various combination therapies, including immunotherapy, have been recently tested [29]. Our data on CM-MSNs might be consistent with the clinical data that hypofractionated RT or stereotactic body RT show better effects with immunotherapy [32]. Furthermore, MSNs may provide tumor antigens for longer periods [21], which is an important condition for successful therapeutic cancer vaccines.

The development of therapeutic nanoparticles has been successfully achieved through recent technical advances. However, clinical translation remains a challenge owing to several issues such as biocompatibility and safety. Fortunately, silica-based nanomaterials have been extensively tested because of their non-toxic nature [33]. After the injection of MSNs, their accumulation was found in the liver and spleen, and MSNs were mainly secreted by the intestine and kidneys [33]. Toxicity was rarely observed, although the properties of MSNs, such as their size, would be related to their safety [33,34]. The FDA approved the first human trial of multimodal silica nanoparticles termed "Cornell dots" in 2011 [35]. Thus, MSNs with novel multifunctionality have great potential to be tested in humans. Although biocompatibility needs to be tested, our study suggests that MSNs are promising for cancer treatment in combination with RT. However, questions still remain about optimal treatment settings, including optimal conditions of MSNs (pore size, injection dose, etc.) and combination with immunotherapy and RT (dose and timing) [15].

In this study, we confirmed the mechanism of stimulating the cancer immune system by MSNs with RT and showed their potential for combination with immunotherapy. Future studies will need to test MSNs combined with RT and immunotherapy.

5. Conclusions

In this study, we evaluated the combined effect of MSNs and RT on local tumor control and the abscopal effect using syngeneic murine HCC models. Our findings suggest that MSNs may capture tumor antigens released after RT, which is followed by DC maturation in TDLNs and the infiltration of cytotoxic T cells in tumors, thereby leading to systemic tumor regression. MSNs could be applied to in situ cancer vaccines with RT in the future.

Author Contributions: Conceptualization, N.L. and H.C.P.; methodology, W.-G.A. and H.C.; validation, S.-Y.K., S.-W.S., Y.K. and T.J.; formal analysis, W.-G.A. and S.-W.S.; investigation, K.Y.; resources, N.L.; data curation, C.C. and S.-W.S.; writing—original draft preparation, K.Y. and C.C.; writing—review and editing, N.L. and H.C.P.; visualization, H.C., W.-G.A., S.-W.S. and T.J.; supervision, H.C.P.; project administration, C.C.; funding acquisition, N.L. and H.C.P. All authors have read and agreed to the published version of the manuscript.

Funding: This research was supported by grants from the National Research Foundation of Korea (NRF), funded by the Korean government (2017M3A9G5082642, 2018R1A2B2002835, and 2019R1A2C1008021).

Institutional Review Board Statement: The animal experiments were reviewed and approved by the Institutional Animal Care and Use Committee of the Samsung Biomedical Research Institute (No. 20181227001).

Informed Consent Statement: Not applicable.

Data Availability Statement: Not applicable.

Conflicts of Interest: The authors declare no conflict of interest.

References

1. Twomey, J.D.; Zhang, B. Cancer Immunotherapy Update: FDA-Approved Checkpoint Inhibitors and Companion Diagnostics. *AAPS J.* **2021**, *23*, 39. [CrossRef]
2. Postow, M.A.; Callahan, M.K.; Barker, C.A.; Yamada, Y.; Yuan, J.; Kitano, S.; Mu, Z.; Rasalan, T.; Adamow, M.; Ritter, E.; et al. Immunologic Correlates of the Abscopal Effect in a Patient with Melanoma. *N. Engl. J. Med.* **2012**, *366*, 925–931. [CrossRef]
3. McGlynn, K.A.; Petrick, J.L.; El-Serag, H.B. Epidemiology of Hepatocellular Carcinoma. *Hepatology* **2021**, *73* (Suppl. 1), 4–13. [CrossRef]
4. El-Khoueiry, A.B.; Sangro, B.; Yau, T.; Crocenzi, T.S.; Kudo, M.; Hsu, C.; Kim, T.-Y.; Choo, S.-P.; Trojan, J.; Welling, T.H.; et al. Nivolumab in patients with advanced hepatocellular carcinoma (CheckMate 040): An open-label, non-comparative, phase 1/2 dose escalation and expansion trial. *Lancet* **2017**, *389*, 2492–2502. [CrossRef]
5. Zhu, A.X.; Finn, R.S.; Edeline, J.; Cattan, S.; Ogasawara, S.; Palmer, D.; Verslype, C.; Zagonel, V.; Fartoux, L.; Vogel, A.; et al. Pembrolizumab in patients with advanced hepatocellular carcinoma previously treated with sorafenib (KEYNOTE-224): A non-randomised, open-label phase 2 trial. *Lancet Oncol.* **2018**, *19*, 940–952. [CrossRef]
6. Khan, A.A.; Liu, Z.-K.; Xu, X. Recent advances in immunotherapy for hepatocellular carcinoma. *Hepatobiliary Pancreat. Dis. Int.* **2021**. [CrossRef] [PubMed]
7. Bian, J.; Lin, J.; Long, J.; Yang, X.; Yang, X.; Lu, X.; Sang, X.; Zhao, H. T lymphocytes in hepatocellular carcinoma immune microenvironment: Insights into human immunology and immunotherapy. *Am. J. Cancer Res.* **2020**, *10*, 4585–4606. [PubMed]
8. Sangro, B.; Sarobe, P.; Hervás-Stubbs, S.; Melero, I. Advances in immunotherapy for hepatocellular carcinoma. *Nat. Rev. Gastroenterol. Hepatol.* **2021**, *18*, 525–543. [CrossRef]
9. Choi, C.; Yoo, G.S.; Cho, W.K.; Park, H.C. Optimizing radiotherapy with immune checkpoint blockade in hepatocellular carcinoma. *World J. Gastroenterol.* **2019**, *25*, 2416–2429. [CrossRef]
10. Yu, J.I.; Lee, S.J.; Lee, J.; Lim, H.Y.; Paik, S.W.; Yoo, G.S.; Choi, C.; Park, H.C. Clinical significance of radiotherapy before and/or during nivolumab treatment in hepatocellular carcinoma. *Cancer Med.* **2019**, *8*, 6986–6994. [CrossRef]
11. Yoo, G.S.; Ahn, W.-G.; Kim, S.-Y.; Kang, W.; Choi, C.; Park, H.C. Radiation-induced abscopal effect and its enhancement by programmed cell death 1 blockade in the hepatocellular carcinoma: A murine model study. *Clin. Mol. Hepatol.* **2021**, *27*, 144–156. [CrossRef]
12. Lurje, I.; Werner, W.; Mohr, R.; Roderburg, C.; Tacke, F.; Hammerich, L. In Situ Vaccination as a Strategy to Modulate the Immune Microenvironment of Hepatocellular Carcinoma. *Front. Immunol.* **2021**, *12*, 650486. [CrossRef]
13. Chen, F.; Hableel, G.; Zhao, E.R.; Jokerst, J.V. Multifunctional nanomedicine with silica: Role of silica in nanoparticles for theranostic, imaging, and drug monitoring. *J. Colloid Interface Sci.* **2018**, *521*, 261–279. [CrossRef]
14. Thakur, N.; Thakur, S.; Chatterjee, S.; Das, J.; Sil, P.C. Nanoparticles as Smart Carriers for Enhanced Cancer Immunotherapy. *Front. Chem.* **2020**, *8*, 8. [CrossRef]
15. Narayan, R.; Nayak, U.Y.; Raichur, A.M.; Garg, S. Mesoporous Silica Nanoparticles: A Comprehensive Review on Synthesis and Recent Advances. *Pharmaceutics* **2018**, *10*, 118. [CrossRef]
16. Barui, S.; Cauda, V. Multimodal Decorations of Mesoporous Silica Nanoparticles for Improved Cancer Therapy. *Pharmaceutics* **2020**, *12*, 527. [CrossRef]
17. Lee, J.E.; Lee, N.; Kim, H.; Kim, J.; Choi, S.H.; Kim, J.H.; Kim, T.; Song, I.-C.; Park, S.P.; Moon, W.K.; et al. Uniform Mesoporous Dye-Doped Silica Nanoparticles Decorated with Multiple Magnetite Nanocrystals for Simultaneous Enhanced Magnetic Resonance Imaging, Fluorescence Imaging, and Drug Delivery. *J. Am. Chem. Soc.* **2010**, *132*, 552–557. [CrossRef]
18. Shin, S.-W.; Yang, K.; Lee, M.; Moon, J.; Son, A.; Kim, Y.; Choi, S.; Kim, D.-H.; Choi, C.; Lee, N.; et al. Manganese Ferrite Nanoparticles Enhance the Sensitivity of Hepa1-6 Hepatocellular Carcinoma to Radiation by Remodeling Tumor Microenvironments. *Int. J. Mol. Sci.* **2021**, *22*, 2637. [CrossRef]
19. Min, Y.; Roche, K.C.; Tian, S.; Eblan, M.J.; McKinnon, K.P.; Caster, J.; Chai, S.; Herring, L.E.; Zhang, L.; Zhang, T.; et al. Antigen-capturing nanoparticles improve the abscopal effect and cancer immunotherapy. *Nat. Nanotechnol.* **2017**, *12*, 877–882. [CrossRef]
20. Wang, X.; Li, X.; Yoshiyuki, K.; Watanabe, Y.; Sogo, Y.; Ohno, T.; Tsuji, N.M.; Ito, A. Comprehensive Mechanism Analysis of Mesoporous-Silica-Nanoparticle-Induced Cancer Immunotherapy. *Adv. Health Mater.* **2016**, *5*, 1169–1176. [CrossRef]
21. Hong, X.; Zhong, X.; Du, G.; Hou, Y.; Zhang, Y.; Zhang, Z.; Gong, T.; Zhang, L.; Sun, X. The pore size of mesoporous silica nanoparticles regulates their antigen delivery efficiency. *Sci. Adv.* **2020**, *6*, eaaz4462. [CrossRef]
22. Cha, B.G.; Jeong, J.H.; Kim, J. Extra-Large Pore Mesoporous Silica Nanoparticles Enabling Co-Delivery of High Amounts of Protein Antigen and Toll-like Receptor 9 Agonist for Enhanced Cancer Vaccine Efficacy. *ACS Central Sci.* **2018**, *4*, 484–492. [CrossRef]
23. Fehres, C.M.; Unger, W.W.J.; Egarcia-Vallejo, J.J.; Kooyk, Y.E. Understanding the Biology of Antigen Cross-Presentation for the Design of Vaccines Against Cancer. *Front. Immunol.* **2014**, *5*, 149. [CrossRef] [PubMed]
24. Schuler, G. Dendritic cells in cancer immunotherapy. *Eur. J. Immunol.* **2010**, *40*, 2123–2130. [CrossRef] [PubMed]
25. Jarosz-Biej, M.; Smolarczyk, R.; Cichoń, T.; Kulach, N. Tumor Microenvironment as A "Game Changer" in Cancer Radiotherapy. *Int. J. Mol. Sci.* **2019**, *20*, 3212. [CrossRef] [PubMed]
26. Comiskey, M.C.; Dallos, M.C.; Drake, C.G. Immunotherapy in Prostate Cancer: Teaching an Old Dog New Tricks. *Curr. Oncol. Rep.* **2018**, *20*, 75. [CrossRef] [PubMed]

27. Rizvi, N.A.; Hellmann, M.D.; Snyder, A.; Kvistborg, P.; Makarov, V.; Havel, J.J.; Lee, W.; Yuan, J.; Wong, P.; Ho, T.S.; et al. Mutational landscape determines sensitivity to PD-1 blockade in non–small cell lung cancer. *Science* **2015**, *348*, 124–128. [CrossRef] [PubMed]
28. Devi, K.S.P.; Anandasabapathy, N. The origin of DCs and capacity for immunologic tolerance in central and peripheral tissues. *Semin. Immunopathol.* **2016**, *39*, 137–152. [CrossRef]
29. Saxena, M.; van der Burg, S.H.; Melief, C.J.M.; Bhardwaj, N. Therapeutic cancer vaccines. *Nat. Rev. Cancer* **2021**, *21*, 360–378. [CrossRef]
30. Wang, Z.; Cao, Y.J. Adoptive Cell Therapy Targeting Neoantigens: A Frontier for Cancer Research. *Front. Immunol.* **2020**, *11*, 176. [CrossRef]
31. Garg, A.D.; Agostinis, P. Cell death and immunity in cancer: From danger signals to mimicry of pathogen defense responses. *Immunol. Rev.* **2017**, *280*, 126–148. [CrossRef]
32. Chen, Y.; Gao, M.; Huang, Z.; Yu, J.; Meng, X. SBRT combined with PD-1/PD-L1 inhibitors in NSCLC treatment: A focus on the mechanisms, advances, and future challenges. *J. Hematol. Oncol.* **2020**, *13*, 1–17. [CrossRef]
33. Tarn, D.; Ashley, C.E.; Xue, M.; Carnes, E.C.; Zink, J.I.; Brinker, C.J. Mesoporous Silica Nanoparticle Nanocarriers: Biofunctionality and Biocompatibility. *Accounts Chem. Res.* **2013**, *46*, 792–801. [CrossRef]
34. Iturrioz-Rodríguez, N.; A Correa-Duarte, M.; Fanarraga, M.L. Controlled drug delivery systems for cancer based on mesoporous silica nanoparticles. *Int. J. Nanomed.* **2019**, *14*, 3389–3401. [CrossRef] [PubMed]
35. Benezra, M.; Medina, O.P.; Zanzonico, P.B.; Schaer, D.; Ow, H.; Burns, A.; DeStanchina, E.; Longo, V.; Herz, E.; Iyer, S.; et al. Multimodal silica nanoparticles are effective cancer-targeted probes in a model of human melanoma. *J. Clin. Investig.* **2011**, *121*, 2768–2780. [CrossRef]

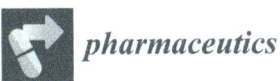

Article

Sulfonated Amphiphilic Poly(α)glutamate Amine—A Potential siRNA Nanocarrier for the Treatment of Both Chemo-Sensitive and Chemo-Resistant Glioblastoma Tumors

Adva Krivitsky [1], Sabina Pozzi [1], Eilam Yeini [1], Sahar Israeli Dangoor [1], Tal Zur [1], Sapir Golan [1], Vadim Krivitsky [2], Nitzan Albeck [1,3], Evgeny Pisarevsky [1], Paula Ofek [1], Asaf Madi [4] and Ronit Satchi-Fainaro [1,3,*]

1. Department of Physiology and Pharmacology, Sackler Faculty of Medicine, Tel Aviv University, Tel Aviv 69978, Israel; advashy@gmail.com (A.K.); sabina.pozzi26@gmail.com (S.P.); eilamyeini@gmail.com (E.Y.); sahardang@gmail.com (S.I.D.); kwaifeh@gmail.com (T.Z.); sapir5050@gmail.com (S.G.); nitzan.albeck@gmail.com (N.A.); jalchemic@gmail.com (E.P.); Paula.Ofek@gmail.com (P.O.)
2. School of Chemistry, The Raymond and Beverly Sackler Faculty of Exact Sciences, Tel Aviv University, Tel Aviv 69978, Israel; vadimkri777@gmail.com
3. Sagol School of Neuroscience, Tel Aviv University, Tel Aviv 69978, Israel
4. Department of Pathology, Sackler Faculty of Medicine, Tel Aviv University, Tel Aviv 69978, Israel; asafmadi@tauex.tau.ac.il
* Correspondence: ronitsf@tauex.tau.ac.il; Tel.: +972-3-6407427

Citation: Krivitsky, A.; Pozzi, S.; Yeini, E.; Israeli Dangoor, S.; Zur, T.; Golan, S.; Krivitsky, V.; Albeck, N.; Pisarevsky, E.; Ofek, P.; et al. Sulfonated Amphiphilic Poly(α)glutamate Amine—A Potential siRNA Nanocarrier for the Treatment of Both Chemo-Sensitive and Chemo-Resistant Glioblastoma Tumors. *Pharmaceutics* 2021, 13, 2199. https://doi.org/10.3390/pharmaceutics13122199

Academic Editors: Yu Seok Youn and Marina Santiago Franco

Received: 28 November 2021
Accepted: 15 December 2021
Published: 20 December 2021

Publisher's Note: MDPI stays neutral with regard to jurisdictional claims in published maps and institutional affiliations.

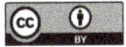

Copyright: © 2021 by the authors. Licensee MDPI, Basel, Switzerland. This article is an open access article distributed under the terms and conditions of the Creative Commons Attribution (CC BY) license (https://creativecommons.org/licenses/by/4.0/).

Abstract: Development of chemo-resistance is a major challenge in glioblastoma (GB) treatment. This phenomenon is often driven by increased activation of genes associated with DNA repair, such as the alkyl-removing enzyme O^6-methylguanine-DNA methyltransferase (MGMT) in combination with overexpression of canonical genes related to cell proliferation and tumor progression, such as Polo-like kinase 1 (Plk1). Hereby, we attempt to sensitize resistant GB cells using our established amphiphilic poly(α)glutamate (APA): small interfering RNA (siRNA) polyplexes, targeting Plk1. Furthermore, we improved brain-targeting by decorating our nanocarrier with sulfonate groups. Our sulfonated nanocarrier showed superior selectivity towards P-selectin (SELP), a transmembrane glycoprotein overexpressed in GB and angiogenic brain endothelial cells. Self-assembled polyplexes of sulfonated APA and siPlk1 internalized into GB cells and into our unique 3-dimensional (3D) GB spheroids inducing specific gene silencing. Moreover, our RNAi nanotherapy efficiently reduced the cell viability of both chemo-sensitive and chemo-resistant GB cells. Our developed sulfonated amphiphilic poly(α)glutamate nanocarrier has the potential to target siRNA to GB brain tumors. Our findings may strengthen the therapeutic applications of siRNA for chemo-resistant GB tumors, or as a combination therapy for chemo-sensitive GB tumors.

Keywords: nanocarrier; polyplexes; siRNA delivery; glioblastoma therapy; amphiphilic poly(α)glutamate; P-selectin

1. Introduction

Glioblastoma (GB) is the most common and the deadliest type of malignant primary brain tumor in adults, with an annual age-adjusted incidence rate of 4.4 per 100,000 population. GB patient prognosis is extremely poor, with a 5-year survival rate of only 5.5% [1]. The current treatment regimen includes maximal surgical resection, followed by radiation and chemotherapy with alkylating agents, such as temozolomide (TMZ) [2]. This regimen increases patients' median survival of 3 to 14 months [3,4]. Complete surgical removal is nearly impossible, due to the invasive nature of GB tumors; therefore, tumor relapse frequently occurs. Recurrence developed in more than 90% of patients within several years, and often displays enhanced resistance to initial chemotherapy treatment [5]. One of the most investigated mechanisms for TMZ chemotherapy-resistance in GB is the activation of the O^6-methylguanine–DNA methyltransferase (MGMT) enzyme. This enzyme, highly active in GB tumors, is responsible for removing the methyl group from the O^6 position in guanine nucleotides, thus resolving DNA damage induced following TMZ treatment. The lack of DNA methylation directs the cells to DNA damage repair and rescues them from apoptosis. The activity of the MGMT enzyme can be "switched off" by inducing methylation on the MGMT promoter itself. High levels of MGMT promoter methylation have been shown to correlate with prolonged survival in TMZ treated-GB patients [6]. Therefore, targeting the MGMT gene may sensitize tumor cells to TMZ and increase treatment efficiency in TMZ-resistant patients [7–9]. In order to investigate the naturally developed resistance towards TMZ, we have established a resistant clone of U251 human GB cells by culturing the U251 TMZ-sensitive cells (referred to in here as "U251") in the presence of increasing doses of TMZ for a period of over 6 months (referred to in here as TMZ resistant or "TMZ-R"). Nonetheless, treatments targeting alternative cellular pathways which can potentially overcome TMZ-resistance are still lacking. Gene therapy in general, and RNA therapies in particular, have emerged as a promising approach for the downregulation of oncogenic pathways in GB [10–13]. In particular, RNA interference (RNAi) is known for its ability to selectively silence upregulated genes at the mRNA level. Among the oncogene-activated pathways that sustain GB progression, we focused on Polo-like kinase 1 (Plk1), traditionally not linked to upregulation of TMZ-resistance genes, which may however attenuate GB aggressiveness and may provide an alternative to GB patients that do not respond to TMZ [14]. This serine/threonine kinase has a pronounced role in mitotic regulation and cell cycle progression. It is overexpressed in various cancers, including GB, and associated with poor prognosis and high risk of cancer metastasis [15–17]. We have previously shown that silencing the expression of Plk1 efficiently reduced tumor growth rate and prolonged survival of mice bearing ovarian cancer [18]. In addition, in a mouse model of pancreatic ductal adenocarcinoma (PDAC), Plk1 silencing was shown to synergize with microRNA 34a (miR-34a), via the downregulation of the activated pathway, resulting in tumor growth inhibition [19]. Systemic delivery of RNAi is known to be challenging since short oligonucleotides (OLN) are subjected to rapid renal clearance, degradation while circulating in the body, poor cellular penetration, short half-life, and aggregation in the blood [20–22]. In order to overcome these hurdles, a delivery system needs to be developed. Using a well-designed nanocarrier enabled enhanced tumor accumulation, taking advantage of the enhanced permeability and retention (EPR) effect [23,24]. This phenomenon, observed in the tumor vasculature, is defined by high permeability which allows extravasation of macromolecules, as opposed to the tightly bound healthy endothelium. Furthermore, impaired lymphatic drainage associated with cancer may increase drugs accumulation [23]. We have previously developed a polymeric nanocarrier based on poly(α)glutamic acid (PGA), a biodegradable and water-soluble polymer further modified with physiologically-protonated amine groups. Electrostatic-based complexation with the negatively-charged siRNA formed a defined population of nanoparticles with the ability to internalize into cancer cells via endocytosis [25] and induce gene silencing [26]. Furthermore, we introduced a modification with alkyl groups forming inner hydrophobic core exposing the positively-charged moieties outwards in a micellar-like structure [26,27]. Our active polymeric micelles demonstrated biocompatibility and preferential accumulation in several tumor types when systemically injected, leading to an anticancer therapeutic effect. Furthermore, these micelles selectively delivered siRNA to mammary adenocarcinoma tumors without accumulating in the liver and crossed the dense stroma of PDAC, internalizing into tumor cells and achieving silencing of the target [19]. However, delivery of drugs to the central nervous system (CNS) is extremely difficult since the brain is protected by a highly selective mechanism of capillaries, called the blood–brain barrier (BBB) [28]. Even though brain tumors often display compromised BBB and permeable endothelium, the latter varies with tumor type, location, and prior treatment [29]. The inflamed cerebral endothelium often expresses P-selectin (SELP) protein, a transmembrane adhesive glycoprotein that facilitates leukocytes and platelets adhesion [30]. We have previously shown that SELP enhances GB progression by promoting tumor cell proliferation and invasion and immunosuppression via microglia/macrophages anti-inflammatory polarization [31,32]. Recently, we have shown that targeting SELP by the addition of sulfonate moieties on dendritic polyglycerol nanocarrier facilitated nanoparticles accumulation into tumors and enhanced the anticancer activity of Paclitaxel (PTX) in a mouse model of GB [33]. Therefore, we have modified our previously designed amphiphilic poly(α)glutamate amine (APA) [19,27] with sulfonate groups, in order to mimic the tyrosine sulfate moieties of P-selectin glycoprotein ligand-1 (PSGL-1), the natural ligand of SELP [34], and improve drug targeting to the brain. This chemical modification resulted in increased accumulation of the polyplexes into 3D spheroids of U251 TMZ-sensitive or -resistant cells, compared to untargeted nanocarrier. These results highlight the great potential of our nanocarrier as a parenteral injectable, non-toxic, and efficient delivery vehicle for siRNA, now being evaluated for its potential in reaching brain tumors and reducing GB tumorigenesis. We hypothesize that our treatment can serve as combination therapy for chemo-resistant and chemo-sensitive GB tumors.

2. Materials and Methods

2.1. Materials

All chemicals and solvents were A.R. or HPLC grade. Chemical reagents were purchased from Merck (White House Station, NJ, USA) and Sigma–Aldrich (St. Louis, MO, USA). O-benzyl protected glutamic acid (H-Glu(OBzl)-OH) was purchased from Chemimpex (Dillon Drive, IL, USA). HPLC grade solvents were purchased from BioLab (Jerusalem, Israel). Dulbecco's modified Eagle medium (DMEM) and fetal bovine serum (FBS) were purchased from Gibco (Crofton Rd, Dún Laoghaire, Dublin, Ireland). All other tissue culture reagents were purchased from Biological Industries Ltd. (Kibbutz Beit Haemek, Israel). MGMT siRNA (siMGMT) was purchased from Ambion (Invitrogen, Waltham, MA, USA). Plk1 siRNA (siPlk1) and green fluorescent protein (GFP) siRNA (siGFP) were purchased from Biospring (Frankfurt am Main, Germany). Cy5-labeled negative control siRNA (Cy5-siNC) was purchased from Sigma–Aldrich (St. Louis, MO, USA). TMZ was purchased from Petrus chemicals (Herzeliya, Israel).

2.2. Cell Culture

Glioblastoma (GB) cell lines. Human U251 cells were purchased from the European Collection of Authenticated Cell Cultures (ECACC). Murine GL261 cells were purchased from the National Cancer Institute (Frederick, MD, USA). All GB cells were cultured in DMEM supplemented with 10% FBS, 100 µg/mL of streptomycin, 12.5 U/mL of nystatin, 100 U/mL of penicillin, and 2 mM of L-glutamine. All cells were tested for mycoplasma with a mycoplasma detection kit (Biological Industries Ltd., Beit Haemek, Israel). Cells were grown at 37 °C; 5% CO_2.

2.2.1. Establishment of mCherry and iRFP Stably-Expressing U251 Cells

mCherry/iRFP infecting viral particles were produced as described previously [35,36]. Briefly, HEK 293T cells were transfected with pQC mCherry [35] and with the compatible packaging plasmids pCMV-VSV-G (#8454, Addgene, Watertown, MA, USA) and pUMVC (#8449, Addgene, Watertown, MA, USA), or with pLVX-iRFP [37] together with pCMV-VSV-G (#8454, Addgene, Watertown, MA, USA) and psPAX2 (#12260, Addgene, Watertown, MA, USA). Viral particle-containing media were collected after 48 h. For cell infection, U251 cells were incubated with viral particles and polybrene (8 µg/mL) (hexadimethrine bromide) for 8–16 h prior medium replacement. Following 48 h, mCherry-infected cells were selected by puromycin and iRFP infected cells by hygromycin.

2.2.2. Establishment of mCherry U251 Chemo-Resistant Cell Line (U251 TMZ-R)

U251 cells were cultured with increasing doses of temozolomide (TMZ 1 µM to 10 µM) over a period of 6 months.

2.3. IC$_{50}$ Determination Assay

U251 or U251 TMZ-R cells were plated onto 96-well plates at a density of 2.5×10^4 cells/well. Twenty-four hours later, cells were treated with TMZ at increasing concentrations (0.001–1000 µM). Following 5 days, cells were counted using Beckman Coulter counter (Beckman Coulter Life Sciences, Indianapolis, IN, USA). Results are presented as the percentage of confluence compared to untreated cells.

2.4. RNA Isolation and Quantitative Real-Time RT-PCR (qRT-PCR)

RNA was isolated using EZ-RNA II total RNA isolation kit (Biological Industries, Kibbutz Beit Haemek, Israel) according to the manufacturer's protocol. Actin was used for normalization as a house-keeping gene. Primers used: PLK1 FOR:5′-CACAGTTTCGAGGTGG ATGT-3′, PLK1 REV:5′-ATCCGGAGGTAGGTCTCTTT-3′. MGMT FOR:5′-GTTTGCGACTT GGTACTTGG-3′, MGMT REV:5′-TGCCCAGGAGCTTTATTTCG-3′. Actin FOR: 5′-CCAAC CGCGAGAAGATGA-3′, Actin REV: 5′-CCAGAGGCGTACAGGGATAG-3′.

2.5. Animal Models

In order to assess Plk1 and SELP expression in GB tumors by histology, 6-week-old male SCID mice (Envigo CRS, Ness-Ziona, Israel) were anesthetized by ketamine (150 mg/kg) and xylazine (12 mg/kg) injected intraperitoneally (IP). Then, iRFP-labeled U251 human GB cells (5×10^4 cells) were stereotactically implanted into the brain striatum (N = 10) as previously described [32]. Tumor development was followed by MRI (MR Solutions Ltd., Guildford, UK) and Maestro™ imaging system (CRI Inc., Woburn, MA, USA) as previously described [10].

Animals Ethics Statement

Animals were housed in the Tel Aviv University animal facility. All experiments received ethical approval by the animal care and use committee (IACUC) of Tel Aviv University (approval no. 01-19-097, Approval and expiry dates 15 December 2019–15 December 2023) and conducted in accordance with NIH guidelines.

2.6. Frozen OCT Tissue Fixation

Tumor-bearing mice were anesthetized by IP injection of ketamine (100 mg/kg) and xylazine (12 mg/kg), followed by PBS perfusion and 4% paraformaldehyde (PFA). Brains were harvested, then incubated with 4% PFA for 4 h and with 0.5 M of sucrose (BioLab Ltd., Jerusalem, Israel) for 1 h, and 1 M of sucrose for overnight (ON). Brains were embedded in optimal cutting temperature (OCT) compound (Scigen, Thermo Fisher Scientific, Waltham, MA, USA) on dry ice, then stored at $-80\ °C$.

2.7. Immunostaining

OCT-embedded tumor samples were cryo-sectioned (5 µm thick sections), and stained using BOND RX autostainer (Leica Microsystems, Wetzlar, Germany). Cryo-sections were immunostained for: Plk1- using rabbit anti-human/mouse Plk1 antibody (Cat. No. BS-3535R dilution 1:50, Bioss Antibodies, Woburn, MA, USA) and Alexa Fluor 488-goat anti-rabbit secondary antibody (Cat. No. ab150077, dilution 1:300, Abcam, Cambridge, UK); SELP- using mouse anti-human SELP antibody (Cat. No. BBA1, Clone BBIG-E, dilution 1:30, R&D systems, McKinley, MN, USA) and Alexa Fluor 568-goat anti-mouse secondary antibody (Cat. No. ab175473, dilution 1:300, Abcam, Cambridge, UK). Slides were blocked by incubating with 10% goat serum in PBS containing 0.02% Tween-20, for 30 min. Then, slides were incubated with primary antibodies for 1 h, washed, and incubated with secondary antibodies for 1 h at room temperature. Then, slides were washed using BOND Wash Solution (Leica Microsystems, Wetzlar, Germany) and treated with ProLong® Gold mounting with DAPI (Thermo Fisher Scientific, Waltham, MA, USA). Then slides were covered with coverslips. Images were obtained using the EVOS FL Auto cell imaging system (Thermo Fisher Scientific, Waltham, MA, USA).

2.8. Survival Analysis Based on TCGA Data

For survival analysis we used OSgbm, which assesses the prognostic value of our selected genes [38]. Briefly, OSgbm contains 684 samples with transcriptome profiles and clinical information from The Cancer Genome Atlas (TCGA), Gene Expression Omnibus (GEO), and Chinese Glioma Genome Atlas (CGGA). Survival analysis data were presented by Kaplan–Meier (KM) plot with hazard ratio (HR) and log-rank p value.

2.9. Synthesis of APA-Sulfonate (APAS)

APA was synthesized by conjugating ethylenediamine and hexylamine groups to a poly(α)glutamate backbone via the pending carboxylic acid moieties as was previously described [19,27]. To a solution of APA (130 mg, 0.592 mmol per monomer) in dry dimethylformamide (DMF) (5 mL), tributylamine was added (270 µL, 1.14 mmol, 1.93 equiv. per monomer), and the reaction was left to stir for 20 min. Then, the reaction mixture was stirred for 1.5 h at 25 °C, under Argon atmosphere ($Ar_{(g)}$). Propanesultone (20 µL, 0.237 mmol, 0.4 equiv. per monomer) was added, and the reaction was left to stir for ON under $Ar_{(g)}$. DMF was removed under vacuum. The remaining residue was suspended in water (30 mL). pH was adjusted to 3.0 with HCl, and the remaining solution was dialyzed against water (8 L), freeze-dried, and lyophilized to obtain a white powder at a yield of 70%.

2.10. Multi-Angle Static Light Scattering (MALS)

The molecular weight of APA was determined using Agilent 1200 series HPLC system (Agilent Technologies Santa Clara, CA, USA), equipped with a multi-angle light scattering detector (Wyatt Technology, Santa Barbara, CA, USA). APA was separated using Kw404-4F column (Showa Denko America Inc., New York, NY, USA) and a mixture of 0.5 M AcOH in ACN: double distilled water (DDW) 4:6 ($v/v\%$) as a mobile phase. Sample was prepared at a concentration of 4 mg/mL in the mobile phase buffer, then filtered using a 0.2-µm filter prior to the analysis. Sample was ran at a flow of 0.5 mL/min. Molecular weight (Mw) was analyzed using the ASTRA software (Wyatt Technology, Santa Barbara, CA, USA).

2.11. Scanning Electron Microscope (SEM)

APA:siPlk1 sample was prepared in DDW at 0.1 mg/mL concentration (APA equiv.). The sample was dropped on a silicon wafer and allowed to dry. SEM images were obtained using Quanta 200 FEG Environmental SEM (FEI, Hillsboro, OR, USA) at high vacuum and 3.0 KV. Images were collected using secondary electrons detector.

2.12. Dynamic Light Scattering (DLS) and Phase Analysis Light Scattering (PALS)

Samples were prepared at a polymer concentration of 0.1 mg/mL in 15 mM of HEPES. Size and zeta potential measurements were made with a Mobius DLS/PALS instrument (Wyatt Technology, Santa Barbara, CA, USA). Sixty µL of the sample was loaded into the dip cell. Data were analyzed according to the isotropic sphere method, and were measured as intensity distribution. Average values were calculated based on 3–5 independent measurements. All measurements were performed at 25 °C.

2.13. Elemental Analysis (EDS)

APA and APAS samples were prepared in DDW at a concentration of 10 mg/mL, then, dropped on a silicon wafer, allowed to dry, and dropped again several times. EDS was performed by an LN Oxford thin window detector of 138 eV resolution and ISIS software using Quanta 200 FEG Environmental SEM (FEI, Hillsboro, OR, USA) at high vacuum and 20.0 KV.

2.14. Proliferation Assay

U251 and U251 TMZ-R cells were plated onto 96-well plates at densities of 7.5×10^4 and 5×10^4 cells/well, respectively. Twenty four hours later, cells were treated with APA:siPlk1 or APA:siGFP at 5 N/P ratio and 250/500 nM. Following 20 h, cells were imaged using IncuCyte ZOOM™ (Satorius, Goettingen, Germany). Red channel images were taken using a 10× objective. Results were calculated by the IncuCyte™ Software. Results were presented as confluence percentage compared with untreated cells.

2.15. Multicellular Tumor Spheroids (MCTS)

MCTS were prepared from GL261 cells, mCherry-labeled U251, or U251 TMZ-R cells by a modified hanging-drop method [33]. Briefly, cells were seeded in droplets (2500 cells/25 µL for staining/internalization assay and 8000 cells/25 µL for flow cytometry analysis) in 4:1 DMEM:methylcellulose. Following 72 h, spheroids were embedded in Cultrex® Reduced Growth Factor Basement Membrane Matrix (R&D systems, McKinley, MN, USA) and incubated for 48 h. The matrix was then dissolved using Cell Recovery Solution (Corning, Watertown, NY, USA) and spheroids were transferred to Eppendorf tubes for further treatment with APA:Cy5-siRNA, APAS:Cy5-siRNA, or Cy5-siRNA alone. For SELP staining, spheroids were incubated with mouse anti-human SELP primary antibody for ON (Cat. No. BBA1, Clone BBIG-E, dilution 1:50, R&D systems, McKinley, MN, USA), then washed and incubated with mouse IgG kappa binding protein (m-IgGκ BP) conjugated to CruzFluor™ 488 (CFL 488) (Cat. No. sc-516176, dilution 1:300, Santa Cruz Biotechnology Inc., Dallas, TX, USA) secondary antibody for 3 h. SELP inhibitor (KF38789, Cat. No. 2748, Tocris BioScience, Bristol, UK) was added 1 h prior to treatment at a concentration of 2 µM to the relevant tubes. For confocal imaging, spheroids were collected, washed, fixed with 4% PFA in PBS solution, and mounted on coverslips. The Leica SP8 imaging system (Leica Microsystems, Wetzlar, Germany) was used for imaging. For FACS analysis, recovered spheroids were dismantled to create a single-cell suspension. Cells were incubated with mouse anti-human SELP primary antibody (BBA1, R&D) for 1 h on ice. Then, cells were washed and incubated with mouse IgG kappa binding protein (m-IgGκ BP) conjugated to CruzFluor™ 488 (CFL 488) (sc-516176, Santa Cruz Biotechnology, Inc., Dallas, TX, USA) for 1 h on ice. Cells were then washed with PBS supplemented with 5 mM of EDTA, 1% sodium azide, and 1% FBS. Fluorescent intensity was analyzed by flow cytometry using Attune NxT cytometer (Thermo Fisher Scientific, Waltham, MA, USA) and analyzed by Kaluza 2.1 software (Beckman Coulter, Brea, CA, USA).

2.16. SELP Expression in 3D vs. 2D Cell Culture

To assess SELP expression, iRFP-labeled U251 GB cells were grown in 10-cm^2 petri-dish (1×10^6 cells) or as 3D spheroids (as detailed above in the MCTS section) for 48 h. Cells from 2D cell culture were harvested using a cell scraper, whereas cell suspension from 3D spheroids was obtained by matrix digestion using Cell Recovery Solution, as previously described. SELP expression was evaluated using flow cytometry analysis as described above.

2.17. Infra-Red Spectroscopy

ATR-IR spectroscopy was performed using TENSOR 27 spectrometer (BRUKER, Billerica, MA, USA).

2.18. Electrophoretic Shift Assay (EMSA)

Evaluation of polymer:siRNA complexation at N/P ratios between 1 and 25 was performed by mixing 50 pmol of siRNA and APA/APAS polymers at different concentrations in DDW and incubate for 20 min at room temperature. Mobility of free and nanocarrier-complexed siRNA was then analyzed by agarose-gel electrophoresis.

2.19. Western Blot

Cells were seeded in 6-well plates at a density of 3×10^5 cells/well. After 24 h, cells were treated with 100 nM of siRNA-equivalent dose. Following 48 h, cells were harvested and lysed using NP40 reagent. Lysates were loaded and ran into a 12% acrylamide gel under 120 V for ~2 h. Proteins were transferred to nitrocellulose membrane under a current of 250 mA for 2 h. The nitrocellulose membrane was blocked with 5% skim milk in TBST

(15 mM of NaCl, 1 mM of Trisma base, pH = 8.0, 0.1% Tween 20) for 1 h, and incubated with rabbit MT3.1 anti-MGMT antibody (Abcam, Cambridge, UK) (1:1000 in TBST), or mouse anti-HSC 70 antibody (Cat. Sc-7298, Clone B6, Santa Cruz Biotechnology, Dallas, TX, USA) (1:40,000 in TBST) ON at 4 °C. Secondary horseradish peroxidase (HRP)-conjugated goat anti-rabbit, or goat anti-mouse antibodies (Jackson Immunoresearch, Baltimore, PA, USA; Abcam, Cambridge, UK) were incubated with nitrocellulose membrane at 1:10,000 in TBST for 1 h. Blots were developed using Westar Supernova ECL kit (Cyanagen, Bologna, Italy) in accordance with the manufacturer's protocol.

2.20. H-Nuclear Magnetic Resonance (NMR)

APA/APAS samples were dissolved in deuterium oxide. NMR spectroscopy was obtained using 400 MHz Avance, (Bruker, Billerica, MA, USA).

2.21. Internalization of APA/APAS:Cy5-siRNA Polyplexes into U251 Cells (2D)

Cells were seeded (5×10^4 cells/well) on 13-mm cover glasses in a 24-well plate and incubated for 24 h. Cells were treated with 100 nM of siRNA-equivalent concentration alone or complexed with APA/APAS for 20 min, then washed several times with PBS, fixed with 4% PFA for 30 min at room temperature, and washed with PBS again. Cells were then mounted on slides using ProLong®® Gold antifade reagent with DAPI (Thermo Fisher Scientific, Waltham, MA, USA). Internalization was followed using Leica SP8 confocal imaging systems (X60 Magnification) (Leica Microsystems GmbH, Wetzlar, Germany).

2.22. Statistical Analysis

Data were presented as mean ± standard deviation (represented graphically as error bars). Statistical significance was analyzed by Student's *t*-test.

3. Results and Discussion

3.1. TMZ-Induced Resistance in U251 GB Cells Enhances MGMT mRNA Levels but Does Not Alter Plk1 mRNA Levels

To establish a correlation between the expression levels of MGMT or Plk1 and GB patient's survival, we obtained data from the OSgbm database [38]. Survival data of 684 GB patients (25% long term and 25% short term survivors) revealed that high expression of both MGMT and Plk1 significantly correlated with short-term survival, while low expression of both proteins significantly correlated with long-term survival of GB patients (Figure 1A). In order to investigate the expression levels of these two proteins in the context of TMZ-resistance, we first evaluated the establishment of a TMZ- resistant (U251 TMZ-R) clone. Hence, the proliferation assay performed on U251 and U251 TMZ-R cells showed that cell viability was reduced to 50% following 72 h incubation with 30 and 300 µM TMZ in U251 and U251 TMZ-R cells, respectively (Figure 1B,C). Furthermore, the expression levels of MGMT and Plk1 mRNA in both U251 and the U251 TMZ-R clone were evaluated by real-time qPCR (Figure 1D). The obtained results confirmed that in comparison to parental U251, TMZ-R cells express significantly higher levels of MGMT, while Plk1's expression remained unchanged following the acquirement of TMZ resistance. Therefore, we concluded that the inhibition of Plk1 could be an additional and attractive strategy to use in combination with TMZ in order to improve the survival of GB patients, whether sensitive or resistant to chemotherapy. Figure 1D shows low expression of MGMT in U251 compared with U251 TMZ-R cells (~230-fold change), while Plk1 expression in both cell lines was similar. Furthermore, cryosection of U251 tumors, obtained in intracranially injected SCID mice, confirmed the expression of Plk1 in our GB mouse model (Figure 1E).

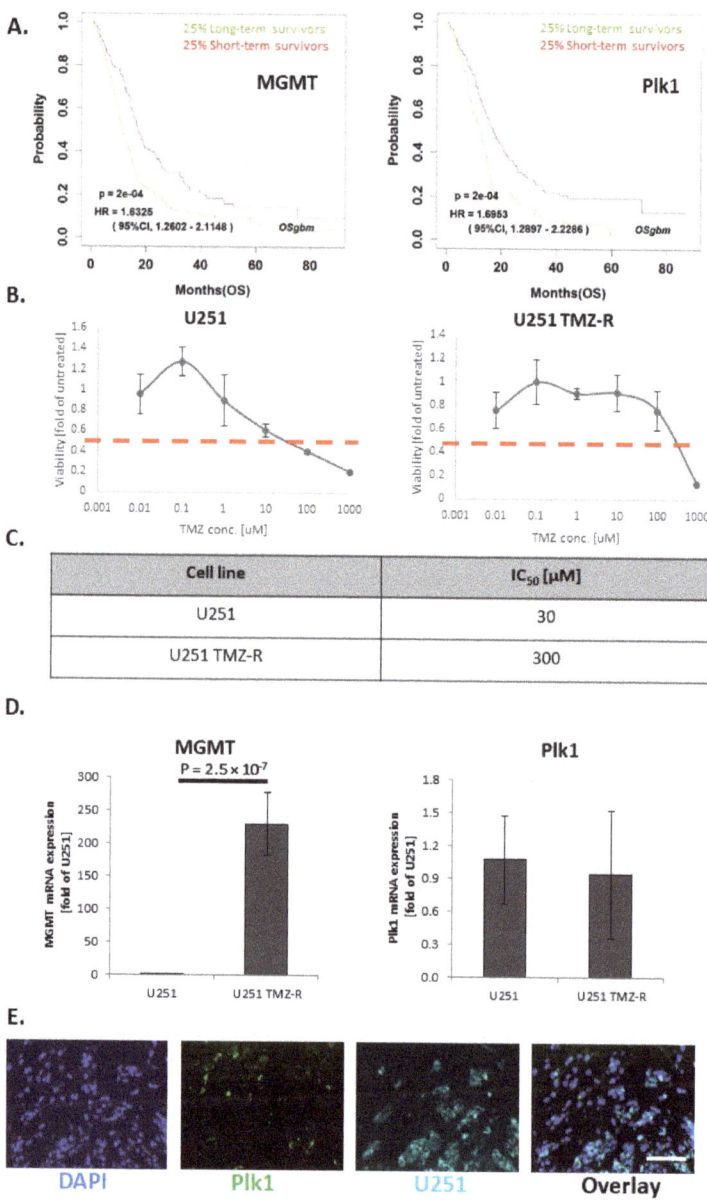

Figure 1. The development of resistance to TMZ enhances MGMT expression without altering Plk1 oncogene levels in GB. (**A**) Survival analysis performed on OSgbm database comparing MGMT expression (left panel) and Plk1 expression (right panel) of the top 25% longest GB survivors versus the bottom 25% shortest survivors. (**B**) Inhibitory concentration 50% (IC_{50}) plot of parental U251 glioblastoma cells vs. TMZR clone. (**C**) Table summarizing the IC_{50} of wild-type U251 cells versus U251 TMZ-R cells. (**D**) TMZ resistance in U251 occurred via upregulation of MGMT, without changing Plk1 levels. (**E**) Intracranial U251 GB tumors show Plk1 expression (scale = 100 μm).

3.2. APA:siPlk1 Complexes Efficiently Silence Plk1 Expression in Both U251 and U251 TMZ-R Cells

RNAi therapeutics have the potential to silence "undruggable targets" such as Plk1. To overcome the multiple barriers associated with RNAi delivery, we used our previously published APA RNAi nanocarrier [19,27]. MALS analysis showed APA bears the Mw of 17,870 g/mol, ascribed to 70 repeating units, and have Mw/Mn of 1.29 (Figure 2A). APA was complexed with Plk1 siRNA at N/P ratio of 5, to yield a main population of nanoparticles with a hydrodynamic diameter of 133 ± 7 nm (79.3 ± 1.15% of the nanoparticles by intensity distribution) and an almost neutral zeta potential of 0.75 ± 0.97 mV (Figure 2C, Supplementary Materials Figure S1). Furthermore, the polydispersity index (PDI) of this main population was narrow (0.05 ± 0.005). SEM images of the dry droplet of complexes matched the DLS diameter (110 ± 15 nm) and showed spherical morphology. Similar properties were exhibited by APA:siGFP polyplexes, used in this study as a negative control. The hydrodynamic diameter of the main population (82.6 ± 12.5%) of APA:siGFP polyplexes was 115 ± 32 nm, and its zeta potential was 0.52 ± 0.17 mV (Supplementary Materials Figure S1B,C). Polyplexes at the size range of ~10–150 nm were previously shown to benefit from selective accumulation at the tumor site due to the EPR effect [10,18,36]. Elemental analysis of APA:siPlk1 and APA:siGFP polyplexes confirmed that both complexes contained similar weight percentages of nitrogen and phosphorus (15.14 ± 3.14% of nitrogen and 2.8 ± 0.15% phosphorus in APA:siPlk1 and 13.29 ± 3.02% of nitrogen and 3.11 ± 0.2% phosphorus in APA:siGFP, respectively) (Supplementary Materials Figure S1D). These data verified the fact that the same N/P ratio was used for the two polyplexes to treat GB cells. The ability of APA:siPlk1 polyplexes to induce specific gene silencing in both U251 and U251 TMZ-R cells was evaluated at the mRNA level by RT-PCR. Cells were treated with APA:siPlk1, APA:siGFP, or siPlk1 alone at a concentration of 100 nM siRNA for 48 h. APA:siPlk1 reduced Plk1 mRNA level by ~95% in U251 cells and by ~90% in U251 TMZ-R cells compared to untreated cells, while siPlk1 alone did not induce any silencing in both cell lines examined. APA:siGFP did not significantly reduce Plk1 mRNA levels, showing ~35% and ~13% silencing in U251 and U251 TMZ-R cells, respectively (Figure 2D).

3.3. Treatment with APA:siPlk1 Polyplexes Reduces the Viability of Both U251 Cells and U251 TMZ-R Clone

Next, the effect of treatment with APA:siPlk1 polyplexes on the viability of U251 and U251 TMZ-R cells was evaluated. Cells were treated with APA:siPlk1, APA:siGFP, or siPlk1 alone at siRNA concentrations of 100, 250, and 500 nM for 20 h. Representative images at 20 h are presented (Figure 3A), and bar graphs of cell viability are presented (Figure 3B). While treating U251 and U251 TMZ-R with 100 nM APA:siPlk1, APA:siGFP polyplexes, or siPlk1 alone, did not affect the viability of the cells, 250 nM of APA:siPlk1 polyplexes reduced the viability of U251 and TMZ-R cells by ~40%. On the other hand, treating U251 and U251 TMZ-R with 250 nM APA:siGFP or siPlk1 alone did not cause any cell toxicity. When U251 and U251 TMZ-R cells were exposed to 500 nM of APA:siPlk1 polyplexes, the viability of U251 and U251 TMZ-R cells was reduced by ~80% compared to untreated cells, while siPlk1 alone did not affect the cell viability. Nonetheless, such a high concentration of APA:siGFP polyplexes induced cell toxicity, therefore reducing the cell viability by ~70% and ~60% in U251 and U251 TMZ-R, respectively, compared to untreated cells. The specific and selective activity of APA:siPlk1 polyplexes at 250 nM siRNA equivalent treatment dose demonstrated to be an efficient treatment that affected the proliferation of GB cells.

A.

	Mn [g/mol]	Mw/Mn	DP
APA	17,870	1.29	70

B.

C.

	N/P	Diameter by DLS [nm, Mean ± SD]	PDI [Mean ± SD]	Zeta potential [mV, Mean ± SD]	Diameter by SEM [nm, Mean ± SD]
APA:siPlk1	5	133 ± 7	0.05 ± 0.005	0.75 ± 0.97	110 ± 15

D.

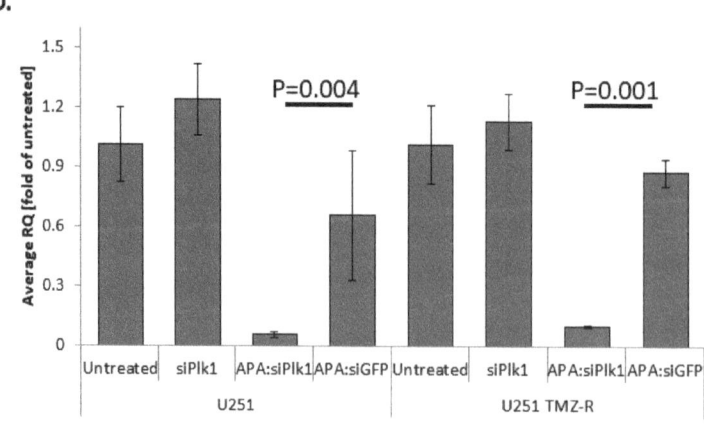

Figure 2. Physico-chemical characteristics and silencing activity of APA:siPlk1 polyplexes. (**A**) Table summarizing the Mw (Mn), PDI (Mw/Mn), and theoretical degree of polymerization (DP) as obtained by multi-angle light scattering (MALS). (**B**) Scanning electron microscope (SEM) image of the dry droplet of polyplexes (scale = 500 nm). (**C**) Table summarizing the hydrodynamic diameter, polydispersity index (PDI) and zeta potential of the main population of polyplexes, obtained by Mobius and PALS instruments, and the average diameter obtained by SEM. (**D**) Specific mRNA silencing obtained by RT-PCR, performed on U251 and U251 TMZ-R GB cells following treatment with APA:siPlk1 polyplexes.

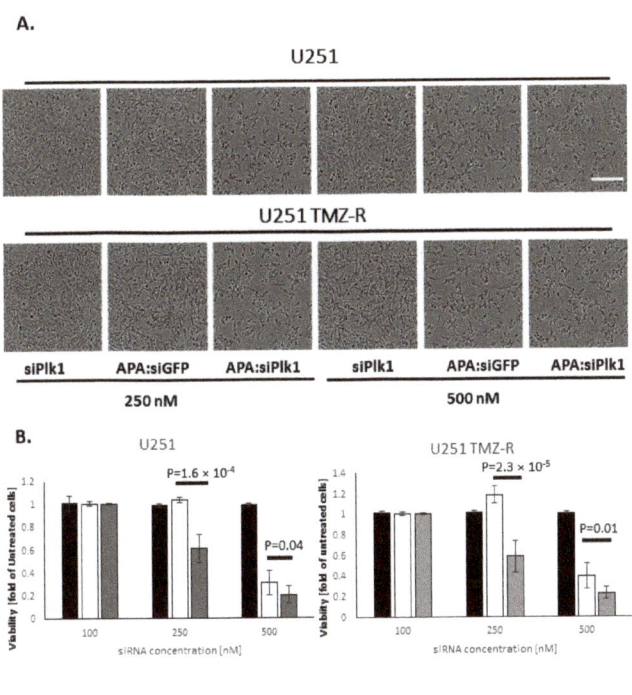

Figure 3. APA:siPlk1 treatment reduced the viability of U251 and U251 TMZ-R cells. (**A**) Representative phase-contrast images of the cells following 20 h of treatment. (**B**) Bar graph of cells viability following 20 h of treatment based on red-channel images (scale = 20 μm).

3.4. SELP Is Expressed on the Membranes of GB Cells and Represents a Suitable Candidate for Active Targeting for the Delivery of siRNA Polyplexes

SELP was previously found to be upregulated on both GB tumors and inflamed cerebral endothelium at the tumor site, as opposed to its basal expression in healthy brain tissue. Aiming to optimize our APA:siPlk1 by the addition of active targeting, we evaluated the relevance of targeting SELP using U251 GB cells. We first assessed the expression of SELP in U251 and U251 TMZ-R GB spheroids, and in U251 tumor slices (Figure 4). Immunostaining of SELP in U251 and U251 TMZ-R spheroids demonstrated that 3D cultures of GB cells expressed SELP (Figure 4A). Interestingly, flow cytometry analysis for SELP on spheroids of U251 and U251 TMZ-R revealed slightly higher expression of SELP in the TMZ-R cells (34% in U251 compared with 39% positive cells in U251 TMZ-R clone). These findings suggest that targeting SELP would be effective for GB tumors, whether sensitive or resistant to chemotherapy (Figure 4B). Furthermore, flow cytometry analysis for SELP expression in U251 cells grown in 2D monolayer or 3D spheroids demonstrated a remarkable increased expression of SELP in the 3D culture (Supplementary Materials Figure S2A). This highlights the importance and the relevance of using SELP as active targeting for the delivery of our polyplexes to GB tumors [28]. The BBB represents a challenge for the delivery of drugs to the brain. Hence, targeting SELP that is normally expressed on brain endothelium and is upregulated in cancer can facilitate accumulation in GB tumors, as previously observed [33]. Furthermore, the expression of SELP in in vivo settings was validated on slices of U251 intracranial tumors resected from SCID mice (Figure 4C, Supplementary Materials Figure S2B). Immunostaining demonstrated high expression of SELP, nearby to the expression of both the endothelial marker CD31 (Supplementary

Materials Figure S2B) and Plk1 (Figure 4C), emphasizing the rationale for targeting SELP in combination with specific Plk1-downregulating therapeutic modality.

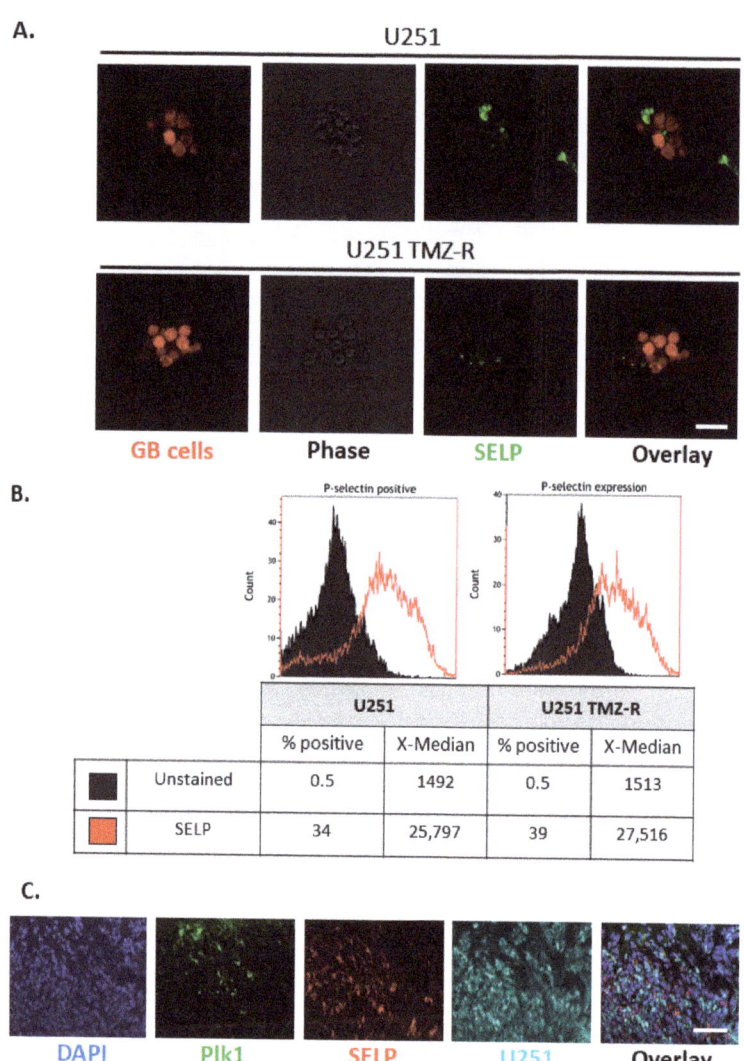

Figure 4. SELP expression on U251 and U251 TMZ-R 3D spheroids. (**A**) Imaged by confocal microscopy (scale = 20 μm) and (**B**) analyzed by fluorescence activated cell sorting (FACS). (**C**) SELP expression on slices of U251 intracranial tumors and co-localization with Plk1 (scale = 100 μm).

3.5. Sulfonation of Amphiphilic Poly(α)glutamate Amine (APA)

In order to improve the delivery of our polyplexes to brain tumors, APA was conjugated with sulfonate groups. These groups were shown before to enhance brain uptake and to accumulate in GB tumors due to mimicry of the natural ligand of SELP [33]. APA was modified with sulfonate groups using propanesultone reagent (Figure 5A). Ten equivalents of base (tributylamine) per propanesultone were required for the substitution of 15% of the amine groups. The product was characterized by ^{1}H-NMR and the addition of sulfonate groups was validated by the appearance of 2 peaks at the regions of 3.6 and 2.9 ppm

(Figure 5B). Furthermore, infrared (IR) spectrum demonstrated the addition of a band at the region of 1000–1050 cm^{-1} characteristic to sulfonic acid group [39] (Supplementary Materials Figure S3). Elemental analysis approved sulfonation ratio of ~15%, corresponding to Sulfur weight % of 1.53 ± 0.07, while APA did not have a detectable amount of Sulfur (0.04 ± 0.04, Figure 5C).

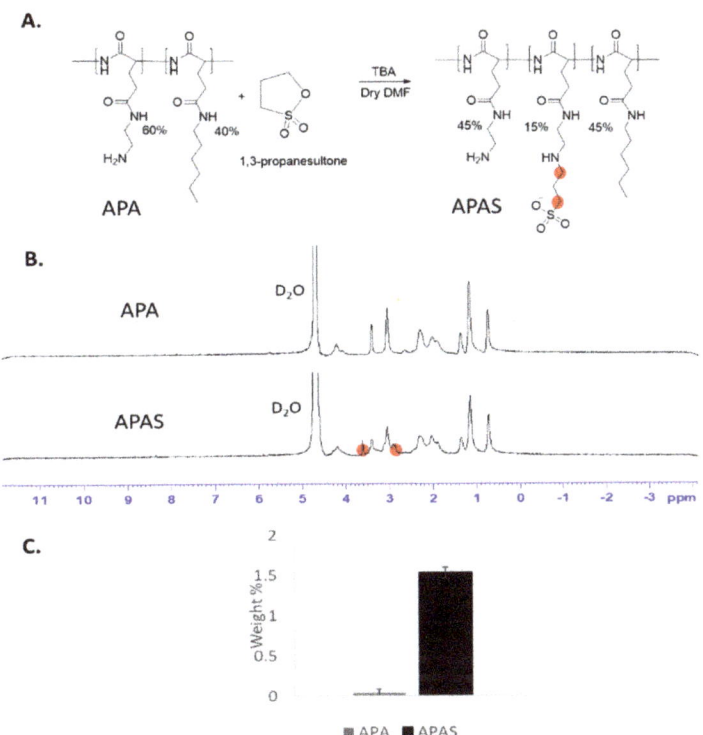

Figure 5. Synthesis and characterization of APAS. (**A**) Modification of APA with sulfonate groups using propanesultone. (**B**) ^{1}H-NMR spectrum of APA and APAS in D$_2$O. (**C**) Elemental analysis demonstrating the weight percent of Sulfur (S) in dry samples of APA and APAS, as obtained by energy-dispersive X-ray spectroscopy (EDS) analysis.

3.6. APAS forms Active Complexes with siRNA and Enables Silencing of GB-Relevant Genes

We further evaluated complexes formed by self-assembly of APAS and siRNA and compared them with APA:siRNA polyplexes. Hence, we complexed either APA or APAS polymers with siRNA at increasing N/P ratios. Complexes were loaded on an agarose gel supplemented with ethidium bromide, and allowed to run under 100 V for 15 min. Retardation of migration of the free siRNA following neutralization of its negative charge by complexing with the positively charged polymer was evaluated under UV light (Figure 6A). As shown, while APA neutralized the charge of siRNA already at N/P ratio of 5, a higher N/P ratio was required to complex siRNA in the case of APAS. Full complexation between APAS and siRNA was shown only at N/P ratio of 15, due to the extra negative charge of sulfonate groups in physiological pH. Therefore, polyplexes at N/P ratio of 15 were selected for additional characterization and silencing evaluation (Figure 6B,C, Supplementary Materials Figure S4). DLS measurements demonstrated a hydrodynamic diameter of 113 ± 35 nm (80.3 ± 12.5% of the population by intensity distribution) similar to APA:siPlk1 polyplexes, and a slightly higher polydispersity (0.2 ± 0.3) compared to APA:siPlk1 polyplexes. Surface charge was negligibly higher compared to APA:siRNA polyplexes (1.5 ±

0.3 mV), due to the higher N/P ratio used for the complexation of APAS:siRNA polyplexes. Next, selective silencing of APAS:siPlk1 polyplexes was evaluated at the mRNA level in U251 and U251 TMZ-R cells (Figure 6C). While APAS:siGFP did not silence Plk1 mRNA, APAS:siPlk1 reduced Plk1 mRNA levels to ~25% compared to untreated cells in both U251 and U251 TMZ-R cells. To demonstrate silencing of MGMT in TMZ resistant GB cells, U251 TMZ-R cells were treated with APAS:siMGMT, and the mRNA and protein levels were evaluated (Figure 6D,E). The highly MGMT-expressing U251 TMZ-R cells were treated with polyplexes of APAS:siMGMT, APAS:siGFP, or siMGMT alone for 48 h. RT-PCR analysis demonstrated that treatment with APAS:siMGMT reduced the mRNA levels to ~15% of untreated cells, while APAS:siGFP or siMGMT alone did not affect MGMT mRNA levels. Furthermore, western blot analysis corroborated our previous results, showing a reduction of MGMT at the protein level following APAS:siMGMT treatment (Figure 6E).

3.7. Sulfonate Modification Facilitated Internalization of Cy5-siRNA into U251 and U251 TMZ-R Spheroids

Next, the effect of the SELP targeting on internalization was evaluated using 3D settings of U251 and U251 TMZ-R 3D spheroids. 3D spheroids were treated with APA:Cy5-siRNA, APAS:Cy5-siRNA, or Cy5-siRNA alone for 20 min. While Cy5-siRNA alone was unable to internalize to the 3D spheroids, APA:Cy5-siRNA internalized to both U251 and U251 TMZ-R 3D spheroids. Strikingly, much higher internalization into the 3D spheroids was shown by the APAS:Cy5-siRNA polyplexes (Figure 7). Supplementary Materials Figure S5A shows internalization of APA/S:cy5-siRNA polyplexes into U251 cells grown in 2D culture. As the expression of SELP is much lower in 2D settings compared with the 3D spheroids (Supplementary Materials Figure S2), the effect of targeting SELP in 2D is less pronounced, and the internalization into the cells was only slightly higher following treatment with APAS:Cy5-siRNA compared to APA:Cy5-siRNA (Figure 7). Furthermore, Cy5-siRNA was unable to enter into U251 cells seeded in 2D monolayer as well. To validate the specific targeting of SELP, GL261 murine GB 3D spheroids were disintegrated and treated with either APA:Cy5-siRNA, APAS:Cy5-siRNA or Cy5-siRNA alone in the presence of 2 µM of the SELP inhibitor KF38789 (Supplementary Materials Figure S5B). APAS:Cy5-siRNA polyplexes demonstrated higher internalization into GL261 spheroids-derived cells within 5 min post-treatment (median fluorescence intensity of 3536 compared with 2931, respectively). Furthermore, the addition of SELP inhibitor reduced the internalization of APAS:Cy5-siRNA polyplexes to the level of 2016, while it did not alter the internalization of APA:Cy5-siRNA polyplexes (median fluorescence intensity = 2847, Supplementary Materials Figure S5).

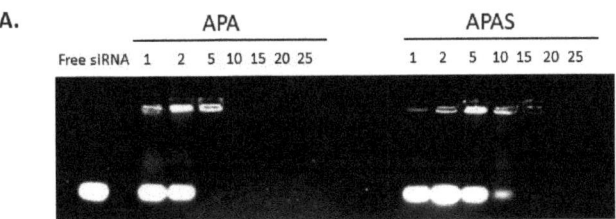
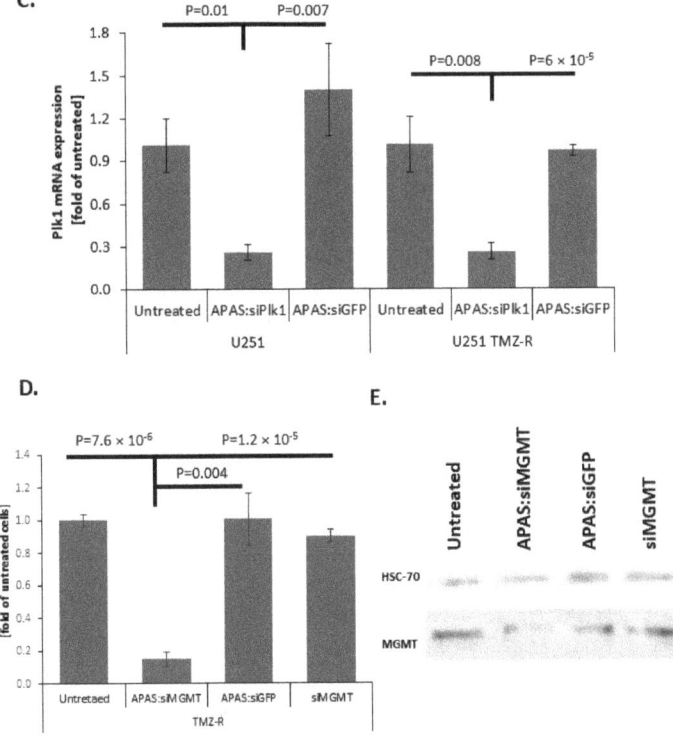

Figure 6. Sulfonate modification maintained size and activity of APA complexes. (A) Electrophoretic shift assay (EMSA) of polyplexes of APA and APAS with siRNA at increasing N/P ratios. (B) Table summarizing the hydrodynamic diameter, polydispersity index (PDI), and zeta potential of the main population of APAS:siPlk1 polyplexes as obtained by Mobius and PALS instruments. (C) Specific Plk1 mRNA silencing obtained by RT-PCR, performed on U251 and U251 TMZ-R GB cells following treatment with APAS:siPlk1 polyplexes. (D,E) Specific MGMT mRNA silencing obtained by RT-PCR (D) and western Blot (E) performed on U251 and U251 TMZ-R GB cells following treatment with APAS:siMGMT polyplexes.

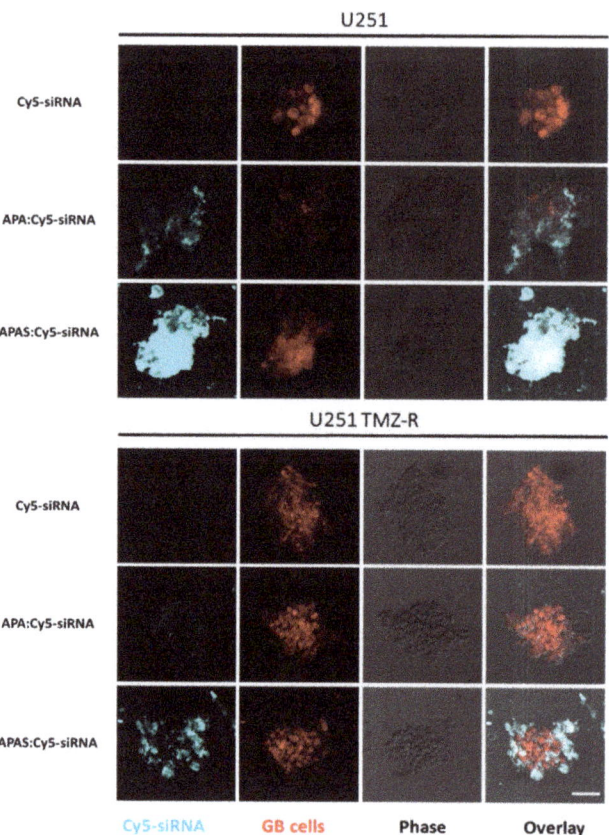

Figure 7. Sulfonate modification of APA facilitated internalization of Cy5-siRNA carrying polyplexes into both U251 and U251 TMZ-R spheroids (scale = 50 µm).

4. Conclusions

Resistance to chemotherapy is frequently observed in GB patients that undergo surgical resection and radiotherapy; hence, alternative therapeutic approaches are in need. While targeting signaling pathways that are associated with resistance may improve the outcome of TMZ treatment, silencing oncogenes that are not related to developing chemotherapy resistance such as Plk1, may be an alternative treatment suitable for both chemo-sensitive and chemo-resistant tumors. APA complexed with siPlk1 formed size-controlled, injectable, and non-toxic polyplexes that were able to induce specific gene silencing and affected the proliferation of U251 and U251 TMZ-R cells. In order to maximize the therapeutic benefit, APA was modified with sulfonate groups targeting the siRNA to SELP overexpressed on GB endothelial and tumor cells which led to higher internalization into U251 3D spheroids. Our results highlight the therapeutic potential of sulfonated APA as RNAi nanocarrier, for maximal therapeutic response in chemo-resistant and chemo-sensitive GB brain tumors, which should be further evaluated in vivo.

Supplementary Materials: The following are available online at https://www.mdpi.com/article/10.3390/pharmaceutics13122199/s1, Figure S1: Physicochemical characteristics of APA:siGFP polyplexes. Figure S2: A. High expression of SELP on U251 spheroids (3D) compared with tissue culture (2D) as obtained by fluorescence activated cell sorting (FACS). B. Co-localization of SELP with CD31 in U251 intracranial tumors. Figure S3: IR spectrum of APA and APAS. Figure S4: APAS:siPlk1 representative histogram of the main population of polyplexes as obtained by Mobius DLS instrument.

Figure S5: A. Sulfonate modification had minor effect on internalization of Cy5-siRNA carrying polyplexes into U251 cells (2D). B. Inhibition of SELP reduced internalization of APAS:Cy5-siRNA polyplexes into GL261 spheroids, but did not alter the internalization of APA:Cy5-siRNA polyplexes, as obtained by fluorescence activated cell sorting (FACS).

Author Contributions: Conceptualization, A.K. and R.S.-F.; methodology, A.K., S.P., E.Y., P.O., T.Z., E.P., V.K., S.G., S.I.D. and N.A.; formal analysis, A.K., S.P., E.Y., V.K., S.G., S.I.D. and A.M.; investigation, A.K., R.S.-F., S.P. and E.Y.; writing—original draft preparation, A.K., and R.S.-F.; writing—review and editing, A.K., R.S.-F., S.P., E.Y., P.O. and S.I.D.; visualization, A.K.; supervision, R.S.-F.; project administration, A.K., and R.S.-F.; funding acquisition, R.S.-F. All authors have read and agreed to the published version of the manuscript.

Funding: This research was funded by Rimonim Consortium and the MAGNET Program of the Office of the Chief Scientist of the Israel Ministry of Industry, Trade and Labor for supporting this research, the European Research Council (ERC) Advanced Grant (835227; 3DBrainStrom); ERC Proof of Concept (PoC) Grant (862580; 3DCanPredict); the Israel Science Foundation (Grant no. 1969/18); the Israel Cancer Research Fund (PROF-18-682); the Nancy and Peter Brown friends of the Israel Cancer Association (ICA) USA, in memory of Kenny and Michael Adler (20150909); and from the Morris Kahn Foundation. The APC was funded by the Sackler Faculty of Medicine, Tel Aviv University.

Institutional Review Board Statement: The study was conducted according to the guidelines of the Declaration of Helsinki, and approved by the the animal care and use committee (IACUC) of Tel Aviv University (approval no. 01-19-097, Approval and expiry dates 15 December 2019–15 December 2023).

Data Availability Statement: The GBM patient sequencing data analyzed are available in the OSgbm database (http://bioinfo.henu.edu.cn/GBM/GBMList.jsp) (accessed on 27 November 2021).

Acknowledgments: A.K. thanks the Marian Gertner Institute for granting her the Outstanding Achievements Award for research conducted in the field of nano-systems for medical applications at Tel Aviv University. P.O. thanks the Naomi Foundation for the Global Research and Training Fellowship in Medical and Life Sciences. We would like to thank the Sackler Cellular & Molecular Imaging Center (SCMIC) for the imaging service, and special thanks to Sasha Lichtenstein, for her kind and professional assistance.

Conflicts of Interest: R.S.-F. is a Board Director at Teva Pharmaceutical Industries Ltd. All other authors declare no conflict of interest.

References

1. Gittleman, H.; Boscia, A.; Ostrom, Q.T.; Truitt, G.; Fritz, Y.; Kruchko, C.; Barnholtz-Sloan, J.S. Survivorship in adults with malignant brain and other central nervous system tumor from 2000–2014. *Neuro-Oncology* **2018**, *20* (Suppl. 7), vii6–vii16.
2. Castro, M.G.; Cowen, R.; Williamson, I.K.; David, A.; Jimenez-Dalmaroni, M.J.; Yuan, X.; Bigliari, A.; Williams, J.C.; Hu, J.; Lowenstein, P.R. Current and future strategies for the treatment of malignant brain tumors. *Pharmacol. Ther.* **2003**, *98*, 71–108. [CrossRef]
3. Stupp, R.; Mason, W.P.; van den Bent, M.J.; Weller, M.; Fisher, B.; Taphoorn, M.J.; Belanger, K.; Brandes, A.A.; Marosi, C.; Bogdahn, U. Radiotherapy plus concomitant and adjuvant temozolomide for glioblastoma. *N. Engl. J. Med.* **2005**, *352*, 987–996. [CrossRef] [PubMed]
4. Schapira, A.H. *Neurology and Clinical Neuroscience*; Elsevier: Amsterdam, The Netherlands, 2007.
5. Rommelaere, J.; Raykov, Z.; Grekova, S.; Kiprijanova, I.; Geletneky, K.; Koch, U.; Apraliamian, M. Oncolytic Virotherapy for Prevention of Tumor Recurrence. U.S. Patent No. 9,861,669, 9 January 2018.
6. Hegi, M.E.; Diserens, A.-C.; Gorlia, T.; Hamou, M.-F.; de Tribolet, N.; Weller, M.; Kros, J.M.; Hainfellner, J.A.; Mason, W.; Mariani, L. MGMT gene silencing and benefit from temozolomide in glioblastoma. *N. Engl. J. Med.* **2005**, *352*, 997–1003. [CrossRef]
7. Papachristodoulou, A.; Signorell, R.D.; Werner, B.; Brambilla, D.; Luciani, P.; Cavusoglu, M.; Grandjean, J.; Silginer, M.; Rudin, M.; Martin, E. Chemotherapy sensitization of glioblastoma by focused ultrasound-mediated delivery of therapeutic liposomes. *J. Control. Release* **2019**, *295*, 130–139. [CrossRef] [PubMed]
8. Sloan, A.E.; Roger, L.; Murphy, C.; Reese, J.; Lazarus, H.M.; Dropulic, B.; Gerson, S.L. A phase I study of MGMT-P140K transfected hematopoetic progenitor cells (HPC) combined with TMZ/O^6BG dose escalation for newly diagnosed, MGMT unmethylated glioblastoma: Tolerance and evidence of survival benefit. *Am. Soc. Clin. Oncol.* **2019**, *37*, 2062. [CrossRef]
9. Yu, W.; Zhang, L.; Wei, Q.; Shao, A. O^6-methylguanine-DNA Methyltransferase (MGMT): Challenges and New Opportunities in Glioma Chemotherapy. *Front. Oncol.* **2020**, *9*, 1547. [CrossRef]

10. Ofek, P.; Calderon, M.; Mehrabadi, F.S.; Krivitsky, A.; Ferber, S.; Tiram, G.; Yerushalmi, N.; Kredo-Russo, S.; Grossman, R.; Ram, Z.; et al. Restoring the oncosuppressor activity of microRNA-34a in glioblastoma using a polyglycerol-based polyplex. *Nanomedicine* **2016**, *12*, 2201–2214. [CrossRef]
11. Tiram, G.; Ferber, S.; Ofek, P.; Eldar-Boock, A.; Ben-Shushan, D.; Yeini, E.; Krivitsky, A.; Blatt, R.; Almog, N.; Henkin, J.; et al. Reverting the molecular fingerprint of tumor dormancy as a therapeutic strategy for glioblastoma. *FASEB J.* **2018**, *32*, 5835–5850. [CrossRef]
12. Zafir-Lavie, I.; Sherbo, S.; Goltsman, H.; Badinter, F.; Yeini, E.; Ofek, P.; Miari, R.; Tal, O.; Liran, A.; Shatil, T.; et al. Successful intracranial delivery of trastuzumab by gene-therapy for treatment of HER2-positive breast cancer brain metastases. *J. Control. Release* **2018**, *291*, 80–89. [CrossRef]
13. Shatsberg, Z.; Zhang, X.; Ofek, P.; Malhotra, S.; Krivitsky, A.; Scomparin, A.; Tiram, G.; Calderón, M.; Haag, R.; Satchi-Fainaro, R. Functionalized nanogels carrying an anticancer microRNA for glioblastoma therapy. *J. Control. Release* **2016**, *239*, 159–168. [CrossRef]
14. Higuchi, F.; Fink, A.L.; Kiyokawa, J.; Miller, J.J.; Koerner, M.V.; Cahill, D.P.; Wakimoto, H. PLK1 inhibition targets Myc-activated malignant glioma cells irrespective of mismatch repair deficiency–mediated acquired resistance to temozolomide. *Mol. Cancer Ther.* **2018**, *17*, 2551–2563. [CrossRef]
15. Strebhardt, K.; Ullrich, A. Targeting polo-like kinase 1 for cancer therapy, Nature reviews. *Cancer* **2006**, *6*, 321–330. [PubMed]
16. Pezuk, J.; Brassesco, M.; Morales, A.; de Oliveira, J.; Queiroz, R.d.; Machado, H.; Carlotti, C.; Neder, L.; Scrideli, C.; Tone, L. Polo-like kinase 1 inhibition causes decreased proliferation by cell cycle arrest, leading to cell death in glioblastoma. *Cancer Gene Ther.* **2013**, *20*, 499–506. [CrossRef]
17. Lerner, R.G.; Grossauer, S.; Kadkhodaei, B.; Meyers, I.; Sidorov, M.; Koeck, K.; Hashizume, R.; Ozawa, T.; Phillips, J.J.; Berger, M.S. Targeting a Plk1-controlled polarity checkpoint in therapy-resistant glioblastoma-propagating cells. *Cancer Res.* **2015**, *75*, 5355–5366. [CrossRef]
18. Polyak, D.; Krivitsky, A.; Scomparin, A.; Eliyahu, S.; Kalinski, H.; Avkin-Nachum, S.; Satchi-Fainaro, R. Systemic delivery of siRNA by aminated poly(α)glutamate for the treatment of solid tumors. *J. Control. Release* **2017**, *257*, 132–143. [CrossRef]
19. Gibori, H.; Eliyahu, S.; Krivitsky, A.; Ben-Shushan, D.; Epshtein, Y.; Tiram, G.; Blau, R.; Ofek, P.; Lee, J.S.; Ruppin, E.; et al. Amphiphilic nanocarrier-induced modulation of PLK1 and miR-34a leads to improved therapeutic response in pancreatic cancer. *Nat. Commun* **2018**, *9*, 16. [CrossRef]
20. Scomparin, A.; Polyak, D.; Krivitsky, A.; Satchi-Fainaro, R. Achieving successful delivery of oligonucleotides—From physico-chemical characterization to in vivo evaluation. *Biotechnol. Adv.* **2015**, *33 Pt 3*, 1294–1309. [CrossRef] [PubMed]
21. Ben-Shushan, D.; Markovsky, E.; Gibori, H.; Tiram, G.; Scomparin, A.; Satchi-Fainaro, R. Overcoming obstacles in microRNA delivery towards improved cancer therapy. *Drug Deliv. Transl. Res.* **2014**, *4*, 38–49. [CrossRef] [PubMed]
22. Tiram, G.; Scomparin, A.; Ofek, P.; Satchi-Fainaro, R. Interfering cancer with polymeric siRNA nanomedicines. *J. Biomed. Nanotechnol.* **2014**, *10*, 50–66. [CrossRef]
23. Maeda, H.; Wu, J.; Sawa, T.; Matsumura, Y.; Hori, K. Tumor vascular permeability and the EPR effect in macromolecular therapeutics: A review. *J. Control. Release* **2000**, *65*, 271–284. [CrossRef]
24. Markovsky, E.; Baabur-Cohen, H.; Eldar-Boock, A.; Omer, L.; Tiram, G.; Ferber, S.; Ofek, P.; Polyak, D.; Scomparin, A.; Satchi-Fainaro, R. Administration, distribution, metabolism and elimination of polymer therapeutics. *J. Contr. Release* **2012**, *161*, 446–460. [CrossRef]
25. Krivitsky, A.; Polyak, D.; Scomparin, A.; Eliyahu, S.; Ori, A.; Avkin-Nachum, S.; Krivitsky, V.; Satchi-Fainaro, R. Structure–function correlation of aminated poly (α) glutamate as siRNA nanocarriers. *Biomacromolecules* **2016**, *17*, 2787–2800. [CrossRef]
26. Krivitsky, A.; Krivitsky, V.; Polyak, D.; Scomparin, A.; Eliyahu, S.; Gibori, H.; Yeini, E.; Pisarevsky, E.; Blau, R.; Satchi-Fainaro, R. Molecular weight-dependent activity of aminated poly (α) glutamates as siRNA nanocarriers. *Polymers* **2018**, *10*, 548. [CrossRef]
27. Krivitsky, A.; Polyak, D.; Scomparin, A.; Eliyahu, S.; Ofek, P.; Tiram, G.; Kalinski, H.; Avkin-Nachum, S.; Gracia, N.F.; Albertazzi, L.; et al. Amphiphilic poly(alpha)glutamate polymeric micelles for systemic administration of siRNA to tumors. *Nanomedicine* **2018**, *14*, 303–315. [CrossRef] [PubMed]
28. Yeini, E.; Ofek, P.; Albeck, N.; Ajamil, D.R.; Neufeld, L.; Eldar-Boock, A.; Kleiner, R.; Vaskovich, D.; Koshrovski-Michael, S.; Israeli, S.D. Targeting Glioblastoma: Advances in Drug Delivery and Novel Therapeutic Approaches. *Adv. Ther.* **2020**, *4*, 2000124. [CrossRef]
29. Muldoon, L.L.; Soussain, C.; Jahnke, K.; Johanson, C.; Siegal, T.; Smith, Q.R.; Hall, W.A.; Hynynen, K.; Senter, P.D.; Peereboom, D.M. Chemotherapy delivery issues in central nervous system malignancy: A reality check. *J. Clin. Oncol.* **2007**, *25*, 2295–2305. [CrossRef]
30. Lorant, D.E.; Topham, M.K.; Whatley, R.E.; McEver, R.P.; McIntyre, T.M.; Prescott, S.M.; Zimmerman, G.A. Inflammatory roles of P-selectin. *J. Clin. Investig.* **1993**, *92*, 559–570. [CrossRef]
31. Läubli, H.; Borsig, L. *Selectins Promote Tumor Metastasis*; Seminars in Cancer Biology; Elsevier: Amsterdam, The Netherlands, 2010; pp. 169–177.
32. Yeini, E.; Ofek, P.; Pozzi, S.; Albeck, N.; Ben-Shushan, D.; Tiram, G.; Golan, S.; Kleiner, R.; Sheinin, R.; Dangoor, S.I.; et al. P-selectin axis plays a key role in microglia immunophenotype and glioblastoma progression. *Nat. Commun.* **2021**, *12*, 1912. [CrossRef] [PubMed]

33. Ferber, S.; Tiram, G. Co-targeting the tumor endothelium and P-selectin-expressing glioblastoma cells leads to a remarkable therapeutic outcome. *eLife* **2017**, *6*, e25281. [CrossRef] [PubMed]
34. Wilkins, P.P.; Moore, K.L.; McEver, R.P.; Cummings, R.D. Tyrosine sulfation of P-selectin glycoprotein ligand-1 is required for high affinity binding to P-selectin. *J. Biol. Chem.* **1995**, *270*, 22677–22680. [CrossRef] [PubMed]
35. Segal, E.; Pan, H.; Ofek, P.; Udagawa, T.; Kopeckova, P.; Kopecek, J.; Satchi-Fainaro, R. Targeting angiogenesis-dependent calcified neoplasms using combined polymer therapeutics. *PLoS ONE* **2009**, *4*, e5233. [CrossRef] [PubMed]
36. Santana-Magal, N.; Farhat-Younis, L.; Gutwillig, A.; Gleiberman, A.; Rasoulouniriana, D.; Tal, L.; Netanely, D.; Shamir, R.; Blau, R.; Feinmesser, M.; et al. Melanoma-Secreted Lysosomes Trigger Monocyte-Derived Dendritic Cell Apoptosis and Limit Cancer Immunotherapy. *Cancer Res.* **2020**, *80*, 1942–1956. [CrossRef] [PubMed]
37. Tiram, G.; Segal, E.; Krivitsky, A.; Shreberk-Hassidim, R.; Ferber, S.; Ofek, P.; Udagawa, T.; Edry, L.; Shomron, N.; Roniger, M. Identification of dormancy-associated microRNAs for the design of osteosarcoma-targeted dendritic polyglycerol nanopolyplexes. *ACS Nano* **2016**, *10*, 2028–2045. [CrossRef] [PubMed]
38. Dong, H.; Wang, Q.; Li, N.; Lv, J.; Ge, L.; Yang, M.; Zhang, G.; An, Y.; Wang, F.; Xie, L. OSgbm: An online consensus survival analysis web server for Glioblastoma. *Front. Genet.* **2020**, *10*, 1378. [CrossRef]
39. Kim, J.-G.; Sim, S.J.; Kim, J.-H.; Kim, S.H.; Kim, Y.H. Synthesis and polymerization of methacryloyl-PEG-sulfonic acid as a functional macromer for biocompatible polymeric surfaces. *Macromol. Res.* **2004**, *12*, 379–383. [CrossRef]

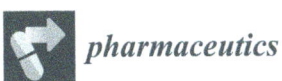

Article

Cathepsin B-Overexpressed Tumor Cell Activatable Albumin-Binding Doxorubicin Prodrug for Cancer-Targeted Therapy

Hanhee Cho [1,2,†], Man Kyu Shim [1,†], Suah Yang [1,3], Sukyung Song [1,4], Yujeong Moon [1,5], Jinseong Kim [1,3], Youngro Byun [6], Cheol-Hee Ahn [2,*] and Kwangmeyung Kim [1,3,*]

[1] Biomedical Research Institute, Korea Institute of Science and Technology (KIST), Seoul 02792, Korea; ricky@kist.re.kr (H.C.); mks@kist.re.kr (M.K.S.); haehwan@kist.re.kr (S.Y.); t17192@kist.re.kr (S.S.); phoenix0310@kist.re.kr (Y.M.); 218843@kist.re.kr (J.K.)
[2] Department of Materials Science and Engineering, Seoul National University, Seoul 08826, Korea
[3] KU-KIST Graduate School of Converging Science and Technology, Korea University, Seoul 02841, Korea
[4] Department of Biosystems & Biotechnology, Korea University, Seoul 02841, Korea
[5] Department of Bioengineering, Korea University, Seoul 02841, Korea
[6] Research Institute of Pharmaceutical Sciences, College of Pharmacy, Seoul National University, Seoul 08826, Korea; yrbyun@snu.ac.kr
* Correspondence: chahn@snu.ac.kr (C.-H.A.); kim@kist.re.kr (K.K.)
† These authors contributed equally to this work.

Abstract: Prodrugs are bioreversible medications that should undergo an enzymatic or chemical transformation in the tumor microenvironment to release active drugs, which improve cancer selectivity to reduce toxicities of anticancer drugs. However, such approaches have been challenged by poor therapeutic efficacy attributed to a short half-life and low tumor targeting. Herein, we propose cathepsin B-overexpressed tumor cell activatable albumin-binding doxorubicin prodrug, Al-ProD, that consists of a albumin-binding maleimide group, cathepsin B-cleavable peptide (FRRG), and doxorubicin. The Al-ProD binds to in situ albumin, and albumin-bound Al-ProD indicates high tumor accumulation with prolonged half-life, and selctively releases doxorubicin in cathepsin B-overexpressed tumor cells, inducing a potent antitumor efficacy. Concurrently, toxicity of Al-ProD toward normal tissues with innately low cathepsin B expression is significantly reduced by maintaining an inactive state, thereby increasing the safety of chemotherapy. This study offers a promising approach for effective and safe chemotherapy, which may open new avenues for drug design and translational medicine.

Keywords: prodrug; albumin; drug delivery; targeted therapy; chemotherapy

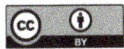

1. Introduction

Chemotherapy is still the first-line treatment option owing to its high sensitivity against wide range of cancers, but it is often accompanied by serious side effects attributed to a lack of cancer selectivity [1]. The risk of side effects by chemotherapy restricts drug dosage, which may limit the tumors from being exposed to sufficiently high drug concentrations, eventually leading to treatment failure [2]. Thus, many endeavors have been made to overcome these issues by improving the cancer selectivity of anticancer drugs to tumors. One of the promising approaches, prodrug, involves bioreversible medications that should undergo an enzymatic or chemical transformation in the tumor microenvironment to release active drugs, which greatly improve the cancer selectivity to reduce the off-target toxicity of anticancer drugs [3–5]. Selective activation of prodrugs can be achieved by intrinsic differences of enzyme expression between tumor and normal tissues [6]. Many designed prodrugs that selectively release active drugs by overexpressed enzymes in the tumor microenvironment, including caspases, cathepsins, and matrix metalloproteinases

(MMPs), have greatly increased the safety of chemotherapy with minimal side effects [7–10]. However, such approaches have been challenged by unfavorable pharmacokinetics (PK), indicating a short in vivo half-life and poor tumor targeting owing to their small molecule structure, resulting in limited antitumor efficacy [11].

Albumin is the most abundant protein in the blood and has 17 disulphide bonds with one free thiol from unpaired cysteine (Cys34), which has emerged as a versatile protein carrier to improve the PK profile of anticancer drugs for tumor targeting [12]. The underlying mechanism of albumin-based drug delivery is that anticancer drugs containing thiol-reactive molecules selectively bind to accessible free thiol on Cys34 of endogenous albumins, and thus enhance the half-lives of drugs [13]. This long half-life is attributable mainly to its macromolecular size, being above the kidney filtration threshold, as well as receptor-mediated salvage mechanism, preventing degradation, facilitated by the neonatal Fc receptor (FcRn) [14]. Therefore, anticancer drugs bound to albumin accumulate within tumors via the enhanced permeability and retention (EPR) effect that is shown in the macromolecular complex by the increased vascular permeability and low lymphatic drainage [15,16]. In clinics, albumin-bound doxorubicin, Aldoxorubicin, has shown potent antitumor efficacy with significantly prolonged patient survival [17]. However, the delivery efficiency to tumors of even the effective drug carriers was, unexpectedly, found to be less than 1~3% in many preclinical studies [18]. This means that a considerable amount of drugs inevitably localized in the off-target tissues and blood stream, which can increase the risk of systemic toxicity. Thus, albumin-based drug delivery of aldoxorubicin still indicated representative side effects of chemotherapy in patients at various stages [19].

2. Materials and Methods

2.1. Materials

Phe-Arg-Arg-Gly (NH$_2$-FRRG-COOH) peptide was synthesized from Peptron (Daejeon, Republic of Korea). Cathepsin B-inhibitory siRNA, γ-maleimidobutyric acid, and Monoclonal anti-mouse cathepsin B antibody were purchased from Santa Cruz Biotechnology (Dallas, TX, USA). Cell counting kit-8 (CCK-8) was purchased from Vitascientific (Beltsville, MD, USA). TUNEL assays kit, recombinant cathepsin B, cathepsin E, cathepsin D, caspase-9, and caspase-3 were purchased from R&D systems (Minneapolis, MN, USA). BCA protein quantification kit was purchased from Thermo Fisher scientific (Oakville, ON, USA). Maleimide-PEG$_2$-NHS, human serum albumin (HSA), mouse serum albumin (MSA), bovine serum albumin (BSA), hematoxylin and eosin (H&E) staining kit, and doxorubicin hydrochloride were purchased from Sigma Aldrich (Oakville, ON, USA). Fetal bovine serum (FBS), RPMI 1640 medium, Dulbecco's modified Eagle medium (DMEM) high glucose medium, streptomycin, and penicillin were purchased from WELGENE Inc. (Daegu, Korea). Anti-β-actin antibody was purchased from Abcam (Hanam, Republic of Korea). MDA-MB231 (human breast cancer cells) and H9C2 (rat BDIX heart myoblasts) cell lines were purchased from American Type Culture Collection (ATCC; Manassas, VA, USA). Six-week-old female Balb/c nude mice were purchased from NaraBio, Inc. (Seoul, Korea).

2.2. Synthesis of Cathepsin B-Overexpressed Tumor Cell Activatable Albumin-Binding Doxorubicin Prodrug (Al-ProD)

Al-ProD was synthesized via a two-step reaction. At first, maleimide-PEG$_2$-NHS (100 mg, 1 equiv) was reacted with NH$_2$-FRRG-COOH (251.4 mg, 2 equiv) in anhydrous DMF (10 mL) at 37 °C for 12 h, and maleimide-PEG$_2$-FRRG-COOH was purified using HPLC. Second, subsequent synthesis of maleimide-PEG$_2$-FRRG-DOX (Al-ProD) was performed by dissolving maleimide-PEG$_2$-FRRG-COOH (150 mg, 2 equiv), doxorubicin (DOX; 48.2 mg, 1 equiv), EDC (44.1 mg, 4 equiv), and NHS (40.9 mg, 4 equiv) in anhydrous 10 mL DMF, while stirring at 37 °C for 24 h. Then, Al-ProD was further purified via HPLC, and lyophilized at −90 °C to obtain a red powder (Freeze Dryer, ilShinBioBase, Republic of Korea). After preparation, successful synthesis of Al-ProD was confirmed by measuring purity and molecular weight via HPLC and MALDI-TOF mass spectrometer, respectively.

2.3. Characterization of Al-ProD

The albumin-binding property of Al-ProD was firstly evaluated. Briefly, to a human serum albumin (HSA), mouse serum albumin (MSA), or bovine serum albumin (BSA; 700 µM in PBS; pH 7.4), Al-ProD (100 µM) was added and incubated for 0, 5, and 60 min at room temperature. As a control, the HSA solution was pre-incubated with γ-maleimidobutyric acid for 1 h before adding Al-ProD. After incubation, samples were analyzed via native 12% SDS-PAGE gel. The gels were observed by trans-UV using the iBright^{TM} Imaging System (Invitrogen by Thermo Fisher Scientiric), and then stained with coomassie blue for visualizing proteins. The albumin-binding property of Al-ProD was further analyzed using reverse-phased high performance liquid chromatography (RP-HPLC; Agilent cary 300; Agilent Technologies) with ACN/H_2O gradient from 80:20 to 20:80 for 30 min under a fluorescence detector (Ex/Em: 530/590 nm). In addition, mass shift after incubation of HSA with Al-ProD for 5 min was confirmed by a matrix-assisted laser desorption/ionization time of flight (MALDI-TOF, AB Sciex TOF/TOF 5800 System, Annapolis, MD, USA) mass spectrometer with a cyano-4-hydroycinnamic acid (CHCA) matrix. Next, cathepsin B-specific cleavage of Al-ProD that was pre-incubated with HSA for 5 min (HSA-bound Al-ProD; 10 µM) was assessed by incubating with cathepsin B, cathepsin E, cathepsin D, cathepsin L, caspase-9, or caspase-3 (50 µg) at 37 °C for 24 h, followed by an analysis using HPLC with ACN/H_2O gradient from 20:80 to 80:20 for 30 min.

2.4. Cellular Uptake

To assess intracellular behavior of Al-ProD via fluorescence imaging, 3×10^5 MDA-MB231 and H9C2 cells were seeded in confocal dishes. After 24 h stabilization, each cell was incubated with free DOX or HSA-bound Al-ProD (2 µM) for 48 h at 37 °C. As a control, MDA-MB231 cells were pre-incubated for 2 h with cathepsin B-inhibitory siRNA that was pre-incubated with Lipofectamine 2000 for 40 min at room temperature. Then, cells were washed twice with DPBS, fixed with 5% paraformaldehyde for 15 min, and stained with 4′,6-diamidino-2-phenylindole (DAPI) for 10 min. Fluorescence imaging was performed using a Leica TCS SP8 confocal laser-scanning microscope (Leica Microsystems GmbH; Wetzlar, Germany). The DOX fluorescence in images was quantitatively analyzed using an Image Pro software (Media Cybernetic, Rockville, MD, USA).

2.5. Cytotoxicity Assay

The cytotoxicity of Al-ProD was assessed via cell counting kit-8 (CCK) assays. First, 5×10^3 MDA-MB231 or H9C2 cells were seeded in 96-well cell culture plates. After 24 h stabilization, the free DOX or HSA-bound Al-ProD were added to each well and incubated for 48 h. Then, the cells were additionally incubated with culture medium containing 10% CCK solution for 30 min. The cell viability was measured using a microplate reader (VERSAmaxTM; Molecular Devices Corp., San Jose, CA, USA) with 450 nm of wavelength.

2.6. Western Blot

Cathepsin B expression in MDA-MB231 and H9C2 cells was analyzed via Western blot [20]. Briefly, 2×10^5 MDA-MB231 or H9C2 cells were seeded in six-well cell culture plates. After 24 h incubation, MDA-MB231 and H9C2 cells were solubilized using lysis buffer including 1% protease inhibitors, and the resulting lysates were centrifuged at 3000 rpm for 40 min to remove debris. The proteins in lysates were quantified by BCA protein quantification kit, and then separated using sodium dodecyl sulfate-polyacrylamide (SDS-PAGE) gel electrophoresis and transferred onto PVDF membranes. Then, membranes were incubated with TBS-T containing 5% bovine serum albumin (BSA) for 1 h to block non-specific IgG binding and incubated with anti-cathepsin B primary antibody for 12 h at 4 °C. Finally, membranes were incubated with HRP-conjugated anti-mouse IgG antibody for 2 h at room temperature and immunoreactive bands were observed via an enhanced chemiluminescence (ECL) system.

2.7. Pharmacokinetics (PK)

Mice were bred under pathogen-free conditions at the Korea Institute of Science and Technology (KIST). All experiments with live animals were performed in compliance with the relevant laws and institutional guidelines of Institutional Animal Care and Use Committee (IACUC) in Korea Institute of Science and Technology (KIST), and IACUC approved the experiment (approved number of 2020-123). To assess pharmacokinetic (PK) profiles in vivo, BALB/c nude mice were intravenously injected with free DOX (3 mg/kg) or Al-ProD (3 mg/kg based on DOX contents), and blood samples were collected from mice at pre-determined times (0, 3 h, 6 h, 9 h, 12 h, 24 h, 48 h, 72 h, 96 h, 120 h, and 144 h). Then, each drug in the blood samples was extracted with DMSO by intense vortex and the samples were centrifuged at 2000 rpm for 40 min to obtain as a blood plasma. Finally, amount of free DOX and Al-ProD in samples was analyzed by IVIS Lumina Series III system (PerkinElmer; Waltham, MA, USA).

2.8. Biodistribution in Breast Tumor Models

The biodistribution of Al-ProD was assessed in breast tumor models, which were prepared by subcutaneous inoculation of 1×10^7 MBA-MB231 cells into the left flank of BALB/c nude mice. When the tumor volumes were approximately 200–250 mm^3, the mice were intravenously injected with free DOX (3 mg/kg) or Al-ProD (3 mg/kg based on DOX contents). Then, noninvasive near-infrared fluorescence (NIRF) imaging was performed using an IVIS Lumina Series III system after 0 h, 3 h, 6 h, 12 h, 24 h, 48 h, and 72 h of injection. Fluorescence intensities in tumor regions were quantified via Living Image software. Mice were sacrificed after 12 h of injection for ex vivo imaging, followed by the collection of lung, liver, kidney, spleen, heart, and tumor tissues. Tumor tissues were also cut into 10 μm thick sections for histological assays. Slide-mounted tumor sections were analyzed by Leica TCS SP8 confocal laser-scanning microscope.

2.9. Antitumor Efficacy and Toxicity Evaluation

To evaluate the antitumor efficacy, MDA-MB231 tumor-bearing mice were randomly divided into three groups: (i) saline; (ii) free DOX; and (iii) Al-ProD. Then, mice were treated once every three days with free DOX (3 mg/kg) or Al-ProD (3 mg/kg based on DOX contents), at which time tumor volumes were approximately 60–80 mm^3. Antitumor efficacy was assessed by measuring tumor volumes once every two days, calculated as largest diameter $\times$ smallest diameter^2 $\times$ 0.53, once every 2 days. The body weights of mice were also measured once every two days to assess in vivo toxicity. The in vivo toxicity of Al-ProD was further assessed by histological analyses. At 20 days after treatment, major organs were collected from mice and samples were stained with H&E following the manufacturer's protocol. Then, organ sections were observed using an optical microscope.

2.10. Statistics

The statistical significance between two groups was analyzed using Student's t-test. One-way analysis of variance (ANOVA) was performed for comparisons of more than two groups, and multiple comparisons were analyzed using Tukey–Kramer post-hoc test. Survival data were plotted as Kaplan–Meier curves and analyzed using log-rank test. Statistical significance was indicated with an asterisk (* $p < 0.05$, ** $p < 0.01$, and *** $p < 0.001$) in the figures.

2.11. Data Availability

All relevant data are available with the article and its Supplementary Information files, or available from the corresponding authors upon reasonable request.

3. Results

3.1. Albumin-Binding and Selective Activation of Al-ProD

Herein, we propose cathepsin B-overexpressed tumor cell activatable albumin-binding doxorubicin prodrug, Al-ProD, which can effectively deliver anticancer drugs by in situ albumin-mediated passive targeting with minimal side effects. The Al-ProD was prepared by conjugating doxorubicin (DOX) to C-terminus of cathepsin B-cleavable peptide (NH$_2$-FRRG-COOH; NH$_2$-*Phe-Arg-Arg-Gly*-COOH) and introducing a maleimide group to the N-terminus of peptide (Figure 1a). The maleimide group in the Al-ProD selectively bound to the thiol in physiological pH, thereby allowing the covalent binding with in situ circulating albumin (Figure 1b). Moreover, FRRG peptide is a well-known substrate of cathepsin B, which is associated with tumor invasion and metastasis as a promising cancer biomarker overexpressed in malignant tumors compared with normal tissues in clinical studies [21,22]. Compared with other substrate peptide of cathepsin B, FRRG peptide exhibited high specificity against the target enzyme without non-specific cleavage and, especially, it was reported that G-DOX cleaved from FRRG-DOX by enzymatic cleavage was additionally metabolized into free DOX by intracellular proteases [23,24]. Therefore, the in situ albumin-bound Al-ProD greatly enhances tumor accumulation with prolonged in vivo half-life and induces a potent antitumor efficacy by selectively releasing free DOX in cathepsin B-overexpressed tumor cells (Figure 1c). Concurrently, toxicity toward normal tissues with innately low cathepsin B expression is significantly reduced by maintaining a non-toxic inactive state, thereby increasing the safety of chemotherapy (Figure 1d). In the present study, albumin-binding of Al-ProD was confirmed on human serum albumin (HSA), mouse serum albumin (MSA), and bovine serum albumin (BSA). Selective action of Al-ProD was studied in breast cancer cells and cardiomyocytes, indicating differential levels of cathepsin B. The in vivo pharmacokinetics and tumor regression effect with minimal toxicity were also carried out in breast cancer models.

The cathepsin B-overexpressed tumor cell activatable albumin-binding doxorubicin prodrug, Al-ProD, which consists of albumin-binding maleimide group, cathepsin B-cleavable peptide (NH$_2$-FRRG-COOH; NH$_2$-*Phe-Arg-Arg-Gly*-COOH), and doxorubicin (DOX), was designed for cancer-targeted therapy with minimal side effects. The Al-ProD was synthesized by conjugating DOX to C-terminus of FRRG peptide and introducing a maleimide group to the N-terminus of peptide (Figure S1). After the reaction, 99% of Al-ProD was purified with HPLC (Figure S2). The successful synthesis was also confirmed via matrix-assisted laser desorption ionization time-of-flight (MALDI-TOF) mass spectrometer, wherein the exact molecular weight of Al-ProD was calculated to be 1370.44 Da for $C_{64}H_{83}N_{13}O_{21}$, and measured to be 1370.616 m/z [M] (Figure S3). First, the plasma albumin-binding ability of Al-ProD was assessed by various in vitro studies. The Al-ProD and albumin from different species of human (human serum albumin; HSA), mouse (mouse serum albumin; MSA), and bovine (bovine serum albumin; BSA) were clearly observed via the doxorubicin absorbance and coomassie blue staining in SDS-PAGE gel, respectively (Figure 2a). Importantly, the band of Al-ProD was detected below 7 kDa, but the band shifted to 50–75 kDa after incubation with HSA, BSA, or MSA for 1 h. MALDI-TOF mass spectrometer further confirmed the molecular weight shift of the HSA from 66,409 to 67,780 m/z when incubated with Al-ProD, showing a mass difference comparable to that of Al-ProD (1370.616 m/z), indicating the successful albumin-binding (Figure S4). In contrast, the Al-ProD band was not shifted when each albumin (HSA, MSA, and BSA) was pre-incubated with 4-maleimido butyric acid to block the thiol group. As a control, FRRG-DOX with the absence of a maleimide group and free DOX were also not bound to all types of albumin, only showing the band below 7 kDa. The HSA-binding of Al-ProD was further analyzed by HPLC (Figure 2b). Binding of Al-ProD with HSA in HPLC spectrum was confirmed by a shift of the Al-ProD peak (14 min) to a broad peak at 16 min that appeared to be a free HSA peak, wherein the binding was accomplished within 5 min. However, Al-ProD did not bound to HSA for 60 min when the thiol group of HSA was blocked.

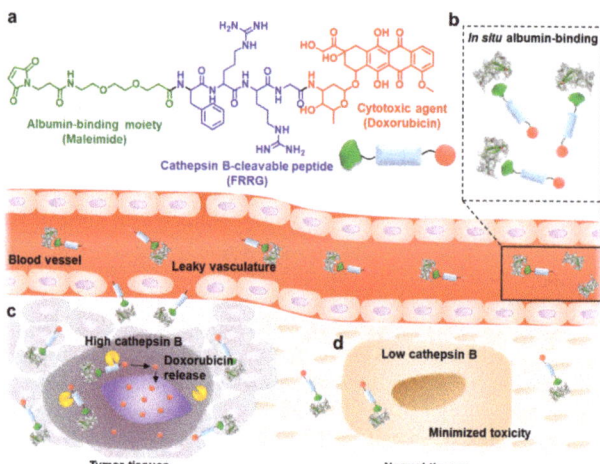

Figure 1. In situ albumin-mediated cancer-targeted therapy by Al-ProD. (a) The Al-ProD is prepared by conjugating doxorubicin (DOX) to the C-terminus of cathepsin B-cleavable peptide (FRRG) and introducing a maleimide group to the N-terminus of peptide. (b) Intravenously injected Al-ProD efficiently binds to in situ circulating albumin in blood vessels. (c) Albumin-bound Al-ProD greatly enhances tumor accumulation via albumin-mediated passive tumor targeting and induces a potent antitumor efficacy by selectively releasing free DOX in cathepsin B-overexpressed tumor cells. (d) Concurrently, Al-ProD significantly reduced toxicity toward normal tissues with innately low cathepsin B expression by maintaining a non-toxic inactive state, thereby increasing the safety of chemotherapy.

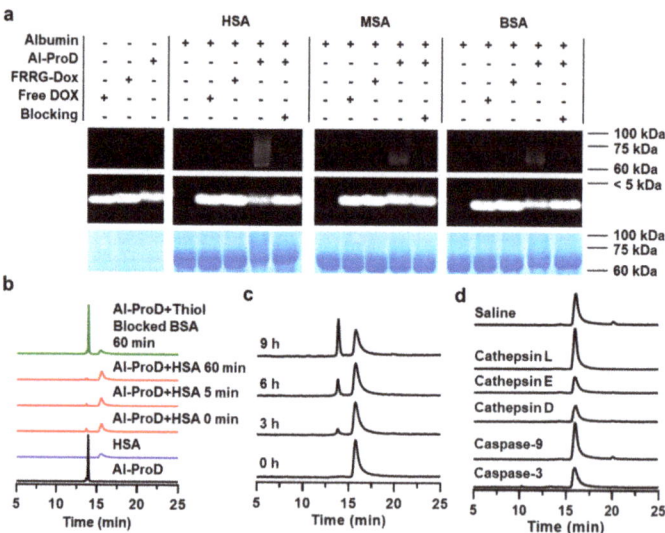

Figure 2. Albumin binding and selective activation of Al-ProD. (a,b) Albumin-binding of Al-ProD. Al-ProD was incubated with human serum albumin (HSA), mouse serum albumin (MSA), or bovine serum albumin at room temperature. As a control, the HSA solution was pre-incubated with γ-maleimidobutyric acid to block thiol in HSA. In addition, free DOX or FRRG-DOX with the absence of a maleimide group were also incubated with three types of serum albumin. After incubation, samples were analyzed via (a) SDS-PAGE gel and (b) RP-HPLC. (c,d) HPLC chromatograms when Al-ProD was incubated with (c) cathepsin B or (d) other enzymes.

Next, we assessed the cathepsin B-specific cleavage of Al-ProD by incubation with various enzymes. As the Al-ProD releases the DOX molecules via enzymatic degradation in the presence of cathepsin B, it is major of concern whether the cathepsin B can recognize and cleave FRRG peptide without interference by albumin adjacent when Al-ProD was bound to albumin. To address this concern, HSA-bound Al-ProD was incubated with enzyme reaction buffer containing cathepsin B (MES buffer; 50 µg/mL). The result showed that HSA-bound Al-ProD began to be cleaved to glycine-conjugated doxorubicin (G-DOX) after 3 h incubation and G-DOX release was gradually increased for 9 h incubation (Figure 2c). These results were clearly supported by MALDI-TOF analysis, which confirm the molecular weight of G-DOX (calculated mass: 600.58 Da, measured mass: 601.2019 m/z [M+H], 623.184 [M+Na], and 639.1573 [M+K]) at a newly appeared peak (14 min) after incubation with cathepsin B in the HPLC spectrum (Figure S5). It was already reported that G-DOX cleaved from FRRG-DOX by cathepsin B enzymatic cleavage are efficiently metabolized into free DOX by intracellular proteases [23,24]. In contrast, HSA-bound Al-ProD was not cleaved by other enzymes, such as caspase-3, caspase-9, cathepsin D, cathepsin E, and cathepsin L, or saline (hydrolysis; Figure 2d). These results clearly demonstrate that Al-ProD successfully binds to albumin via a maleimide group and selectively releases DOX molecules in the presence of cathepsin B enzyme.

3.2. Cancer Cell-Selective Cytotoxicity of Al-ProD

The in vitro selective activation of Al-ProD premised on differential expression levels of cathepsin B was assessed in breast cancer cells (MDA-MB231) and rat BDIX cardiomyocytes (H9C2). As expected, MDA-MB231 cells expressed a 24.26 ± 3.08-fold high amount of cathepsin B compared with H9C2 cells (Figure S6). Each cell showed a robust uptake of HSA-bound Al-ProD (red color) after 48 h of incubation, as confirmed by confocal laser scanning microscope (CLSM; Figure 3a). However, DOX fluorescence was limited to the cytoplasm of H9C2 cells, whereas that in MDA-MB231 cells was observed in nuclei. The HSA-bound Al-ProD also remained in the cytoplasm of cathepsin B-suppressed MDA-MB231 cells, which are pre-treated with cathepsin B-inhibitory siRNA for 24 h. Quantitatively, DOX fluorescence in nuclei was 2.48–2.89-fold stronger in HSA-bound Al-ProD-treated MDA-MB231 cells than H9C2 and cathepsin B-suppressed MDA-MB231 cells (Figure 3b). In contrast, intracellular free DOX was clearly observed at the nuclei in both MDA-MB231 and H9C2 cells, regardless of cathepsin B expression (Figure 3c). As the mode of action of DOX is intercalation into DNA base pairs, inducing breakage of DNA strand and inhibition of DNA and RNA replication, the DOX moleucle inside the nuclei of cells is an important indicator of its cytotoxicity. As a result, this differential cellular uptake of Al-ProD resulted in cancer cell-selective cytotoxicity [25]. The IC_{50} value of HSA-bound Al-ProD in MDA-MB231 was measured to be 7.33 µM, while it was >200 µM in H9C2 cells after 48 h incubation, which showed about a 30-fold difference that indicates cancer cell-selective cytotoxicity (Figure 3d). In contrast, free DOX exhibited indiscriminate cytotoxicity in both MDA-MB231 and H9C2 cells with nearly similar IC_{50} values (Figure 3e). These results suggest that Al-ProD can efficiently eradicate cancers with minimal off-target toxicities toward normal tissues by selective activation in cancer cells.

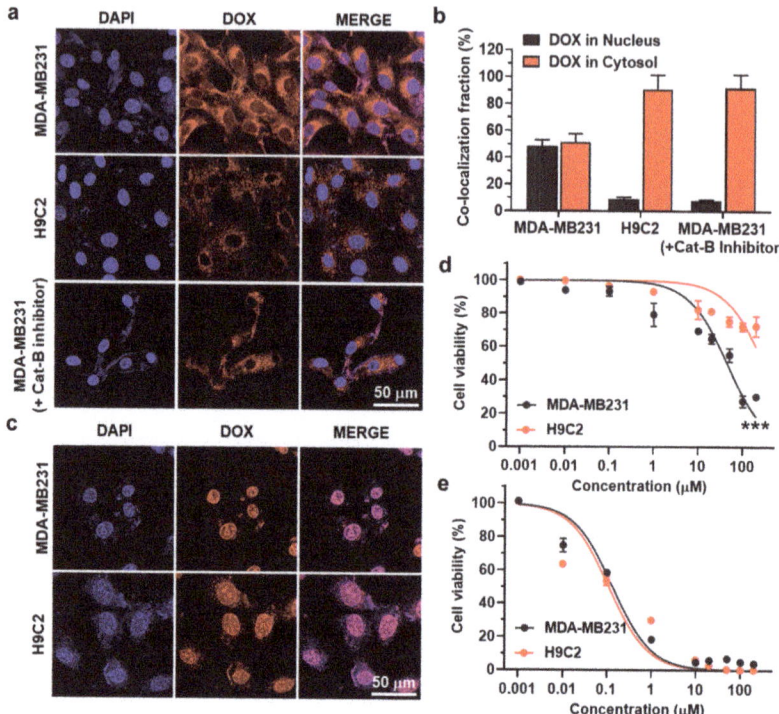

Figure 3. Cellular uptake and cytotoxicity of Al-ProD. (**a**) Fluorescence images of MDA-MB231 and H9C2 cells treated with Al-ProD. As a control, MDA-MB231 cells were pre-incubated with cathepsin B-inhibitory siRNA. (**b**) Quantification analysis of DOX fluorescence in nuclei or cytosol of Al-ProD- or free DOX-treated MDA-MB231, H9C2, and cathepsin B-inhibitory siRNA-treated MDA-MB231 cells. (**c**) Fluorescence images of MDA-MB231 and H9C2 cells treated with free DOX. (**d**,**e**) Cytotoxicity of (**d**) Al-ProD or (**e**) free DOX in MDA-MB231 and H9C2 cells. Significance (*** $p < 0.001$) was determined by Student's t-test (**d**).

3.3. Pharmecokinetics and Tumor Targeting of Al-ProD

To evaluate the high tumor accumulation of albumin-binding Al-ProD by extended in vivo half-life, the pharmacokinetics (PK) of Al-ProD and free DOX was firstly compared in BALB/c nude mice after intravenous injection at a dose of molar equivalent to 3 mg/kg of doxorubicin. In contrast to free DOX, showing fast in vivo clearance with a half-life of 15 min, Al-ProD showed a significantly extended half-life of more than 3 h (Figure 4a). In addition, a detectable amount of the Al-ProD remained for 144 h in the body, indicating the dramatically extended residence time in vivo. As a result, the area under the curve (AUC) of Al-ProD was approximately sevenfold increased compared with that of free DOX. The tumor accumulation of Al-ProD by extended in vivo half-life was further assessed via noninvasive near-infrared fluorescence (NIRF) imaging in breast tumor models. The breast tumor-bearing mice were prepared by subcutaneous inoculation of MDA-MB231 cells (1×10^7) into BALB/c nude mice, and free DOX (3 mg/kg) or Al-ProD (3 mg/kg based on DOX contens) were intravenously injected into mice. In the case of free DOX, the DOX fluorescence in tumor tissues was rapidly decreased for 6 h owing to its rapid in vivo clearance by a short half-life (Figure 4b). However, DOX fluorescence of Al-ProD in tumor tissues was significantly stronger than free DOX at all time points and was retained for 72 h of injection, which indicates high tumor accumulation by albumin-mediated passive targeting effect. The DOX fluorescence from tumor tissues was quantitatively 3.33–4.08-fold stronger in mice treated with Al-ProD than free DOX after 12 h injection (Figure 4c). Ex vivo imaging after 12 h of injection further confirmed the high tumor accumulation of Al-ProD, wherein the DOX fluorescence in tumor tissues was 3.41–4.92-fold stronger than the free DOX group (Figure 4d). Finally, histological analyses also indicated strong DOX fluorescence (red color) in whole tumor tissues from mice treated with Al-ProD compared with free DOX (Figure 4e). In contrast, only a small quantity of free DOX was observed in tumor tissues. These results demonstrate that the abumin-binding property of Al-ProD greatly extended the in vivo half-life of drugs, leading to high tumor accumulation via a passive targeting effect.

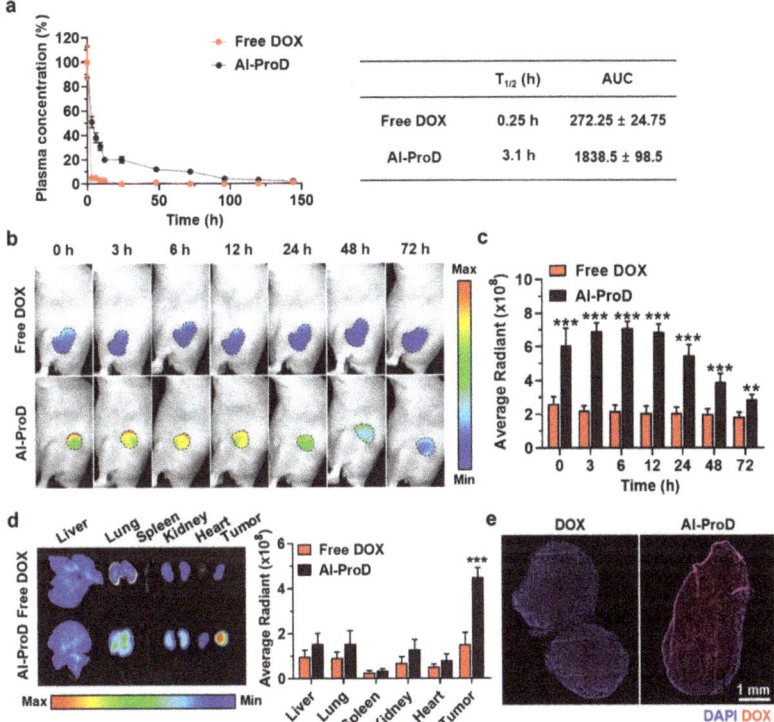

Figure 4. Pharmacokinetics and biodistribution of Al-ProD. (a) PK profiles of Al-ProD and free DOX. Area under the curve (AUC) was calculated by Origin 2020 software. (b) NIRF images of MDA-MB231 tumor-bearing mice treated with Al-ProD of free DOX. (c) Quantification analysis on the DOX fluorescence at tumor tissues in NIRF images. (d) Ex vivo imaging of organs from mice treated with Al-ProD or free DOX after 12 h injection. (e) Quantification analysis of the DOX fluorescence at major organs in ex vivo imaging. (e) Fluorescence images of whole tumor tissues after 12 h of Al-ProD or free DOX treatment. Significance (** $p < 0.01$, *** $p < 0.001$) was determined by Student's t-test (c,d).

3.4. Antitumor Efficacy and Toxicity Studies of Al-ProD in Breast Tumor Models

To evaluate the antitumor efficacy, MDA-MB231 tumor-bearing mice prepared by same protocol as in Figure 4b were treated with free DOX (3 mg/kg) or Al-ProD (3 mg/kg based on DOX contens) once every three days. Importantly, Al-ProD (347.42 ± 25.9 mm^3) significantly decreased the tumor volume compared with free DOX (580.25 ± 139.92 mm^3; $p < 0.05$) and saline (1810.98 ± 544.56 mm^3; $p < 0.001$) groups on day 20 after treatment (Figure 5a). Tumor tissues stained with H&E and TUNEL also showed greatly elevated damaged areas and apoptosis in the Al-ProD group compared with the free DOX and saline groups, which clearly indicated the potent antitumor efficacy by albumin-mediated passive targeting of Al-ProD (Figure 5b). Next, we assessed the reduced off-target toxicity of Al-ProD by high cancer selectivity during treatment. Body weights of mice in the free DOX group gradually decreased during treatment owing to severe systemic toxicity, while those in the Al-ProD group showed no significant body weight loss, similar to the saline group (Figure 5c). Furthermore, normal organs stained with H&E exhibited structural abnormalities in the free DOX group, whereas only negligible toxicity was observed in organs of the Al-ProD group on day 20 after treatment (Figure 5d). In agreement with the above results, the mice in free DOX group were all dead within 18 days, with a median survival of 16 days, whereas Al-ProD-treated mice survived over 25 days (Figure 5e). As a control, median survial of the saline group was measured to be 20 days, wherein the mice were dead as a result of tumor progression. Collectively, our findings demonstrate that Al-ProD effectively inhibits tumor growth without side effects, thereby allowing effective and safe chemotherapy.

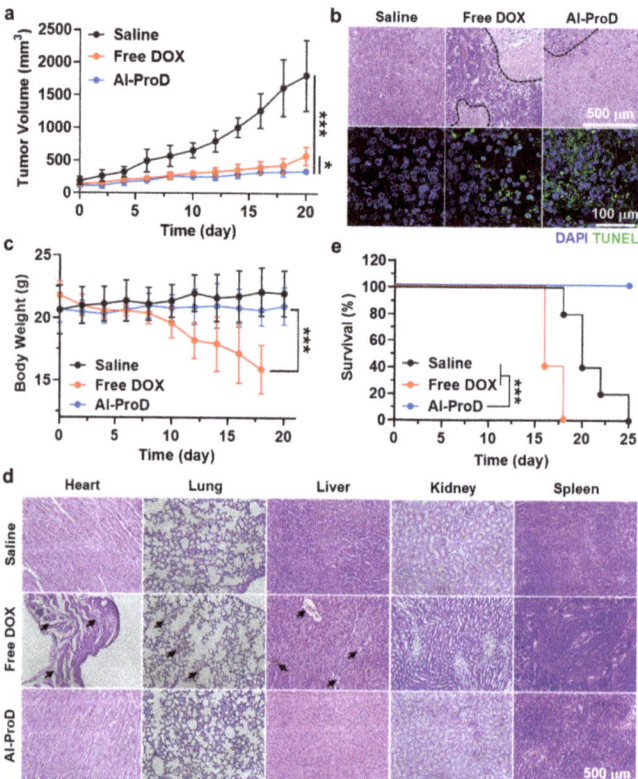

Figure 5. Antitumor efficacy and toxicity evaluation of Al-ProD. (a) Tumor growth curves of MDA-MB231 tumor-bearing mice after saline, free DOX, or Al-ProD treatment once every three days. (b) Tumor tissues stained with H&E or TUNEL to assess antitumor efficacy on day 20 after treatment. (c) Body weights during treatment. (d) Major organs stained with H&E to assess structural abnormalities on day 20 after treatment. (e) Mice survival during treatment. Significance (* $p < 0.05$ and *** $p < 0.001$) was determined by one-way ANOVA with the Tukey–Kramer post-hoc test (a,c) or log-rank test (e).

4. Conclusions

In summary, we proposed achieving the effective and safe chemotherapy with cathepsin B-overexpressed tumor cell activatable albumin-binding doxorubicin prodrug (Al-ProD) via albumin-mediated drug delivery. Al-ProD, which consists of albumin-binding maleimide, cathepsin B-cleavable peptide, and doxorubicin, efficiently bound to plasma albumin, thereby dramatically extending the in vivo half-life of doxorubicin. Importantly, highly accumulated Al-ProD in the tumor tissues via albumin-mediated passive targeting selectively released doxorubicin in cathepsin B-overexpressed cancer cells, which provoked potent antitumor efficacy. Concurrently, Al-ProD significantly reduced the toxicity against normal tissues with innately low cathepsin B by maintaining an inactive state. As a result, localized tumor delivery of doxorubicin by Al-ProD greatly inhibited the breast tumor progression with minimized side effects. Compared with the conventional drug delivery system that encapsultes active drugs into nanoparticles, Al-ProD can prevent the off-target toxicities by accidental drug leakage during circulation. In addition, this system also reduces the risk of potential side effects from carrier materials by using the natural delivery carrier. Finally, presice and consice structures allow the simple preparation protocol, thereby overcoming the fundamental problems of targeted drugs for clinical translation, such as difficulty in quality control (QC) and mass production. Therefore, this study provides a promising approach for effective and safe chemotherapy, which may open new avenues for drug design and provide significant advances for translational nanomedicine. However, unexpectedly low delivery efficiency of targeted drugs is still a common limitation of current drug delivery systems. Thus, many researchers are making efforts to develop the advanced formulation and to increase the understanding of the complex tumor microenvironment that reduces the delivery efficiency of targeted drugs. Considering the clinical success of albumin-mediated drug delivery to improve the pharmacokinetics and tumor targeting of drugs as well as ongoing pipelines like Al-ProD will further move albumin-binding drugs from bench to bedside.

Supplementary Materials: The following are available online at https://www.mdpi.com/article/10.3390/pharmaceutics14010083/s1, Figure S1. Synthetic scheme to prepare cathepsin B-overexpressed tumor cell activatable albumin-binding doxorubicin prodrug (Al-ProD). Figure S2. The purity (>99%) of Al-ProD was confirmed by high performance liquid chromatography (HPLC). Figure S3. The molecular weight of Al-ProD was confirmed via MALDI-TOF mass spectrometer. Figure S4. MALDI-TOF analysis results of human serum albumin and human serum albumin-bound Al-ProD. Figure S5. Metabolite assay of Al-ProD. Glycine-conjugated doxorubicin (G-DOX) release from Al-ProD was confirmed via MALDI-TOF mass spectrometer. Figure S6. Cathepsin B expression levels of MDA-MB231 and H9C2 cells. (left) Western blot analysis of cathepsin B of MDA-MB231 cancer cells and H9C2 normal cells. (right) Relative expression levels of cathepsin B in each cell.

Author Contributions: Conceptualization, M.K.S. and K.K.; methodology, M.K.S. and H.C.; validation, H.C.; formal analysis, H.C. and Y.B.; investigation, H.C., S.Y., S.S., Y.M. and J.K.; resources, C.-H.A. and K.K.; data curation, H.C. and M.K.S.; writing—original draft preparation, M.K.S., C.-H.A. and K.K.; visualization, H.C.; supervision, C.-H.A. and K.K.; project administration, C.-H.A. and K.K.; funding acquisition, K.K. All authors have read and agreed to the published version of the manuscript.

Funding: This work was supported from the National Research Foundation (NRF) of South Korea, funded by the Ministry of Science (NRF-2019R1A2C3006283 and NRF-2021R1C1C2005460) of the Republic of Korea, the KU-KIST Graduate School of Converging Science and Technology (Korea University), and the Intramural Research Program of KIST.

Institutional Review Board Statement: The study was conducted according to the guidelines of the Declaration of Helsinki and approved by the Institutional Review Board (or Ethics Committee) of Korea Institute of Science and Technology (approved number of 2020-123).

Informed Consent Statement: Not applicable.

Data Availability Statement: Not applicable.

Conflicts of Interest: The authors declare no conflict of interest.

References

1. Zhong, L.; Li, Y.; Xiong, L.; Wang, W.; Wu, M.; Yuan, T.; Yang, W.; Tian, C.; Miao, Z.; Wang, T.; et al. Small Molecules in Targeted Cancer Therapy: Advances, Challenges, and Future Perspectives. *Signal Transduct. Target. Ther.* **2021**, *6*, 201. [CrossRef] [PubMed]
2. Senapati, S.; Mahanta, A.K.; Kumar, S.; Maiti, P. Controlled Drug Delivery Vehicles for Cancer Treatment and Their Performance. *Signal Transduct. Target. Ther.* **2018**, *3*, 7. [CrossRef] [PubMed]
3. Liu, B.-Y.; Yang, X.-L.; Xing, X.; Li, J.; Liu, Y.-H.; Wang, N.; Yu, X.-Q. Trackable Water-Soluble Prodrug Micelles Capable of Rapid Mitochondrial-Targeting and Alkaline pH-Responsive Drug Release for Highly Improved Anticancer Efficacy. *ACS Macro Lett.* **2019**, *8*, 719–723. [CrossRef]
4. Sun, H.; Zhong, Z. 100th Anniversary of Macromolecular Science Viewpoint: Biological Stimuli-Sensitive Polymer Prodrugs and Nanoparticles for Tumor-Specific Drug Delivery. *ACS Macro Lett.* **2020**, *9*, 1292–1302. [CrossRef]
5. Kim, J.; Shim, M.K.; Yang, S.; Moon, Y.; Song, S.; Choi, J.; Kim, J.; Kim, K. Combination of Cancer-Specific Prodrug Nanoparticle with Bcl-2 Inhibitor to Overcome Acquired Drug Resistance. *J. Control. Release* **2021**, *330*, 920–932. [CrossRef]
6. Wu, L.; Qu, X. Cancer Biomarker Detection: Recent Achievements and Challenges. *Chem. Soc. Rev.* **2015**, *44*, 2963–2997. [CrossRef]
7. Lock, L.L.; Tang, Z.; Keith, D.; Reyes, C.; Cui, H. Enzyme-Specific Doxorubicin Drug Beacon as Drug-Resistant Theranostic Molecular Probes. *ACS Macro Lett.* **2015**, *4*, 552–555. [CrossRef]
8. Wang, Y.; Cheetham, A.G.; Angacian, G.; Su, H.; Xie, L.; Cui, H. Peptide–Drug Conjugates as Effective Prodrug Strategies for Targeted Delivery. *Adv. Drug Deliv. Rev.* **2017**, *110–111*, 112–126. [CrossRef]
9. Um, W.; Park, J.; Ko, H.; Lim, S.; Yoon, H.Y.; Shim, M.K.; Lee, S.; Ko, Y.J.; Kim, M.J.; Park, J.H.; et al. Visible light-induced apoptosis activatable nanoparticles of photosensitizer-DEVD-anticancer drug conjugate for targeted cancer therapy. *Biomaterials* **2019**, *224*, 119494. [CrossRef]
10. Choi, J.; Shim, M.K.; Yang, S.; Hwang, H.S.; Cho, H.; Kim, J.; Yun, W.S.; Moon, Y.; Kim, J.; Yoon, H.Y.; et al. Visible-Light-Triggered Prodrug Nanoparticles Combine Chemotherapy and Photodynamic Therapy to Potentiate Checkpoint Blockade Cancer Immunotherapy. *ACS Nano* **2021**, *15*, 12086–12098. [CrossRef]
11. Wong, B.S.; Yoong, S.L.; Jagusiak, A.; Panczyk, T.; Ho, H.K.; Ang, W.H.; Pastorin, G. Carbon Nanotubes for Delivery of Small Molecule Drugs. *Adv. Drug Deliv. Rev.* **2013**, *65*, 1964–2015. [CrossRef]
12. Chung, S.W.; Cho, Y.S.; Choi, J.U.; Kim, H.R.; Won, T.H.; Kim, S.Y.; Byun, Y. Highly Potent Monomethyl Auristatin E Prodrug Activated by Caspase-3 for the Chemoradiotherapy of Triple-Negative Breast Cancer. *Biomaterials* **2019**, *192*, 109–117. [CrossRef]
13. Chaudhury, C.; Mehnaz, S.; Robinson, J.M.; Hayton, W.L.; Pearl, D.K.; Roopenian, D.C.; Anderson, C.L. The Major Histocompatibility Complex-related Fc Receptor for IgG (FcRn) Binds Albumin and Prolongs Its Lifespan. *J. Exp. Med.* **2003**, *197*, 315–322. [CrossRef]
14. Elsadek, B.; Kratz, F. Impact of albumin on drug delivery—New applications on the horizon. *J. Control. Release* **2012**, *157*, 4–28. [CrossRef]
15. Torchilin, V. Tumor Delivery of Macromolecular Drugs Based on the EPR Effect. *Adv. Drug Deliv. Rev.* **2011**, *63*, 131–135. [CrossRef]
16. Lim, S.; Park, J.; Shim, M.K.; Um, W.; Yoon, H.Y.; Ryu, J.H.; Lim, D.-K.; Kim, K. Recent advances and challenges of repurposing nanoparticle-based drug delivery systems to enhance cancer immunotherapy. *Theranostics* **2019**, *9*, 7906–7923. [CrossRef]
17. Eilber, F.C.; Sankhala, K.K.; Chawla, S.P.; Chua-Alcala, V.S.; Gordon, E.M.; Quon, D.; Kim, K.; Chawla, S.; Wu, N.; Wieland, S.; et al. Administration of Aldoxorubicin and 14 Days Continuous Infusion of Ifosfamide/Mesna in Metastatic or Locally Advanced Sarcomas. *J. Clin. Oncol.* **2017**, *35*, 11051. [CrossRef]
18. Hare, J.I.; Lammers, T.; Ashford, M.B.; Puri, S.; Storm, G.; Barry, S.T. Challenges and Strategies in Anti-Cancer Nanomedicine Development: An Industry Perspective. *Adv. Drug Deliv. Rev.* **2017**, *108*, 25–38. [CrossRef]
19. Sachdev, E.; Sachdev, D.; Mita, M. Aldoxorubicin for the Treatment of Soft Tissue Sarcoma. *Expert Opin. Investig. Drugs* **2017**, *26*, 1175–1179. [CrossRef]
20. Shim, M.K.; Yoon, H.Y.; Ryu, J.H.; Koo, H.; Lee, S.; Park, J.H.; Kim, J.-H.; Lee, S.; Pomper, M.G.; Kwon, I.C.; et al. Cathepsin B-Specific Metabolic Precursor for In Vivo Tumor-Specific Fluorescence Imaging. *Angew. Chem. Int. Ed.* **2016**, *55*, 14698–14703. [CrossRef]
21. Shim, M.K.; Park, J.; Yoon, H.Y.; Lee, S.; Um, W.; Kim, J.-H.; Kang, S.-W.; Seo, J.-W.; Hyun, S.-W.; Park, J.H.; et al. Carrier-Free Nanoparticles of Cathepsin B-Cleavable Peptide-Conjugated Doxorubicin Prodrug for Cancer Targeting Therapy. *J. Control. Release* **2019**, *294*, 376–389. [CrossRef]
22. Shim, M.K.; Moon, Y.; Yang, S.; Kim, J.; Cho, H.; Lim, S.; Yoon, H.Y.; Seong, J.-K.; Kim, K. Cancer-specific drug-drug nanoparticles of pro-apoptotic and cathepsin B-cleavable peptide-conjugated doxorubicin for drug-resistant cancer therapy. *Biomaterials* **2020**, *261*, 120347. [CrossRef]
23. Yang, S.; Shim, M.K.; Kim, W.J.; Choi, J.; Nam, G.-H.; Kim, J.; Kim, J.; Moon, Y.; Kim, H.Y.; Park, J.; et al. Cancer-activated doxorubicin prodrug nanoparticles induce preferential immune response with minimal doxorubicin-related toxicity. *Biomaterials* **2021**, *272*, 120791. [CrossRef]

24. Kim, J.; Shim, M.K.; Cho, Y.-J.; Jeon, S.; Moon, Y.; Choi, J.; Kim, J.; Lee, J.; Lee, J.-W.; Kim, K. The safe and effective intraperitoneal chemotherapy with cathepsin B-specific doxorubicin prodrug nanoparticles in ovarian cancer with peritoneal carcinomatosis. *Biomaterials* **2021**, *279*, 121189. [CrossRef]
25. Yang, F.; Teves, S.S.; Kemp, C.J.; Henikoff, S. Doxorubicin, DNA torsion, and chromatin dynamics. *Biochim. Biophys. Acta (BBA) Rev. Cancer* **2014**, *1845*, 84–89. [CrossRef]

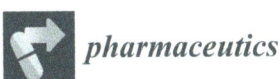

Article

Novel Selectively Targeted Multifunctional Nanostructured Lipid Carriers for Prostate Cancer Treatment

Lital Cohen [1], Yehuda G. Assaraf [2,*] and Yoav D. Livney [1,*]

[1] The Laboratory of Biopolymers for Food and Health, Department of Biotechnology and Food Engineering, Technion–Israel Institute of Technology, Haifa 3200003, Israel; litalco@campus.technion.ac.il
[2] The Fred Wyszkowski Cancer Research Laboratory, Department of Biology, Technion–Israel Institute of Technology, Haifa 3200003, Israel
* Correspondence: assaraf@technion.ac.il (Y.G.A.); livney@technion.ac.il (Y.D.L.)

Abstract: Prostate cancer (PC) is the most common cancer in men over 50 and the 4th most prevalent human malignancy. PC treatment may include surgery, androgen deprivation therapy, chemotherapy, and radiation therapy. However, the therapeutic efficacy of systemic chemotherapy is limited due to low drug solubility and insufficient tumor specificity, inflicting toxic side effects and frequently provoking the emergence of drug resistance. Towards the efficacious treatment of PC, we herein developed novel selectively PC-targeted nanoparticles (NPs) harboring a cytotoxic drug cargo. This delivery system is based upon PEGylated nanostructured lipid carriers (NLCs), decorated with a selective ligand, targeted to prostate-specific membrane antigen (PSMA). NPs loaded with cabazitaxel (CTX) displayed a remarkable loading capacity of 168 ± 3 mg drug/g SA-PEG, encapsulation efficiency of $67 \pm 1\%$, and an average diameter of 159 ± 3 nm. The time-course of in vitro drug release from NPs revealed a substantial drug retention profile compared to the unencapsulated drug. These NPs were selectively internalized into target PC cells overexpressing PSMA, and displayed a dose-dependent growth inhibition compared to cells devoid of the PSMA receptor. Remarkably, these targeted NPs exhibited growth-inhibitory activity at pM CTX concentrations, being markedly more potent than the free drug. This selectively targeted nano-delivery platform bears the promise of enhanced efficacy and minimal untoward toxicity.

Keywords: prostate cancer; nanoparticles; nanostructured lipid carriers; prostate-specific membrane antigen; targeted delivery; encapsulation; cabazitaxel

1. Introduction

Cancer is one of the leading causes of morbidity and mortality worldwide. In this respect, prostate cancer (PC) is the most common cancer in men over the age of 50 and the 4th most prevalent human malignancy [1]. The current modalities to treat early-stage PC include surgery, radiation therapy, and for some men, androgen deprivation therapy [2,3]. Unfortunately, however, PC cells frequently acquire resistance to therapy, resulting in local relapse, progression, and metastasis [2,3]. This latter phase of the disease is referred to as castration-resistant prostate cancer (CRPC) or metastatic CRPC (mCRPC), which can further become a lethal disease (see Figure 1 in reference [4]) [2,3,5]. The most common metastases reside in lymph nodes and bone [6]. The current treatment of CRPC includes systemic second-generation endocrine treatment, followed by combination chemotherapy, where docetaxel (DTX) and cabazitaxel (CTX) are the cytotoxic drugs approved for the treatment of this stage of the disease [6,7]. Like the parent drug paclitaxel (PTX), DTX and CTX are taxanes that promote microtubule assembly and inhibit microtubule depolymerization, thereby causing an antimitotic cytotoxic effect [8–10]. This treatment is limited by low drug bioavailability due to the poor solubility of these therapeutic agents in the blood and the side effects to healthy tissues, causing reduced quality of life [2,3,5–7]. The goal of cancer therapeutics is to achieve a curative targeted treatment which also reduces systemic toxicity [11].

One of the strategies to overcome these serious therapeutic hurdles and limitations is selective targeting using nanoparticles (NPs). The mode of drug accumulation and cytotoxicity relies on passive targeting, which depends on the enhanced permeability and retention (EPR) effect [11–15]. This effect is characterized by structural abnormalities in tumor vasculature and lack of lymphatic drainage. Thereby, it enables extravasation of NPs from the tumor's leaky blood vessels into the tumor and results in marked accumulation in the internal tumor microenvironment (TME) [11–15]. The EPR effect provides favorable conditions for the use of long-circulating nanocarriers that can evade immune surveillance and interaction with the reticuloendothelial system (RES) [11–15]. The RES is a global system of macrophages, mainly in the liver and spleen, aimed at engulfing and eliminating foreign particles that are recognized by antibodies, a process known as opsonization [11–15]. Thereafter, actively targeted NPs interact with, and undergo, internalization into target cells via receptor-mediated endocytosis [11–17]. The mechanism underlying endocytosis is based upon the interaction between ligand-decorated NPs, and a tumor-specific antigen, or defined receptor, selectively overexpressed on the surface of PC cells.

Various cell surface antigens were used for the targeting of PC cells via selective receptor-mediated endocytosis (see Figure 2 in reference [4]). One of the most highly selective and well-characterized biomarker antigens of PC is prostate-specific membrane antigen (PSMA), also known as glutamate carboxypeptidase II (GCP-II), N-acetyl-α-linked acidic dipeptidase I, or folate hydrolase [2,3]. PSMA is a surface receptor overexpressed by a factor of 100–1000 in 94% of PC cells, compared to normal tissues including healthy prostate epithelial tissues [2,3,18]. Moreover, its expression increases with cancer progression, aggressiveness, and metastasis [2,3,18]. Therefore, PSMA has been extensively used as a bona fide target antigen for both diagnostic imaging and targeted drug delivery in the treatment of PC [19–24]. Compounds based on a urea linkage between two amino acids were found to have comparable affinities for PSMA and a strong interaction with the active site of GCP-II via hydrogen bonds [25–27].

As NPs undergo internalization into target cells, intracellular drug release occurs, thereby achieving a specific therapeutic effect [11–17]. Furthermore, uptake via receptor-mediated endocytosis is usually followed by lysosomal degradation of the NPs, thus facilitating the release of the encapsulated drug cargo into the cytoplasm, hence achieving a potent therapeutic effect [11–17].

The selective internalization of targeted NPs is an effective strategy to overcome cancer multidrug resistance (MDR), which remains a primary impediment towards efficacious cancer therapy [15,28–35]. This selective targeting constitutes a major advantage to evade MDR efflux pumps including P-glycoprotein (Pgp/ABCB1), multidrug resistance-associated protein 1 (MRP1/ABCC1), and breast cancer resistance protein (BCRP/ABCG2); these ATP-driven transmembrane efflux pumps extrude a multitude of chemotherapeutic drugs which are structurally and mechanistically distinct, resulting in a broad spectrum resistance to multiple anticancer drugs known as MDR [15,36–40].

Several important physicochemical properties should be optimized to establish an effective nanocarrier system with regards to: (a) permeation out of the leaky blood vessels and accumulation in the TME through the EPR effect, and (b) specific interaction with target cells and intracellular release of the encapsulated drug. The size and zeta-potential of NPs are some of the most important factors to be considered. A size range of 50–200 nm was found to be suitable for efficient extravasation from the tumor blood vessels, avoiding filtration by the kidney and minimal capture by the liver [11,13]. NPs with negative or neutral zeta-potential, as an indicator for anionic or neutral surface charge, respectively, are less subjected to opsonization and are unlikely to undergo electrostatic interaction followed by non-specific uptake by the negatively charged cellular membranes [13].

As part of the innovative development of pharmaceutical drug carriers, nanostructured lipid carriers (NLCs) constitute an effective option for stable and controlled drug delivery. NLCs consist of a nanostructured lipid matrix, made of a mixture of solid and liquid lipids, surface-stabilized by a surfactant or a mixture of surfactants [41–43]. The incorporation of liquid lipids with solid lipids generates liquid domains within the crystalline structure of the solid lipid lattice, which in turn enables the stable entrapment of the lipophilic drug cargo for the enhancement of drug loading capacity and minimization of premature outward diffusion [41–47]. In the current study, we developed NLCs which are composed of biocompatible and biodegradable components, including an oleic acid liquid core, surface-stabilized by solidifying stearic acid (SA), conjugated to polyethylene glycol (SA-PEG). Coating the surface of NLCs with PEG, a process called PEGylation, provides stealth functionality (i.e., immune system "transparency") that contributes to a markedly prolonged blood circulation time and is known to attenuate the clearance of the NPs from the circulation by hindering the otherwise dominant uptake by the RES [48]. This is critical for maximizing the passive uptake into the tumor and improving the pharmacokinetic and pharmacodynamic profiles of the nanocarriers. PEG is conjugated via an amide linkage to the targeting ligand (TL) Glutamate-Urea-Lysine (Glu-Urea-Lys), a small molecule urea-derivative which is an established ligand for specific binding to the PSMA receptor [25–27,49,50].

We undertook a thorough literature and patent review to confirm the novelty of the current nanodelivery system and delineate the differences of our nanomedicine system compared to other previously described NPs for prostate cancer treatment. A variety of nanocarrier drug delivery systems have been studied for the potential treatment of prostate cancer, including lipid-based NPs [51–57], inorganic NPs [58–61], and polymeric NPs [62–68]. Lipid NPs, including the NPs developed in our present study, have several advantages over other nanodelivery systems. The most compelling advantages of lipidic nanocarriers are their ease of scalability, low untoward toxicity, and more controllable release patterns [69]. Various lipidic NPs for prostate cancer treatment have been studied, and perhaps the most common lipidic drug delivery vehicles are liposomes. The major advantage of NLCs over liposomes is that the distinctive nanostructure of NLCs allows for a markedly enhanced loading capacity and sustained drug release profile. Hence, we chose NLCs for the current study.

We herein developed a targeted nanodelivery platform for the encapsulation of the therapeutic agent CTX. CTX is a novel second-generation anti-microtubule agent of the taxane family, with enhanced anti-tumor activity in MDR cancer cells, as, advantageously, it is a relatively poor efflux substrate of P-gp [70,71]. The current study aimed to construct a novel targeted drug nanodelivery system, characterize it, and evaluate the selective uptake and cytotoxicity to prostate cancer cells.

2. Materials and Methods

2.1. Materials

SA conjugated to polyethylene glycol (PEG) (2KDa) (SA-PEG) and SA-PEG with a carboxylic end group at the PEG terminus were custom-synthesized (Creative PEGWorks, Durham, NC). Glu-Urea-Lys with protecting groups of tert-Butyl esters was purchased from ABX advanced biochemical compounds (Radeberg, Germany). Cyanine7 with amine modification (Cy7-NH2) was purchased from Moshe Stauber Biotech Applications (Lod, Israel). All other chemicals were obtained from Sigma-Aldrich (Merck, Rehovot, Israel).

2.2. Cell Cultures

Human prostate cancer cell lines LNCaP (overexpressing the PSMA receptor) and PC-3 (devoid of PSMA expression), human non-small cell lung cancer (NSCLC) 1975 cells, human embryonic kidney HEK-293 cells, and normal human bronchial epithelial BEAS2B cells were cultured in an RPMI-1640 medium, supplemented with 10% fetal bovine serum (FBS), 2 mM glutamine, 100 µg/mL penicillin, and streptomycin (Biological Industries, Beit-HaEmek, Israel). The growth medium of LNCaP cells was supplemented with 5 µg/mL insulin (Sigma-Aldrich, Merck, Rehovot, Israel). Neonatal foreskin fibroblast FSE cells were cultured in a DMEM medium, supplemented with 10% FBS, 2 mM glutamine, 100 µg/mL penicillin, and streptomycin. Cells were incubated at 37 °C in a humidified atmosphere of 5% CO_2. NSCLC 1975, HEK-293, BEAS2B, and FSE cells were obtained from ATCC [72]. LNCaP and PC-3 cells were generously provided by Prof. David (Dedi) Meiri (Technion, Haifa, Israel) and were also originally obtained from ATCC. The actual surface expression of the PSMA receptor by LNCaP and PC-3 cells was determined by immunohistochemistry, conducted by the department of pathology in Rambam Health Care Campus, Haifa, Israel.

2.3. Methods

2.3.1. Preparation of NLCs

Self-assembled NLCs were prepared by a surfactant-free nanoprecipitation method [72–74] with several modifications for the stabilization of the nanocarriers system, as follows: For the unloaded NPs, SA-PEG (20 mg/mL) was dissolved in distilled water (DW) that was filtered through a 0.22 µm syringe filter prior to the addition of SA-PEG. The aqueous phase remained at 70 °C in order for the SA to be in its liquid state, as the melting point of SA was reported to be 69.6 °C [75]. A liquid lipid phase dissolved in ethanol (EtOH) was then added dropwise into the preheated aqueous phase under magnetic stirring of 600 rpm. The mixture was agitated at room temperature for 10 min to reach equilibrium. Different liquid lipids were used in the lipid phase including α-pinene, oleic acid (OA), orange oil, lemon oil, and jasmine oil. Samples were then transferred to a cold-water bath at 4 °C under stirring for another 10 min, for the solidification of the SA in the SA-PEG shell of the NPs, and in order to reach a final equilibrium.

2.3.2. Synthesis of SA-PEG-TL and Preparation of Targeted NLCs

SA-PEG conjugated to PSMA targeting ligand (SA-PEG-TL) was synthesized by covalent coupling of SA-PEG-COOH with the amine group in the side chain of lysine in the PSMA TL, Glu-Urea-Lys (Figure 1) [76]. The carboxylic groups of Glu-Urea-Lys were masked by protecting groups of *tert*-Butyl esters. Briefly, SA-PEG-COOH (0.02 mmol), equal molar ratio of Glu-Urea-Lys TL (0.02 mmol), reagents 1-Ethyl-3-(3-dimethylaminopropyl) carbodiimide (EDC, 0.027 mmol), and 4-Dimethylaminopyridine (DMAP, 0.002 mmol) were dissolved in dimethylformamide (DMF, 1 mL), with continuous stirring at room temperature for 24 h. DMF was evaporated and ^{1}H-NMR spectroscopy was conducted on a Bruker AVENCE II 400 MHz (^{1}H at 400 MHz) instrument in DMSO-d_6 as a solvent to validate the conjugation process [77]. Elimination of impurities was achieved by dialysis (molecular weight cutoff of 500–1000Da, BDL (Beith Dekel) Ltd., Raanana, Israel) against DW for 24 h. After conjugation and elimination of impurities, the SA-PEG-TL conjugation product was quantified using back titration. The excess of SA-PEG-COOH that did not react with the amine group on the PSMA TL was measured by titration with 0.01 M NaOH. The molarity of the SA-PEG-TL was calculated by the difference between the original molarity of SA-PEG-COOH and the molarity obtained by the acid-base titration. Thereafter, the PSMA TL protecting groups were removed under acidic conditions using trifluoroacetic acid (TFA) (Figure 1) and the isobutylene by-product was evaporated together with the solvents. ^{1}H-NMR spectroscopy was conducted on a Bruker AVENCE 200 MHz (^{1}H at 200 MHz) instrument in DMSO-d_6 as a solvent to confirm the exposure of the carboxylic groups of the PSMA TL in the final SA-PEG-TL conjugation product [77]. For the preparation of targeted NLCs, SA-PEG-TL was added to the aqueous phase with SA-PEG at 70 °C. OA dissolved in EtOH was then added dropwise into the preheated aqueous phase under magnetic stirring of 600 rpm at room temperature for 10 min. Samples were then transferred to a cold-water bath at 4 °C under stirring for another 10 min.

2.3.3. Preparation of Drug-Loaded NPs

Drug-loaded NPs were prepared as described in Section 2.3.1, with the addition of CTX dissolved in EtOH in the OA liquid lipid phase. The mixture was added dropwise to the water phase, containing SA-PEG and SA-PEG-TL. Samples were stirred at room temperature for 10 min and transferred to 4 °C for another 10 min. Samples were then centrifuged at 10,000× g at 4 °C for 20 min to sediment the unbound excess drug aggregates [72–74]. It was verified that under these centrifugation conditions the sediment does not contain any significant amount of the NPs, but only the crystalline drug excess.

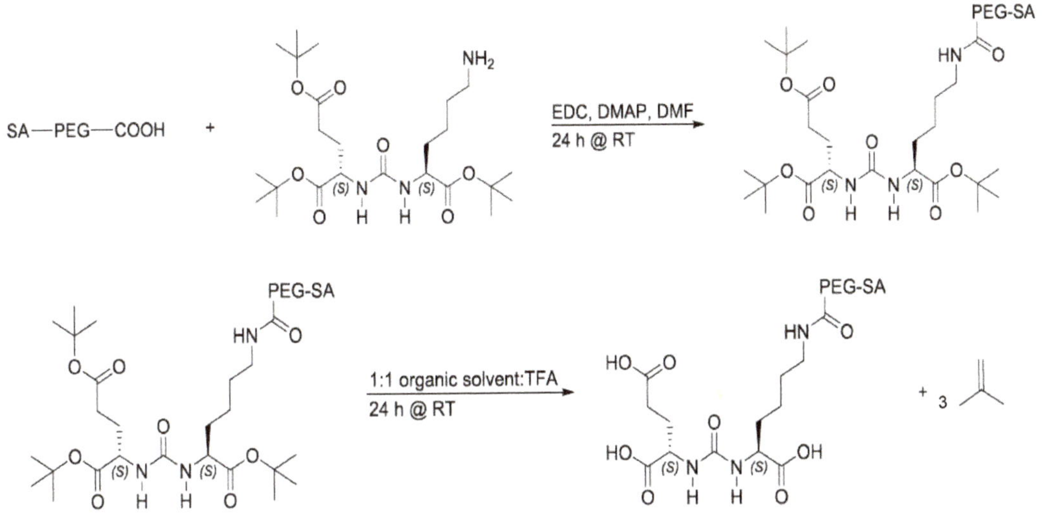

Figure 1. Synthesis of SA-PEG with PSMA TL Glu-Urea-Lys. SA-PEG-COOH was conjugated to Glu-Urea-Lys with protecting groups of tert-Butyl esters. The SA-PEG-TL was subjected to acidic conditions for the removal of the protecting groups, hence regaining the carboxylic groups of the PSMA TL.

2.3.4. Particle Size Distribution and Zeta-Potential Analyses

The colloidal stability of the NLCs and the drug-loaded NPs was studied according to volume-weighted particle size distribution and zeta-potential using a dynamic light scattering (DLS)/zeta-potential analyzer, Zetasizer Ultra (Malvern Instruments Ltd., Worcestershire, UK). Samples were prepared by the nanoprecipitation method as described above and size distribution and zeta-potential measurements were carried out. Zeta-potential was calculated based on the Smoluchowski model [78]. Measurements from two independent experiments, each performed in triplicates, are presented as means ± standard error (SE).

2.3.5. Analysis of Drug Loading Capacity and Encapsulation Efficiency

To quantify the amount of drug loaded into the NPs, NLCs were prepared at increasing drug to SA-PEG molar ratios [72,79]. The drug-loaded NPs were prepared and centrifuged as mentioned in Section 2.3.3 [72–74]. Quantification of the encapsulated drug in the supernatant was performed by lyophilizing the supernatant and dissolving it in EtOH to extract the CTX from the NLCs. Thereafter, the samples were filtered through a 0.45μm membrane. The concentration of drugs was determined using reversed-phase HPLC (RP-HPLC) and analyzed using a linear calibration curve [80,81]. RP-HPLC was conducted using a 4.6 × 250 mm C18 Kromasil RP-HPLC column and a UV detector at 234 nm for CTX detection. The mobile phase consisted of acetonitrile (ACN) and water (50:50, v/v). The injection volume was 20 μL, at a flow rate of 1ml/min. The column temperature was kept at 25 °C, and the HPLC run was set for 25 min [80,81] with a 6 min ACN rinse between runs.

Calculation of the loading capacity (LC, i.e., the mass ratio of drug to carrier) and encapsulation efficiency (EE) (i.e., the percent of encapsulated drug from the added drug) of the NPs was performed using Equations (1) and (2) [72–74]:

$$LC \text{ (mg drug/g SA-PEG)} = W_{ED}/W_{SA\text{-}PEG} \quad (1)$$

$$EE \text{ (\%)} = (W_{ED}/W_{TD}) \times 100\% \quad (2)$$

W_{ED} is the amount of encapsulated drug; $W_{SA\text{-}PEG}$ is the total amount of SA-PEG in the sample; W_{TD} is the total amount of drug in the sample.

Results from two independent experiments, each performed in duplicates, are presented as means ± SE.

2.3.6. Cryogenic-Transmission Electron Microscopy Imaging (Cryo-TEM)

Cryo-TEM (Philips CM120 microscope) analysis was used for the imaging of NLCs and NPs loaded with 0.6:1 CTX: SA-PEG molar ratio. Samples were prepared as described and images were taken at 4 °C. A Gatan Multi Scan 791 cooled CCD camera was used to acquire the images, using the Digital Micrograph 3.1 software package [72]. NPs size was determined using ImageJ software.

2.3.7. Time-Course of In Vitro Drug Release

The time-course of in vitro release of drugs from the loaded NPs as compared to free drugs was studied by the dialysis method [72,73]. One ml of drug-loaded NPs or free drugs (both systems in DDW) were placed in dialysis tubes (molecular weight cutoff of 3.5 kDa, Sigma-Aldrich, Merck, Rehovot, Israel) and incubated in 30 mL of buffer comprising phosphate-buffered saline (PBS, 10 mM, pH 7.4) containing 0.1% wt Tween 80 for 72 h at 37 °C, with continuous gentle agitation (100 rpm). At defined time intervals (0, 2, 4, 6, 10, 23, 29, 36, 47, 58, 72 h), the dialysate was collected and replaced by the same volume of fresh release buffer. To calculate the cumulative release of drugs, the dialysates from each time point were freeze-dried, dissolved in EtOH for CTX extraction, filtered through 0.45 μm membrane, and quantified using RP-HPLC, as described in Section 2.3.5 above. The results are presented as the means of two independent experiments ± SE.

2.3.8. Determination of NPs Concentration by Nanosight

NPs concentration was determined using Nanosight instrument (NS300, Malvern Instruments Ltd., Worcestershire, UK). Samples were prepared as described above, diluted with DW, and measured at 25 °C. Results are presented as the means of two independent experiments ± SE.

2.3.9. Characterization of NPs Specificity by Confocal Laser Microscopy

Fluorescent NPs were formed as described above, with the addition of SA-PEG conjugated to the fluorophore Cy7 (SA-PEG-Cy7) in the aqueous phase during the NPs' preparation. The conjugation between Cy7-NH$_2$ and SA-PEG-COOH was performed using the EDC and N-hydroxysuccinimide (NHS) conjugation method as previously described [82]. SA-PEG-COOH (0.0125 mmol) was incubated with excess of EDC and NHS (at a 1:2 EDC: NHS molar ratio) for 15 min at room temperature with gentle shaking. The resulting NHS-activated SA-PEG was covalently linked to Cy7-NH$_2$ (0.0125 mmol). The sample was allowed to react for 2 h with constant mixing at room temperature, and the final conjugate was dialyzed against DW (molecular weight cutoff of 3.5kDa, Sigma-Aldrich, Merck, Rehovot, Israel) for 24 h with five replacements of the dialysate to remove unreacted fluorophore.

Selective internalization of Cy7-labeled NPs was studied using confocal fluorescence microscopy (inverted confocal microscope, Zeiss LSM 710) [72,79]. Prior to the experiments, cells were seeded on μ-slides VI 0.4 (Ibidi, Martinsried, Germany) at 50% confluence and incubated overnight. Cells were then washed with PBS and incubated with 1 μg/mL

Hoechst 33342 in growth medium for 10 min to achieve nuclear DNA staining. Thereafter, cells were incubated with different fluorescent NPs.

For selective internalization of targeted NPs as a function of the concentration of the PSMA TL, LNCaP target cells were incubated for 2 h at 37 °C, with non-targeted NPs and NPs decorated with increasing TL concentrations of 15 nM, 30 nM, and 80 nM (diluted 1:400 (v/v) in FBS-free medium). Thereafter, cells were washed twice with PBS to remove free fluorescent NPs. Two fluorescence channels were used during image capture: (1) blue for the viable DNA-dye Hoechst 33342 (Excitation/Emission: 350/461 nm); and (2) deep red for the Cy7-labeled NPs (Excitation/Emission: 720/750 nm).

To explore the internalization specificity of the NPs, LNCaP and PC-3 cells were incubated with non-targeted fluorescent NPs or 30 nM TL-decorated fluorescent NPs (diluted 1:400 (v/v) in FBS-free medium) for 2 h at 37 °C. In addition, NSCLC 1975, HEK293, BEAS2B, and FSE cells, were incubated with targeted fluorescent NPs (diluted 1:400 (v/v) in FBS-free medium) for 2 h at 37 °C. Then, cells were washed twice with PBS to remove free fluorescent NPs, and confocal microscope images were captured with the same fluorescence channels as mentioned above.

For characterization of the active internalization of NPs, LNCaP cells were incubated with a serum-free medium containing targeted NPs (diluted 1:400 (v/v)) for 1 h, at two different temperatures: 4 °C and 37 °C. Following incubation, cells were washed twice with PBS and the cellular fluorescence pattern was examined. Images were analyzed with IMARIS software.

2.3.10. Growth Inhibition Assays

The selective growth inhibition of CTX-loaded NPs was studied in LNCaP target cells and PC-3 non-target cells, using an XTT (2,3-bis-(2-methoxy-4-nitro-5-sulfophenyl)-2H-tetrazolium-5-carboxanilide)-based colorimetric cell proliferation kit as previously described [72,79,83]. The preparation of CTX-loaded NPs was performed as described above and the NPs had undergone 24 h dialysis before cell exposure, to simulate conditions in the human body. The dialysis was conducted as described in Section 2.3.7, but with the use of 10% FBS to capture the released CTX [83]. Prior to the experiment, 96-well plates were coated with poly-L-Lysine before cell plating. LNCaP and PC-3 cells were seeded in 96-well plates at 5×10^4 and 2.5×10^4 cells/mL, respectively, and incubated overnight to allow for cell attachment. Following exposure of the cells to CTX-loaded NPs at increasing CTX concentrations of 0.001–100 nM for 24 h, cells were incubated for an additional 72 h with a fresh growth medium. Cellular growth inhibition was determined by adding the XTT reagent. Data were plotted using a nonlinear curve fitting of a sigmoidal model (Hill1) with OriginPro 9.0 to obtain a dose-response curve according to Equation (3) [72,79,83]:

$$P = P_\infty + (P_0 - P_\infty) \times ([D]^n / ((IC_{50})^n + [D]^n)) \tag{3}$$

P stands for the percentage of live cells; P∞ represents the minimal percent of live cells at infinite drug concentration; P0 is the maximal percent of surviving cells in the absence of drug (100% = control), [D] stands for the drug concentration; IC50 stands for the drug concentration exerting 50% inhibition of cell growth; n indicates the abruptness of the dose-response curve.

Cells grown with free CTX at the same concentrations or medium with the addition of non-encapsulating NLCs served as the controls. Results shown are the means of two independent experiments, each performed in triplicates ± SE.

3. Results and Discussion

3.1. Self-Assembly of the Delivery System

NLCs are typically composed of a mixture of solid and liquid lipids at different ratios, designed to obtain stable core-shell (or multi-core-shell) structured spherical particles. We examined different formulations, and a mixture of 60% SA-PEG and 40% liquid lipid was selected for further characterization. Self-assembled NLCs were prepared as described in Section 2.3.1.

Various liquid lipids were studied for NP size distribution, as an assessment of the compatibility between the crystalline shell created by solidifying SA and the liquid lipid core (Figure 2).

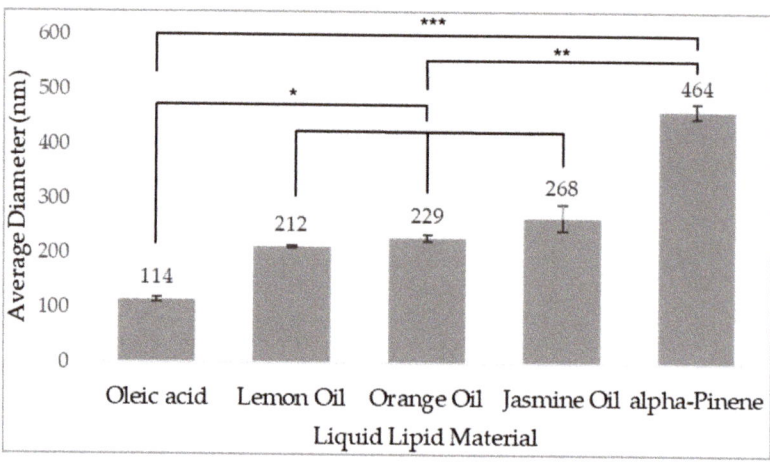

Figure 2. Mean diameter of monomodal distribution of NLCs with various liquid lipids. NLCs formulations of 60% SA-PEG and 40% of different liquid lipids were examined for size distribution. Values presented are means ± SE, n = 2 (two independent experiments each performed in triplicates). Significant differences between liquid lipids are marked as follows: * ($p < 0.0080$); ** ($p < 0.0009$); *** ($p < 0.0005$).

To form a stable colloidal system of NPs suitable for effective accumulation in the TME and internalization into target cancer cells via endocytosis, we aimed at forming NPs with a mean diameter of 50–200 nm and a zeta-potential below −30mV (17, 19, 37). NPs with 40% oleic acid displayed a monomodal distribution with a mean size of less than 200 nm and were therefore selected as the formulation for further experiments.

To generate NPs that will selectively target PC cells, the PSMA TL, Glu-Urea-Lys, was conjugated via an amide linkage to SA-PEG. SA-PEG with a carboxylic end group at the PEG terminus and the amine group in the lysine side chain of the Glu-Urea-Lys TL with protecting groups of *tert*-Butyl esters, were conjugated for the synthesis of SA-PEG-TL (Figure 1). Following the conjugation and elimination of unwanted impurities, the protecting groups were removed to yield three carboxylic groups, constituting the binding motif to the PSMA receptor (Figure 1). NLCs with the PSMA TL (Targeted-NLCs) were slightly enlarged with an average diameter of 129 ± 3 nm, and a zeta-potential of −36.3 ± 0.3 mV. This negative surface charge of NPs was achieved thanks to the reduction of the carboxylic protecting groups of *tert*-Butyl esters, as shown in the H-NMR spectroscopy (Figure 3), thus exposing the negative charge of the TL at physiological pH. It is known that PEGylation (even without charge) provides good colloidal stability by steric repulsion of the NPs [84]. Moreover, the negative zeta potential provides additional colloidal stability by electrostatic repulsion, and it is also known that zeta potential that is more negative than (−30 mV), provides good colloidal stability [85] (even in the absence of PEGylation). Therefore, these results indicate that we have successfully formed colloidally stable NPs that could serve as a nanocarrier system that is decorated with a specific targeting ligand. This system was subjected to further analyses.

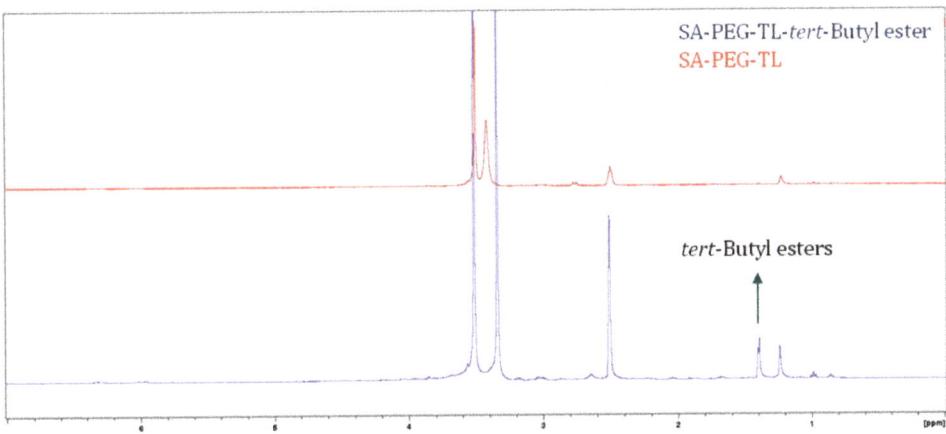

Figure 3. H-NMR spectroscopy. Tracings represent SA-PEG-TL with tert-Butyl esters protecting groups (blue) compared to the final conjugation product SA-PEG-TL (red). The H-NMR spectroscopy confirms that the tert-Butyl ester protecting groups were removed, thus revealing the carboxylic groups of the TL. Measurements were performed in duplicates.

3.2. Physicochemical Characterization of NPs

The size distribution and zeta-potential of targeted-NLCs were determined at increasing drug to SA-PEG molar ratios using DLS/zeta-potential analyzer [72–74,79]. CTX was dissolved in the liquid lipid phase together with the OA and loaded into the targeted NLCs by physical encapsulation. Following centrifugal sedimentation of the unbound excess drug, CTX-loaded NPs were studied for size distribution and displayed a monomodal distribution (Figure 4).

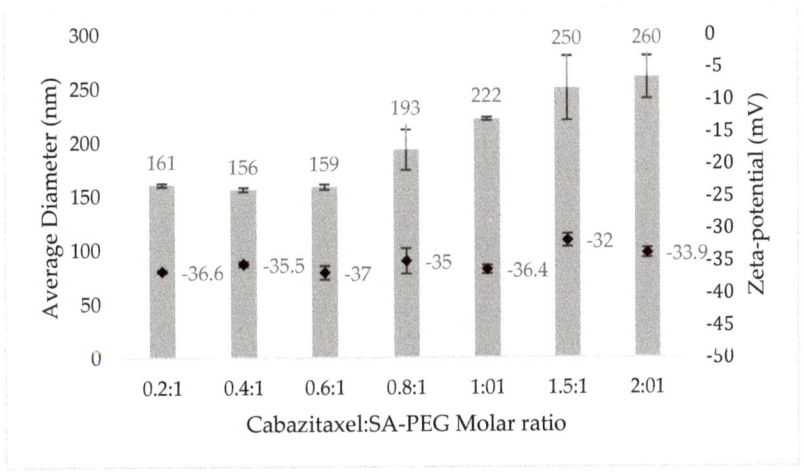

Figure 4. Mean diameter and zeta-potential of NPs at increasing CTX: SA-PEG molar ratios. Columns represent the mean diameter and black diamonds represent the zeta-potential. Values presented are means ± SE, n = 2 (two independent experiments, each performed in triplicates).

Expectedly, at increasing drug to SA-PEG molar ratios, there was an increase in the average diameter of NPs. This is due to the encapsulation of molecules that are characterized by a hydrophobic taxadiene core, as in the case of CTX. As the drug: SA-PEG ratio increased, the volume-to-surface ratio increased and thus the average diameter of the NPs increased. In contrast, the zeta-potential of the NPs remained negative and in the range of -35 ± 3 mV. As we aimed to obtain NPs with an average size of less than 200 nm, a CTX: SA-PEG molar ratio of 0.2–0.6:1 appeared to be suitable, and the drug loading capacity was hence studied.

3.3. Drug Loading Capacity (LC) and Encapsulation Efficiency (EE)

The LC and EE of CTX at increasing drug to SA-PEG molar ratios were determined by centrifugal sedimentation of unbound excess drug and quantification of the encapsulated drug in the supernatant by RP-HPLC (Figure 5). Expectedly, at increasing drug to SA-PEG molar ratios, the EE decreased, whereas the LC increased. It is evident from Figure 5 that increased concentrations of CTX led to a significant increase in LC, up to 0.6:1 CTX to SA-PEG molar ratio. However, at higher drug concentrations, the increase in LC became more moderate. These results are consistent with the DLS data showing a major increase in the average diameter of NPs between 0.6:1 to 0.8:1 CTX: SA-PEG molar ratio (159 $\pm$ 3 nm and 193 $\pm$ 19 nm, respectively). Taken collectively, the formulation displaying the optimal relation between LC, EE, and particle size was 0.6:1 CTX: SA-PEG, with an average diameter of 159 $\pm$ 3 nm, LC of 168 $\pm$ 3 mg CTX/g SA-PEG, and EE of 67% $\pm$ 1%.

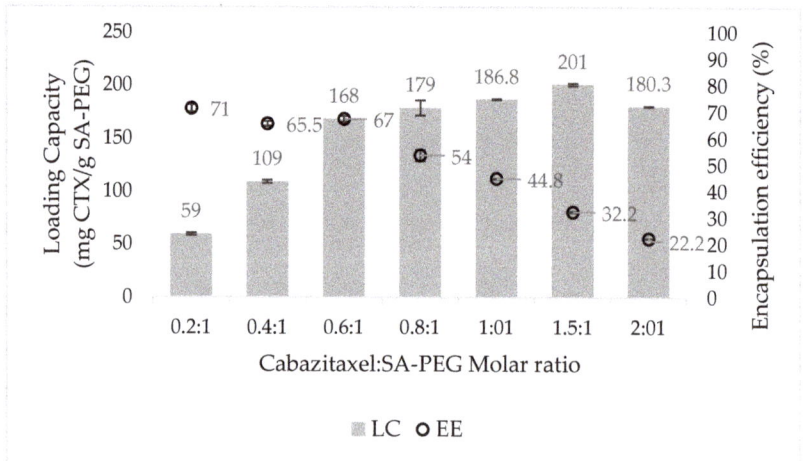

Figure 5. CTX loading capacity (LC) and encapsulation efficiency (EE) at increasing CTX: SA-PEG molar ratios. Columns represent the LC, whereas circles denote EE. Values shown are means $\pm$ SE, n = 2 (two independent experiments, each performed in triplicates).

3.4. The Morphology of Drug-Loaded NPs

The morphology of the NPs was examined by analyzing cryogenic transmission electron microscopy (Cryo-TEM) images (Figure 6). NPs loaded with CTX (Figure 6A) appear as spherical particles with an average diameter, which agrees with the DLS measurements. As it was previously found that spherical particles are able to undergo faster internalization than non-spherical NPs, this result contributes to the efficiency of the delivery system [86]. Additionally, non-encapsulated NLCs (Figure 6B) displayed a similar morphology, supporting the incorporation of drugs into the NLCs nanocapsules.

3.5. In Vitro Profile of CTX Release from the NPs

The time-course of in vitro release of CTX from NPs was assessed by dialysis in a large volume of a PBS buffer pH 7.4 containing 0.1% wt Tween 80 for 72 h at 37 °C, with continuous mixing. We used a buffer containing Tween 80 so that the hydrophobic drug released from the NPs was efficiently bound and solubilized by Tween 80%, mimicking human serum albumin binding of hydrophobic drugs. The above conditions were used to simulate the systemic circulation of NPs in the blood over 24–48 h, assuming this was a typical time for circulating NPs to accumulate in the tumor via the EPR effect [87]. At defined time intervals, the dialysate was replaced with fresh buffer, and the drug was quantified using RP-HPLC [72,73]. The complete replacement of fresh release buffer caused a stronger release driving force and constituted stringent release conditions [72,73].

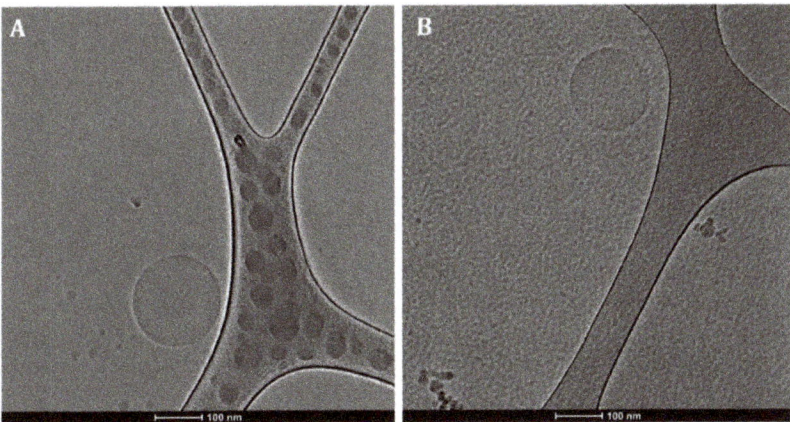

Figure 6. Analysis of the morphology of NPs by Cryo-TEM. Cryo-TEM images of (**A**) 0.6:1 CTX: SA-PEG NPs; and (**B**) NLCs not encapsulating a drug, in water. The scale bars denote 100 nm. Note that the CryoTEM images only show examples of the morphology of typical NPs. For size statistics, please refer to the DLS data.

The in vitro release profile of CTX from NPs showed substantial drug retention, as opposed to a burst-release of the unencapsulated drug during the first 10 h (Figure 7). These results were affected by the ratio between the liquid and solid lipids in the NPs formulation. As previously reported [41–43], the solid lipids of NLCs form a crystalline shell that acts as a barrier, and the liquid lipids form a cohesive hydrophobic inner core with strong interaction with the drugs loaded. Thus, a substantial reduction in drug release from the NPs was observed. However, the initial release of the drug from the NPs, possibly of some unencapsulated drug, or drug particles that were weakly adsorbed to the outer shell of the NPs, was slightly more rapid.

3.6. Selective Targeting and Internalization of NPs into LNCaP Target Cells

The selective internalization of targeted NPs labeled with the deep red fluorescent dye, Cy7, was studied using confocal laser microscopy. The cell lines that were examined were LNCaP, PC cells overexpressing PSMA that were used as the target cells; PC-3, rare PC cells lacking PSMA expression; NSCLC 1975 cells; human embryonic kidney HEK-293 cells; normal human bronchial epithelial BEAS2B cells; and neonatal foreskin fibroblast FSE cells.

First, the actual surface expression of PSMA by the above PC cell lines was determined by immunohistochemistry, conducted by the department of pathology in Rambam Health Care Campus, Haifa, Israel. Expectedly, LNCaP cells displayed PSMA overexpression (Figure 8A), whereas PC-3 cells were devoid of PSMA (Figure 8B). These results are shown by the brown immunohistochemistry staining of the PSMA receptor that was largely confined to the plasma membrane of LNCaP cells.

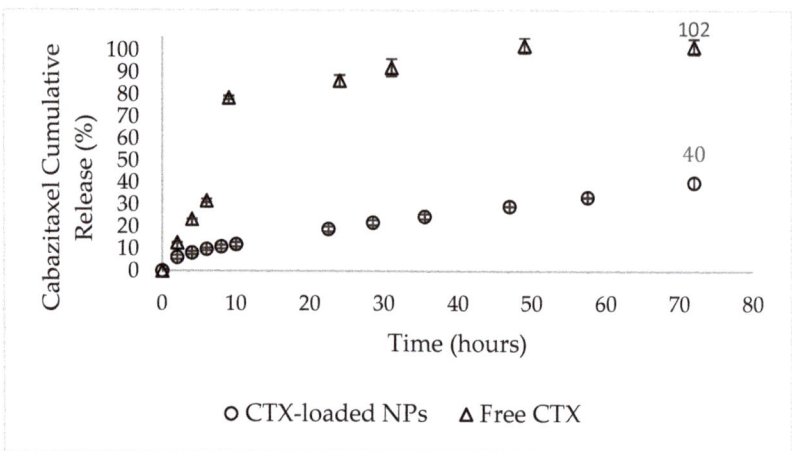

Figure 7. Time-course of CTX drug release. In vitro drug release profiles of CTX-loaded NPs (circles) compared to unencapsulated CTX (triangles). The values shown are means ± SE, n = 2 (two independent experiments).

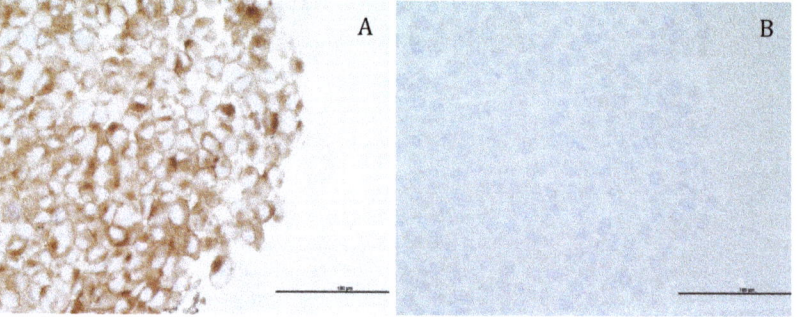

Figure 8. Immunohistochemistry analysis of PSMA expression. PSMA expression (shown as a brown diaminobenzidine immunohistochemistry staining) was examined in: (**A**) LNCaP; (**B**) PC-3 cell lines by the department of pathology in Rambam Health Care Campus. Scale bars denote 100 μm.

The optimal amount of the TL conjugated to the NPs was examined by evaluation of the fluorescence signal in LNCaP target cells (Figure 9). The NPs were decorated with TL concentrations of 15 nM, 30 nM, and 80 nM, or no TL at all. We found that the internalization of NPs into LNCaP target cells is dependent on the concentration of TL decorating the NPs surface. Following 2 h incubation with NPs decorated with increasing TL concentrations at 37 °C, LNCaP cells displayed some cellular internalization upon 15 nM TL decoration and maximal internalization at 30 nM TL. The possible reasons for the result that optimal internalization of NPs occurred at 30 nM TL decoration, and only decreased at higher TL concentrations are: (a) A large number of TLs on the NPs surface may facilitate over-binding of a single NP to multiple PSMA receptors [88], thereby impairing proper internalization; (b) The large number of TLs sterically hindered these ligands from binding to the cell surface PSMA receptors [89]; (c) The negative surface charge of the NPs, caused by the large number of dissociated carboxylic groups on the PSMA TLs, resulted in an extensive repulsion between NPs and the negatively charged outer leaflet of the plasma membrane [13].

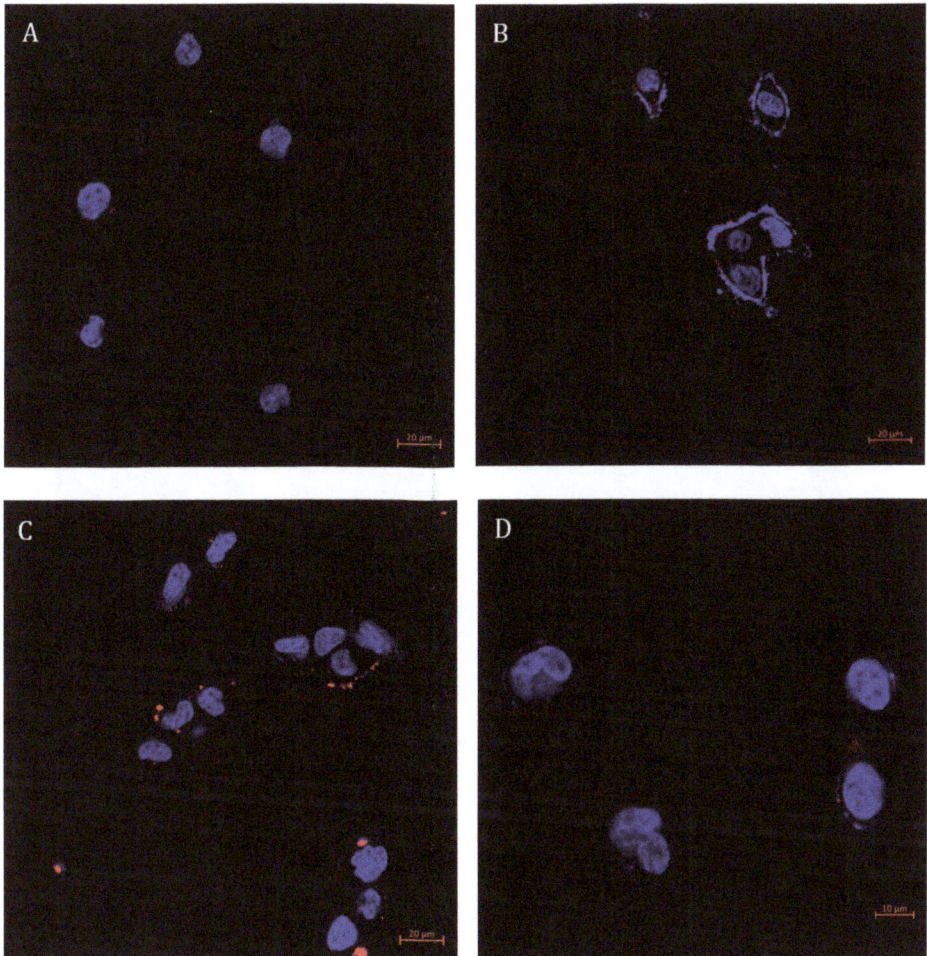

Figure 9. Selective targeting of NPs decorated with increasing concentrations of the TL, to PSMA-overexpressing LNCaP cells. Confocal laser microscopy images of LNCaP cells, following 2 h incubation with: (**A**) NPs lacking TL decoration; (**B**) NPs decorated with 15 nM of TL; (**C**) with 30 nM of TL; and (**D**) with 80 nM of TL (at 37 °C; samples were diluted 1:400 (v/v) in FBS-free medium). Nuclear DNA staining was achieved with Hoechst 33342 (1 µg/mL) and is marked in blue, whereas NPs labeled with Cy7 are marked in red. Scale bars denote 20 µm in (**A–C**), and 10 µm in (**D**).

The observation of the complete lack of internalization upon exposure of target cells to non-targeted NPs confirmed that the targeting properties were specifically attributable to the PSMA TL, Glu-Urea-Lys. In conclusion, the targeted NPs selected for further studies were those decorated with 30 nM PSMA.

Determination of NPs concentration by Nanosight enabled to calculate the number of TL molecules on the NPs surface. NPs concentration was found to be 0.28894 ± 0.00007 nM, thus decoration of NPs with 30 nM TL resulted in ~100 TL molecules/NP.

To verify the specific internalization of targeted NPs to LNCaP target cells via the PSMA receptor, different cell lines were examined including PC-3, NSCLC 1975, HEK-293, BEAS2B, and FSE cell lines (Figure 10).

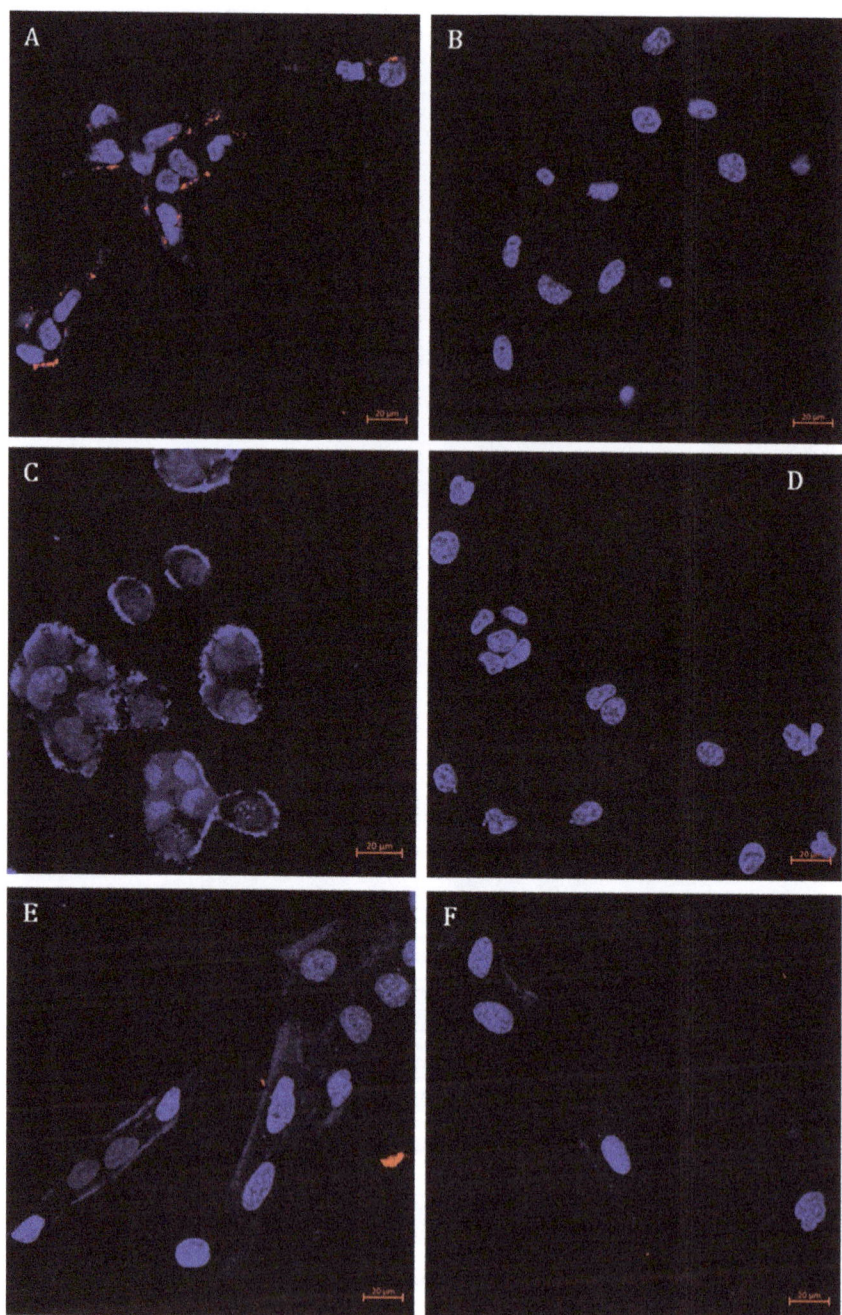

Figure 10. Specific internalization of targeted NPs. Confocal microscopy images of: (**A**) LNCaP; (**B**) PC-3; (**C**) NSCLC 1975; (**D**) HEK293; (**E**) BEAS2B; and (**F**) FSE cells, following 2 h incubation with targeted NPs labeled with Cy7 (at 37 °C; Samples were diluted 1:400 (v/v) in FBS-free medium). Nuclear DNA staining achieved with Hoechst 33342 (1 µg/mL) is marked in blue, whereas NPs labeled with Cy7 are marked in red. Scale bars denote 20 µm.

Neither binding nor internalization were observed in non-target cells, demonstrating absolute specificity and enhanced internalization of NPs by PSMA-expressing PC cells. Moreover, the accumulation of targeted NPs within LNCaP cells appeared as perinuclear punctate staining. This suggests internalization via receptor-mediated endocytosis and intracellular accumulation in endolysosomes [90].

For the characterization of active internalization by endocytosis, cells were incubated at two different temperatures: 4 °C and 37 °C. As endocytosis is an energy-dependent process, we assumed there will be higher accumulation at 37 °C, while at 4 °C only cell surface binding to the PSMA receptor may occur [90]. Confocal microscopy analysis (Figure 11) revealed that the uptake of targeted NPs was based on an endocytic process, with 17 red fluorescent dots per target LNCaP cell and an average intensity of 120 ± 60 (A.U.) at 37 °C compared to 4 dots per target cell and average intensity of 63 ± 30 (A.U.) at 4 °C. It should be noted that cellular processes other than endocytosis, such as diffusion, are also impeded at low temperatures and it is possible that TL binding to the PSMA receptor encouraged the diffusion of the NPs into the cell [91].

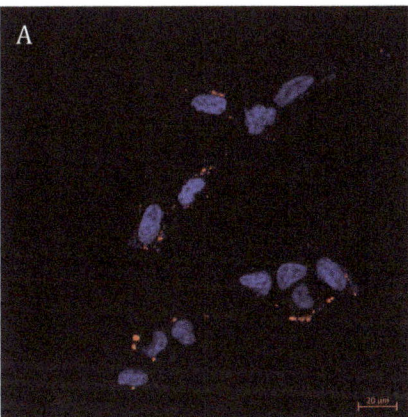 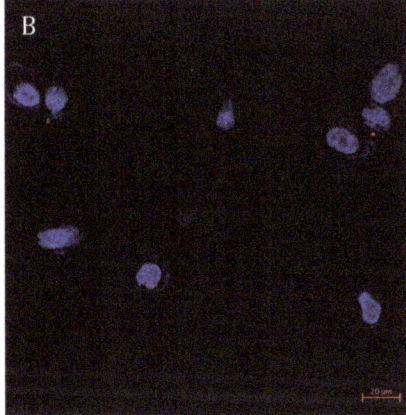

Figure 11. Characterization of active internalization of targeted NPs by LNCaP cells. Confocal laser microscopy images of LNCaP cells, following 1 h incubation with targeted NPs labeled with Cy7 (samples were diluted 1:400 (v/v) in FBS-free medium) at two different temperatures: (**A**) 37 °C; (**B**) 4 °C. Nuclear DNA staining achieved with Hoechst 33342 (1 µg/mL) is marked in blue, whereas NPs labeled with Cy7 are marked in red. Scale bars denote 20 µm.

3.7. Selective Growth Inhibition of CTX-Loaded NPs In Vitro

Cytotoxicity assays were performed using an XTT-based colorimetric cell proliferation kit with PSMA-positive LNCaP cells and compared to PSMA-negative PC cells (PC-3). It is evident from Figure 12 that CTX loaded NPs displayed a remarkable dose-dependent growth inhibitory effect on target LNCaP cells which overexpress PSMA, with an outstanding half-maximal inhibitory concentration (IC_{50}) of 4.0 ± 2.0 pM. In contrast, these NPs did not exhibit any substantial growth inhibitory effect on PC-3 which lacked PSMA expression.

Cells exposed to free CTX in a growth medium for 72 h served as control and IC_{50} values obtained with LNCaP and PC-3 cells were similar: 0.25 ± 0.04 nM and 0.18 ± 0.04 nM, respectively (Figure 13).

The ratio of 62.5-fold between the IC_{50} values of free CTX and CTX-loaded NPs towards target LNCaP cells can be explained by the different exposure times and the targeting ability of the CTX-loaded NPs. The active targeting of CTX-loaded NPs enables the accumulation of NPs in target PC cells and thus a more potent anti-tumor activity. As a result, even at shorter exposure times (24 h, compared to 72 h of free CTX), the cytotoxic effect of the NPs was more significant against LNCaP target cells, as evident from the lower IC$_{50}$ value. Moreover, it has been reported that the IC$_{50}$ of free CTX exposure for 48 h towards LNCaP cells is 2.6–3.1 nM, which supports this conclusion [92,93]. Another important aspect that was achieved in the current study is the remarkable LC of 168 ± 3 mg CTX/g SA-PEG. In this respect, based on the concentration of NPs that was determined by Nanosight, we calculated that each NP carries a cargo of as much as ~700,000 CTX drug molecules. This remarkably large amount of potent cytotoxic drug molecules that are efficiently and specifically internalized by target PC cells, not only eliminate these tumor cells but may also kill neighbor PC cells upon apoptotic and lytic cell death. It is important to emphasize that drug-free NLCs were found to be non-toxic to cells.

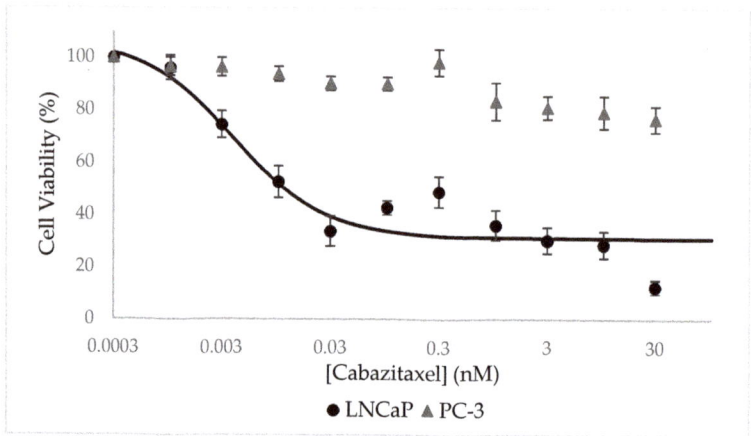

Figure 12. Selective growth inhibition of LNCaP target cells by CTX-loaded NPs. Cell growth inhibition as a function of the concentration of CTX encapsulated within NPs (0.6:1 CTX:SA-PEG molar ratio) in LNCaP target cells (circles) and non-target PC-3 cells (triangle). Values presented are means ± SE, n = 3 (three independent experiments, each performed in triplicates). The sigmoidal model curve of LNCaP cells was fitted using Equation (3).

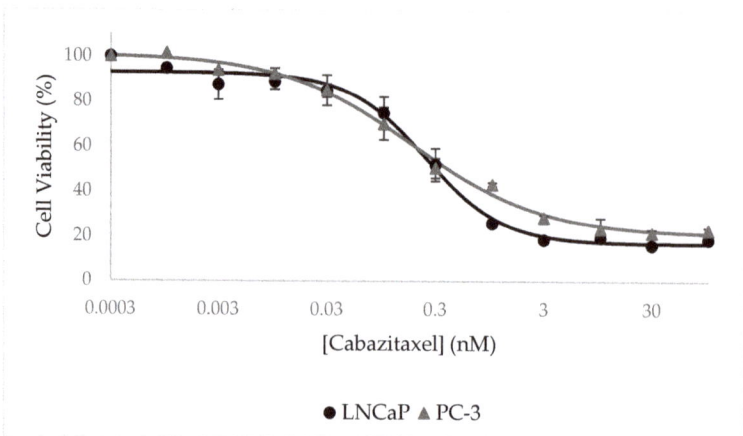

Figure 13. Inhibitory effect of free CTX. Cell viability as a function of free CTX concentration of LNCaP target cells (circles) and PC-3 non-target cells (triangle). Values presented are means ± SE, n = 3 (three independent experiments, each performed in triplicates). Sigmoidal model curves were fitted using Equation (3).

4. Conclusions

Towards the efficacious treatment of PC, CRPC, and mCRPC, we herein developed novel selectively PC-targeted NPs harboring a cytotoxic drug cargo. These targeted NPs demonstrated efficient encapsulation of CTX, high specificity to, and potent eradication of, PSMA-positive target PC cells. Moreover, targeting NPs to the PSMA receptor resulted in uptake via receptor-mediated endocytosis, thus facilitating the intracellular release of the drug cargo, enabling the therapeutic activity. Another important aspect of selective internalization of these targeted NPs is the potential to overcome cancer MDR by evading MDR efflux pumps that extrude a broad spectrum of anticancer drugs from multidrug-resistant cancer cells. This selectively targeted nano-delivery platform should be able to enhance the efficacy of PC treatment, while reducing drug doses and minimizing untoward toxicity. Hence, these novel findings bear promise towards the improvement of patient survival rates and quality of life. Future in vivo studies are warranted that should assess the therapeutic efficacy of the targeted NPs against human PC in a xenograft murine model.

Author Contributions: Investigation, L.C.; writing—original draft preparation, L.C.; writing—review and editing, Y.G.A. and Y.D.L.; supervision, Y.G.A. and Y.D.L. All authors have read and agreed to the published version of the manuscript.

Funding: This research received no external funding.

Institutional Review Board Statement: Not applicable.

Informed Consent Statement: Not applicable.

Data Availability Statement: The data presented in this study are available on request from the corresponding author.

Acknowledgments: We wish to thank Nitsan Dahan for his expert assistance with confocal laser microscopy. Moreover, we thank Moris Eisen, and Kseniya Kulbitski, Technion-Israel Institute of Technology, Haifa, Israel, for professional assistance with the SA-PEG-TL conjugation process. We also wish to thank O. Ben-Izhak from the department of Pathology at the Rambam Medical Center, Haifa, Israel for performing the immunohistochemistry analysis of PSMA expression.

Conflicts of Interest: The authors declare no conflict of interest.

References

1. Henley, S.J.; Ward, E.M.; Scott, S.; Ma, J.; Anderson, R.N.; Firth, A.U.; Thomas, C.C.; Islami, F.; Weir, H.K.; Lewis, D.R.; et al. Annual report to the nation on the status of cancer, part I: National cancer statistics. *Cancer* **2020**, *126*, 2225–2249. [CrossRef] [PubMed]
2. Jin, W.; Qin, B.; Chen, Z.; Liu, H.; Barve, A.; Cheng, K. Discovery of PSMA-specific peptide ligands for targeted drug delivery. *Int. J. Pharm.* **2016**, *513*, 138–147. [CrossRef]
3. Barve, A.; Jin, W.; Cheng, K. Prostate cancer relevant antigens and enzymes for targeted drug delivery. *J. Control. Release* **2014**, *187*, 118–132. [CrossRef] [PubMed]
4. Cohen, L.; Livney, Y.D.; Assaraf, Y.G. Targeted nanomedicine modalities for prostate cancer treatment. *Drug Resist. Updates* **2021**, *56*, 100762. [CrossRef] [PubMed]
5. Fujita, K.; Nonomura, N. Role of Androgen Receptor in Prostate Cancer: A Review. *World J. Men's Health* **2018**, *37*, 288–295. [CrossRef]
6. Karantanos, T.; Evans, C.P.; Tombal, B.; Thompson, T.C.; Montironi, R.; Isaacs, W.B. Understanding the mechanisms of androgen deprivation resistance in prostate cancer at the molecular level. *Eur. Urol.* **2015**, *67*, 470–479. [CrossRef] [PubMed]
7. Chen, Y.; Clegg, N.J.; Scher, H.I. Anti-androgens and androgen-depleting therapies in prostate cancer: New agents for an established target. *Lancet Oncol.* **2009**, *10*, 981–991. [CrossRef]
8. Gelmon, K. The taxoids: Paclitaxel and docetaxel. *Lancet* **1994**, *344*, 1267–1272. [CrossRef]
9. Singla, A.K.; Garg, A.; Aggarwal, D. Paclitaxel and its formulations. *Int. J. Pharm.* **2002**, *235*, 179–192. [CrossRef]
10. Haldar, S.; Chintapalli, J.; Croce, C.M. Taxol induces bcl-2 phosphorylation and death of prostate cancer cells. *Cancer Res.* **1996**, *56*, 1253–1255.
11. Danhier, F.; Feron, O.; Préat, V. To exploit the tumor microenvironment: Passive and active tumor targeting of nanocarriers for anti-cancer drug delivery. *J. Control. Release* **2010**, *148*, 135–146. [CrossRef] [PubMed]

12. Muhamad, N.; Plengsuriyakarn, T.; Na-Bangchang, K. Application of active targeting nanoparticle delivery system for chemotherapeutic drugs and traditional/herbal medicines in cancer therapy: A systematic review. *Int. J. Nanomedicine* **2018**, *13*, 3921–3935. [CrossRef]
13. Ernsting, M.J.; Murakami, M.; Roy, A.; Li, S.-D.D. Factors controlling the pharmacokinetics, biodistribution and intratumoral penetration of nanoparticles. *J. Control. Release* **2013**, *172*, 782–794. [CrossRef] [PubMed]
14. Torchilin, V.P. Passive and active drug targeting: Drug delivery to tumors as an example. *Handb. Exp. Pharmacol.* **2010**, *197*, 3–53. [CrossRef]
15. Bar-Zeev, M.; Livney, Y.D.; Assaraf, Y.G. Targeted nanomedicine for cancer therapeutics: Towards precision medicine overcoming drug resistance. *Drug Resist. Updates* **2017**, *31*, 15–30. [CrossRef] [PubMed]
16. Maeda, H.; Wu, J.; Sawa, T.; Matsumura, Y.; Hori, K. Tumor vascular permeability and the EPR effect in macromolecular therapeutics: A review. *J. Control. Release* **2000**, *65*, 271–284. [CrossRef]
17. Belfiore, L.; Saunders, D.N.; Ranson, M.; Thurecht, K.J.; Storm, G.; Vine, K.L. Towards clinical translation of ligand-functionalized liposomes in targeted cancer therapy: Challenges and opportunities. *J. Control. Release* **2018**, *277*, 1–13. [CrossRef]
18. Minner, S.; Wittmer, C.; Graefen, M.; Salomon, G.; Steuber, T.; Haese, A.; Huland, H.; Bokemeyer, C.; Yekebas, E.; Dierlamm, J.; et al. High level PSMA expression is associated with early psa recurrence in surgically treated prostate cancer. *Prostate* **2011**, *71*, 281–288. [CrossRef]
19. Mayor, N.; Sathianathen, N.J.; Buteau, J.; Koschel, S.; Juanilla, M.A.; Kapoor, J.; Azad, A.; Hofman, M.S.; Murphy, D.G. Prostate-specific membrane antigen theranostics in advanced prostate cancer: An evolving option. *BJU Int.* **2020**, *126*, 525–535. [CrossRef]
20. Jones, W.; Griffiths, K.; Barata, P.C.; Paller, C.J. PSMA theranostics: Review of the current status of PSMA-targeted imaging and radioligand therapy. *Cancers.* **2020**, *12*, 1367. [CrossRef]
21. Niaz, M.O.; Sun, M.; Ramirez-Fort, M.; Niaz, M.J. Prostate-specific Membrane Antigen Based Antibody-Drug Conjugates for Metastatic Castration-resistance Prostate Cancer. *Cureus* **2020**, *12*, e7147. [CrossRef]
22. Niaz, M.O.; Sun, M.; Ramirez-Fort, M.; Niaz, M.J. Review of Lutetium-177-labeled Anti-prostate-specific Membrane Antigen Monoclonal Antibody J591 for the Treatment of Metastatic Castration-resistant Prostate Cancer. *Cureus* **2020**, *12*, e7107. [CrossRef] [PubMed]
23. Iravani, A.; Violet, J.; Azad, A.; Hofman, M.S. Lutetium-177 prostate-specific membrane antigen (PSMA) theranostics: Practical nuances and intricacies. *Prostate Cancer Prostatic Dis.* **2020**, *23*, 38–52. [CrossRef]
24. Chandran, S.S.; Ray, S.; Pomper, M.G.; Denmeade, S.R.; Mease, R.C. Prostate Specific Membrane Antigen (PSMA) Targeted Nanoparticles for Therapy of Prostate Cancer. U.S. Patent Application No. US9422234B2, 23 August 2016.
25. Kozikowski, A.P.; Zhang, J.; Nan, F.; Petukhov, P.A.; Grajkowska, E.; Wroblewski, J.T.; Yamamoto, T.; Bzdega, T.; Wroblewska, B.; Neale, J.H. Synthesis of Urea-Based Inhibitors as Active Site Probes of Glutamate Carboxypeptidase II: Efficacy as Analgesic Agents. *J. Med. Chem.* **2004**, *47*, 1729–1738. [CrossRef]
26. Harada, N.; Kimura, H.; Ono, M.; Saji, H. Preparation of asymmetric urea derivatives that target prostate-specific membrane antigen for SPECT imaging. *J. Med. Chem.* **2013**, *56*, 7890–7901. [CrossRef]
27. Chandran, S.S.; Banerjee, S.R.; Mease, R.C.; Pomper, M.G.; Denmeade, S.R. Characterization of a targeted nanoparticle functionalized with a urea-based inhibitor of prostate-specific membrane antigen (PSMA). *Cancer Biol. Ther.* **2008**, *7*, 974–982. [CrossRef]
28. Lepeltier, E.; Rijo, P.; Rizzolio, F.; Popovtzer, R.; Petrikaite, V.; Assaraf, Y.G.; Passirani, C. Nanomedicine to target multidrug resistant tumors. *Drug Resist. Updates* **2020**, *52*, 100704. [CrossRef]
29. Long, L.; Assaraf, Y.G.; Lei, Z.N.; Peng, H.; Yang, L.; Chen, Z.S.; Ren, S. Genetic biomarkers of drug resistance: A compass of prognosis and targeted therapy in acute myeloid leukemia. *Drug Resist. Updates* **2020**, *52*, 100703. [CrossRef] [PubMed]
30. Nassir, A.M.; Ibrahim, I.A.A.; Md, S.; Waris, M.; Tanuja; Ain, M.R.; Ahmad, I.; Shahzad, N. Surface functionalized folate targeted oleuropein nano-liposomes for prostate tumor targeting: In vitro and in vivo activity. *Life Sci.* **2019**, *220*, 136–146. [CrossRef]
31. Kopecka, J.; Trouillas, P.; Gašparović, A.Č.; Gazzano, E.; Assaraf, Y.G.; Riganti, C. Phospholipids and cholesterol: Inducers of cancer multidrug resistance and therapeutic targets. *Drug Resist. Updates* **2020**, *49*, 100670. [CrossRef] [PubMed]
32. Assaraf, Y.G.; Brozovic, A.; Gonçalves, A.C.; Jurkovicova, D.; Linē, A.; Machuqueiro, M.; Saponara, S.; Sarmento-Ribeiro, A.B.; Xavier, C.P.R.; Vasconcelos, M.H. The multi-factorial nature of clinical multidrug resistance in cancer. *Drug Resist. Updates* **2019**, *46*, 100645. [CrossRef] [PubMed]
33. Leonetti, A.; Wever, B.; Mazzaschi, G.; Assaraf, Y.G.; Rolfo, C.; Quaini, F.; Tiseo, M.; Giovannetti, E. Molecular basis and rationale for combining immune checkpoint inhibitors with chemotherapy in non-small cell lung cancer. *Drug Resist. Updates* **2019**, *46*, 100644. [CrossRef]
34. Cui, Q.; Wang, J.Q.; Assaraf, Y.G.; Ren, L.; Gupta, P.; Wei, L.; Ashby, C.R.; Yang, D.H.; Chen, Z.S. Modulating ROS to overcome multidrug resistance in cancer. *Drug Resist. Updates* **2018**, *41*, 1–25. [CrossRef]
35. Jiang, W.; Xia, J.; Xie, S.; Zou, R.; Pan, S.; Wang, Z.W.; Assaraf, Y.G.; Zhu, X. Long non-coding RNAs as a determinant of cancer drug resistance: Towards the overcoming of chemoresistance via modulation of lncRNAs. *Drug Resist. Updates* **2020**, *50*, 100683. [CrossRef] [PubMed]
36. Li, W.; Zhang, H.; Assaraf, Y.G.; Zhao, K.; Xu, X.; Xie, J.; Yang, D.H.; Chen, Z.S. Overcoming ABC transporter-mediated multidrug resistance: Molecular mechanisms and novel therapeutic drug strategies. *Drug Resist. Updates* **2016**, *27*, 14–29. [CrossRef] [PubMed]

37. Livney, Y.D.; Assaraf, Y.G. Rationally designed nanovehicles to overcome cancer chemoresistance. *Adv. Drug Deliv. Rev.* **2013**, *65*, 1716–1730. [CrossRef]
38. Gottesman, M.M.; Lavi, O.; Hall, M.D.; Gillet, J.P. Toward a Better Understanding of the Complexity of Cancer Drug Resistance. *Annu. Rev. Pharmacol. Toxicol.* **2016**, *56*, 85–102. [CrossRef]
39. Shapira, A.; Livney, Y.D.; Broxterman, H.J.; Assaraf, Y.G. Nanomedicine for targeted cancer therapy: Towards the overcoming of drug resistance. *Drug Resist. Updates* **2011**, *14*, 150–163. [CrossRef]
40. Zhang, H.; Xu, H.; Ashby, C.R.; Assaraf, Y.G.; Chen, Z.S.; Liu, H.M. Chemical molecular-based approach to overcome multidrug resistance in cancer by targeting P-glycoprotein (P-gp). *Med. Res. Rev.* **2020**, *41*, 525–555. [CrossRef]
41. Beloqui, A.; Solinís, M.Á.; Rodríguez-Gascón, A.; Almeida, A.J.; Préat, V. Nanostructured lipid carriers: Promising drug delivery systems for future clinics. *Nanomed. Nanotechnol. Biol. Med.* **2016**, *12*, 143–161. [CrossRef] [PubMed]
42. Selvamuthukumar, S.; Velmurugan, R. Nanostructured Lipid Carriers: A potential drug carrier for cancer chemotherapy. *Lipids Health Dis.* **2012**, *11*, 159–166. [CrossRef] [PubMed]
43. Haider, M.; Abdin, S.M.; Kamal, L.; Orive, G. Nanostructured lipid carriers for delivery of chemotherapeutics: A review. *Pharmaceutics* **2020**, *12*, 288. [CrossRef]
44. Emami, J.; Rezazadeh, M.; Varshosaz, J.; Tabbakhian, M.; Aslani, A. Formulation of LDL Targeted Nanostructured Lipid Carriers Loaded with Paclitaxel: A Detailed Study of Preparation, Freeze Drying Condition, and In Vitro Cytotoxicity. *J. Nanomater.* **2012**, *2012*, 358782. [CrossRef]
45. Chen, Y.; Pan, L.; Jiang, M.; Li, D.; Jin, L. Nanostructured lipid carriers enhance the bioavailability and brain cancer inhibitory efficacy of curcumin both in vitro and in vivo. *Drug Deliv.* **2016**, *23*, 1383–1392. [CrossRef]
46. Jiang, H.; Geng, D.; Liu, H.; Li, Z.; Cao, J. Co-delivery of etoposide and curcumin by lipid nanoparticulate drug delivery system for the treatment of gastric tumors. *Drug Deliv.* **2016**, *23*, 3665–3673. [CrossRef]
47. Bin, Z.; Yueying, Z.; Yu, D. Lung cancer gene therapy: Transferrin and hyaluronic acid dual ligand-decorated novel lipid carriers for targeted gene delivery. *Oncol. Rep.* **2017**, *37*, 937–944. [CrossRef]
48. Lin, W.J.; Juang, L.W.; Lin, C.C. Stability and release performance of a series of pegylated copolymeric micelles. *Pharm. Res.* **2003**, *20*, 668–673. [CrossRef]
49. Zhang, Z.; Zhu, Z.; Yang, D.; Fan, W.; Wang, J.; Li, X.; Chen, X.; Wang, Q.; Song, X. Preparation and affinity identification of glutamic acid-urea small molecule analogs in prostate cancer. *Oncol. Lett.* **2016**, *12*, 1001–1006. [CrossRef]
50. Maresca, K.P.; Hillier, S.M.; Femia, F.J.; Keith, D.; Barone, C.; Joyal, J.L.; Zimmerman, C.N.; Kozikowski, A.P.; Barrett, J.A.; Eckelman, W.C.; et al. A Series of Halogenated Heterodimeric Inhibitors of Prostate Specific Membrane Antigen (PSMA) as Radiolabeled Probes for Targeting Prostate Cancer. *J. Med. Chem.* **2009**, *52*, 347–357. [CrossRef] [PubMed]
51. Pereira, S.G.T.; Hudoklin, S.S.; Kreft, M.E.; Kostevsek, N.; Stuart, M.C.A.; Al-Jamal, W.T. Intracellular Activation of a Prostate Specific Antigen-Cleavable Doxorubicin Prodrug: A Key Feature toward Prodrug-Nanomedicine Design. *Mol. Pharm.* **2019**, *16*, 1573–1585. [CrossRef]
52. Wang, L.; Qu, M.; Huang, S.; Fu, Y.; Yang, L.; He, S.; Li, L.; Zhang, Z.; Lin, Q.; Zhang, L. A novel α-enolase-targeted drug delivery system for high efficacy prostate cancer therapy. *Nanoscale* **2018**, *10*, 13673–13683. [CrossRef]
53. Ikemoto, K.; Shimizu, K.; Ohashi, K.; Takeuchi, Y.; Shimizu, M.; Oku, N. Bauhinia purprea agglutinin-modified liposomes for human prostate cancer treatment. *Cancer Sci.* **2016**, *107*, 53–59. [CrossRef]
54. Cao, Y.; Zhou, Y.; Zhuang, Q.; Cui, L.; Xu, X.; Xu, R.; He, X. Anti-tumor effect of RGD modified PTX loaded liposome on prostatic cancer. *Int. J. Clin. Exp. Med.* **2015**, *8*, 12182–12191.
55. Zhang, L.; Shan, X.; Meng, X.; Gu, T.; Lu, Q.; Zhang, J.; Chen, J.; Jiang, Q.; Ning, X. The first integrins β3-mediated cellular and nuclear targeting therapeutics for prostate cancer. *Biomaterials* **2019**, *223*, 119471. [CrossRef] [PubMed]
56. Patil, Y.; Shmeeda, H.; Amitay, Y.; Ohana, P.; Kumar, S.; Gabizon, A. Targeting of folate-conjugated liposomes with co-entrapped drugs to prostate cancer cells via prostate-specific membrane antigen (PSMA). *Nanomedicine* **2018**, *14*, 1407–1416. [CrossRef] [PubMed]
57. EP3799888A1—Liposomes Comprising Anti-Lox Antibody. Available online: https://www.patentguru.com/EP3799888A1 (accessed on 26 October 2021).
58. Saroj, S.; Rajput, S.J. Etoposide encased folic acid adorned mesoporous silica nanoparticles as potent nanovehicles for enhanced prostate cancer therapy: Synthesis, characterization, cellular uptake and biodistribution. *Artif. Cells Nanomed. Biotechnol.* **2018**, *46*, 1115–1130. [CrossRef]
59. Tambe, P.; Kumar, P.; Paknikar, K.M.; Gajbhiye, V. Decapeptide functionalized targeted mesoporous silica nanoparticles with doxorubicin exhibit enhanced apoptotic effect in breast and prostate cancer cells. *Int. J. Nanomed.* **2018**, *13*, 7669–7680. [CrossRef] [PubMed]
60. Rivero-Buceta, E.; Vidaurre-Agut, C.; Vera-Donoso, C.D.; Benlloch, J.M.; Moreno-Manzano, V.; Botella, P. PSMA-Targeted Mesoporous Silica Nanoparticles for Selective Intracellular Delivery of Docetaxel in Prostate Cancer Cells. *ACS Omega* **2019**, *4*, 1281–1291. [CrossRef]
61. Kumar, A.; Huo, S.; Zhang, X.; Liu, J.; Tan, A.; Li, S.; Jin, S.; Xue, X.; Zhao, Y.; Ji, T.; et al. Neuropilin-1-targeted gold nanoparticles enhance therapeutic efficacy of platinum(IV) drug for prostate cancer treatment. *ACS Nano* **2014**, *8*, 4205–4220. [CrossRef] [PubMed]

62. Hrkach, J.; Von Hoff, D.; Ali, M.M.; Andrianova, E.; Auer, J.; Campbell, T.; De Witt, D.; Figa, M.; Figueiredo, M.; Horhota, A.; et al. Preclinical development and clinical translation of a PSMA-targeted docetaxel nanoparticle with a differentiated pharmacological profile. *Sci. Transl. Med.* **2012**, *4*, 128ra39. [CrossRef]
63. Von Hoff, D.D.; Mita, M.M.; Ramanathan, R.K.; Weiss, G.J.; Mita, A.C.; Lorusso, P.M.; Burris, H.A.; Hart, L.L.; Low, S.C.; Parsons, D.M.; et al. Phase I study of PSMA-targeted docetaxel-containing nanoparticle BIND-014 in patients with advanced solid tumors. *Clin. Cancer Res.* **2016**, *22*, 3157–3163. [CrossRef]
64. Autio, K.A.; Dreicer, R.; Anderson, J.; Garcia, J.A.; Alva, A.; Hart, L.L.; Milowsky, M.I.; Posadas, E.M.; Ryan, C.J.; Graf, R.P.; et al. Safety and Efficacy of BIND-014, a Docetaxel Nanoparticle Targeting Prostate-Specific Membrane Antigen for Patients with Metastatic Castration-Resistant Prostate Cancer: A Phase 2 Clinical Trial. *JAMA Oncol.* **2018**, *4*, 1344–1351. [CrossRef]
65. Autio, K.A.; Garcia, J.A.; Alva, A.S.; Hart, L.L.; Milowsky, M.I.; Posadas, E.M.; Ryan, C.J.; Summa, J.M.; Youssoufian, H.; Scher, H.I.; et al. A phase 2 study of BIND-014 (PSMA-targeted docetaxel nanoparticle) administered to patients with chemotherapy-naïve metastatic castration-resistant prostate cancer (mCRPC). *J. Clin. Oncol.* **2016**, *34*, 233. [CrossRef]
66. Bharali, D.J.; Sudha, T.; Cui, H.; Mian, B.M.; Mousa, S.A. Anti-CD24 nano-targeted delivery of docetaxel for the treatment of prostate cancer. *Nanomed. Nanotechnol. Biol. Med.* **2017**, *13*, 263–273. [CrossRef] [PubMed]
67. Chen, Z.; Tai, Z.; Gu, F.; Hu, C.; Zhu, Q.; Gao, S. Aptamer-mediated delivery of docetaxel to prostate cancer through polymeric nanoparticles for enhancement of antitumor efficacy. *Eur. J. Pharm. Biopharm.* **2016**, *107*, 130–141. [CrossRef] [PubMed]
68. Karandish, F.; Haldar, M.K.; You, S.; Brooks, A.E.; Brooks, B.D.; Guo, B.; Choi, Y.; Mallik, S. Prostate-Specific Membrane Antigen Targeted Polymersomes for Delivering Mocetinostat and Docetaxel to Prostate Cancer Cell Spheroids. *ACS Omega* **2016**, *1*, 952–962. [CrossRef]
69. Ghasemiyeh, P.; Mohammadi-Samani, S. Solid lipid nanoparticles and nanostructured lipid carriers as novel drug delivery systems: Applications, advantages and disadvantages. *Res. Pharm. Sci.* **2018**, *13*, 288. [CrossRef]
70. Yin, X.; Luo, L.; Li, W.; Yang, J.; Zhu, C.; Jiang, M.; Qin, B.; Yuan, X.; Yin, H.; Lu, Y.; et al. A cabazitaxel liposome for increased solubility, enhanced antitumor effect and reduced systemic toxicity. *Asian J. Pharm. Sci.* **2019**, *14*, 658–667. [CrossRef]
71. Sun, B.; Straubinger, R.M.; Lovell, J.F. Current taxane formulations and emerging cabazitaxel delivery systems. *Nano Res.* **2018**, *11*, 5193–5218. [CrossRef]
72. Engelberg, S.; Netzer, E.; Assaraf, Y.G.; Livney, Y.D. Selective eradication of human non-small cell lung cancer cells using aptamer-decorated nanoparticles harboring a cytotoxic drug cargo. *Cell Death Dis.* **2019**, *10*, 702. [CrossRef]
73. Zhao, X.; Tang, D.; Yang, T.; Wang, C. Facile preparation of biocompatible nanostructured lipid carrier with ultra-small size as a tumor-penetration delivery system. *Colloids Surf. B Biointerfaces* **2018**, *170*, 355–363. [CrossRef]
74. Ding, X.; Xu, X.; Zhao, Y.; Zhang, L.; Yu, Y.; Huang, F.; Yin, D.; Huang, H. Tumor targeted nanostructured lipid carrier co-delivering paclitaxel and indocyanine green for laser triggered synergetic therapy of cancer. *RSC Adv.* **2017**, *7*, 35086–35095. [CrossRef]
75. Severino, P.; Pinho, S.C.; Souto, E.B.; Santana, M.H.A. Polymorphism, crystallinity and hydrophilic–lipophilic balance of stearic acid and stearic acid–capric/caprylic triglyceride matrices for production of stable nanoparticles. *Colloids Surf. B Biointerfaces* **2011**, *86*, 125–130. [CrossRef]
76. Malhotra, M.; Tomaro-Duchesneau, C.; Prakash, S. Synthesis of TAT peptide-tagged PEGylated chitosan nanoparticles for siRNA delivery targeting neurodegenerative diseases. *Biomaterials* **2013**, *34*, 1270–1280. [CrossRef] [PubMed]
77. Fulmer, G.R.; Miller, A.J.M.; Sherden, N.H.; Gottlieb, H.E.; Nudelman, A.; Stoltz, B.M.; Bercaw, J.E.; Goldberg, K.I. NMR chemical shifts of trace impurities: Common laboratory solvents, organics, and gases in deuterated solvents relevant to the organometallic chemist. *Organometallics* **2010**, *29*, 2176–2179. [CrossRef]
78. Delgado, A.V.; González-Caballero, F.; Hunter, R.J.; Koopal, L.K.; Lyklema, J. Measurement and Interpretation of Electrokinetic Phenomena (IUPAC Technical Report). *Pure Appl. Chem.* **2005**, *77*, 1753–1805. [CrossRef]
79. Edelman, R.; Assaraf, Y.G.; Levitzky, I.; Shahar, T.; Livney, Y.D. Hyaluronic acid-serum albumin conjugate-based nanoparticles for targeted cancer therapy. *Oncotarget* **2017**, *8*, 24337–24353. [CrossRef]
80. Xin, H.; Chen, L.; Gu, J.; Ren, X.; Wei, Z.; Luo, J.; Chen, Y.; Jiang, X.; Sha, X.; Fang, X. Enhanced anti-glioblastoma efficacy by PTX-loaded PEGylated poly(ε-caprolactone) nanoparticles: In vitro and in vivo evaluation. *Int. J. Pharm.* **2010**, *402*, 238–247. [CrossRef] [PubMed]
81. Qu, N.; Lee, R.J.; Sun, Y.; Cai, G.; Wang, J.; Wang, M.; Lu, J.; Meng, Q.; Teng, L.; Wang, D.; et al. Cabazitaxel-loaded human serum albumin nanoparticles as a therapeutic agent against prostate cancer. *Int. J. Nanomedicine* **2016**, *11*, 3451–3459. [CrossRef]
82. Aravind, A.; Varghese, S.H.; Veeranarayanan, S.; Mathew, A.; Nagaoka, Y.; Iwai, S.; Fukuda, T.; Hasumura, T.; Yoshida, Y.; Maekawa, T.; et al. Aptamer-labeled PLGA nanoparticles for targeting cancer cells. *Cancer Nanotechnol.* **2012**, *3*, 1–12. [CrossRef]
83. Engelberg, S.; Lin, Y.; Assaraf, Y.G.; Livney, Y.D. Targeted nanoparticles harboring jasmine-oil-entrapped paclitaxel for elimination of lung cancer cells. *Int. J. Mol. Sci.* **2021**, *22*, 1019. [CrossRef]
84. Qian, W.; Murakami, M.; Ichikawa, Y.; Che, Y. Highly efficient and controllable PEGylation of gold nanoparticles prepared by femtosecond laser ablation in water. *J. Phys. Chem. C* **2011**, *115*, 23293–23298. [CrossRef]
85. Standard, A. *ASTM D4187-82: Zeta Potential of Colloids in Water and Waste Water*; American Society for Testing and Materials: West Conshohocken, PA, USA, 1985.
86. Champion, J.A.; Mitragotri, S. Role of target geometry in phagocytosis. *Proc. Natl. Acad. Sci. USA* **2006**, *103*, 4930–4934. [CrossRef] [PubMed]

87. Yaari, Z.; Da Silva, D.; Zinger, A.; Goldman, E.; Kajal, A.; Tshuva, R.; Barak, E.; Dahan, N.; Hershkovitz, D.; Goldfeder, M.; et al. Theranostic barcoded nanoparticles for personalized cancer medicine. *Nat. Commun.* **2016**, *7*, 13325. [CrossRef]
88. Zhao, H.; Yung, L.Y.L. Selectivity of folate conjugated polymer micelles against different tumor cells. *Int. J. Pharm.* **2008**, *349*, 256–268. [CrossRef] [PubMed]
89. Wang, M.; Thanou, M. Targeting nanoparticles to cancer. *Pharmacol. Res.* **2010**, *62*, 90–99. [CrossRef]
90. Harush-Frenkel, O.; Debotton, N.; Benita, S.; Altschuler, Y. Targeting of nanoparticles to the clathrin-mediated endocytic pathway. *Biochem. Biophys. Res. Commun.* **2007**, *353*, 26–32. [CrossRef] [PubMed]
91. Dreifuss, T.; Ben-Gal, T.-S.; Shamalov, K.; Weiss, A.; Jacob, A.; Sadan, T.; Motiei, M.; Popovtzer, R. Uptake mechanism of metabolic-targeted gold nanoparticles. *Nanomedicine* **2018**, *13*, 1535–1549. [CrossRef] [PubMed]
92. Sekino, Y.; Han, X.; Kawaguchi, T.; Babasaki, T.; Goto, K.; Inoue, S.; Hayashi, T.; Teishima, J.; Shiota, M.; Yasui, W.; et al. TUBB3 Reverses Resistance to Docetaxel and Cabazitaxel in Prostate Cancer. *Int. J. Mol. Sci.* **2019**, *20*, 3936. [CrossRef] [PubMed]
93. Al Nakouzi, N.; Le Moulec, S.; Albigès, L.; Wang, C.; Beuzeboc, P.; Gross-Goupil, M.; De La Motte Rouge, T.; Guillot, A.; Gajda, D.; Massard, C.; et al. Cabazitaxel Remains Active in Patients Progressing After Docetaxel Followed by Novel Androgen Receptor Pathway Targeted Therapies. *Eur. Urol.* **2015**, *68*, 228–235. [CrossRef] [PubMed]

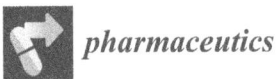

Article

Combined Antitumor Therapy Using In Situ Injectable Hydrogels Formulated with Albumin Nanoparticles Containing Indocyanine Green, Chlorin e6, and Perfluorocarbon in Hypoxic Tumors

Woo Tak Lee [1], Johyun Yoon [1], Sung Soo Kim [1], Hanju Kim [1], Nguyen Thi Nguyen [1], Xuan Thien Le [1], Eun Seong Lee [2], Kyung Taek Oh [3], Han-Gon Choi [4] and Yu Seok Youn [1,*]

[1] School of Pharmacy, Sungkyunkwan University, 2066 Seobu-ro, Jangan-gu, Suwon 16419, Gyeonggi-do, Korea; wtak94@naver.com (W.T.L.); morningbright96@gmail.com (J.Y.); alsajls417@gmail.com (S.S.K.); gkswn4564@naver.com (H.K.); ngtnguyen1710@gmail.com (N.T.N.); lexuanthien.dkh@gmail.com (X.T.L.)
[2] Department of Biotechnology and Department of Biomedical-Chemical Engineering, The Catholic University of Korea, 43 Jibong-ro, Bucheon-si 14662, Gyeonggi-do, Korea; eslee@catholic.ac.kr
[3] College of Pharmacy, Chung-Ang University, 84 Heukseok-ro, Dongjak-gu, Seoul 06974, Korea; kyungoh@cau.ac.kr
[4] College of Pharmacy, Hanyang University, 55 Hanyangdaehak-ro, Sangnok-gu, Ansan 15588, Gyeonggi-do, Korea; hangon@hanyang.ac.kr
* Correspondence: ysyoun@skku.edu; Tel.: +82-31-290-7785

Citation: Lee, W.T.; Yoon, J.; Kim, S.S.; Kim, H.; Nguyen, N.T.; Le, X.T.; Lee, E.S.; Oh, K.T.; Choi, H.-G.; Youn, Y.S. Combined Antitumor Therapy Using In Situ Injectable Hydrogels Formulated with Albumin Nanoparticles Containing Indocyanine Green, Chlorin e6, and Perfluorocarbon in Hypoxic Tumors. *Pharmaceutics* **2022**, *14*, 148. https://doi.org/10.3390/pharmaceutics14010148

Academic Editor: Jun Dai

Received: 29 November 2021
Accepted: 6 January 2022
Published: 8 January 2022

Publisher's Note: MDPI stays neutral with regard to jurisdictional claims in published maps and institutional affiliations.

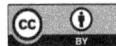

Copyright: © 2022 by the authors. Licensee MDPI, Basel, Switzerland. This article is an open access article distributed under the terms and conditions of the Creative Commons Attribution (CC BY) license (https://creativecommons.org/licenses/by/4.0/).

Abstract: Combined therapy using photothermal and photodynamic treatments together with chemotherapeutic agents is considered one of the most synergistic treatment protocols to ablate hypoxic tumors. Herein, we sought to fabricate an in situ-injectable PEG hydrogel system having such multifunctional effects. This PEG hydrogel was prepared with (i) nab^{TM}-technique-based paclitaxel (PTX)-bound albumin nanoparticles with chlorin-e6 (Ce6)-conjugated bovine serum albumin (BSA-Ce6) and indocyanine green (ICG), named ICG/PTX/BSA-Ce6-NPs (~175 nm), and (ii) an albumin-stabilized perfluorocarbon (PFC) nano-emulsion (BSA-PFC-NEs; ~320 nm). This multifunctional PEG hydrogel induced moderate and severe hyperthermia (41−42 °C and >48 °C, respectively) at the target site under two different 808 nm laser irradiation protocols, and also induced efficient singlet oxygen ($^1O_2$) generation under 660 nm laser irradiation supplemented by oxygen produced by ultrasound-triggered PFC. Due to such multifunctionality, our PEG hydrogel formula displayed significantly enhanced killing of three-dimensional 4T1 cell spheroids and also suppressed the growth of xenografted 4T1 cell tumors in mice (tumor volume: 47.7 ± 11.6 and 63.4 ± 13.0 mm^3 for photothermal and photodynamic treatment, respectively, vs. PBS group (805.9 ± 138.5 mm^3), presumably based on sufficient generation of moderate heat as well as $^1O_2/O_2$ even under hypoxic conditions. Our PEG hydrogel formula also showed excellent hyperthermal efficacy (>50 °C), ablating the 4T1 tumors when the irradiation duration was extended and output intensity was increased. We expect that our multifunctional PEG hydrogel formula will become a prototype for ablation of otherwise poorly responsive hypoxic tumors.

Keywords: photothermal therapy; photodynamic therapy; combined antitumor effect; oxygenation; hydrogel; hypoxic tumor

1. Introduction

Photodynamic therapy (PDT) has become a prominent therapeutic modality for cancer treatment [1–3]. Briefly, PDT is based on the clinical use of reactive oxygen species (ROS) such as singlet oxygen ($^1O_2$) or hydroxyl radicals (OH) generated from oxygen (O_2) using photosensitizers (PS) and light energy. The intracellularly generated ROS are able to damage cancer cells and tumor vasculature and also induce immune-mediated tumor suppression [3]. To date, several PDT agents, such as Photofrin®, Foscan®, and Visudyne®, etc., have been approved by the U.S. FDA, and the therapeutic availability of PDT has expanded toward cancer therapy. However, the clinical application of PDT is often restricted because most PS agents are effective only under focused laser illumination (650–900 nm) in the presence of sufficient oxygen. Unlike normal tissues, oxygenation in primary tumors is not regulated, and thus the partial oxygen pressure of tumors is often heterogeneous and can be remarkably low [4]. Interestingly, the O_2 concentration within human tumors is known to be 1.3%~3.9% (mostly less than 0.33%), in comparison with 3.1%~8.7% within normal tissues [4,5]. The efficacy of many PDT and chemotherapeutic agents is seriously impaired by low oxygen concentrations within hypoxic tumors, which causes hypoxia-induced resistance of tumors to antitumor therapy [6]. Therefore, increasing the oxygen concentration in hypoxic tumors can be an effective method to overcome hypoxia-induced resistance of tumors to PDT [7–9].

Photothermal therapy (PTT) is also a promising antitumor modality that acts by raising tissue temperature [10]. Cancer cells are susceptible to temperature elevation and are often killed as a result of irreversible damage and subsequent induction of apoptosis even after exposure to temperatures >48 °C for only 5 min [11]. Many organic PTT agents emit heat in response to focused near-infrared (NIR) laser irradiation at wavelengths of 650−900 nm [10,12]. Because the hyperthermia can be concentrated within the area targeted by the NIR irradiation, PTT may create relatively little damage to surrounding healthy tissues [10,13]. Moreover, PTT can also be used to induce moderate local hyperthermia (39–42 °C) that promotes the delivery of oxygen as well as chemotherapeutics into tumor tissues due to elevated tumor blood flow [14,15]. This moderate PTT is useful in clinical settings because it attenuates the tumor hypoxic state and improves the efficacy of chemotherapeutic agents [16,17].

Albumin is a versatile carrier due to its excellent pharmaceutical advantages, such as biodegradability, biocompatibility, high stability, and solubility [18,19]. It has been used as a building material to fabricate a great number of therapeutic and diagnostic drug delivery systems, including nanoconjugates [20,21], nano-/micro-particles [22–25], and hydrogels of various sizes [26–29]. In practice, the nab™ (nanoparticle albumin-bound)-based paclitaxel formulation Abraxane® (Celgene Corp.) has displayed enhanced antitumor efficacy over the conventional paclitaxel formulation of Taxol®. In particular, this prototypical nab™ formula has sufficient flexibility and expandability to entrap various hydrophobic drugs, is better able to target the tumor gp60-mediated transcytosis pathway [18], and has been extensively used as a biocompatible component of injectable hydrogels [26–29].

In this study, we developed a multifunctional in situ-forming PEG-albumin hydrogel that was able to generate oxygen (O_2) and singlet oxygen ($^1O_2$) and emit moderate or severe heat for the combination treatment of hypoxic tumors using chemotherapeutic, photodynamic, and photothermal therapy. This PEG hydrogel formula was designed to include (i) albumin nanoparticles containing paclitaxel (PTX), chlorin e6 (Ce6), and indocyanine green (ICG), and (ii) an albumin-stabilized perfluorocarbon (PFC) nano-emulsion (NE). The capability of this PEG hydrogel formula to generate heat and oxygen/singlet oxygen was carefully evaluated. The physicochemical and photo-induced properties of this multifunctional PEG hydrogel were also assessed by using relevant analyses. Finally, the combined chemotherapeutic, photodynamic and photothermal effects of this PEG hydrogel formula were carefully evaluated in 4T1 cell spheroids under hypoxic conditions and in 4T1 tumor-bearing mice.

2. Materials and Methods

2.1. Materials

Paclitaxel (PTX) was obtained from JW Pharmaceutical Corporation (Dangjin, South Korea). Indocyanine green (ICG) and icosafluoro-15-crown-5-ether (PFC) were purchased from Tokyo Chemical Industry Co., LTD. (Tokyo, Japan). Chlorin e6 (Ce6) was supplied by Frontier Scientific (Salt Lake City, UT, USA). Bovine serum albumin (BSA) and

2-iminothiolane (2-IT; Traut's reagent) were purchased from Sigma-Aldrich (St. Louis, MO, USA). Four-arm polyethylene glycol maleimide (4-arm PEG-MAL; Mw 20 kDa) was purchased from NOF Corporation (Tokyo, Japan). The 4T1 breast cancer cells were obtained from the American Type Culture Collection (ATCC; Rockville, MD, USA). LIVE/DEAD™ viability/cytotoxicity assay kits, Singlet Oxygen Sensor Green reagent (SOSG), and Cell-ROX™ Deep Red reagent were purchased from Thermo Fisher Scientific (Waltham, MA, USA). Anti-HIF-1α primary and Alexa Fluor®-488-conjugated goat anti-rabbit secondary antibodies were purchased from Abcam (Cambridge, MA, USA). Trypsin-EDTA and penicillin-streptomycin (P/S) solution were purchased from Corning (Somerville, NY, USA). Dulbecco's Modified Eagle Medium (DMEM) and fetal bovine serum (FBS) were purchased from Capricorn (Ebsdorfergrund, Hesse, Germany). All other reagents were obtained from Sigma-Aldrich unless otherwise indicated.

2.2. Animals

The animals were cared for in accordance with the Guide for the Care and Use of Laboratory Animals published by the United States National Institutes of Health. The protocols were also approved by the Institutional Animal Care and Use Committee (IACUC) of Sungkyunkwan University (IACUC number: 202106291, approval date 15 July 2021). The BALB/c *nu/nu* mice (female, 6 weeks old) were purchased from ORIENT BIO (Seongnam, South Korea). Mice were housed in microisolator cages on individually ventilated cage racks with ad libitum access to an autoclaved standard rodent diet (LabDiet 5008, Purina, St. Louis, MO, USA) and were kept under a 12 h light/dark cycle.

2.3. Synthesis of Ce6-Conjugated BSA (BSA-Ce6)

The BSA was covalently modified with Ce6 using a slight modification of the previous method [2]. Briefly, Ce6 (1 mmol), N-dicyclohexylcarbodiimide (DCC, 4 mmol), and N-hydroxysuccinimide (NHS, 5 mmol) were dissolved in 10 mL anhydrous dimethyl sulfoxide (DMSO) in a glass tube. Triethylamine (TEA, 4 mmol) was added to the mixture, and the reaction was performed in the dark at ambient temperature for 24 h. After removing the precipitate, the NHS-activated Ce6 was stored at −70 °C until required. Separately, 1.5 mL of Ce6-NHS (150 µmol) in DMSO was mixed dropwise with 50 mL of BSA (7.5 µmol; 0.1 M sodium borate buffer, pH 8.5) at a feeding ratio of 20:1 (Ce6:BSA). The reaction was allowed to continue at 450 rpm in the dark condition for 24 h. Unreacted Ce6 and DMSO were removed by using a dialysis membrane (MwCO: 10 kDa; Spectrum Labs, Rancho Dominguez, CA, USA) against 60% ethanol and deionized water (DW) for 48 and 24 h, respectively 24 h. Finally, Ce6-BSA was concentrated in DW using a centrifugal concentrator (MwCO: 30 kDa, Amicon® Ultra, Millipore, Burlington, MA, USA) and then lyophilized and stored at −20 °C for further use.

2.4. Preparation of ICG/PTX/BSA-Ce6-NPs

The ICG/PTX/BSA-Ce6-NPs were prepared as previously described using the nanoparticle albumin-bound (nab™) technology with some adjustments [2,30–34]. In brief, 45 mg BSA, 5 mg BSA-Ce6, and 0.75 mg ICG were dissolved in 5 mL DW. Then, 5 mg PTX was dissolved in 0.1 mL of a 9:1 solution (chloroform:ethanol). These two solutions were gently shaken and homogenized by using a high-speed homogenizer (WiseTis® HG-15D: DAI-HAN Scientific Co., Seoul, South Korea) at 14,500 rpm for 3 min, and then passed through a high-pressure homogenizer (EmulsiFlex-B15 device, Avestin, Ottawa, ON, Canada) for nine cycles at 20,000 psi. The resulting dispersion was rotary evaporated for 15 min under reduced pressure at 40 °C to remove chloroform and ethanol. The nanoparticle fraction was centrifuged at 6000 rpm, and the supernatant was collected. The resulting suspension was lyophilized and stored at −20 °C until required.

2.5. Fabrication of BSA-Stabilized PFC Nano-Emulsion

The BSA-PFC nano-emulsion (BSA-PFC-NEs) was fabricated using a slight modification of the previous method [35]. A 300 µL aliquot of icosafluoro-15-crown-5-ether (PFC) was mixed with 4 mL of PBS containing 40 mg of BSA. The mixture was held in an ice bath and ultrasonicated (operation 8 s, interval 2 s) at an amplitude of 20% for 400 s. The resulting nano-emulsion was centrifuged (8000 rpm, 3 min), and the resulting nano-emulsion pellets were re-dispersed in 0.1 mL PBS.

2.6. Characterization of ICG/PTX/BSA-Ce6-NPs and BSA-PFC-NEs

The particle size and zeta potential of ICG/PTX/BSA-Ce6-NPs and BSA-PFC-NEs (DW) were measured by using a Zetasizer Nano ZS90 instrument (Malvern Instruments, Worcestershire, U.K.) at a dynamic light scattering mode. The surface morphology of the NPs was observed by transmission electron microscopy (TEM: JEM-3010, JEOL, Tokyo, Japan) and field-emission scanning electron microscopy (FE-SEM: JSM7000F, JEOL, Tokyo, Japan). The particle sizes of ICG/PTX/BSA-Ce6-NPs and BSA-PFC-NEs were measured at 0, 1, 2, 4, 8, 12, 24, 48, and 72 h at room temperature. In addition, UV-VIS-NIR spectral scans of ICG/PTX/BSA-Ce6-NPs or free ICG/Ce6 were also recorded over a range of wavelengths (300–900 nm) using a Synergy™ NEO microplate reader (Bio Tek, Winooski, VT, USA).

2.7. Preparation of In Situ-Gelling PEG Hydrogel with ICG/PTX/BSA-Ce6-NPs and BSA-PFC-NEs

The PEG hydrogel with ICG/PTX/BSA-Ce6-NPs and BSA-PFC-NEs (ICG/PTX/BSA-Ce6-NPs~PFC-NEs@Gel) was formulated using an in situ-gelling PEG hydrogel according to the protocol described previously with modifications [26,27,36]. To synthesize thiolated BSA (BSA-SH), BSA (500 mg) was dissolved in 1 mL of 100 mM PBS buffer (pH 8.0) containing 2-iminothiolane (2-IT, 12.5 mg), and the mixture was allowed to react by stirring for 2.5 h. The unreacted 2-IT was removed using a centrifugal concentrator (MwCO: 10 kDa, Amicon® Ultra, Millipore). The formula (1 mL) of the in situ-gelling PEG hydrogel comprised (i) ICG/PTX/BSA-Ce6-NPs (300 µL; 30 mg/mL), (ii) BSA-PFC-NEs (100 µL as a final emulsion), (iii) BSA-SH (150 µL; 500 mg/mL), and (iv) 4-arm PEG-MAL (450 µL; 11.4 mg/mL). Each component was mixed immediately, and gelation was optimized by monitoring the gelation time according to the molar ratio of 4-arm PEG-MAL and BSA-SH (BSA-SH:4-arm PEG-MAL = 1:3.3~4.5). The material was considered to be in a gel state if it did not flow when inverted.

2.8. Characterization of ICG/PTX/BSA-Ce6-NPs~PFC-NEs@Gel

The different PEG hydrogel formulas (Z1~Z6) with ICG/PTX/BSA-Ce6-NPs and BSA-PFC-NEs were designated as follows: (i) Z1 = PEG hydrogel; (ii) Z2 = PTX/BSA-NPs@Gel; (iii) Z3 = BSA-PFC-NEs@Gel; (iv) Z4 = PTX/BSA-Ce6-NPs@Gel; (v) Z5 = ICG/PTX-BSA-NPs@Gel; (vi) Z6 = ICG/PTX/BSA-Ce6-NPs~PFC-NEs@Gel (Table 1). General features of the hydrogel were characterized using photographs, photothermal images (FLIR E85 photothermal camera, FLIR Systems, Inc., Wilsonville, OR, USA), and fluorescence images (FOBI in vivo imaging system, NeoScience, Suwon, Korea).

2.9. In Vitro and In Vivo Photothermal Imaging and Hyperthermia Monitoring

A thermal imaging camera was used to measure the photothermal effect of the ICG/PTX/BSA-Ce6-NPs in vitro and in vivo using a slight modification of the previous method [26]. Naïve PEG hydrogel or ICG/PTX/BSA-Ce6-NPs@Gel in 1.5 mL Eppendorf tubes was irradiated for 5 min with an 808-nm laser (0.8 or 1.2 W/cm^2 to induce mild or severe hyperthermia, respectively). To obtain photothermal images in vivo, naive PEG hydrogel or ICG/PTX/BSA-Ce6-NPs@Gel was injected into the tumors of mice, and the tumor regions were either irradiated or not irradiated with 808 nm laser (0.6–0.8 W/cm^2) for 20 min. Temperature changes within the tumor areas were recorded and observed using a FLIR E85 photothermal camera (FLIR Systems, Inc., Wilsonville, USA).

Table 1. Formulations and treatment groups used in this study.

Hydrogel Formulation Groups	Characteristics	Abbreviation	Laser Irradiation	Ultrasound
Z1	PEG hydrogel	-	-	-
Z2	PEG hydrogel with PTX/BSA-NPs	PTX/BSA-NPs@Gel	-	-
Z3	PEG hydrogel with BSA-PFC-NEs	BSA-PFC-NEs@Gel	-	-
Z4	PEG hydrogel with PTX/BSA-Ce6-NPs	PTX/BSA-Ce6-NPs@Gel	-	-
Z5	PEG hydrogel with ICG/PTX-BSA-NPs	ICG/PTX-BSA-NPs@Gel	-	-
Z6	PEG hydrogel with ICG/PTX/BSA-Ce6-NPs and BSA-PFC-NEs	ICG/PTX/BSA-Ce6-NPs~PFC-NEs@Gel	-	-
Animal Group	Intratumor Treatment Groups		Laser Irradiation	Ultrasound
G1	PBS	-	-	-
G2	PEG hydrogel with PTX-BSA-NPs	PTX/BSA-NPs@Gel	-	-
G3	PEG hydrogel with ICG/PTX/BSA-Ce6-NPs	ICG/PTX/BSA-Ce6-NPs@Gel	660 nm (+)	-
G4			808 nm (+)	-
G5	PEG hydrogel with ICG/PTX/BSA-Ce6-NPs and BSA-PFC-NEs	ICG/PTX/BSA-Ce6-NPs~PFC-NEs@Gel	660 nm/808 nm (+)	US (+)

2.10. Singlet Oxygen Generation by ICG/PTX/BSA-Ce6-NPs

Singlet Oxygen Sensor Green (SOSG) reagent was used to assess singlet oxygen generation from ICG/PTX/BSA-Ce6-NPs. Free Ce6 and ICG/PTX/BSA-Ce6-NPs were mixed with the SOSG reagent (final concentration 10 μM) in a 24-well plate. A 660-nm laser (10 mW/cm^2) irradiated the respective sample wells for free Ce6 and ICG/PTX/BSA-Ce6-NPs under either normoxic or hypoxic conditions. Hypoxia was precisely achieved by incubating the hypoxic chamber in a hypoxic gas stream (5% CO_2:95% N_2 on a volume basis). While irradiating the sample wells with the laser for 60 min, a 100 μL aliquot of each sample was collected every 10 min. The intensity of the green fluorescence emitted from SOSG induced by $^1O_2$ generation was determined using a multi-mode microplate reader (excitation 485 nm; emission 538 nm).

2.11. Encapsulation Efficiency and Release Profiles of PTX, ICG, and BSA-Ce6

The encapsulation efficiency (EE) of PTX, BSA-Ce6, and ICG into ICG/PTX/BSA-Ce6-NPs was examined. Briefly, 5 mg of the lyophilized ICG/PTX/BSA-Ce6-NPs was dissolved in 0.5 mL DW, and then 4.5 mL acetonitrile (ACN) was added to the NPs solution, followed by sonication for 30 min and centrifugation for 15 min (14,500 rpm). Subsequently, the supernatant was withdrawn for the quantification of PTX and ICG. The EE of BSA-Ce6 was calculated by measuring the supernatant concentration of BSA-Ce6 after the nanoparticle preparation. For the release test, a 5 mL ICG/PTX/BSA-Ce6-NPs solution (10 mM PBS, pH 7.4) was loaded into the PEG hydrogel. The drug release from the hydrogel was carried out using a gently rotated bench-top rotator (150 rpm, 37 °C). At predetermined times, a 0.15 mL aliquot was withdrawn and centrifuged (14,500 rpm, 10 min), and the fluorescence intensities of the supernatants were measured by using a fluorescence spectrometer (FluoroMax Plus; HORIBA Scientific, Tokyo, Japan). Three replicates of each sample were prepared and analyzed (n = 3). The excitation/emission wavelengths used for ICG and Ce6 were 420/526 and 405/670 nm, respectively. To determine the loading efficiency of PTX, the supernatant was subjected to reverse-phase high-performance liquid chromatography (RP-HPLC) using a PLRP-S Zorbax 100 RP-18 column (150 × 4.6 mm, 8 μm/300 Å; Agilent

Technologies, Palo Alto, CA, USA). An isocratic elution method was performed at a flow rate of 1.0 mL/min using a mixed solution (DW:ACN = 45:55). Eluates were monitored at 220 nm. Drug loading efficiency (%) was calculated as amount of drug entrapped/amount of drug loaded × 100.

2.12. Cytotoxicity of ICG/PTX/BSA-Ce6-NPs in 4T1 Cell Spheroids Using LIVE/DEAD^{TM} Cell Assay

Three-dimensional culture of 4T1 cells to form spheroids was performed by a slight modification of previously described methods [2,26,30]. LIVE/DEAD™ viability/cytotoxicity kits were used to visualize the death and viability of the 4T1 cells. Briefly, the 4T1 cells were cultured in DMEM media containing 10% (v/v) fetal bovine serum and 1% penicillin/streptomycin in a 5% CO_2, 95% RH incubator at 37 °C. A 100 µL sample containing 4000 cells was seeded into each well of V-bottom cell plates (Shimadzu, Kyoto, Japan) designed to induce the formation of 3D multicellular spheroids. The 4T1 cell spheroids were then allowed to become established over three days before further experiments. The spheroids previously incubated with ICG/PTX/BSA-Ce6-NPs@Gel for 6 h were assigned to groups with or without laser irradiation (808 nm for 10 min or 660 nm for 60 min, respectively) and/or with or without an ultrasound (US) scan (US for 15 min) according to the previously described oxygen conditions (normoxic, hypoxic or oxygenated). The degree of hyperthermia induced was determined irradiation at 0.8 and 1.2 W/cm^2 for mild and severe hyperthermia, respectively, where the target temperatures were set to 41–42 °C or >48 °C, respectively. The hypoxic condition was precisely achieved by incubating the hypoxic chamber in a hypoxic gas stream (5% CO_2:95% N_2 on a volume basis). The plates for samples were washed three times with DPBS, and the medium was replenished with fresh medium before laser or ultrasound treatment. After laser or ultrasound treatment, the cells were stained with Calcein-AM (for live cells) and Ethidium Homodimer-1 (for dead cells). Subsequently, the stained cells were observed by CLSM (excitation/emission wavelengths of 494/517 nm for Calcein-AM and 528/617 nm for Ethidium Homodimer-1, respectively).

2.13. ROS Deep Assay at 4T1 Cell Spheroids

The 4T1 cell spheroids were plated into each well of an 8-well chamber (Ibidi, Martinsried, Germany) and incubated with ICG/PTX/BSA-Ce6-NPs for 6 h. Cell spheroids were replenished with fresh DMEM (1% FBS) prior to laser irradiation (660 nm) and a US scan performed under normoxic, hypoxic, or oxygenated conditions. CellROX® Reagent was added to the cell spheroids at a final concentration of 20 µM and the plates were incubated at 37 °C for 2 h. Spheroids were washed three times with DPBS and stained with DAPI. The intracellular distribution of ROS in the spheroid cells was visualized using confocal laser scanning microscopy (CLSM; Carl Zeiss, Jena, Germany).

2.14. HIF-1α Visualization at 4T1 Cell Spheroids

The 4T1 cell spheroids were plated into each well of an 8-well chamber (Ibidi, Martinsried, Germany) and incubated with BSA-PFC-NEs for 1 h. The cell spheroids were subjected to a US scan under normoxic, hypoxic, or oxygenated conditions. Hypoxic conditions were achieved by incubating the hypoxic chamber in a hypoxic gas stream (5% CO_2:95% N_2 on a volumetric basis). The spheroids were fixed with 4% formaldehyde for 60 min and incubated for 90 min with 0.1% Triton X-100, and then incubated with 1% BSA, 22.52 mg/mL glycine in PBST (PBS + 0.1% Tween 20) for 2 h to block unspecific binding of the antibodies. The resulting spheroids were further incubated with the diluted antibody solution (anti-HIF-1 alpha antibody-Alexa Fluor 488; 1/25) in 1% BSA in PBST in a humidified chamber for 1 h at room temperature. After removing the supernatant, the cell spheroids were washed three times in PBS, incubated with DAPI (DNA stain) for 4 h, and further rinsed with PBS. Samples were observed using CSLM.

2.15. In Vivo Imaging of ICG/PTX/BSA-Ce6-NPs

The in situ-gelling ICG/PTX/BSA-Ce6-NPs~PFC-NEs@Gel (100 µL) were directly injected into 4T1-cell-xenografted tumors on mice. At predetermined times, the fluorescence signals of Ce6 and ICG originating from the tumors were visualized at 630 and 730 nm, respectively, and at predetermined times using a FOBI in vivo imaging system (NeoScience, Suwon, Korea).

2.16. In Vivo Photoacoustic Imaging

Photoacoustic (PA) imaging was used to determine the saturation/distribution of oxygen or PFC gas inside the xenografted 4T1 tumors. When the tumors reached ~150 mm^3 volumes, the mice were treated with (i) PBS; (ii) ICG/PTX/BSA-Ce6-NPs~PFC-NEs@Gel + US(+); (iii) ICG/PTX/BSA-Ce6-NPs~PFC-NEs@Gel + US(−). At before and after (30 min) intratumor injections, tumor oxygenation (as the oxyhemoglobin:HbO$_2$ ratio) was visualized and recorded using a Vevo® LAZR-X Multimodal Imaging System (FujiFilm, VisualSonics Inc., Minato, Tokyo, Japan) set to the Oxy-hem mode (750 and 850 nm) at predetermined times.

2.17. In Vivo Antitumor Efficacy in 4T1 Cell-Xenograft Mice

The 4T1 cells (100 µL; 3 × 10^6 cells) were injected subcutaneously into the dorsal flanks of the mice. When the volume of the tumors reached ~150 mm^3, the mice were randomly divided into five groups (G1−G5) as follows: (I) control: PBS; (II) chemotherapeutic = PTX/BSA-NPs@Gel (100 µg PTX (0.1 mL/mouse); (III) deoxy-photodynamic = ICG/PTX/BSA-Ce6-NPs@Gel + 660 nm (+); (IV) severe hyperthermia = ICG/PTX/BSA-Ce6-NPs@Gel + 808 nm(+); and (V) oxy-photodynamic plus moderate hyperthermia = ICG/PTX/BSA-Ce6-NPs~PFC-NEs@Gel + 660 nm (+) + 808 nm(+) + US(+) (Table 1). All treatments were injected intratumorally. Tumor volume and body weight of the mice were measured every day. Tumor volume (V) was calculated using the equation V = 0.5 × A × B^2, where A is length (longest diameter) and B is width (shortest diameter). On day 14, the mice were sacrificed, and their tumors were harvested and photographed. The tumors were stored in formalin for further experiment.

2.18. Data Analyses

All data are presented as the mean ± standard deviation (SD). The significance of differences between treatment group results was determined using Student's t-test, and p-values < 0.05 were considered statistically significant.

3. Results

3.1. Preparation and Characterization of ICG/PTX/BSA-Ce6-NPs and BSA-PFC-NEs

The ICG/PTX/BSA-Ce6-NPs and BSA-PFC-NEs were fabricated using a high-pressure homogenizer based on the nab^{TM} technology and ultrasonication, respectively (Figure 1). The sizes of the prepared ICG/PTX/BSA-Ce6-NPs and BSA-PFC-NEs were 175.8 ± 5.8 and 323.4 ± 6.6 nm, respectively (Figure 2A). Their zeta potentials were shown to be −40.3 ± 0.3 and −32.2 ± 1.2, respectively (Figure 2B). The ICG/PTX/BSA-Ce6-NPs were highly homogeneous and spherical, whereas the BSA PFC NEs appeared to be rather irregular and less homogeneous (Figure 2C). These solutions of ICG/PTX/BSA-Ce6-NPs and BSA-PFC-NEs showed the typical characteristics of a colloid or nano-emulsion (Figure 2D). In particular, the particle sizes of both the ICG/PTX/BSA-Ce6-NPs and BSA-PFC-NEs remained stable over a three-day evaluation period (Figure 2E). When observed at wavelengths ranging between 300 and 900 nm, the ICG/PTX/BSA-Ce6-NPs were found to have typical absorption profiles of indocyanine green and chlorin e6 of around ~800 nm and 660 nm, respectively. The Ce6-BSA, BSA-BC-NPs, and Ce6-BSA-BC-NPs were investigated (Figure 2F). In addition, the loading efficiency of PTX, ICG, and BSA-Ce6 was found to be ~73.0%, 53.2%, and 82.1%, respectively.

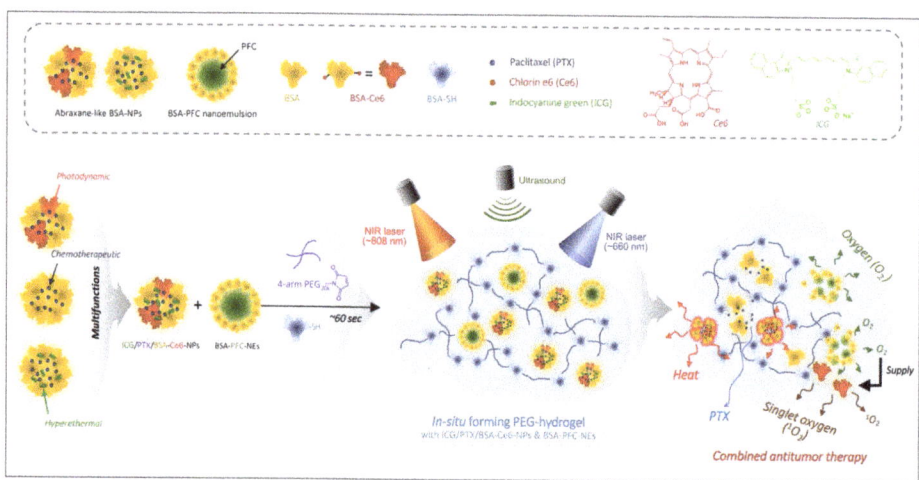

Figure 1. Schematic illustration of combined photothermal and photodynamic therapy for hypoxic tumors using ICG/PTX/BSA-Ce6-NPs~PFC-NEs@Gel under laser irradiation (660/808 nm) and ultrasound trigger.

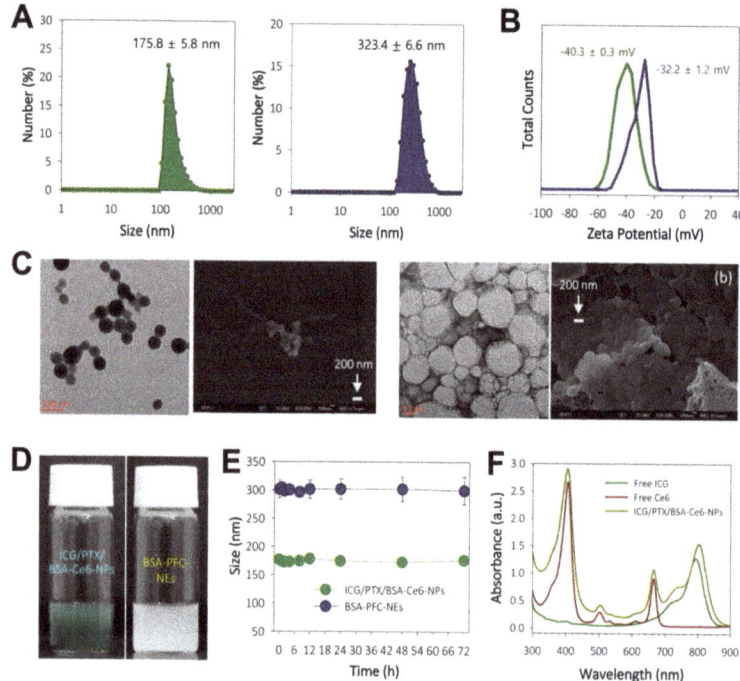

Figure 2. (**A**) Histograms of particle sizes of ICG/PTX/BSA-Ce6-NPs and BSA-PFC-Nes. (**B**) Zeta potentials of ICG/PTX/BSA-Ce6-NPs and BSA-PFC-NEs. (**C**) TEM and FE-SEM images of ICG/PTX/BSA-Ce6-NPs (left: a) and BSA-PFC-NEs (right: b). (**D**) Photographs showing colloidal solution state for ICG/PTX/BSA-Ce6-NPs and BSA-PFC-NEs. (**E**) Physical stability of ICG/PTX/BSA-Ce6-NPs and BSA-PFC-NEs based on size changes over 3 days. (**F**) UV-VIS spectroscopic analyses for free ICG, free Ce6, and ICG/PTX/BSA-Ce6-NPs at 300–900 nm wavelengths.

3.2. Preparation, Characterization, and Drug Release Profiles of ICG/PTX/BSA-Ce6-NPs~PFC-NEs@Gel

Given that the gelation process depends on a rapid thiol-maleimide reaction, in situ gelling of the PEG hydrogel was evaluated by monitoring the relationship between the gelation time and the molar ratio of 4-arm PEG-MAL to BSA-SH. As shown in Figure 3A, reducing the 4-arm PEG-MAL to BSA-SH molar ratio sharply reduced the gelation time, with the PEG hydrogel becoming solid in approximately 1 min at a 4-arm PEG-MAL to BSA-SH ratio of 4.4:1.0, which was considered optimal to perform a series of related steps (i.e., material mixing, syringe filling, and injection). The in vitro release profiles of Ce6 (as a BSA-Ce6 conjugate), ICG, and PTX from ICG/PTX/BSA-Ce6-NPs~PFC-NEs@Gel were observed over 168 h. As shown in Figure 3B, >90% amount of BSA-Ce6 and ICG was released over 24 h with initial burst-out, and the remaining amount of both BSA-Ce6 and ICG appeared to be completely released from the PEG hydrogel after 144 h, which was appropriate for the in vivo laser irradiation protocol. In contrast, PTX displayed a gradual linear release pattern consisting without significant initial fast release until 168 h, which was presumably due to the hydrophobic property, tight binding to albumin molecules, and low solubility/diffusion of PTX. Thus, PTX seemed to have considerable time to be released from the PEG hydrogel. Subsequently, the hydrophobicity difference between PTX, ICG, and BSA-Ce6 led to a great discrepancy in the release pattern.

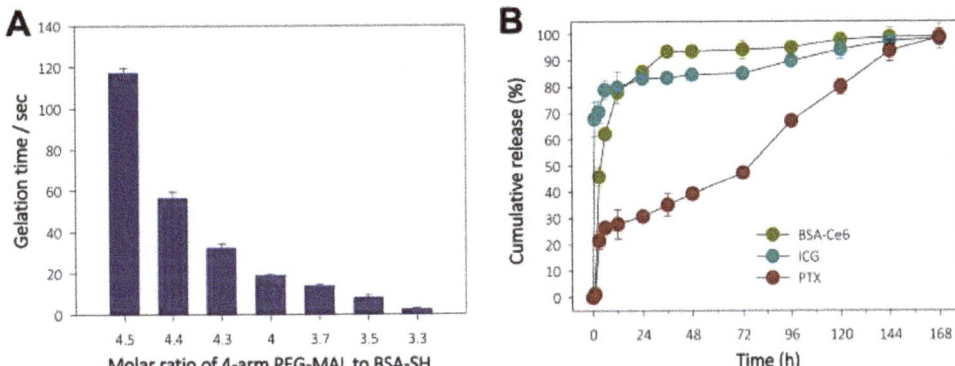

Figure 3. (**A**) Monitoring of gelation time for in situ-forming PEG hydrogel according to the 4-arm PEG-MAL:BSA-SH molar ratio. (**B**) Release profiles for BSA-Ce6, ICG, and PTX from ICG/PTX/BSA-Ce6-NPs@Gel.

Separately, the various hydrogel formulations (Z1–Z6) had distinct colors, ranging from transparent to milky, khaki green, or dark green, depending on ICG, Ce6, and PFC concentrations (Figure 4A). All formulas gelled easily within ~60 s and did not flow or drop when turned upside-down. As shown in Figure 4B,C, PEG hydrogels containing ICG (Z5 and Z6) produced significant hyperthermia, and those containing both ICG and Ce6 emitted strong fluorescence at the relevant emission wavelengths. The FE-SEM images showed that the PEG hydrogels contained considerable amounts of nanoparticles having sizes of ~150 and >300 nm, presumably corresponding to ICG/PTX/BSA-Ce6-NPs and BSA-PFC-NEs (Figure 4D).

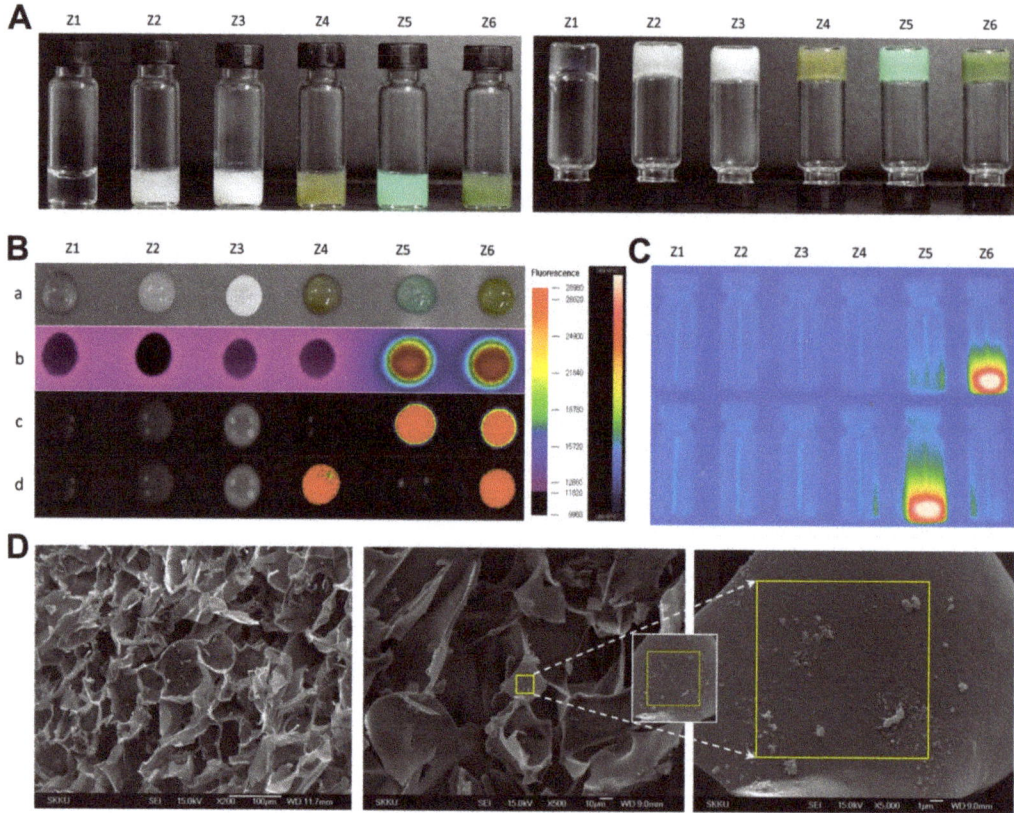

Figure 4. (**A**) Photographs of PEG hydrogel formulation groups (Z1–Z6) in the regular (left) and upside-down (right) state. (**B**) Various images of PEG hydrogel formulation groups (Z1–Z6) (a) photograph at 10 min after gelation, (b) thermal images, (c) fluorescence images of ICG, (d) fluorescence images of Ce6. (**C**) Thermal images of glass vials containing the Z1–Z6 PEG hydrogel formulations during laser irradiation at 420/526 and 405/670 nm, excitation/emission wavelengths to identify ICG and Ce6, respectively. (**D**) FE-SEM images for the morphology of inner structures of ICG/PTX/BSA-Ce6-NPs@Gel.

3.3. Photothermal and Photodynamic Activity of ICG/PTX/BSA-Ce6-NPs

The induction of hyperthermia by ICG/PTX/BSA-Ce6-NPs@Gel when irradiated by the 808 nm laser was evaluated. As shown in Figure 5A,E, the temperature of the ICG/PTX/BSA-Ce6-NPs@Gel quickly increased from 26 to 56 °C within 5 min of initiation of 808-nm laser irradiation (1.2 W/cm^2), whereas the temperature of the plain PEG hydrogel increased by only 3 °C. However, the temperature of ICG/PTX/BSA-Ce6-NPs@Gel increased to 42 °C in response to 808 nm laser irradiation (0.8 W/cm^2) (Figure 5B). As shown in Figure 5C, when 808-nm laser irradiation (0.8 W/cm^2) was applied intermittently in 3 min on/off cycles, the gel temperature reached ~41 °C after 30 s irradiation and returned to the basal temperature before additional irradiation. Separately, ICG/PTX/BSA-Ce6-NPs were clearly able to induce singlet oxygen generation, as evaluated by the fluorescence intensity caused by SOSG. Overall, the SOSG fluorescence appeared to increase with the duration of irradiation (Figure 5D). Singlet oxygen generation by ICG/PTX/BSA-Ce6-NPs appeared comparable to that of free Ce6, and much less singlet oxygen was generated under hypoxic conditions than under normoxic conditions. Furthermore, the tumor temperature of 4T1 tumor-bearing mouse treated with ICG/PTX/BSA-Ce6-NPs@Gel plus 808-nm laser irradiation (0.8 W/cm^2) maintained around ~41 °C for 20 min, whereas that of mouse treated with the naïve PEG hydrogel at the same condition did not significantly increase (Figure 5F).

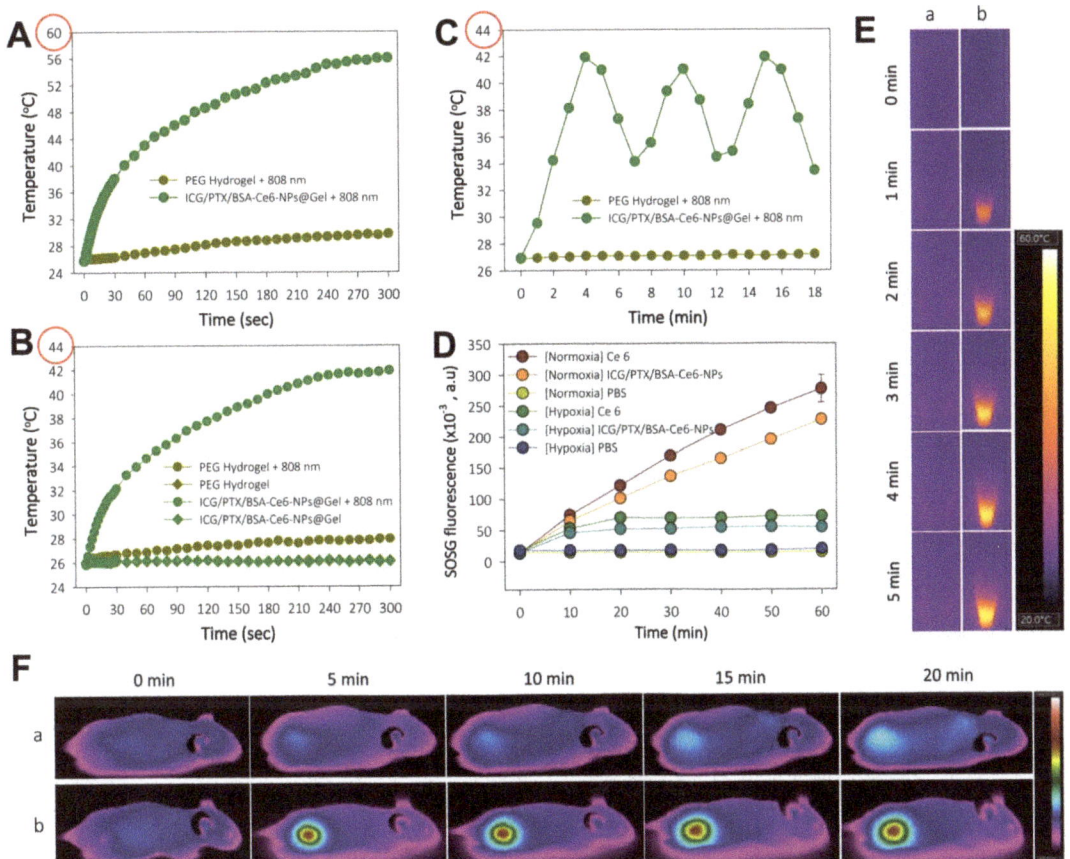

Figure 5. (**A**) Temperature change profile for naïve PEG hydrogel and ICG/PTX/BSA-Ce6-NPs@Gel after targeted 808-nm laser irradiation (1.2 W/cm^2) to induce severe hyperthermia with. (**B**) Temperature change profile for naïve PEG hydrogel and ICG/PTX/BSA-Ce6-NPs@Gel with or without targeted 808-nm laser irradiation (0.8 W/cm^2) to induce moderate hyperthermia. (**C**) Temperature adjustment profile for ICG/PTX/BSA-Ce6-NPs@Gel during alternating on and off 808-nm laser irradiation (0.8 W/cm^2) for 3 min cycles. (**D**) SOSG fluorescence profiles of Ce6 and ICG/PTX/BSA-Ce6-NPs in response to continuous 660 nm-irradiation (10 mW/cm^2) as assessed by singlet oxygen generation under normoxic and hypoxic conditions. (**E**) Thermal images of (a) naïve PEG hydrogel and (b) ICG/PTX/BSA-Ce6-NPs@Gel during 808 nm laser irradiation (1.2 W/cm^2). (**F**) In vivo whole-body thermal images of mice bearing 4T1 tumor injected with (a) naïve PEG hydrogel or (b) ICG/PTX/BSA-Ce6-NPs@Gel plus 808-nm laser irradiation (0.8 W/cm^2) over 20 min.

3.4. Cytotoxicity Evaluation of 4T1 Cell Spheroids Based on LIVE/DEAD™ Assay

With regard to photothermal effects, when irradiated with the 808 nm laser at 1.2 W/cm^2 for 10 min, 4T1 cell spheroids appeared to be absolutely dead, showing clear red fluorescence color, whereas 4T1 spheroids were almost all alive after irradiation with the 808 nm laser at 0.8 W/cm² for 10 min, showing mostly green fluorescence color (Figure 6A). With regard to photodynamic effects, the 4T1 cell spheroids cultured with PBS and ICG/PTX/BSA-Ce6-NPs/BSA-PFC-NEs seemed all alive when held under hypoxic conditions, irrespective of 660 nm laser irradiation. However, the 4T1 cell spheroids cultured with ICG/PTX/BSA-Ce6-NPs and irradiated with the 660 nm laser for 60 min were obviously dead when held under normoxic conditions, whereas non-irradiated 4T1 cell spheroids cultured under the same condition showed negligible cytotoxicity. Furthermore, the 4T1 cell spheroids incubated with ICG/PTX/BSA-Ce6-NPs/BSA-PFC-NEs and irradiated with the 660 nm laser (60 min) and also subjected to a US scan (15 min) were mostly dead because oxygen release from the BSA-PFC-NEs was induced by ultrasound scan energy, whereas the 4T1 cell spheroids cultured under the same conditions but without the US scan clearly remained alive (Figure 6B).

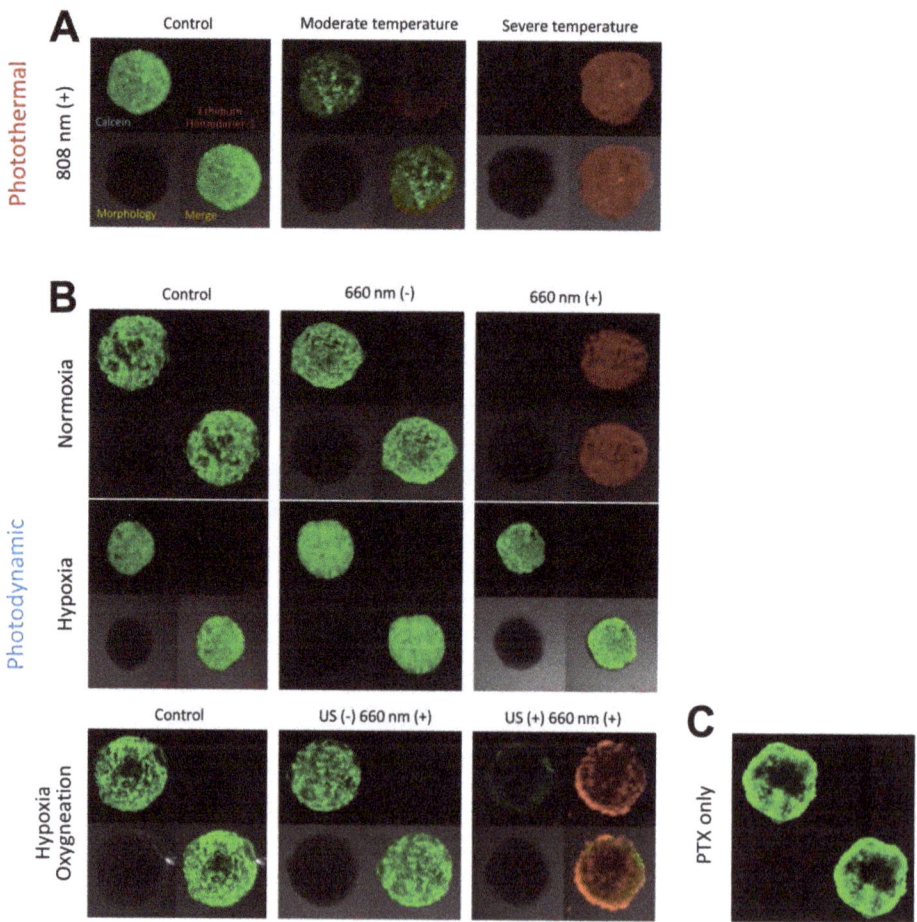

Figure 6. (**A**) CLSM images for 4T1 cell spheroids incubated with ICG/PTX/BSA-Ce6-NPs@Gel under 808 nm laser irradiation specifically adjusted to induce regular, moderate, or severe temperature. (**B**) CLSM images for 4T1 cell spheroids incubated with ICG/PTX/BSA-Ce6-NPs@Gel with or without 660 nm laser irradiation under normoxic, hypoxic, or oxygenated conditions. (**C**) CLSM images for 4T1 cell spheroids incubated with PTX/BSA-NPs@Gel. Green and red colors represent live and dead cells, respectively.

3.5. Visualization of Hypoxia in 4T1 Cell Spheroids

Hypoxic conditions were precisely achieved at the hypoxic chamber in a hypoxic gas stream (5% CO_2:95% N_2 on a volumetric basis), and the resulting hypoxia was demonstrated by visualizing the hypoxia-inducible factor (HIF)-1α at 4T1 cell spheroids. As shown in Figure 7A, spheroids treated at hypoxia were strongly stained with anti-HIF-1α antibody, displaying green fluorescence. On the other hand, spheroids treated at normoxia was not stained with anti-HIF-1α antibody because HIF-1α was negligibly expressed. However, 4T1 cell spheroids incubated with ICG/PTX/BSA-Ce6-NPs/BSA-PFC-NEs that were not subjected to a US scan displayed strong green fluorescence when cultured under hypoxic conditions. In contrast, the same 4T1 cell spheroids oxygenated by a US scan did not show the typical hypoxic fluorescence signal.

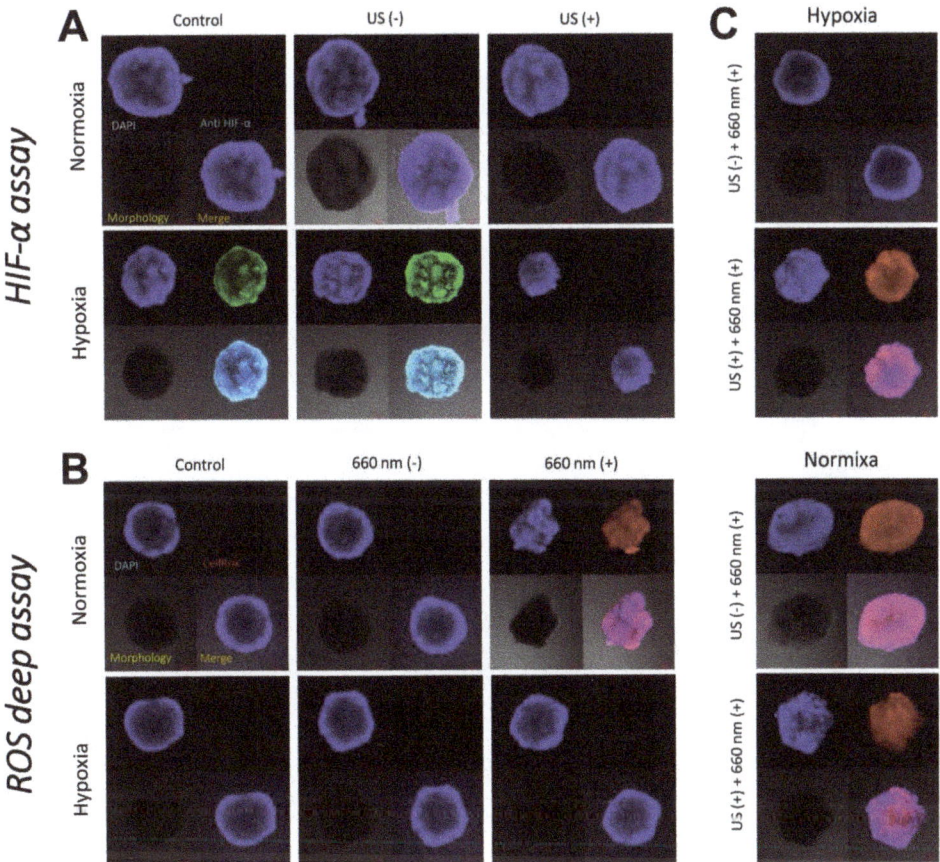

Figure 7. (**A**) CLSM images of 4T1 cell spheroids incubated with ICG/PTX/BSA-Ce6-NEs@Gel with or without US guidance under normoxic or hypoxic conditions in order to assess consequent HIF-1α production. (**B**) CLSM images of 4T1 cell spheroids incubated with ICG/PTX/BSA-Ce6-NPs~PFC-NEs@Gel with or without 660 nm laser irradiation under normoxic or hypoxic conditions in order to assess consequent intracellular ROS (singlet oxygen) production. (**C**) CLSM images of 4T1 cell spheroids incubated with ICG/PTX/BSA-Ce6-NPs~PFC-NEs@Gel with or without US guidance and irradiated with a 660 nm laser under normoxic or hypoxic conditions in order to assess consequent intracellular ROS production.

3.6. Visualization of Singlet Oxygen Generation in 4T1 Cell Spheroids

The intracellular ROS levels/distributions were visualized in each group of 4T1 cell spheroids by CLSM. When cultured under hypoxic conditions, all test groups of 4T1 cells incubated with ICG/PTX/BSA-Ce6-NPs~PFC-NEs@Gel did not exhibit strong red signals indicating significant intracellular ROS production, as detected by the ROS-sensitive dye CellROX® Deep Red, regardless of the use of 660 nm laser irradiation (Figure 7B). In contrast, when cultured under normoxic conditions, all 4T1 cell spheroids incubated with the various hydrogels and irradiated with the 660 nm laser displayed strong red fluorescence signals, and this phenomenon appeared even when the spheroids were cultured under hypoxic conditions but oxygenated by a US scan of the PEG hydrogel samples (Figure 7C).

3.7. In Vivo Tumor Localization of ICG/PTX/BSA-Ce6-NPs~PFC-NEs@Gel in 4T1 Tumor-Bearing Mice

After intratumor injection of ICG/PTX/BSA-Ce6-NPs~PFC-NEs@Gel, ICG and Ce6 fluorescence were visualized in xenografted 4T1 tumor-bearing mice. The ICG and BSA-Ce6 from the PEG hydrogel were diffusely distributed within the tumors. The considerable fluorescence levels were maintained until 12 h, but their NIR-fluorescence signals gradually decreased and then faded out 72 h after intratumor injection (Figure 8).

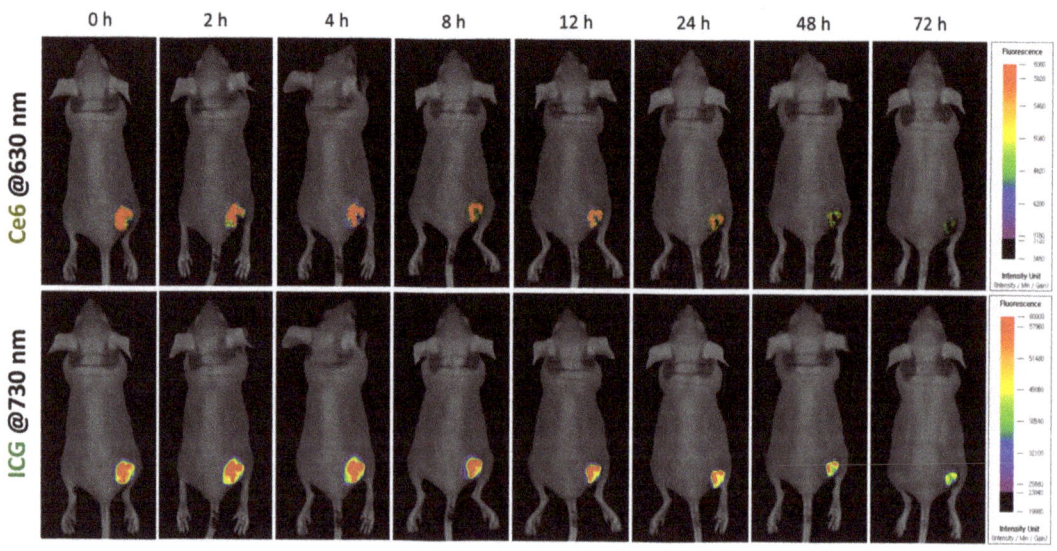

Figure 8. In vivo visualization of 4T1 tumor-bearing mouse after intratumor injection of ICG/PTX/BSA-Ce6-NPs~PFC-NEs@Gel based on Ce6 and ICG fluorescence, at 630 and 730 nm, respectively.

3.8. Photoacoustic Imaging of 4T1 Cell-Xenograft Tumors

The accumulation of oxygen (as HbO_2) produced in 4T1 tumors xenografted onto mice was visualized using photoacoustic (PA) analyses with high resolution and deep imaging depth (Figure 9). Groups were designated as either the PBS control or ICG/PTX/BSA-Ce6-NPs~PFC-NEs@Gel (G5 formula) with or without a US scan. The PEG hydrogel group (G5) with US scan under mild heat (41–42 °C) clearly displayed the greatest oxygen distribution (red signal) throughout the tumors on PA imaging: the HbO_2 percentage was measured as 25.0% to 42.7% at before and after US, respectively, compared with the negligible HbO_2-level changes (around 23.1%~29.6%) for PBS control and G5 + US(−). This result demonstrated that our ICG/PTX/BSA-Ce6-NPs~PFC-NEs@Gel had a significant ability to supply oxygen to the hypoxic breast tumors.

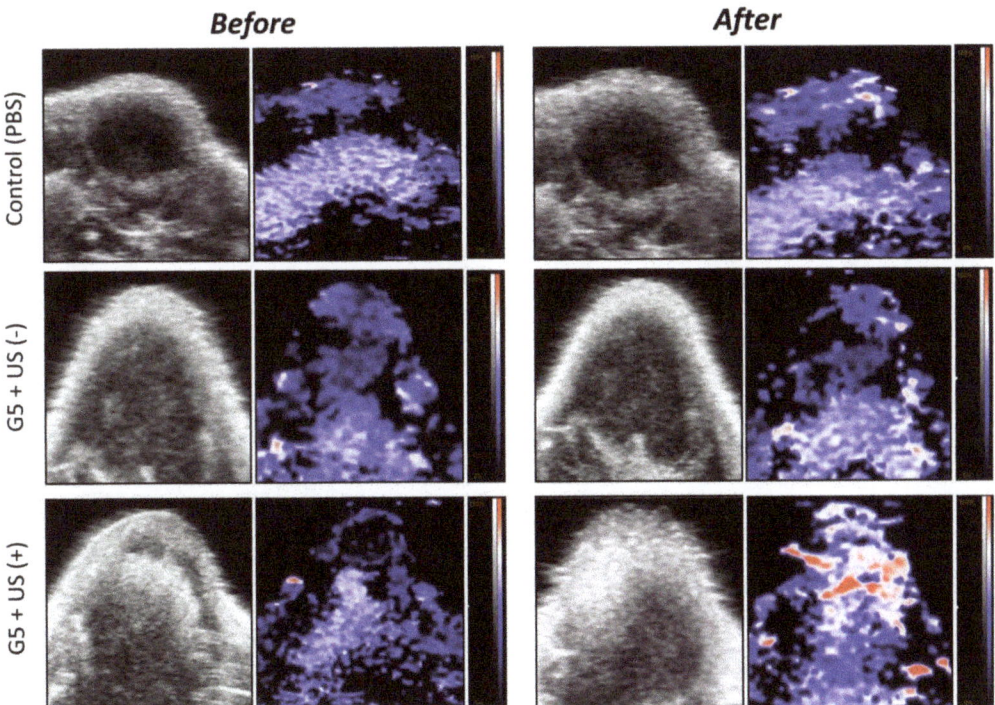

Figure 9. Photoacoustic images of 4T1 cell tumors of mice before and after (at 20 min) intratumor injection of PBS or ICG/PTX/BSA-Ce6-NPs~PFC-NEs@Gel with or without US trigger.

3.9. Antitumor Efficacy in 4T1 Tumor-Bearing Mice

The antitumor effects of ICG/PTX/BSA-Ce6-NPs~PFC-NEs@Gel were evaluated in 4T1 tumor-bearing mice. The tumor volumes for each group of mice were measured for 14 days after treatment (Figure 10A): the final tumor volumes for the G1 to G5 groups were 805.9 ± 138.5, 565.5 ± 41.6, 424.2 ± 90.6, 47.7 ± 11.6, and 63.4 ± 13.0 mm^3, respectively. The G4 formulation with severe heat-induced regression of almost the entire tumor in each xenografted mouse due to the hyperthermal effect. In addition, the G5 formulation (with oxygen provided by the US scan and mild heat induced by the 808 nm laser and singlet oxygen generated by 660 nm laser irradiation) noticeably suppressed the tumors as compared to the G3 group that did not receive oxygen induced by the US scan. The body weight of the mice in the five treatment groups was maintained without significant change over 14 days, indicating that all mice were well cared for without deleterious effects during the entire therapy period (Figure 10E).

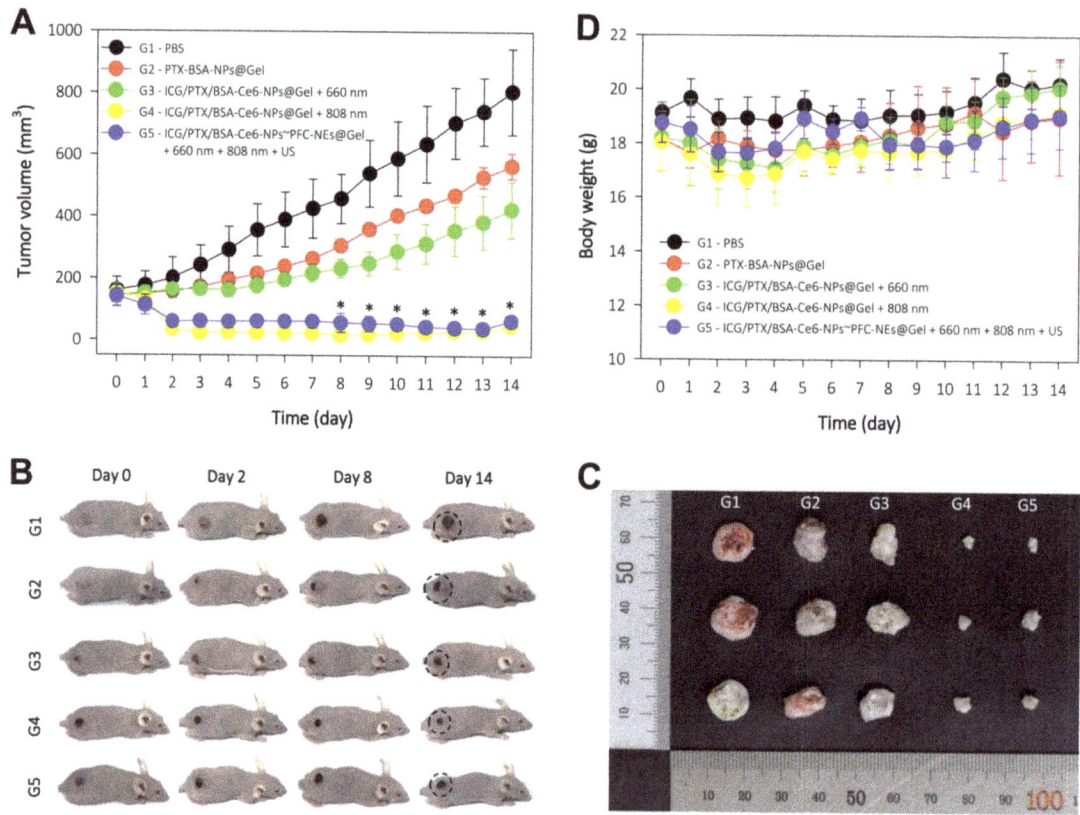

Figure 10. In vivo antitumor efficacy of each PEG hydrogel formulation in five treatment groups of 4T1 tumor-bearing mice (G1–G5): (I) control = PBS; (II) chemotherapeutic = PTX/BSA-NPs@Gel (100 μg PTX (0.1 mL/mouse)); (III) deoxy-photodynamic = ICG/PTX/BSA-Ce6-NPs@Gel + 660 nm (+); (IV) severe hyperthermia = ICG/PTX/BSA-Ce6-NPs@Gel + 808 nm(+); (V) oxy-photodynamic plus moderate hyperthermia = ICG/PTX/BSA-Ce6-NPs@Gel + BSA-PFC-NEs + 660 nm (+) + 808 nm(+) + US(+). All treatments were injected intratumorally. (**A**) Tumor volumes in each group over 14 days. (**B**) Representative photographs of 4T1-tumor-bearing mice at the indicated days after treatment. (**C**) Photographs of tumors excised from each treatment group. (**D**) Body weight change of 4T1-tumor-bearing mice in the different treatment groups over 14 days post treatment.

4. Discussion

Combined anticancer treatment using different therapeutic modalities has attracted great attention as an effective way of suppressing malignant tumors [37]. In particular, co-therapy using PDT and PTT may accomplish synergistic efficacy based on different modes of anticancer treatment [26,38]. While PDT is a well-established technique that is commonly used clinically, is minimally invasive, and produces few side effects [39], PTT is used for two distinct purposes in practice: (i) independent treatment to suppress tumors by severe hyperthermia and (ii) supportive treatment to improve the delivery of chemotherapeutics and oxygen into tumors by increasing tumor blood flow due to moderate hyperthermia. Moreover, concurrent use of chemotherapeutics could accelerate tumor ablation [40]. To this end, we focused on enhancing hypoxia-induced tumor suppression by the use of intratumorally injectable PEG hydrogel formulations based on combined effects of chemotherapeutic, photodynamic, and photothermal modalities plus an oxygen-generation system.

For photodynamic therapy, Ce6 was chosen because it is one of the most efficient and safe second-generation PSs that is approved by the FDA for clinical use. It is sensitive to the light of a wide range of wavelengths (red to NIR: 650–900 nm), which penetrates relatively deep into tumors (presumably hypoxic regions) [39]. However, Ce6 is difficult to formulate on account of its poor solubility in both water and chloroform/dichloromethane; hence, albumin conjugates of Ce6 have been used to surmount this difficulty [2,41]. On the other hand, PFC formulated in albumin-stabilized nano-emulsion can be used to potentiate the photodynamic activity of Ce6 in hypoxic tumors by providing oxygen. Several methods have been introduced to supply or generate extra-/intracellular oxygen (i.e., CaO_2/catalase [7], MnO_2/H_2O_2 [9,42], and a PFC oxygen shuttle/US [35,43]). Among these, PFC is chemically inert and has been explored as an artificial blood substitute due to its high affinity for oxygen. Indocyanine green (ICG) was considered the first option considered for photothermal therapy because it is a deep-penetrating NIR dye approved by the US FDA; in addition, ICG is multifunctional and is also used as a diagnostic and photodynamic agent [44]. However, ICG has several undesirable properties, including concentration-dependent aggregation, poor aqueous stability, and rapid renal elimination from the body, which limit its clinical use [45,46].

The primary aim of this study was to fabricate an in situ-injectable "one-pot" delivery system optimal for including Ce6, ICG, PFC, and PTX in an attempt to achieve concurrent photodynamic, photothermal, and chemotherapeutic effects as a result of improved oxygenation of hypoxic tumors. Previously, we developed a simple method to prepare an in situ-gelling albumin-cross-linked PEG hydrogel system. This hydrogel system comprised only two components (thiolated albumin and 4-arm PEG-maleimide (20 kDa)) and is easily gelled within ~60 s in situ [26,27,36]. If required, the gelation time could be easily adjusted from approximately 15 s to 5 min according to the intended purpose [27]. Likewise, as shown in Figures 3 and 4, all formulations of our ICG/PTX/BSA-Ce6-NPs~PFC-NEs@Gel appeared to be gelled well within 60 s and to have acceptable elastic gel characters: all PEG hydrogel formulations (Z1–Z6) did not flow or drop when held upside-down for 60 s. In clinical settings, this 60 sec period can be critical to allow medical doctors or nurses to complete a series of injection steps: (i) mixing/dissolving powder materials with sterile water for injection, (ii) filling a syringe with the resulting solution, and (iii) immediately injecting the hydrogel into relevant sites before gelation occurs. Likewise, the gelation time for our PEG hydrogels, including those with added ICG/PTX/BSA-Ce6-NPs and BSA-PFC-NEs, was flexibly controlled for 30–120 s depending upon the BSA-SH:4-arm PEG-MAL molar ratio (=1:4.3–4.5). The prepared PEG hydrogel was confirmed to contain ICG/PTX/BSA-Ce6-NPs and BSA-PFC-NEs and displayed moderate to severe hyperthermal and photodynamic effects as measured by a photothermal camera and SOSG fluorescence (Figure 5). In addition, formation of the PEG hydrogel was the result of a specific reaction between artificially driven thiol groups in BSA and maleimide groups of the 4-arm PEG-MAL, and thus the delay or interruption of the release of BSA-Ce6, ICG, or PTX/PFC due to conjugation with PEG frames could be theoretically excluded. Consequently, BSA-Ce6, ICG, and PTX were almost released within 24~36 h (Figure 3B), and oxygen release from BSA-PFC-NEs seemed to be triggered by ultrasound and contributed to the creation of normoxic conditions.

Albumin nanoparticles/nano-emulsions conjugated with Ce6, ICG, and PFC were used as nano-systems inside the PEG hydrogel. Owing to problems with the solubility and stability of Ce6 and ICG, nab^{TM}-technique-based albumin nanoparticles were considered to be an optimal formulation to stably load both Ce6 and ICG into the hydrogels. Previously, our group has optimized albumin nanoparticle formulations for Ce6 and ICG [2,30]. Basically, the strongly hydrophobic chemotherapeutic agent PTX played a role in physically cross-linking albumin molecules, and Ce6-conjugated BSA (BSA-Ce6) was embedded within the resulting ICG/PTX/BSA-Ce6-NPs during their preparation. Despite high water solubility, ICG is known to strongly bind to albumin and thus is highly encapsulated into albumin nanoparticles because the aromatic and heteroaromatic rings of ICG interact strongly with hydrophobic pockets within albumin molecules [45,47]. As shown in Figure 2A,C, these two photothermal and photodynamic agents were simultaneously incorporated into albumin nanoparticles of ~175 nm diameter, and the resulting ICG/PTX/BSA-Ce6-NPs were able to provide both activities in response to the laser irradiations (660 and 808 nm). On the other hand, liquid PFC was easily formed through ultrasonication as a nano-emulsion (BSA-PFC-NEs) stabilized by surrounding albumin molecules, showing ~320 nm emulsion size, and thus appeared to be loaded into the PEG hydrogel. Importantly, the entrapped ICG/PTX/BSA-Ce6-NPs and BSA-PFC-NEs appeared not to undergo sudden release from the PEG hydrogel because the hydrogel mesh formed by four-arm PEG (Mn 5–20 kDa) is thought to be ~5 to 15 nm as estimated using the Flory–Rehner equation or rubber elasticity theory [48]. However, ICG and BSA-Ce6 of relatively small size (<6 nm) may be released through the mesh pores and move (in)to target cancer cells.

Our PEG hydrogel formulated with added ICG/PTX/BSA-Ce6-NPs and BSA-PFC-NEs had significant ability to kill 4T1 cell spheroids due to both 808 nm laser-induced hyperthermia and 660 nm laser-induced photodynamic cell death, accompanied by oxygen release from US-triggered BSA-PFC-NEs. Whereas cell death induced by PTX alone seemed insignificant, the production of naïve oxygen and singlet oxygen from our PEG formulations was clearly observed in anti-HIF-1α and ROS deep assays, respectively (Figures 7 and 8). In addition, our ICG/PTX/BSA-Ce6-NPs~PFC-NEs@Gel unambiguously increased oxygen supply to the tumor region as shown in the photoacoustic imaging (Figure 9), and the PEG hydrogel was retained within the area of the injection site for more than three days. This indicated that additional laser irradiation or US scanning might result in much better tumor suppression/regression. Overall, the severe hyperthermal tumor ablation effect of our formula combined with the strengthened photodynamic activity due to oxygenation and moderate hyperthermia (41–42 °C) appeared to potentiate hypoxic tumor ablation in 4T1 tumor-bearing mice.

5. Conclusions

In summary, the in-situ injectable PEG hydrogel with added ICG/PTX/BSA-Ce6-NPs (~175 nm) and BSA-PFC-NEs (~320 nm) was easily and quickly (~60 s) fabricated and displayed photothermal, photodynamic, and oxygen-supplying activity. The hypoxic tumors of mice treated with our PEG hydrogel formula and with 808/660 nm laser irradiation plus ultrasound scanning were unambiguously suppressed in volume compared with those of all other groups. This remarkable tumor size reduction is attributable to the strengthened photodynamic activity due to oxygenation and moderate hyperthermia (41~42 °C) by the multifunctional effect of loaded Ce6, ICG, and PFC. In addition, our PEG hydrogel formula had sufficient hyperthermal activity to ablate the 4T1 tumors when the irradiation time and output intensity increased. We believe our multifunctional PEG hydrogel formula can be a prototype for ablating otherwise unresponsive hypoxic tumors in coordination with deep-penetrating outer stimuli.

Author Contributions: Conceptualization: Y.S.Y. and W.T.L.; Methodology: W.T.L. and S.S.K.; Software: W.T.L. and N.T.N.; Validation: J.Y. and W.T.L.; Formal analysis: H.K. and W.T.L.; Investigation: E.S.L. and K.T.O.; Resources: H.-G.C.; Data curation: W.T.L., X.T.L. and Y.S.Y.; Writing—original draft preparation: Y.S.Y.; Writing—review and editing: E.S.L., K.T.O., Y.S.Y. and H.-G.C.; Visualization: Y.S.Y.; Supervision: Y.S.Y.; Project administration: Y.S.Y.; Funding acquisition: Y.S.Y. All authors have read and agreed to the published version of the manuscript.

Funding: This work was supported by National Research Foundation of Korea (NRF) grants funded by the Korean government (MSIT) (no. NRF-2019R1A2C2085292 and no. NRF-2019R1A5A2027340).

Institutional Review Board Statement: The study was conducted according to the guidelines of the Declaration of Helsinki and approved by the Institutional Review Board (or Ethics Committee) of Sungkyunkwan University (approved number of 202106291, approval date 15 July 2021).

Informed Consent Statement: Not applicable.

Data Availability Statement: Not applicable.

Conflicts of Interest: The authors declare no conflict of interest.

References

1. Baskaran, R.; Lee, J.; Yang, S.G. Clinical development of photodynamic agents and therapeutic applications. *Biomater. Res.* **2018**, *22*, 25. [CrossRef] [PubMed]
2. Phuong, P.T.T.; Lee, S.; Lee, C.; Seo, B.; Park, S.; Oh, K.T.; Lee, E.S.; Choi, H.G.; Shin, B.S.; Youn, Y.S. Beta-carotene-bound albumin nanoparticles modified with chlorin e6 for breast tumor ablation based on photodynamic therapy. *Colloids Surf. B Biointerfaces* **2018**, *171*, 123–133. [CrossRef] [PubMed]
3. Dolmans, D.E.; Fukumura, D.; Jain, R.K. Photodynamic therapy for cancer. *Nat. Rev. Cancer* **2003**, *3*, 380–387. [CrossRef]
4. Kizaka-Kondoh, S.; Inoue, M.; Harada, H.; Hiraoka, M. Tumor hypoxia: A target for selective cancer therapy. *Cancer. Sci.* **2003**, *94*, 1021–1028. [CrossRef]
5. Hockel, M.; Vaupel, P. Tumor hypoxia: Definitions and current clinical, biologic, and molecular aspects. *J. Natl. Cancer Inst.* **2001**, *93*, 266–276. [CrossRef]
6. Brown, J.M.; Wilson, W.R. Exploiting tumour hypoxia in cancer treatment. *Nat. Rev. Cancer* **2004**, *4*, 437–447. [CrossRef] [PubMed]
7. Huang, C.C.; Chia, W.T.; Chung, M.F.; Lin, K.J.; Hsiao, C.W.; Jin, C.; Lim, W.H.; Chen, C.C.; Sung, H.W. An implantable depot that can generate oxygen in situ for overcoming hypoxia-induced resistance to anticancer drugs in chemotherapy. *J. Am. Chem. Soc.* **2016**, *138*, 5222–5225. [CrossRef] [PubMed]
8. Chen, H.; Tian, J.; He, W.; Guo, Z. H_2O_2-activatable and O_2-evolving nanoparticles for highly efficient and selective photodynamic therapy against hypoxic tumor cells. *J. Am. Chem. Soc.* **2015**, *137*, 1539–1547. [CrossRef]
9. Yang, G.; Xu, L.; Chao, Y.; Xu, J.; Sun, X.; Wu, Y.; Peng, R.; Liu, Z. Hollow MnO_2 as a tumor-microenvironment-responsive biodegradable nano-platform for combination therapy favoring antitumor immune responses. *Nat. Commun.* **2017**, *8*, 902. [CrossRef] [PubMed]
10. Jung, H.S.; Verwilst, P.; Sharma, A.; Shin, J.; Sessler, J.L.; Kim, J.S. Organic molecule-based photothermal agents: An expanding photothermal therapy universe. *Chem. Soc. Rev.* **2018**, *47*, 2280–2297. [CrossRef] [PubMed]
11. Jaque, D.; Maestro, L.M.; del Rosal, B.; Haro-Gonzalez, P.; Benayas, A.; Plaza, J.; Rodríguez, E.M.; Solé, J.G. Nanoparticles for photothermal therapies. *Nanoscale* **2014**, *6*, 9494–9530. [CrossRef]
12. Lee, C.; Hwang, H.S.; Lee, S.; Kim, B.; Kim, J.O.; Oh, K.T.; Lee, E.S.; Choi, H.G.; Youn, Y.S. Rabies virus-inspired silica-coated gold nanorods as a photothermal therapeutic platform for treating brain tumors. *Adv. Mater.* **2017**, *29*, 1605563. [CrossRef] [PubMed]
13. Day, E.S.; Morton, J.G.; West, J.L. Nanoparticles for thermal cancer therapy. *J. Biomech. Eng.* **2009**, *131*, 074001–074005. [CrossRef]
14. Song, C.; Shakil, A.; Osborn, J.; Iwata, K. Tumour oxygenation is increased by hyperthermia at mild temperatures. *Int. J. Hyperthermia* **1996**, *12*, 367–373. [CrossRef] [PubMed]
15. Okajima, K.; Griffin, R.J.; Iwata, K.; Shakil, A.; Song, C.W. Tumor oxygenation after mild-temperature hyperthermia in combination with carbogen breathing: Dependence on heat dose and tumor type. *Radiat. Res.* **1998**, *149*, 294–299. [CrossRef] [PubMed]
16. Wust, P.; Hildebrandt, B.; Sreenivasa, G.; Rau, B.; Gellermann, J.; Riess, H.; Felix, R.; Schlag, P. Hyperthermia in combined treatment of cancer. *Lancet. Oncol.* **2002**, *3*, 487–497. [CrossRef]
17. Mohamed, F.; Marchettini, P.; Stuart, O.A.; Urano, M.; Sugarbaker, P.H. Thermal enhancement of new chemotherapeutic agents at moderate hyperthermia. *Ann. Surg. Oncol.* **2003**, *10*, 463–468. [CrossRef]
18. Kratz, F. Albumin as a drug carrier: Design of prodrugs, drug conjugates and nanoparticles. *J. Control. Release* **2008**, *132*, 171–183. [CrossRef]
19. Elsadek, B.; Kratz, F. Impact of albumin on drug delivery—New applications on the horizon. *J. Control. Release* **2012**, *157*, 4–28. [CrossRef]
20. Kratz, F. DOXO-EMCH (INNO-206): The first albumin-binding prodrug of doxorubicin to enter clinical trials. *Expert. Opin. Investig. Drugs* **2007**, *16*, 855–866. [CrossRef]
21. Kim, I.; Kim, T.H.; Ma, K.; Lee, E.S.; Kim, D.; Oh, K.T.; Lee, D.H.; Lee, K.C.; Youn, Y.S. Synthesis and evaluation of human serum albumin-modified exendin-4 conjugate via heterobifunctional polyethylene glycol linkage with protracted hypoglycemic efficacy. *Bioconjug. Chem.* **2010**, *21*, 1513–1519. [CrossRef] [PubMed]
22. Bae, S.; Ma, K.; Kim, T.H.; Lee, E.S.; Oh, K.T.; Park, E.S.; Lee, K.C.; Youn, Y.S. Doxorubicin-loaded human serum albumin nanoparticles surface-modified with TNF-related apoptosis-inducing ligand and transferrin for targeting multiple tumor types. *Biomaterials* **2012**, *33*, 1536–1546. [CrossRef] [PubMed]
23. Choi, S.H.; Byeon, H.J.; Choi, J.S.; Thao, L.; Kim, I.; Lee, E.S.; Shin, B.S.; Lee, K.C.; Youn, Y.S. Inhalable self-assembled albumin nanoparticles for treating drug-resistant lung cancer. *J. Control. Release* **2015**, *197*, 199–207. [CrossRef] [PubMed]
24. Park, S.; Kim, H.; Lim, S.C.; Lim, K.; Lee, E.S.; Oh, K.T.; Choi, H.G.; Youn, Y.S. Gold nanocluster-loaded hybrid albumin nanoparticles with fluorescence-based optical visualization and photothermal conversion for tumor detection/ablation. *J. Control. Release* **2019**, *304*, 7–18. [CrossRef]
25. Ohta, S.; Hashimoto, K.; Fu, X.; Kamihira, M.; Sakai, Y.; Ito, T. Development of human-derived hemoglobin–albumin microspheres as oxygen carriers using Shirasu porous glass membrane emulsification. *J. Biosci. Bioeng.* **2018**, *126*, 533–539. [CrossRef]

26. Lee, C.; Lim, K.; Kim, S.S.; Lee, E.S.; Oh, K.T.; Choi, H.G.; Youn, Y.S. Chlorella-gold nanorods hydrogels generating photosynthesis-derived oxygen and mild heat for the treatment of hypoxic breast cancer. *J. Control. Release* **2019**, *294*, 77–90. [CrossRef]
27. Kim, I.; Choi, J.S.; Lee, S.; Byeon, H.J.; Lee, E.S.; Shin, B.S.; Choi, H.G.; Lee, K.C.; Youn, Y.S. In situ facile-forming PEG cross-linked albumin hydrogels loaded with an apoptotic TRAIL protein. *J. Control. Release* **2015**, *214*, 30–39. [CrossRef]
28. Hirose, M.; Tachibana, A.; Tanabe, T. Recombinant human serum albumin hydrogel as a novel drug delivery vehicle. *Mater. Sci. Eng. C Mater.* **2010**, *30*, 664–669. [CrossRef]
29. Raja, S.T.K.; Thiruselvi, T.; Mandal, A.B.; Gnanamani, A. pH and redox sensitive albumin hydrogel: A self-derived biomaterial. *Sci. Rep.* **2015**, *5*, 15977. [CrossRef] [PubMed]
30. Pham, P.T.T.; Le, X.T.; Kim, H.; Kim, H.K.; Lee, E.S.; Oh, K.T.; Choi, H.G.; Youn, Y.S. Indocyanine Green and Curcumin Co-Loaded Nano-Fireball-Like Albumin Nanoparticles Based on Near-Infrared-Induced Hyperthermia for Tumor Ablation. *Int. J. Nanomed.* **2020**, *15*, 6469. [CrossRef]
31. Byeon, H.J.; Lee, S.; Min, S.Y.; Lee, E.S.; Shin, B.S.; Choi, H.G.; Youn, Y.S. Doxorubicin-loaded nanoparticles consisted of cationic-and mannose-modified-albumins for dual-targeting in brain tumors. *J. Control. Release* **2016**, *225*, 301–313. [CrossRef]
32. Kim, S.S.; Kim, H.K.; Kim, H.; Lee, W.T.; Lee, E.S.; Oh, K.T.; Choi, H.G.; Youn, Y.S. Hyperthermal paclitaxel-bound albumin nanoparticles co-loaded with indocyanine green and hyaluronidase for treating pancreatic cancers. *Arch. Pharm. Res.* **2021**, *44*, 182–193. [CrossRef]
33. Min, S.Y.; Byeon, H.J.; Lee, C.; Seo, J.; Lee, E.S.; Shin, B.S.; Choi, H.G.; Lee, K.C.; Youn, Y.S. Facile one-pot formulation of TRAIL-embedded paclitaxel-bound albumin nanoparticles for the treatment of pancreatic cancer. *Int. J. Pharm.* **2015**, *494*, 506–515. [CrossRef]
34. Lee, E.S.; Youn, Y.S. Albumin-based potential drugs: Focus on half-life extension and nanoparticle preparation. *J. Pharm. Investig.* **2016**, *46*, 305–315. [CrossRef]
35. Song, X.; Feng, L.; Liang, C.; Yang, K.; Liu, Z. Ultrasound triggered tumor oxygenation with oxygen-shuttle nanoperfluorocarbon to overcome hypoxia-associated resistance in cancer therapies. *Nano Lett.* **2016**, *16*, 6145–6153. [CrossRef] [PubMed]
36. Lee, C.; Lim, K.; Kim, S.S.; Lee, E.S.; Oh, K.T.; Choi, H.G.; Youn, Y.S. Near infrared light-responsive heat-emitting hemoglobin hydrogels for photothermal cancer therapy. *Colloids Surf. B Biointerfaces* **2019**, *176*, 156–166. [CrossRef] [PubMed]
37. Wei, X.; Chen, H.; Tham, H.P.; Zhang, N.; Xing, P.; Zhang, G.; Zhao, Y. Combined photodynamic and photothermal therapy using cross-linked polyphosphazene nanospheres decorated with gold nanoparticles. *ACS Appl. Nano Mater.* **2018**, *1*, 3663–3672. [CrossRef]
38. Vijayaraghavan, P.; Liu, C.H.; Vankayala, R.; Chiang, C.S.; Hwang, K.C. Designing multi-branched gold nanoechinus for NIR light activated dual modal photodynamic and photothermal therapy in the second biological window. *Adv. Mater.* **2014**, *26*, 6689–6695. [CrossRef]
39. Celli, J.P.; Spring, B.Q.; Rizvi, I.; Evans, C.L.; Samkoe, K.S.; Verma, S.; Pogue, B.W.; Hasan, T. Imaging and photodynamic therapy: Mechanisms, monitoring, and optimization. *Chem. Rev.* **2010**, *110*, 2795–2838. [CrossRef]
40. Huang, X.; Wu, J.; He, M.; Hou, X.; Wang, Y.; Cai, X.; Xin, H.; Gao, F.; Chen, Y. Combined cancer chemo-photodynamic and photothermal therapy based on ICG/PDA/TPZ-loaded nanoparticles. *Mol. Pharm.* **2019**, *16*, 2172–2183. [CrossRef]
41. Jeong, H.; Huh, M.; Lee, S.J.; Koo, H.; Kwon, I.C.; Jeong, S.Y.; Kim, K. Photosensitizer-conjugated human serum albumin nanoparticles for effective photodynamic therapy. *Theranostics* **2011**, *1*, 230. [CrossRef] [PubMed]
42. Kim, J.; Cho, H.R.; Jeon, H.; Kim, D.; Song, C.; Lee, N.; Choi, S.H.; Hyeon, T. Continuous O_2-evolving $MnFe_2O_4$ nanoparticle-anchored mesoporous silica nanoparticles for efficient photodynamic therapy in hypoxic cancer. *J. Am. Chem. Soc.* **2017**, *139*, 10992–10995. [CrossRef] [PubMed]
43. Gao, S.; Wang, G.; Qin, Z.; Wang, X.; Zhao, G.; Ma, Q.; Zhu, L. Oxygen-generating hybrid nanoparticles to enhance fluorescent/photoacoustic/ultrasound imaging guided tumor photodynamic therapy. *Biomaterials* **2017**, *112*, 324–335. [CrossRef] [PubMed]
44. Yannuzzi, L.A. Indocyanine green angiography: A perspective on use in the clinical setting. *Am. J. Ophthalmol.* **2011**, *151*, 745–751.e1. [CrossRef] [PubMed]
45. Sheng, Z.; Hu, D.; Zheng, M.; Zhao, P.; Liu, H.; Gao, D.; Gong, P.; Gao, G.; Zhang, P.; Ma, Y. Smart human serum albumin-indocyanine green nanoparticles generated by programmed assembly for dual-modal imaging-guided cancer synergistic phototherapy. *ACS Nano* **2014**, *8*, 12310–12322. [CrossRef]
46. Mundra, V.; Peng, Y.; Rana, S.; Natarajan, A.; Mahato, R.I. Micellar formulation of indocyanine green for phototherapy of melanoma. *J. Control. Release* **2015**, *220*, 130–140. [CrossRef] [PubMed]
47. Chen, Q.; Liang, C.; Wang, C.; Liu, Z. An imagable and photothermal "Abraxane-like" nanodrug for combination cancer therapy to treat subcutaneous and metastatic breast tumors. *Adv. Mater.* **2015**, *27*, 903–910. [CrossRef]
48. Rehmann, M.S.; Skeens, K.M.; Kharkar, P.M.; Ford, E.M.; Maverakis, E.; Lee, K.H.; Kloxin, A.M. Tuning and predicting mesh size and protein release from step growth hydrogels. *Biomacromolecules* **2017**, *18*, 3131–3142. [CrossRef]

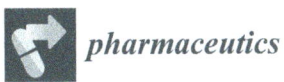

Review

Magnetofection In Vivo by Nanomagnetic Carriers Systemically Administered into the Bloodstream

Artem A. Sizikov [1], Petr I. Nikitin [2,3,*] and Maxim P. Nikitin [1,4,*]

1. Moscow Institute of Physics and Technology, 141701 Dolgoprudny, Russia; aasizikov88@gmail.com
2. Prokhorov General Physics Institute of the Russian Academy of Sciences, 117942 Moscow, Russia
3. National Research Nuclear University "MEPhI", 115409 Moscow, Russia
4. Department of Nanobiomedicine, Sirius University of Science and Technology, 354340 Sochi, Russia
* Correspondence: petr.nikitin@nsc.gpi.ru (P.I.N.); max.nikitin@phystech.edu (M.P.N.)

Abstract: Nanoparticle-based technologies are rapidly expanding into many areas of biomedicine and molecular science. The unique ability of magnetic nanoparticles to respond to the magnetic field makes them especially attractive for a number of in vivo applications including magnetofection. The magnetofection principle consists of the accumulation and retention of magnetic nanoparticles carrying nucleic acids in the area of magnetic field application. The method is highly promising as a clinically efficient tool for gene delivery in vivo. However, the data on in vivo magnetofection are often only descriptive or poorly studied, insufficiently systematized, and sometimes even contradictory. Therefore, the aim of the review was to systematize and analyze the data that influence the in vivo magnetofection processes after the systemic injection of magnetic nanostructures. The main emphasis is placed on the structure and coating of the nanomagnetic vectors. The present problems and future trends of the method development are also considered.

Keywords: magnetofection in vivo; magnetic nanoparticles; iron oxide; gene delivery; gene vectors

1. Introduction

The development of nanosystems that effectively deliver genes into a cell in vivo using magnetofection is a complex and urgent task. A solution to this problem will lead to a significant progress in the creation of drug formulations for gene therapy. In such kind of therapy, nucleic acid molecules delivered into a cell can be used for over-expression of a desired protein, for gene knock down effects, for bypassing or even reparation of genetic mutations, or for activation of the innate immune system [1,2]. There are two main factors limiting biomedical applications of the technology. The first one is not fully understood the process of nucleic acids uptake, their intracellular interactions, intracellular trafficking and regulation of nucleic acid action inside cells at the molecular level. The second one is the direct delivery of nucleic acids to target cells [1,3]. Therefore, choice of the reliable and efficient delivery vectors is very important. When we talk about non-viral vectors, magnetic nanoparticles (MNPs) are often meant. They are considered to be in the center of nanotechnology-based structures for nanomedicine [4,5]. Due to their ability to respond to the magnetic field, MNPs have become very attractive for different theranostic applications [6–8]. When using MNPs, it becomes possible to carry out the magnetically controlled accumulation and release of these particles [9–11], execute the particle tracking by magnetic resonance imaging (MRI) [12–14], imaging of tumors [15,16], precise and quantitative monitoring in vitro [17–19] and in vivo [20,21], by the magnetic particle quantification (MPQ) technique in an extraordinarily wide linear dynamic range (up 7 orders of magnitude). MNPs themselves can be used for tumor therapy [22,23], for targeted drug delivery to a selected part of the body [22–24], or for the magnetic separation of cells [22], as well as for magnetofection [1,25,26]. Magnetofection is defined as method for nucleic acid delivery under the influence of a magnetic field acting on nucleic acid vectors that are associated with magnetic nanoparticles (see scheme in Figure 1) [27,28]. After reaching the cell surface, magnetic nanosystems (usually with polyethylenimine and DNA) are internalized into intracellular vesicles called endosomes as a result of endocytosis. Moreover, for the functional delivery of nucleic acids, so-called endosome escape is required. Otherwise, the magnetic nanoconstructions will be destroyed by the cellular enzyme system. It is believed that PEI–DNA complexes escape from the endosomes due to the so-called proton sponge effect [29]. Magnetic lipoplexes behave in a similar manner [30]. As in the case of nonmagnetic PEI polyplexes [31], a three-step behavior is observed. At the first stage, the magnetic lipoplexes attach to the cell surface and slowly penetrate the cell membrane. Most lipoplexes are internalized through endocytosis during this phase. The second stage is characterized by abnormal and limited diffusion within cells. The third stage is active transport along microtubules inside the cell.

Compared to the commonly used lipid or polymer-based transfection vectors, magnetofection has several advantages, such as higher efficiency, shorter delivery time, a possibility of very local delivery [32–34]. All the above-mentioned advantages of the method are especially relevant when performing magnetofection in vivo. There are several reviews in the literature devoted to various aspects related to in vitro [1,5,27,35–41] and in vivo [42] magnetofection. The latter work considers in vivo delivery of genes using magnetic carriers injected locally to targeted tumors or tissues [42]. In the current work, we provide an overview of the published results on the systemic injection of complex magnetic nanostructures into living organisms. The delivery of drugs/genetic information to the close vicinity of the site of action (tumor, target organ, etc.) is considered to be local. The administration into the circulatory system so that the entire body is affected is regarded as systemic. The main focus is on the magnetic vector structure. We discuss in detail different types of coating of various magnetic particles, give several examples of "unusual" magnetic carriers. Special attention is given to possible ways of development of the existing technology, challenges and prospects of the method.

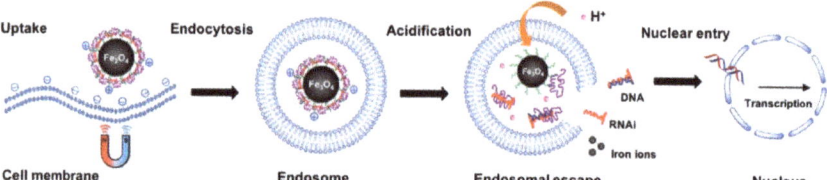

Figure 1. Magnetofection using magnetic nanoparticles. The plasmid DNA is associated with magnetic nanoparticles, which are directed, attracted, and concentrated on the surface of cell membranes, where the endocytosis process brings the nanoparticles into the cell. Adapted with permission from [43].

2. Applications of Nanoscale Carriers for Magnetofection In Vivo

This review is a logical continuation of our previous work [42], where examples of in vivo magnetofection were described in detail for the case of administrating the magnetic vectors directly into a targeted tumor or tissue. Local injections actually allow to avoid such negative effects as undesired interactions with blood components and rapid elimination from the circulation by the reticuloendothelial system (RES). The aim of the present review is to collect and analyze data that influence the processes of magnetofection in vivo after systemic injections of the nucleic acid-bearing magnetic nanoparticles. We have summarized the related results available in various publications on the topic in Table 1.

Table 1. Typical targets, nucleic acid types, magnetic nanoparticle compositions used in published research on magnetofection in different animals after systemic injections of magnetic carriers.

Target (Tissue/Organ)	Animals	Nucleic Acid Type [a]	Magnetic Nanoparticle Composition [b]	References
Subcutaneous tumor/heart	Mouse	shRNA	combiMAG + Lp2000	[44–46]
Subcutaneous tumor	Mouse	pDNA	$Fe_3O_4@SiO_2$–COOH + PEI	[47]
Lungs/heart	Mouse	pDNA	MNBs (Miltenyi Biotec)-PEI	[48]
Right proximal region (subcutaneous tumor)	Mouse	siRNA	LipoMag	[10]
Right testis	Mouse	Antisense ODN	PolyMag	[49]
Liver	Rat	pDNA	MCL	[50]
Hind leg	Mouse	pDNA	PAAIO + CP	[51]
Striatum	Mouse	siRNA	Tf-PEG-PLL/MNP	[52]
Subcutaneous tumor/armpit	Mouse	siRNA	Fe_3O_4 + Chitosan	[53]
dorsal flank (subcutaneous tumor)	Mouse	pDNA	M-MSNs	[54]
Capsule of the liver lobe (transplanted tumor)	Mouse	pDNA	Gal-CMCS-Fe_3O_4-NPs	[55]
Left hepatic lobe	Mouse	siRNA	Gal-PEI-SPIO	[56]
Heart	Mouse	pDNA	MNB/PEI	[57]
Subcutaneous tumor	Mouse	pDNA	TSMCL	[58]
Vessels of the dorsal skin	Mouse	pDNA	MMB	[59]

[a] pDNA = plasmid DNA, Antisense ODN = antisense oligonucleotide, siRNA = small interfering RNA, [b] combiMAG = commercial magnetofection reagent, Lp2000 = Lipofectamine®2000—commercial transfection reagent, PEI = polyethylenimine, MNB = magnetic nanobeads (MiltenyiBiotec, Auburn, CA, USA), LipoMag=commercial transfection kit, PolyMag (Chemicell, Berlin, Germany) = commercial iron oxide nanoparticles, MCL = magnetic cationic liposome, PAAIO = poly(acrylic acid)—bound superparamagnetic iron oxide, CP = polyethylenimine copolymer, Tf = transferrin, PEG = polyethylene glycol, PLL = poly-L-lysine, MNP = magnetic nanoparticle, M-MSNs = magnetic mesoporous silica nanoparticles, Gal = galactose, CMCS = carboxymethyl chitosan, NPs = nanoparticles, SPIO = superparamagnetic iron oxide, TSMCL = magnetic 1,2-dipalmitoyl-sn-glycero-3-phosphocholine (DPPC), 3b-[N-(N',N'-dimethylaminoethane)-carbamoyl]cholesterol (DC-Cholesterol), dimethyldioctadecylammonium bromide (DOAB) and cholesterol liposomes at a molar ratio of 80:5:5:10, MMB = micromagnetobubbles.

The efficiency of the in vivo application of one more magnetic nanocarriers critically depends on the charge and type of the magnetic core coating. Therefore, in this section, we have divided the data into three subsections: magnetic polyplexes (magnetic nanoparticles coated with cationic polymers, Figure 2a), magnetic liposomes (lipid-coated magnetic nanoparticles, Figure 2b), and magnetic nanosystems with an additional active targeting modality (along with the response to the magnetic field, Figure 2c). Furthermore, possible ways of the method evolution are discussed in detail.

2.1. Magnetic Nanoparticles Coated with Cationic Polymers

After the development of a method to synthesize a low aggregated magnetic polyethyleneimine/DNA nanostructures (MPD) and testing these particles when injected locally into a tumor [60], the same authors continued their research on the efficient transfection activity in a serum-containing medium and MPD application in vivo after intravenous injections [47]. The magnetic vector synthesis is described in [60]. Shortly, MNPs were synthesized by two different methods in aqueous [61] and organic media [62] with subsequent modification by ligand exchange or by silane-coupling agents to prepare a negatively charged coating. For this purpose, N-(trimethoxysilylpropyl) ethylenediaminetriacetic acid was used. As a result, the luciferase gene expression in tumors substantially differed for the traditional transfection and magnetofection groups. The luciferase activity effected by the transfection with MPD nanostructures subjected to a magnetic field was about five times stronger compared to that obtained without field application or by the control standard

PEI-DNA complexes. It is also worth noting that a large portion of the particles in all cases settled in the animal's lungs.

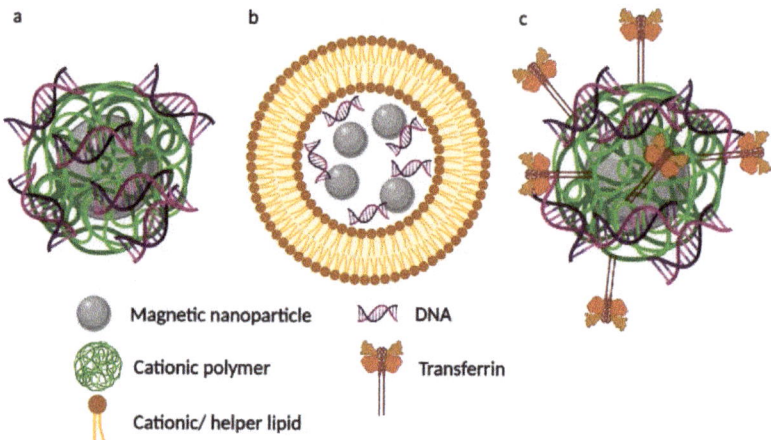

Figure 2. Schematic examples of different magnetic nanocarriers for magnetofection in vivo: (**a**) magnetic polyplex, (**b**) magnetic liposome, (**c**) magnetic polyplex modified with transferrin. Created with BioRender.com (accessed on 7 November 2021).

In contrast, an even higher luciferase activity was recorded, when commercial magnetic nanoparticles were used, namely MNBs (MiltenyiBiotec, Auburn, CA, USA) with an average size of 200 nm [48]. The magnetic polyplex was prepared as follows: biotinylated PEI/DNA complexes were conjugated to MNBs via a sulfo-NHS LC-biotin linker. Two hours after systemic administration of the labeled MNB/Oregon green 488-PEI/pREP4/Luc nanostructures, their accumulation was assessed in vivo by a bioimaging system that detected fluorescence. When using a magnet, the intensity was about 18 times higher in the left side of the animal's chest than without the magnetic field (Figure 3), indicating that the magnet effectively attracted the nanostructures to the left chest (heart and left lung).

Additionally, the magnetic field application caused strong therapeutic gene expression in the left lung and heart. Unfortunately, there was no quantitative assessment as in another publication with similar particles [57], where the level of luciferase gene expression in the heart increased more than three orders of magnitude (!) compared with the control mice without implantation of an epicardial magnet. Another example of work using magnetic vectors based on commercial nanoparticles is discussed in [49]. To investigate whether magnetofection could be a feasible strategy for directing antisense ODN to one specific vascular site after an intra-arterial injection in vivo, the authors infused mice with Cy3-labeled antisense ODN complexed to PolyMAG magnetic particles through a femoral catheter. As a result, solely all large and small arterioles of the cremaster muscle exposed to the magnetic field after the injection of the ODN-MP mixture showed a high level of fluorescence. That was not the case in the vessels of the cremaster muscle of the contralateral testis in the same animals. In these control vessels, similar to the control animal, which was injected with a magnetic vector without applying a magnetic field, only a few large arterioles and none of the small arterioles showed fluorescence, which qualitatively indicated that magnetofection is a working method for active targeting.

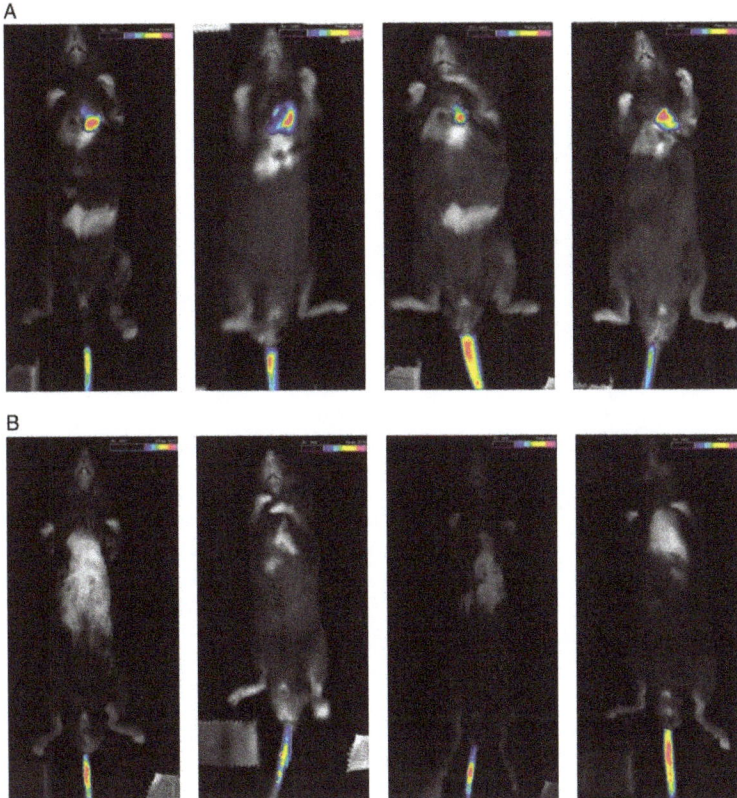

Figure 3. Non-invasive in vivo trafficking of MNB/PEI/DNA nanostructures 2 h after systemic administration. The fluorescent image (pseudocolor) was overlaid on the photographic image. The intensity of fluorescent signal from MNB/Oregon green 488 labeled-PEI/DNA was stronger in the left chest in group with magnet (**A**) compared to the group without magnet (**B**). Adapted with permission from [48].

The work of [53] aimed at estimating the targeting capacity in vivo under the influence of a magnetic field of angiopoietin-2 small-interfering RNA (Ang-2 siRNA) plasmid/chitosan-coated magnetic nanoparticles in a model of malignant melanoma (MM) in nude mice. The method of obtaining chitosan magnetic nanoparticles was quite interesting. At the first stage, magnetic Fe_3O_4 nanoparticles were dispersed in a chitosan solution (Zhejiang Hisun Chemical Co., Ltd., Taizhou, China) under ultrasound agitation. Subsequently, the mixture was added to a mixed phase solvent of liquid paraffin and petroleum ether supplemented with Span-80. The solution was sufficiently emulsified and agitated, then glutaraldehyde solution was slowly added dropwise. Then, the solution was incubated at 40 °C in a water bath for 30 min followed by adjustment pH to 9.0 with NaOH solution. The resulting solution was heated to 60 °C. After standing for 1 h, the precipitate was produced. Then, successive thorough washings with anhydrous ether, acetone, anhydrous ethanol, and distilled water produced the chitosan magnetic nanoparticles. As a result, it was shown, at a qualitative level, that the targeting group (particles + magnetic field) exhibited aggregation of numerous particles on the capsule of tumor tissues and inside blood vessels and staining with Prussian blue was strictly positive.

Another example of using custom-made magnetic particles is given in [51]. It was proposed to use chondroitin sulfate-polyethylenimine copolymer (CP)-coated superparamagnetic iron oxide nanoparticles as an efficient magneto-gene carrier for microRNA-encoding plasmid DNA delivery. The magnetofection gene carrier was prepared by complexation through electrostatic interactions between CP and self-made [63] poly(acrylic acid)-bound iron oxide nanoparticles (SPIONs) (named CPIO). To evaluate the in vivo magneto-induced uptake of the magnetoplex, a biodistribution of CPIO/Cy5-DNA was studied in nude mice with U87-xenografted tumors on the right and left hind leg regions. As a result, the enhanced permeability and retention (EPR) effect [64] played a greater role in biodistribution than the magnetic field (after 48 h, both tumors glowed, the one above, where the magnet was located, glowed slightly stronger).

Magnetic mesoporous silica nanoparticles (M-MSN) are an unusual example of a magnetic vector for in vivo magnetofection. The research of [54] aimed at creating M-MSNs that differed in shape followed by a comparative study of their efficiency in suicide gene therapy of hepatocellular carcinoma (HCC). As a model, the thymidine kinase/ganciclovir of herpes simplex virus (HSV-TK/GCV) gene therapy system was used. Carboxyl-functionalized M-MSNs were first loaded with GCV. Then, PEG-g-PLL was introduced to ensure a positive surface charge of the resulting nanostructure for electrostatic absorption of the TK plasmid. At the first stage, nanosized magnetite coated with polyacrylic acid was obtained [65]. Then, spherical (S-M-MSNs) and rod-shaped (R-M-MSNs) mesoporous silica nanoparticles were synthesized by a simple sol-gel method using the obtained Fe_3O_4 NPs and cetyltrimethylammonium bromide (CTAB) as a template [66,67]. After that, carboxylate-modified M-MSNs were formed via reactions of M-MSNs with ammonium persulfate (APS) and further with succinic anhydride [68,69]. Finally, PEG-g-PLL and M-MSNs–COOH were covalently conjugated using a modified EDC/NHS reaction according to [70,71]. To evaluate the therapy results, the authors proposed a comparison of the sizes of the respective tumors. Compared to the control group, which was given only saline, tumor growth inhibition was observed in all other cases. In addition, the group that was treated with the magnetic field showed a significant reduction in the relative tumor volume and weight compared to the non-magnetic group. Moreover, if both types of the field (constant and variable) were used, then the tumor was less than under a single field type, while the latter, in turn, was less than without any field.

2.2. Lipid-Coated Magnetic Nanostructures

The use of magnetic lipoplexes via magnetic field-assisted systemic delivery appeared to be a much more popular method compared to the local delivery [42]. A team of authors led by Aiqiang Dong believes that liposomal magnetofection works best when administered systemically and that the magnetic field potentiates gene transfection to concentrate magnetic lipoplexes onto target cells [44–46]. In all three papers, the magnetic nanosystems had the following composition: pGFPshIGF-1Rs/combiMAG/lp2000. In [44], it was shown that the silencing efficiency of shRNAs delivered by the liposomal magnetofection after a pGFPshIGF-1R injection reached 43.4 ± 5.7%, 56.3 ± 9.6%, and 72.2 ± 6.8% at 24, 48 and 72 h, respectively, and reached an average of 43.8 ± 5.3% by lipofection. The biological distribution and target tumor suppression after magnetofection were also studied along with the potential toxicity of the method via combiMAG-carrying plasmids expressing green fluorescent protein (GFP) and short hairpin RNAs (shRNAs) targeting IGF-1R (pGFPshIGF-1Rs) in tumor-bearing mice [45]. In that work, the accumulation and delivery of pGFPshIGF-1R into tumors using magnetic nanoparticles and a magnetic field contributed to a significant decrease in tumor growth compared to the control, the suppression rate was 36% on day 30 after treatment. The same magnetic lipoplex can be used for gene therapy after heart failure [46]. The results showed that the silencing efficiency of shRNAs delivered by liposomal magnetofection reached 72.2 ± 6.8, 80.7 ± 9.6 and 84.5 ± 5.6%, at 24, 48 and 72 h, respectively, after pGFPshIGF1R injection.

Namiki Y. et al. [10] described the development of a new nanoparticle, which consisted of an oleic acid-coated magnetic nanocrystal core and a cationic lipid shell (DOTAP (N-[1-(2,3-dioleoyloxy) propyl]-N,N,N-trimethylammonium chloride) and DOPE (dioleoylphosphatidylethanolamine) (1:1)). The lipid mixture dissolved in chloroform was mixed with chloroform-based magnetic fluid. After the addition of distilled water, the homogeneous mixture was evaporated, sonicated, and purified, finally forming LipoMag. LipoMag/siRNA$^{EGFR\#4-mU}$ (siRNA to efficiently knock down the EGFR mRNA in tumor vessels) treatment under a magnetic field exhibited a ≈50% reduction in the tumor volume compared with the control group on day 28th after the treatment initiation.

It is known that liposomes composed of DC-Chol(3β-[N-(N',N'-dimethylaminoethane)-carbamoyl] cholesterol) and DOPE (Dioleoylphosphatidylethanolamine) have been classified as one of the most efficient vectors for transfection of pDNA into cells and in clinical trials [72–74]. In the work [50], DC-Chol and DOPE (1:1 molar ratio) were chosen as the liposome composition, MAG-T (aqueous dispersion of magnetite Fe_2O_3; tartaric acid matrix; mean diameter of 20 nm) was used as the core, and the MCLs were prepared using reverse-phase evaporation. Since the target organ was the liver, the observed luciferase activity 24 h after injection was only one when using MCLs/pDNA nanoformulations under the influence of a magnetic field and 1.5-fold higher compared to the same particles without the field (Figure 4).

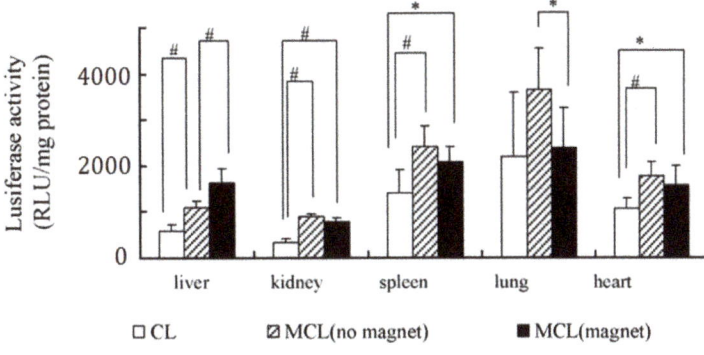

Figure 4. Effect of external magnetic field on the transfection activity of MCLs/pDNA nanoformulations in vivo. The concentration of MAG-T in the MCLs was 1.5 mg/mL and the weight ratio between MCLs and pDNA was 8.0. Luciferase activity was determined 24 h post-injection in the liver, kidney, spleen, lung, and heart, respectively. Each value represented mean ± S.D. (n = 6). * $p < 0.05$, # $p < 0.01$. Adapted with permission from [50].

Another interesting example employing magnetic liposomes is presented in [58]. Here, the delivery system was based on thermosensitive cationic liposomes, which were prepared with a thermosensitive cationic formulation of 1,2-dipalmitoyl-sn-glycero-3-phosphocholine (DPPC), 3b-[N-(N',N'-dimethylaminoethane)-carbamoyl]cholesterol (DC-Cholesterol), dimethyldioctadecylammonium bromide (DOAB) and cholesterol at a molar ratio of 80:5:5:10 (TSCL liposomes). To prepare the magnetic liposomes (TSMCL), a magnetic fluid Fe_3O_4 was used as the core, which was co-encapsulated with ammonium sulfate buffer into the liposomes. The authors of the study [58] designed TSMCL-DOX-shSATB1 as a combined magnetic drug targeting and a magnetofection system to improve the efficiency of simultaneous delivery of DOX and SATB1 shRNAs. Co-delivery of DOX and the shSATB1 vector in an in vivo mouse xenograft model under the influence of a magnetic field resulted in weaker tumor growth compared to control mice.

After studying the behavior of micromagnetobubbles (MMB) through a local injection [75], the same authors continued their research trying systemic administration [59]. The endothelium of the treated dorsal skin clearly showed expression of the dsRed protein 48–72 h after treatment. That expression could not be observed in the vessel wall of mice treated with the plasmid-loaded MMB, where no external magnetic field and ultrasound had been applied, or in the equally treated mice, where only a magnetic field was applied but no ultrasound. Interestingly, although mice treated with only ultrasound but without a magnetic field showed low rates of transfection into the vascular wall in vivo, this effect was more than 60-fold lower than that observed when a magnetic field was added to retain the MMB at the vascular wall.

2.3. Magnetic Nanosystems Possessing an Additional Active Targeting Modality

In order to enhance the penetration of small interference RNA against the polo-like kinase I (siPLK1) across the blood–brain barrier to treat glioblastoma (GBM), magnetic nanoparticles (Tf-PEG-PLL/MNP@siPLK1) modified with transferrin (Tf) were prepared [52] and two types of active targeting were applied. Transferrins are iron-binding blood plasma glycoproteins that control the level of free iron (Fe) in biological fluids [76]. MNPs (Fe_3O_4) were prepared by alkaline co-precipitation [77] with subsequent linking with Tf-PEG-PLL or PEG-PLL. When evaluating in vivo anti-GBM activity, it was found that the tumor inhibition rate raised with increasing the dosage of the magnetic nanocarrier with trans-peptide (no-field conditions were not considered). The biodistributions of another self-luminous siRNA with and without application of the magnetic field were also evaluated (Figure 5).

The fluorescence intensity was significantly higher in the brain upon administration of Tf-PEG-PLL/MNP@Cy5-siPLK1 compared to PEG-PLL/MNP@Cy5-siPLK1 without transferrin. Moreover, it turned out that the magnetic field significantly increased the accumulation of Cy5-siPLK1 in the brain tissues. That, in turn, might contribute to the high activity of Tf-PEG-PLL/MNP @ siPLK1 in vivo against GBM.

The authors of Ref. [55] developed a nanovector with double targeting properties for the efficient delivery of a tumor suppressor gene RASSF1A specifically into hepatocellular carcinoma (HCC) cells by preparing galactosylated-carboxymethyl chitosan-magnetic iron oxide nanoparticles (Gal-CMCS-Fe_3O_4-NPs). It is known that galactose (Gal)-modified magnetic nanoparticles can be discerned specifically by the asialoglycoprotein receptor expressed on the surface of HCC cells and specifically recognized by HCC cells [78]. Fe_3O_4 NPs themselves were obtained in the aforementioned research by alkaline co-precipitation [77], then coated with chitosan [79] followed by the addition of lactose and sodium cyanoborohydride to obtain Gal-CMCS-Fe_3O_4 NPs. The authors studied the biodistribution of the particles loaded with pcDNA6.2mir-EGFP using fluorescent microscopy to visualize GFP expression. They noted green fluorescence in liver and tumor tissues. The average efficiency of pcDNA6.2mir-EGFP transfection in liver tissue was 32.6%. In addition, the average transfection efficiency in tumor tissue was approximately 40.8% and 29.7% when using an external magnetic field and without it, respectively. No overt fluorescence was observed in sections of kidney, spleen, heart, or lung tissues. As for delivery of the RASSF1A gene for HCC treatment, the best results were achieved when a combination of the magnetic vector, external magnetic field, and intra-abdominal administration of mitomycin (MMC—chemotherapy drug) were used for treatment.

The authors of [56] considered magnetic vectors, in which the core consisted of iron oxide modified by galactose (Gal) and polyethylenimine (PEI). The latter acted as shells providing targeted delivery of therapeutic siRNA to the liver cancer. Carboxylate-capped Fe_3O_4 was initially synthesized via the modified oxidative co-precipitation method [80]. Subsequently, PEI was further attached to the surface of Fe_3O_4–COOH via 1-ethyl-3-(3-dimethylaminopropyl)carbodiimide (EDC) followed by the addition of Gal-PEG-NH2. The biodistribution study of the Gal-PEI-SPIO/Cy5-siRNA particles showed rapid accumulation of Cy5-siRNA in the liver and tumor within 8 h. The fluorescence was much more pronounced compared to the case of nano-encapsulated Cy5-siRNA. Fluorescence from Cy5-siRNA was observed within 24 h and decayed significantly over time. With Gal-PEI-SPIO nanoparticles coated with Cy5-miRNA, the fluorescence intensity began gradually decreasing only after 8 h since administration. After 24 h, it was still observable and stronger than that in the control group (RNA only). It was found that the use of a magnetic field did not play a significant role in the inhibition of tumor growth. In general, tumors treated with Gal-PEI-SPIO/si-c-Met showed an obvious decrease in volume. c-Met is a hepatocyte growth factor (HGF) receptor that plays an important role in the proliferation, motility, differentiation, and angiogenesis of HCC [81]. As a result, both groups (with and without magnetic field), in which treatment was used with particles with siRNA, which silenced the expression of c-Met, demonstrated a significant (and almost the same) reduction in tumor volume compared to the control group.

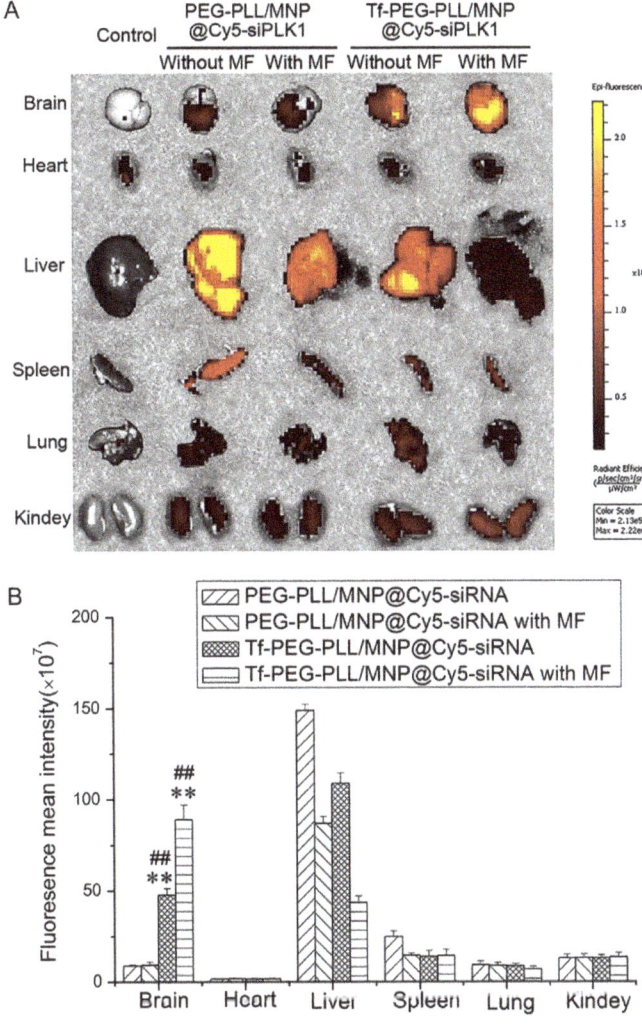

Figure 5. (A) Biodistribution of Cy5-siPLK1 in mice organs at 12 h after the administration of Tf-PEG-PLL/MNP@siPLK1 and PEG-PLL/MNP@siPLK1 by tail vein injection. MF presents the application of magnetic field. (B) The statistic results of panel A. ** $p < 0.01$, vs PEG-PLL/MNP@siPLK1 without MF; ## $p < 0.01$, vs PEG-PLL/MNP@siPLK1 with MF. Data are expressed as the mean ± SD ($n = 3$). Adapted with permission from [52].

3. Conclusions and Outlook

In this review, we have summarized the results of publications devoted to in vivo magnetofection for the case of systemic injection of magnetic nanocarriers and tried to figure out how it works depending on the structure of these magnetic vectors. Judging from the above-cited articles, we can say that the method proved to be a good tool for delivering genetic material (pDNA, siRNA, or antisense ODN, see Table 1) to tumors and tissues via magnetic nanoparticles with various types of coating. Due to the use of a magnetic field, a rather high delivery targeting is achieved at a low loading dose. All this moves magnetofection one step closer to practical applications in gene therapy.

Indeed, it has mentioned in a number of articles that the use of a magnetic field leads to higher gene expression on qualitative [45,49,51] and quantitative [47,48,50,52,56,57] levels. There is also numerical data on a significant decrease in tumor growth compared to control groups [10,45,52,55,56,58], as well as data on silencing efficiency [44,46], which indicate the positive effect of the magnetic field on the transfection process. A logical step would be to compare the results that scientific groups, which study in vivo magnetofection, obtained with the systemic and local routes of injection of magnetic nanostructures based on the same magnetic carriers. This is what the authors of [47,60] carried out. They declared in [47] that transfection by nucleic acid-bearing magnetic nanosystems under a magnetic field produced the highest level of luciferase activity, which was approximately 5-fold higher than that of the magnetic systems without field (when administered locally, the difference was 15-fold [60]). There is also a similar example from a group that has studied the transfection properties of micromagnetobubbles in vivo (local [75] and systemic [59] injections, respectively). Unfortunately, the results of these works could not be directly compared. There are no more examples of such comparisons, probably due to the problems that may be encountered while studying magnetofection in vivo.

The first problem of the precise magnetic guidance of complex magnetic nanostructures is the effect of applied magnetic fields. It is clear that an external magnetic field of higher intensity and gradients contributes to the faster accumulation of the magnetic nanosystems in a target region. On the other hand, an excessively strong magnetic force will result in too intense aggregation of nanoparticles, thus affecting their stability and causing potential cytotoxicity [43]. In turn, a nonlinear decrease in magnetic force with an increasing distance inevitably leads to a weaker response to the external magnetic field, which may become not strong enough to steer the magnetic nanoparticles in the blood flow deep in the body [82]. It would be interesting to study the transgene expression applied with an external magnetic field of stronger gradients, which could penetrate at a larger distance on an intact animal model. In addition, it is difficult, using the current approach, to eliminate completely gene expression in other organs, at least with the commonly used NdFeB magnets. This emphasizes the need for a more focused magnetic field of a higher gradient as, for example, in magnetic systems based on NdFeB micromagnets [83]. In particular, it is reported that the magnetic targeting of deeper situated tissues or of structures situated deeper within organs is weakened, and the enhanced permeability and retention effect, in this case, plays a greater role in biodistribution than the gradient magnetic field [51,84]. To overcome this problem, one of the approaches is to use field-enhancing elements as noted in [85–88], where vascular stents were made magnetic by nickel coating. If implanting these into a deeper situated vessel, these may influence the original magnetic field when magnetized by an external magnetic field and thus may generate strong field gradients deeper into the tissues. Another example of such an invasive technique is the implantation of ferromagnetic wires and exposure of the target area or the whole patient body to an external magnetic field. In this way, strong magnetic field gradients are produced locally and allow capture and concentration of circulating magnetic nanoparticles [89,90]. Alternatively, high gradient [91] or oscillating [92–94] magnetic fields can be used for standard magnetic nanoparticles. Another option is an employment of magnetic materials with higher specific magnetization than iron oxide, but this approach raises biocompatibility concerns. A comparison between magnetite and cobalt nanoparticles (the latter exhibiting a higher magnetization than that of magnetite) of identical sizes and coatings demonstrated similar transfection efficiencies but cobalt cytotoxicity was greater, and the nanoparticles tended to aggregate [38]. For a closer look at modern magnetic systems that allow precise magnetic guiding, we direct the reader to detailed reviews [43,95–97].

The second problem is that in order to further improve the binding of ligands to specific cells, it is necessary to introduce functional ligands such as galactose, folic acid, epithelial cell adhesion molecule and α-fetoprotein that can actively interact with the corresponding binding sites on the cell surfaces [48,55,98]. For example, it is claimed in [48] that conjugation of magnetic nanosystem with a vasculature-permeabilizing agent, such as histamine [99], VEGF [100], or serotonin [101], may further help such complex magnetic nanostructures to cross the endothelial barrier and deliver therapeutic genes to other cell types.

The third problem is that magnetic nanostructures during circulation in the bloodstream inevitably encounter difficulties associated with their interactions with blood components. For example, it is known that cationic nanoparticles attract opsonizing proteins. That causes rapid plasma clearance of the nanocarriers leading to short nanoparticle plasma half-life [102]. Therefore, it is necessary to study in detail the issues related to the factors that affect blood circulation [8,103], as well as elimination [104,105] of nanoparticles for successful applications of in vivo magnetofection, search for new hybrid delivering nanomaterials [106–109] or implementation of more efficient biochemical binding and targeting techniques [110–116]. However, we believe that the magnetofection technique can become a solid option for in vivo targeting combined with improved efficacy of gene delivery, potentially in combination with other physical techniques (electroporation, sonoporation) if appropriate magnetic fields can be generated and if an ideal coating of magnetic particles is found. Still, many questions and problems remain to be addressed before it becomes an efficient and optimized clinical tool for gene therapy.

Author Contributions: Writing—original draft preparation, A.A.S.; writing—review and editing, A.A.S. and P.I.N.; supervision and project administration, M.P.N. All authors have read and agreed to the published version of the manuscript.

Funding: The research was supported by the Ministry of Science and Higher Education of the Russian Federation, contract for the organization and development of world-class research centers No. 075-15-2020-912.

Data Availability Statement: Not applicable.

Conflicts of Interest: The authors declare no conflict of interest.

References

1. Plank, C.; Zelphati, O.; Mykhaylyk, O. Magnetically enhanced nucleic acid delivery. Ten years of magnetofection—Progress and prospects. *Adv. Drug Deliv. Rev.* **2011**, *63*, 1300–1331. [CrossRef]
2. Kawakami, S.; Higuchi, Y.; Hashida, M. Nonviral approaches for targeted delivery of plasmid DNA and oligonucleotide. *J. Pharm. Sci.* **2008**, *97*, 726–745. [CrossRef]
3. Luo, D.; Saltzman, W.M. Enhancement of transfection by physical concentration of DNA at the cell surface. *Nat. Biotechnol.* **2000**, *18*, 893–895. [CrossRef]
4. Pershina, A.G.; Sazonov, A.E.; Filimonov, V.D. Magnetic nanoparticles–DNA interactions: Design and applications of nanobiohybrid systems. *Russ. Chem. Rev.* **2014**, *83*, 299–322. [CrossRef]
5. Sosa-Acosta, J.R.; Iriarte-Mesa, C.; Ortega, G.A.; Díaz-García, A.M. DNA–Iron Oxide Nanoparticles Conjugates: Functional Magnetic Nanoplatforms in Biomedical Applications. *Top. Curr. Chem.* **2020**, *378*, 1–29. [CrossRef]
6. Tregubov, A.A.; Nikitin, P.I.; Nikitin, M.P. Advanced Smart Nanomaterials with Integrated Logic-Gating and Biocomputing: Dawn of Theranostic Nanorobots. *Chem. Rev.* **2018**, *118*, 10294–10348. [CrossRef]
7. Nikitin, M.P.; Shipunova, V.; Deyev, S.; Nikitin, P.I. Biocomputing based on particle disassembly. *Nat. Nanotechnol.* **2014**, *9*, 716–722. [CrossRef]
8. Nikitin, M.P.; Zelepukin, I.; Shipunova, V.O.; Sokolov, I.L.; Deyev, S.M.; Nikitin, P.I. Enhancement of the blood-circulation time and performance of nanomedicines via the forced clearance of erythrocytes. *Nat. Biomed. Eng.* **2020**, *4*, 717–731. [CrossRef]
9. Morozov, V.N.; Kanev, I.L.; Mikheev, A.Y.; Shlyapnikova, E.A.; Shlyapnikov, Y.M.; Nikitin, M.P.; Nikitin, P.; Nwabueze, A.O.; van Hoek, M. Generation and delivery of nanoaerosols from biological and biologically active substances. *J. Aerosol Sci.* **2014**, *69*, 48–61. [CrossRef]
10. Namiki, Y.; Namiki, T.; Yoshida, H.; Ishii, Y.; Tsubota, A.; Koido, S.; Nariai, K.; Mitsunaga, M.; Yanagisawa, S.; Kashiwagi, H.; et al. A novel magnetic crystal–lipid nanostructure for magnetically guided in vivo gene delivery. *Nat. Nanotechnol.* **2009**, *4*, 598–606. [CrossRef]

11. Cho, Y.-S.; Yoon, T.-J.; Jang, E.-S.; Hong, K.S.; Lee, S.Y.; Kim, O.R.; Park, C.; Kim, Y.-J.; Yi, G.-C.; Chang, K. Cetuximab-conjugated magneto-fluorescent silica nanoparticles for in vivo colon cancer targeting and imaging. *Cancer Lett.* **2010**, *299*, 63–71. [CrossRef]
12. Tregubov, A.; Sokolov, I.; Babenyshev, A.; Nikitin, P.; Cherkasov, V.; Nikitin, M. Magnetic hybrid magnetite/metal organic framework nanoparticles: Facile preparation, post-synthetic biofunctionalization and tracking in vivo with magnetic methods. *J. Magn. Magn. Mater.* **2018**, *449*, 590–596. [CrossRef]
13. Motiei, M.; Dreifuss, T.; Sadan, T.; Omer, N.; Blumenfeld-Katzir, T.; Fragogeorgi, E.; Loudos, G.; Popovtzer, R.; Ben-Eliezer, N. Trimodal Nanoparticle Contrast Agent for CT, MRI and SPECT Imaging: Synthesis and Characterization of Radiolabeled Core/Shell Iron Oxide@Gold Nanoparticles. *Chem. Lett.* **2019**, *48*, 291–294. [CrossRef]
14. Lepeltier, E.; Rijo, P.; Rizzolio, F.; Popovtzer, R.; Petrikaite, V.; Assaraf, Y.G.; Passirani, C. Nanomedicine to target multidrug resistant tumors. *Drug Resist. Updat.* **2020**, *52*, 100704. [CrossRef]
15. Medarova, Z.; Pham, W.; Farrar, C.; Petkova, V.; Moore, A.M. In vivo imaging of siRNA delivery and silencing in tumors. *Nat. Med.* **2007**, *13*, 372–377. [CrossRef]
16. Kumar, M.; Yigit, M.; Dai, G.; Moore, A.; Medarova, Z. Image-Guided Breast Tumor Therapy Using a Small Interfering RNA Nanodrug. *Cancer Res.* **2010**, *70*, 7553–7561. [CrossRef]
17. Znoyko, S.L.; Orlov, A.; Pushkarev, A.V.; Mochalova, E.N.; Guteneva, N.V.; Lunin, A.; Nikitin, M.P.; Nikitin, P.I. Ultrasensitive quantitative detection of small molecules with rapid lateral-flow assay based on high-affinity bifunctional ligand and magnetic nanolabels. *Anal. Chim. Acta* **2018**, *1034*, 161–167. [CrossRef]
18. Guteneva, N.V.; Znoyko, S.L.; Orlov, A.V.; Nikitin, M.P.; Nikitin, P.I. Rapid lateral flow assays based on the quantification of magnetic nanoparticle labels for multiplexed immunodetection of small molecules: Application to the determination of drugs of abuse. *Microchim. Acta* **2019**, *186*, 1–9. [CrossRef]
19. Bragina, V.A.; Orlov, A.V.; Znoyko, S.L.; Pushkarev, A.V.; Novichikhin, D.O.; Guteneva, N.V.; Nikitin, M.P.; Gorshkov, B.G.; Nikitin, P.I. Nanobiosensing based on optically selected antibodies and superparamagnetic labels for rapid and highly sensitive quantification of polyvalent hepatitis B surface antigen. *Anal. Methods* **2021**, *13*, 2424–2433. [CrossRef]
20. Nikitin, M.P.; Vetoshko, P.M.; Brusentsov, N.A.; Nikitin, P.I. Highly sensitive room-temperature method of non-invasive in vivo detection of magnetic nanoparticles. *J. Magn. Magn. Mater.* **2009**, *321*, 1658–1661. [CrossRef]
21. Nikitin, M.P.; Orlov, A.V.; Sokolov, I.L.; Minakov, A.A.; Nikitin, P.I.; Ding, J.; Bader, S.D.; Rozhkova, E.A.; Novosad, V. Ultrasensitive detection enabled by nonlinear magnetization of nanomagnetic labels. *Nanoscale* **2018**, *10*, 11642–11650. [CrossRef]
22. Safarik, I.; Safarikova, M. BioMagnetic Research and Technology: A new online journal. *Biomagn. Res. Technol.* **2003**, *1*, 1. [CrossRef]
23. Haimov-Talmoud, E.; Harel, Y.; Schori, H.; Motiei, M.; Atkins, A.; Popovtzer, R.; Lellouche, J.-P.; Shefi, O. Magnetic Targeting of mTHPC To Improve the Selectivity and Efficiency of Photodynamic Therapy. *ACS Appl. Mater. Interfaces* **2019**, *11*, 45368–45380. [CrossRef]
24. Berry, C.C.; Curtis, A.S.G. Functionalisation of magnetic nanoparticles for applications in biomedicine. *J. Phys. D Appl. Phys.* **2003**, *36*, R198–R206. [CrossRef]
25. Jiang, S.; Eltoukhy, A.A.; Love, K.T.; Langer, R.; Anderson, D.G. Lipidoid-Coated Iron Oxide Nanoparticles for Efficient DNA and siRNA delivery. *Nano Lett.* **2013**, *13*, 1059–1064. [CrossRef]
26. Zhang, L.; Wang, T.; Li, L.; Wang, C.; Su, Z.; Li, J. Multifunctional fluorescent-magnetic polyethyleneimine functionalized Fe3O4–mesoporous silica yolk–shell nanocapsules for siRNA delivery. *Chem. Commun.* **2012**, *48*, 8706–8708. [CrossRef]
27. Mykhaylyk, O.; Antequera, Y.S.; Vlaskou, D.; Plank, C. Generation of magnetic nonviral gene transfer agents and magnetofection in vitro. *Nat. Protoc.* **2007**, *2*, 2391–2411. [CrossRef]
28. Plank, C.; Anton, M.; Rudolph, C.; Rosenecker, J.; Krötz, F. Enhancing and targeting nucleic acid delivery by magnetic force. *Expert Opin. Biol. Ther.* **2003**, *3*, 745–758. [CrossRef]
29. Boussif, O.; Lezoualc'H, F.; Zanta, M.A.; Mergny, M.D.; Scherman, D.; Demeneix, B.; Behr, J.P. A versatile vector for gene and oligonucleotide transfer into cells in culture and in vivo: Polyethylenimine. *Proc. Natl. Acad. Sci. USA* **1995**, *92*, 7297–7301. [CrossRef]
30. Sauer, A.; de Bruin, K.; Ruthardt, N.; Mykhaylyk, O.; Plank, C.; Bräuchle, C. Dynamics of magnetic lipoplexes studied by single particle tracking in living cells. *J. Control. Release* **2009**, *137*, 136–145. [CrossRef]
31. de Bruin, K.; Ruthardt, N.; von Gersdorff, K.; Bausinger, R.; Wagner, E.; Ogris, M.; Bräuchle, C. Cellular Dynamics of EGF Receptor–Targeted Synthetic Viruses. *Mol. Ther.* **2007**, *15*, 1297–1305. [CrossRef]
32. Song, H.P.; Yang, J.Y.; Lo, S.L.; Wang, Y.; Fan, W.M.; Tang, X.S.; Xue, J.M.; Wang, S. Gene transfer using self-assembled ternary complexes of cationic magnetic nanoparticles, plasmid DNA and cell-penetrating Tat peptide. *Biomaterials* **2010**, *31*, 769–778. [CrossRef]
33. Plank, C.; Rosenecker, J. Magnetofection: The Use of Magnetic Nanoparticles for Nucleic Acid Delivery. *Cold Spring Harb. Protoc.* **2009**, *2009*, pdb-prot5230. [CrossRef]
34. Castellani, S.; Orlando, C.; Carbone, A.; Di Gioia, S.; Conese, M. Magnetofection Enhances Lentiviral-Mediated Transduction of Airway Epithelial Cells through Extracellular and Cellular Barriers. *Genes* **2016**, *7*, 103. [CrossRef]
35. Plank, C.; Schillinger, U.; Scherer, F.; Bergemann, C.; Remy, J.-S.; Krötz, F.; Anton, M.; Lausier, J.; Rosenecker, J. The Magnetofection Method: Using Magnetic Force to Enhance Gene Delivery. *Biol. Chem.* **2003**, *384*, 737–747. [CrossRef]
36. Schillinger, U.; Brill, T.; Rudolph, C.; Huth, S.; Gersting, S.; Krötz, F.; Hirschberger, J.; Bergemann, C.; Plank, C. Advances in magnetofection—magnetically guided nucleic acid delivery. *J. Magn. Magn. Mater.* **2005**, *293*, 501–508. [CrossRef]

37. Schwerdt, J.I.; Goya, G.F.; Calatayud, M.P.; Herenu, C.B.; Reggiani, P.C.; Goya, R.G. Magnetic field-assisted gene delivery: Achievements and therapeutic potential. *Curr. Gene Ther.* **2012**, *12*, 116–126. [CrossRef]
38. Laurent, N.; Sapet, C.; Le Gourrierec, L.; Bertosio, E.; Zelphati, O. Nucleic acid delivery using magnetic nanoparticles: The Magnetofection™ technology. *Ther. Deliv.* **2011**, *2*, 471–482. [CrossRef]
39. Dobson, J.M. Gene therapy progress and prospects: Magnetic nanoparticle-based gene delivery. *Gene Ther.* **2006**, *13*, 283–287. [CrossRef]
40. Sicard, F.; Sapet, C.; Laurent, N.; Bertosio, E.; Bertuzzi, M.; Zelphati, O. Magnetofection of Minicircle DNA Vectors. In *Minicircle and Miniplasmid DNA Vectors*; Wiley: Hoboken, NJ, USA, 2013; pp. 165–176.
41. Kami, D.; Takeda, S.; Itakura, Y.; Gojo, S.; Watanabe, M.; Toyoda, M. Application of Magnetic Nanoparticles to Gene Delivery. *Int. J. Mol. Sci.* **2011**, *12*, 3705–3722. [CrossRef]
42. Sizikov, A.; Kharlamova, M.; Nikitin, M.; Nikitin, P.; Kolychev, E. Nonviral Locally Injected Magnetic Vectors for In Vivo Gene Delivery: A Review of Studies on Magnetofection. *Nanomaterials* **2021**, *11*, 1078. [CrossRef]
43. Zhang, T.; Xu, Q.; Huang, T.; Ling, D.; Gao, J. New Insights into Biocompatible Iron Oxide Nanoparticles: A Potential Booster of Gene Delivery to Stem Cells. *Small* **2020**, *16*, 2001588. [CrossRef]
44. Wang, C.; Ding, C.; Kong, M.; Dong, A.; Qian, J.; Jiang, D.; Shen, Z. Tumor-targeting magnetic lipoplex delivery of short hairpin RNA suppresses IGF-1R overexpression of lung adenocarcinoma A549 cells in vitro and in vivo. *Biochem. Biophys. Res. Commun.* **2011**, *410*, 537–542. [CrossRef]
45. Kong, M.; Li, X.; Wang, C.; Dong, A.; Duan, Q.; Shen, Z.; Ding, C. Tissue distribution and cancer growth inhibition of magnetic lipoplex-delivered type 1 insulin-like growth factor receptor shRNA in nude mice. *Acta Biochim. Biophys. Sin.* **2012**, *44*, 591–596. [CrossRef]
46. Xu, Y.; Li, X.; Kong, M.; Jiang, D.; Dong, A.; Shen, Z.; Duan, Q. Cardiac-targeting magnetic lipoplex delivery of SH-IGF1R plasmid attenuate norepinephrine-induced cardiac hypertrophy in murine heart. *Biosci. Rep.* **2014**, *34*, 575–582. [CrossRef]
47. Xie, L.; Jiang, Q.; He, Y.; Nie, Y.; Yue, D.; Gu, Z. Insight into the efficient transfection activity of a designed low aggregated magnetic polyethyleneimine/DNA complex in serum-containing medium and the application in vivo. *Biomater. Sci.* **2015**, *3*, 446–456. [CrossRef]
48. Li, W.; Ma, N.; Ong, L.-L.; Kaminski, A.; Skrabal, C.; Ugurlucan, M.; Lorenz, P.; Gatzen, H.-H.; Lützow, K.; Lendlein, A.; et al. Enhanced thoracic gene delivery by magnetic nanobead-mediated vector. *J. Gene Med.* **2008**, *10*, 897–909. [CrossRef]
49. Krötz, F.; de Wit, C.; Sohn, H.-Y.; Zahler, S.; Gloe, T.; Pohl, U.; Plank, C. Magnetofection—A highly efficient tool for antisense oligonucleotide delivery in vitro and in vivo. *Mol. Ther.* **2003**, *7*, 700–710. [CrossRef]
50. Zheng, X.; Lu, J.; Deng, L.; Xiong, Y.; Chen, J. Preparation and characterization of magnetic cationic liposome in gene delivery. *Int. J. Pharm.* **2009**, *366*, 211–217. [CrossRef]
51. Lo, Y.-L.; Chou, H.-L.; Liao, Z.-X.; Huang, S.-J.; Ke, J.-H.; Liu, Y.-S.; Chiu, C.-C.; Wang, L.-F. Chondroitin sulfate-polyethylenimine copolymer-coated superparamagnetic iron oxide nanoparticles as an efficient magneto-gene carrier for microRNA-encoding plasmid DNA delivery. *Nanoscale* **2015**, *7*, 8554–8565. [CrossRef]
52. Liu, D.-Z.; Cheng, Y.; Cai, R.-Q.; Wang, B.W.-W.; Cui, H.; Liu, M.; Zhang, B.-L.; Mei, Q.-B.; Zhou, S.-Y. The enhancement of siPLK1 penetration across BBB and its anti glioblastoma activity in vivo by magnet and transferrin co-modified nanoparticle. *Nanomed. Nanotechnol. Biol. Med.* **2018**, *14*, 991–1003. [CrossRef]
53. Shan, X.-Y.; Xu, T.-T.; Liu, Z.-H.; Shu-Zhong, G.; Zhang, Y.-D.; Guo, S.-Z.; Wang, B. Targeting of angiopoietin 2-small interfering RNA plasmid/chitosan magnetic nanoparticles in a mouse model of malignant melanoma in vivo. *Oncol. Lett.* **2017**, *14*, 2320–2324. [CrossRef]
54. Wang, Z.; Chang, Z.; Lu, M.; Shao, D.; Yue, J.; Yang, D.; Zheng, X.; Li, M.; He, K.; Zhang, M.; et al. Shape-controlled magnetic mesoporous silica nanoparticles for magnetically-mediated suicide gene therapy of hepatocellular carcinoma. *Biomaterials* **2018**, *154*, 147–157. [CrossRef]
55. Xue, W.-J.; Feng, Y.; Wang, F.; Guo, Y.-B.; Li, P.; Wang, L.; Liu, Y.-F.; Wang, Z.-W.; Yang, Y.-M.; Mao, Q.-S. Asialoglycoprotein receptor-magnetic dual targeting nanoparticles for delivery of RASSF1A to hepatocellular carcinoma. *Sci. Rep.* **2016**, *6*, 22149. [CrossRef]
56. Yang, J.; Duan, J.; Wang, J.; Liu, Q.; Shang, R.; Yang, X.; Lu, P.; Xia, C.; Wang, L.; Dou, K. Superparamagnetic iron oxide nanoparticles modified with polyethylenimine and galactose for siRNA targeted delivery in hepatocellular carcinoma therapy. *Int. J. Nanomed.* **2018**, *13*, 1851–1865. [CrossRef]
57. Li, W.; Nesselmann, C.; Zhou, Z.; Ong, L.-L.; Öri, F.; Tang, G.; Kaminski, A.; Lützow, K.; Lendlein, A.; Liebold, A.; et al. Gene delivery to the heart by magnetic nanobeads. *J. Magn. Magn. Mater.* **2007**, *311*, 336–341. [CrossRef]
58. Peng, Z.; Wang, C.; Fang, E.; Lu, X.; Wang, G.; Tong, Q. Co-Delivery of Doxorubicin and SATB1 shRNA by Thermosensitive Magnetic Cationic Liposomes for Gastric Cancer Therapy. *PLoS ONE* **2014**, *9*, e92924. [CrossRef]
59. Mannell, H.; Pircher, J.; Fochler, F.; Stampnik, Y.; Räthel, T.; Gleich, B.; Plank, C.; Mykhaylyk, O.; Dahmani, C.; Wörnle, M.; et al. Site directed vascular gene delivery in vivo by ultrasonic destruction of magnetic nanoparticle coated microbubbles. *Nanomed. Nanotechnol. Biol. Med.* **2012**, *8*, 1309–1318. [CrossRef]
60. Xie, L.; Jiang, W.; Nie, Y.; He, Y.; Jiang, Q.; Lan, F.; Wu, Y.; Gu, Z. Low aggregation magnetic polyethyleneimine complexes with different saturation magnetization for efficient gene transfection in vitro and in vivo. *RSC Adv.* **2013**, *3*, 23571–23581. [CrossRef]

61. Sun, S.; Zeng, H.; Robinson, D.B.; Raoux, S.; Rice, P.M.; Wang, S.X.; Li, G. Monodisperse MFe$_2$O$_4$ (M = Fe, Co, Mn) Nanoparticles. *J. Am. Chem. Soc.* **2004**, *126*, 273–279. [CrossRef]
62. Lu, Z.; Dai, J.; Song, X.; Wang, G.; Yang, W. Facile synthesis of Fe3O4/SiO2 composite nanoparticles from primary silica particles. *Colloids Surf. A Physicochem. Eng. Asp.* **2008**, *317*, 450–456. [CrossRef]
63. Ge, J.; Hu, Y.; Biasini, M.; Dong, C.; Guo, J.; Beyermann, W.P.; Yin, Y. One-Step Synthesis of Highly Water-Soluble Magnetite Colloidal Nanocrystals. *Chem.–A Eur. J.* **2007**, *13*, 7153–7161. [CrossRef]
64. Matsumura, Y.; Maeda, H. A New Concept for Macromolecular Therapeutics in Cancer Chemotherapy: Mechanism of Tumoritropic Accumulation of Proteins and the Antitumor Agent Smancs. *Cancer Res.* **1986**, *46*, 6387–6392.
65. Xia, H.; Zhang, L.; Chen, Q.-D.; Guo, L.; Fang, H.-H.; Li, X.-B.; Song, J.-F.; Huang, X.-R.; Sun, H.-B. Band-Gap-Controllable Photonic Crystals Consisting of Magnetic Nanocrystal Clusters in a Solidified Polymer Matrix. *J. Phys. Chem. C* **2009**, *113*, 18542–18545. [CrossRef]
66. Shao, D.; Wang, Z.; Dong, W.-F.; Zhang, X.; Zheng, X.; Xiao, X.-A.; Wang, Y.-S.; Zhao, X.; Zhang, M.; Li, J.; et al. Facile Synthesis of Core-shell Magnetic Mesoporous Silica Nanoparticles for pH-sensitive Anticancer Drug Delivery. *Chem. Biol. Drug Des.* **2015**, *86*, 1548–1553. [CrossRef] [PubMed]
67. Zhang, L.; Zhang, F.; Dong, W.-F.; Song, J.-F.; Huo, Q.-S.; Sun, H.-B. Magnetic-mesoporous Janus nanoparticles. *Chem. Commun.* **2011**, *47*, 1225–1227. [CrossRef]
68. Shao, D.; Zhang, X.; Liu, W.; Zhang, F.; Zheng, X.; Qiao, P.; Li, J.; Dong, W.-F.; Chen, L. Janus Silver-Mesoporous Silica Nanocarriers for SERS Traceable and pH-Sensitive Drug Delivery in Cancer Therapy. *ACS Appl. Mater. Interfaces* **2016**, *8*, 4303–4308. [CrossRef]
69. Wang, Z.; Wang, Y.-S.; Chang, Z.-M.; Li, L.; Zhang, Y.; Lu, M.-M.; Zheng, X.; Li, M.; Shao, D.; Li, J.; et al. Berberine-loaded Janus nanocarriers for magnetic field-enhanced therapy against hepatocellular carcinoma. *Chem. Biol. Drug Des.* **2016**, *89*, 464–469. [CrossRef]
70. Shao, D.; Zeng, Q.; Fan, Z.; Li, J.; Zhang, M.; Zhang, Y.; Li, O.; Chen, L.; Kong, X.; Zhang, H. Monitoring HSV-TK/ganciclovir cancer suicide gene therapy using CdTe/CdS core/shell quantum dots. *Biomaterials* **2012**, *33*, 4336–4344. [CrossRef]
71. Shao, D.; Li, J.; Xiao, X.; Zhang, M.; Pan, Y.; Li, S.; Wang, Z.; Zhang, X.; Zheng, H.; Zhang, X.; et al. Real-Time Visualizing and Tracing of HSV-TK/GCV Suicide Gene Therapy by Near-Infrared Fluorescent Quantum Dots. *ACS Appl. Mater. Interfaces* **2014**, *6*, 11082–11090. [CrossRef]
72. Liu, C.; Zhang, L.; Zhu, W.; Guo, R.; Sun, H.; Chen, X.; Deng, N. Barriers and Strategies of Cationic Liposomes for Cancer Gene Therapy. *Mol. Ther.-Methods Clin. Dev.* **2020**, *18*, 751–764. [CrossRef] [PubMed]
73. Beltrán-Gracia, E.; López-Camacho, A.; Higuera-Ciapara, I.; Velázquez-Fernández, J.B.; Vallejo-Cardona, A.A. Nanomedicine review: Clinical developments in liposomal applications. *Cancer Nanotechnol.* **2019**, *10*, 1–40. [CrossRef]
74. Bulbake, U.; Doppalapudi, S.; Kommineni, N.; Khan, W. Liposomal Formulations in Clinical Use: An Updated Review. *Pharmaceutics* **2017**, *9*, 12. [CrossRef] [PubMed]
75. Holzbach, T.; Vlaskou, D.; Neshkova, I.; Konerding, M.A.; Wörtler, K.; Mykhaylyk, O.; Gänsbacher, B.; Machens, H.; Plank, C.; Giunta, R.E. Non-viral VEGF165 gene therapy—Magnetofection of acoustically active magnetic lipospheres ('magnetobubbles') increases tissue survival in an oversized skin flap model. *J. Cell. Mol. Med.* **2008**, *14*, 587–599. [CrossRef]
76. Crichton, R.R.; Charloteaux-Wauters, M. Iron transport and storage. *JBIC J. Biol. Inorg. Chem.* **1987**, *164*, 485–506. [CrossRef]
77. Miao, L.; Zhang, K.; Qiao, C.; Jin, X.; Zheng, C.; Yang, B.; Sun, H. Antitumor effect of human TRAIL on adenoid cystic carcinoma using magnetic nanoparticle–mediated gene expression. *Nanomed. Nanotechnol. Biol. Med.* **2013**, *9*, 141–150. [CrossRef]
78. Sato, A.; Takagi, M.; Shimamoto, A.; Kawakami, S.; Hashida, M. Small interfering RNA delivery to the liver by intravenous administration of galactosylated cationic liposomes in mice. *Biomaterials* **2007**, *28*, 1434–1442. [CrossRef] [PubMed]
79. Kou, G.; Wang, S.; Cheng, C.; Gao, J.; Li, B.; Wang, H.; Qian, W.; Hou, S.; Zhang, D.; Dai, J.; et al. Development of SM5-1-conjugated ultrasmall superparamagnetic iron oxide nanoparticles for hepatoma detection. *Biochem. Biophys. Res. Commun.* **2008**, *374*, 192–197. [CrossRef]
80. Bromberg, L.; Diao, Y.; Wu, H.; Speakman, S.A.; Hatton, T.A. Chromium(III) Terephthalate Metal Organic Framework (MIL-101): HF-Free Synthesis, Structure, Polyoxometalate Composites, and Catalytic Properties. *Chem. Mater.* **2012**, *24*, 1664–1675. [CrossRef]
81. A Furge, K.; Zhang, Y.-W.; Woude, G.F.V. Met receptor tyrosine kinase: Enhanced signaling through adapter proteins. *Oncogene* **2000**, *19*, 5582–5589. [CrossRef]
82. Amirfazli, A. Magnetic nanoparticles hit the target. *Nat. Nanotechnol.* **2007**, *2*, 467–468. [CrossRef] [PubMed]
83. Dempsey, N.M.; Le Roy, D.; Marelli-Mathevon, H.; Shaw, G.; Dias, A.; Kramer, R.B.G.; Cuong, L.V.; Kustov, M.; Zanini, L.F.; Villard, C.; et al. Micro-magnetic imprinting of high field gradient magnetic flux sources. *Appl. Phys. Lett.* **2014**, *104*, 262401. [CrossRef]
84. Huang, W.; Liu, Z.; Zhou, G.; Ling, J.; Tian, A.; Sun, N. Silencing Bag-1 gene via magnetic gold nanoparticle-delivered siRNA plasmid for colorectal cancer therapy in vivo and in vitro. *Tumor Biol.* **2016**, *37*, 10365–10374. [CrossRef] [PubMed]
85. Polyak, B.; Fishbein, I.; Chorny, M.; Alferiev, I.; Williams, D.; Yellen, B.; Friedman, G.; Levy, R.J. High field gradient targeting of magnetic nanoparticle-loaded endothelial cells to the surfaces of steel stents. *Proc. Natl. Acad. Sci. USA* **2008**, *105*, 698–703. [CrossRef] [PubMed]
86. Pislaru, S.V.; Harbuzariu, A.; Gulati, R.; Witt, T.; Sandhu, N.P.; Simari, R.D.; Sandhu, G.S. Magnetically Targeted Endothelial Cell Localization in Stented Vessels. *J. Am. Coll. Cardiol.* **2006**, *48*, 1839–1845. [CrossRef]

87. Chorny, M.; Fishbein, I.; Yellen, B.B.; Alferiev, I.S.; Bakay, M.; Ganta, S.; Adamo, R.; Amiji, M.; Friedman, G.; Levy, R.J. Targeting stents with local delivery of paclitaxel-loaded magnetic nanoparticles using uniform fields. *Proc. Natl. Acad. Sci. USA* **2010**, *107*, 8346–8351. [CrossRef]
88. Räthel, T.; Mannell, H.; Pircher, J.; Gleich, B.; Pohl, U.; Krötz, F. Magnetic Stents Retain Nanoparticle-Bound Antirestenotic Drugs Transported by Lipid Microbubbles. *Pharm. Res.* **2011**, *29*, 1295–1307. [CrossRef]
89. Babincová, M.; Babinec, P.; Bergemann, C. High-Gradient Magnetic Capture of Ferrofluids: Implications for Drug Targeting and Tumor Embolization. *Zeitschrift Naturforschung C* **2001**, *56*, 909–911. [CrossRef]
90. Yellen, B.B.; Forbes, Z.G.; Halverson, D.S.; Fridman, G.; Barbee, K.A.; Chorny, M.; Levy, R.; Friedman, G. Targeted drug delivery to magnetic implants for therapeutic applications. *J. Magn. Magn. Mater.* **2005**, *293*, 647–654. [CrossRef]
91. Alexiou, C.; Diehl, D.; Henninger, P.; Iro, H.; Rockelein, R.; Schmidt, W.; Weber, H. A High Field Gradient Magnet for Magnetic Drug Targeting. *IEEE Trans. Appl. Supercond.* **2006**, *16*, 1527–1530. [CrossRef]
92. McBain, S.C.; Griesenbach, U.; Xenariou, S.; Keramane, A.; Batich, C.D.; Alton, E.W.F.W.; Dobson, J. Magnetic nanoparticles as gene delivery agents: Enhanced transfection in the presence of oscillating magnet arrays. *Nanotechnology* **2008**, *19*, 405102. [CrossRef] [PubMed]
93. Kamau, S.W. Enhancement of the efficiency of non-viral gene delivery by application of pulsed magnetic field. *Nucleic Acids Res.* **2006**, *34*, e40. [CrossRef] [PubMed]
94. Pickard, M.; Chari, D. Enhancement of magnetic nanoparticle-mediated gene transfer to astrocytes by 'magnetofection': Effects of static and oscillating fields. *Nanomedicine* **2010**, *5*, 217–232. [CrossRef] [PubMed]
95. Blümler, P. Magnetic Guiding with Permanent Magnets: Concept, Realization and Applications to Nanoparticles and Cells. *Cells* **2021**, *10*, 2708. [CrossRef]
96. Shapiro, B.; Kulkarni, S.; Nacev, A.; Muro, S.; Stepanov, P.Y.; Weinberg, I.N. Open challenges in magnetic drug targeting. *Wiley Interdiscip. Rev. Nanomed. Nanobiotechnol.* **2015**, *7*, 446–457. [CrossRef]
97. Liu, Y.-L.; Chen, D.; Shang, P.; Yin, D.-C. A review of magnet systems for targeted drug delivery. *J. Control. Release* **2019**, *302*, 90–104. [CrossRef]
98. Pilapong, C.; Sitthichai, S.; Thongtem, S.; Thongtem, T. Smart magnetic nanoparticle-aptamer probe for targeted imaging and treatment of hepatocellular carcinoma. *Int. J. Pharm.* **2014**, *473*, 469–474. [CrossRef]
99. Logeart, D.; Hatem, S.; Heimburger, M.; Le Roux, A.; Michel, J.-B.; Mercadier, J.-J. How to Optimize In Vivo Gene Transfer to Cardiac Myocytes: Mechanical or Pharmacological Procedures? *Hum. Gene Ther.* **2001**, *12*, 1601–1610. [CrossRef]
100. Gregorevic, P.; Blankinship, M.J.; Allen, J.M.; Crawford, R.W.; Meuse, L.; Miller, D.; Russell, D.W.; Chamberlain, J. Systemic delivery of genes to striated muscles using adeno-associated viral vectors. *Nat. Med.* **2004**, *10*, 828–834. [CrossRef]
101. Donahue, J.K.; Kikkawa, K.; Thomas, A.D.; Marban, E.; Lawrence, J.H. Acceleration of widespread adenoviral gene transfer to intact rabbit hearts by coronary perfusion with low calcium and serotonin. *Gene Ther.* **1998**, *5*, 630–634. [CrossRef]
102. Weissleder, R.; Bogdanov, A.; Neuwelt, E.A.; Papisov, M. Long-circulating iron oxides for MR imaging. *Adv. Drug Deliv. Rev.* **1995**, *16*, 321–334. [CrossRef]
103. Mirkasymov, A.B.; Zelepukin, I.V.; Nikitin, P.I.; Nikitin, M.P.; Deyev, S.M. In vivo blockade of mononuclear phagocyte system with solid nanoparticles: Efficiency and affecting factors. *J. Control. Release* **2021**, *330*, 111–118. [CrossRef] [PubMed]
104. Zelepukin, I.V.; Yaremenko, A.V.; Yuryev, M.V.; Mirkasymov, A.B.; Sokolov, I.L.; Deyev, S.M.; Nikitin, P.I.; Nikitin, M.P. Fast processes of nanoparticle blood clearance: Comprehensive study. *J. Control. Release* **2020**, *326*, 181–191. [CrossRef] [PubMed]
105. Zelepukin, I.V.; Yaremenko, A.V.; Ivanov, I.N.; Yuryev, M.V.; Cherkasov, V.R.; Deyev, S.M.; Nikitin, P.I.; Nikitin, M.P. Long-Term Fate of Magnetic Particles in Mice: A Comprehensive Study. *ACS Nano* **2021**. [CrossRef] [PubMed]
106. Mukherjee, A.; Waters, A.K.; Kalyan, P.; Achrol, A.S.; Kesari, S.; Yenugonda, V.M. Lipid–polymer hybrid nanoparticles as a next-generation drug delivery platform: State of the art, emerging technologies, and perspectives. *Int. J. Nanomed.* **2019**, *ume 14*, 1937–1952. [CrossRef]
107. Zelepukin, I.V.; Yaremenko, A.V.; Shipunova, V.O.; Babenyshev, A.V.; Balalaeva, I.V.; Nikitin, P.I.; Deyev, S.M.; Nikitin, M.P. Nanoparticle-based drug delivery via RBC-hitchhiking for the inhibition of lung metastases growth. *Nanoscale* **2019**, *11*, 1636–1646. [CrossRef]
108. Ringaci, A.; Yaremenko, A.; Shevchenko, K.; Zvereva, S.; Nikitin, M. Metal-organic frameworks for simultaneous gene and small molecule delivery In vitro and in vivo. *Chem. Eng. J.* **2021**, *418*, 129386. [CrossRef]
109. Lunin, A.V.; Korenkov, E.S.; Mochalova, E.N.; Nikitin, M.P. Green Synthesis of Size-Controlled in Vivo Biocompatible Immunoglobulin-Based Nanoparticles by a Swift Thermal Formation. *ACS Sustain. Chem. Eng.* **2021**, *9*, 13128–13134. [CrossRef]
110. Morachis, J.M.; Mahmoud, E.A.; Almutairi, A. Physical and Chemical Strategies for Therapeutic Delivery by Using Polymeric Nanoparticles. *Pharmacol. Rev.* **2012**, *64*, 505–519. [CrossRef]
111. Cherkasov, V.R.; Mochalova, E.N.; Babenyshev, A.V.; Vasilyeva, A.V.; Nikitin, P.I.; Nikitin, M.P. Nanoparticle Beacons: Supersensitive Smart Materials with On/Off-Switchable Affinity to Biomedical Targets. *ACS Nano* **2020**, *14*, 1792–1803. [CrossRef]
112. Polyak, B.; Friedman, G. Magnetic targeting for site-specific drug delivery: Applications and clinical potential. *Expert Opin. Drug Deliv.* **2009**, *6*, 53–70. [CrossRef] [PubMed]
113. Orlov, A.; Nikitin, M.P.; Bragina, V.A.; Znoyko, S.L.; Zaikina, M.N.; Ksenevich, T.; Gorshkov, B.G.; Nikitin, P. A new real-time method for investigation of affinity properties and binding kinetics of magnetic nanoparticles. *J. Magn. Magn. Mater.* **2015**, *380*, 231–235. [CrossRef]

114. Chorny, M.; Polyak, B.; Alferiev, I.S.; Walsh, K.; Friedman, G.; Levy, R.J. Magnetically driven plasmid DNA delivery with biodegradable polymeric nanoparticles. *FASEB J.* **2007**, *21*, 2510–2519. [CrossRef] [PubMed]
115. Shevchenko, K.G.; Cherkasov, V.R.; Tregubov, A.A.; Nikitin, P.I.; Nikitin, M.P. Surface plasmon resonance as a tool for investigation of non-covalent nanoparticle interactions in heterogeneous self-assembly & disassembly systems. *Biosens. Bioelectron.* **2017**, *88*, 3–8. [CrossRef] [PubMed]
116. Wang, K.; Shang, F.; Chen, D.; Cao, T.; Wang, X.; Jiao, J.; He, S.; Liang, X. Protein liposomes-mediated targeted acetylcholinesterase gene delivery for effective liver cancer therapy. *J. Nanobiotechnol.* **2021**, *19*, 1–15. [CrossRef] [PubMed]

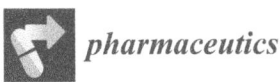

Review

Progress in Nanocarriers Codelivery System to Enhance the Anticancer Effect of Photodynamic Therapy

Yu-Ling Yang †, Ke Lin † and Li Yang *

State Key Laboratory of Biotherapy and Cancer Center/Collaborative Innovation Center for Biotherapy, West China Hospital, Sichuan University, Chengdu 610041, China; yyuling@stu.scu.edu.cn (Y.-L.Y.); linke@stu.scu.edu.cn (K.L.)
* Correspondence: yl.tracy73@scu.edu.cn
† YuLing Yang and Ke Lin contributed equally to the manuscript.

Abstract: Photodynamic therapy (PDT) is a promising anticancer noninvasive method and has great potential for clinical applications. Unfortunately, PDT still has many limitations, such as metastatic tumor at unknown sites, inadequate light delivery and a lack of sufficient oxygen. Recent studies have demonstrated that photodynamic therapy in combination with other therapies can enhance anticancer effects. The development of new nanomaterials provides a platform for the codelivery of two or more therapeutic drugs, which is a promising cancer treatment method. The use of multifunctional nanocarriers for the codelivery of two or more drugs can improve physical and chemical properties, increase tumor site aggregation, and enhance the antitumor effect through synergistic actions, which is worthy of further study. This review focuses on the latest research progress on the synergistic enhancement of PDT by simultaneous multidrug administration using codelivery nanocarriers. We introduce the design of codelivery nanocarriers and discuss the mechanism of PDT combined with other antitumor methods. The combination of PDT and chemotherapy, gene therapy, immunotherapy, photothermal therapy, hyperthermia, radiotherapy, sonodynamic therapy and even multidrug therapy are discussed to provide a comprehensive understanding.

Keywords: codelivery nanocarriers; photodynamic therapy; anticancer therapies; combination therapy

1. Introduction of Photodynamic Therapy and Photosensitizers

1.1. Photodynamic Therapy

Photodynamic therapy (PDT) is a modern noninvasive antitumor technique that has great clinical application potential due to its advantages of simple operation and low systemic toxicity. PDT has been clinically approved for the treatment of some tumors, such as advanced esophageal cancer and advanced lung cancer [1]. Local or systemic photosensitizers (PSs) can be activated to produce cytotoxic reactive oxygen species (ROS) after absorbing light from an appropriate wavelength laser, which can induce tumor cell necrosis and apoptosis or cause angiotoxicity to block tumor cell nutrient supply. In addition, acute inflammatory responses and immunogenic cell death (ICD) induced by PDT have been shown to activate the body's immune system and result in the reconstruction of the tumor microenvironment [2,3].

There are two main mechanisms of the photodynamic reaction. When PSs enter cells, light at a wavelength coinciding with the PS absorption spectrum irradiates the issue, and PSs will be converted from the singlet basic energy state into the excited singlet state because of photon absorption. Part of the energy directs a PS molecule to the excited triplet state. In type I reactions, the PSs in their excited triplet state react with biomolecules and ROS can be generated from radical oxygen species formed by electron transfer reactions such as superoxide ions ($O_2^{\bullet-}$) and hydroxyl radical ($OH^{\bullet}$). In type II reactions, the energy of PSs in their excited triplet state is transferred directly to the oxygen molecule in the basic energetic state, resulting in the generation of singlet oxygen, which is highly

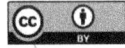

reactive and cytotoxic [2,4]. ROS produced by the two reactions irreversibly damage cells and microvessels, and ROS can fight against cancer by inducing apoptotic cell death, a subroutine mode of active immunity [3,5]. Type II is considered as the most important process affecting PDT efficiency. The balance of the contribution of both reactions depends on many factors, including oxygen concentration and on the structural features of the PSs.

1.2. Photosensitizers

PDT emerged as a tumor treatment in 1907, and the early progression of it is closely related to the development of PSs [4]. The PS types are generally divided into non-porphyrins and porphyrins. The typical non-porphyrin PSs are hypericin, including phenothiazinium dyes, xanthene dyes, phthalimide derivatives, indocyanine green (ICG) etc. Methylene blue (MB), toluidine blue O, Rose Bengal (RB), ICG, as well as the near-infrared dye IR780-iodide have commonly been used in recent years [6–8]. In addition, inorganic materials like graphene oxide (GO) and gold/silver nanoparticles (AuNPs/AgNPs) are also included [9–11], the latter have good biocompatibility and tunable optical properties, and $^1O_2$ can be generated through surface plasmon excitation for PDT of tumors [12]. Metal oxides such as TiO_2 and ZnO_2 NPs can be photoactivated to produce ROS through electron-hole pair interactions with the surrounding $^1O_2$. These nanomaterials generally have the advantages of low toxicity, inertness, good biocompatibility and photostability [13]. Other materials, including black phosphorus nanosheets [14], fullerene [15] and GCNS [16], can also be modified to achieve multifunctionalization.

Porphyrins PSs in the early stage were mainly mixtures obtained from natural porphyrins. For example, hematoporphyrin derivative (HPD), was first used as a PS for bladder cancer in 1970 [17,18]. Unfortunately, Since such PSs had a long half-life and would accumulate excessively in the skin, patients receiving the treatment need to avoid intense light for weeks and their lifestyle is severely affected [19,20]. The second generation are substances with a pure structure, including porphyrins, chlorins, benzoporphyrins and phthalocyanines [9,10]. The common one is 5-aminolevulinic acid (5-ALA), a prodrug of protoporphyrin IX (PpIX), also the current FDA-approved standard for brain tumor visualization. Chlorin e6 (Ce6) is photoactivated at near-infrared wavelengths (664–665 nm) [21–23], has a high efficiency of singlet oxygen generation, and can penetrate deep tissue [24]. Visudyne, the active ingredient of which is verteporfin (benzoporphyrin derivative, BPD), is the only FDA-approved NIR PS for intravenous injection with high singlet oxygen yield and a low skin phototoxicity [25]. Verteporfin has poor solubility and rapid clearance speed in vivo [26], so nanocarriers (liposomes) or cosolvents are used to ameliorate these limitations [27]. Phthalocyanines have two main UV-vis absorption wavelengths: 350 nm and 680 nm, whose high intensity is one of the main characteristics of these dyes. Due to the presence of a high Q band at 680 nm, these dyes can be activated by red light with strong tissue penetration [28]. They have low toxicity and rapid elimination properties [29]. The photophysical properties of phthalocyanines are strongly dependent on central metal ions, and complexes with diamagnetic metal ions such as Zn^{2+} and Al^{3+} help to enhance PDT, including zinc phthalocyanine (ZnPc), zinc hexadecafluorophthalocyanine ($ZnF_{16}Pc$), aluminum chloride phthalocyanine (ClAlPc), etc. At present, there have been a variety of phthalocyanine-based PSs in clinical trials, such as CGP55847, Photosens and so on [30]. The third generation of PSs currently under investigation is designed to synthesize substances that have a higher affinity for tumor tissue, in the form of former drugs or those based on novel drug delivery systems (liposome, polymer, or micelle) [17–19].

The way PDT induces cell death (apoptosis, necrosis, autophagy cell death, or a combination of them) is related to the localization of PSs in subcellular components. Many reports indicate that mitochondria are important targets of PDT, and PSs targeting mitochondria has been proved to induce apoptosis more effectively, which may be related to the loss of mitochondrial membrane potential, inhibition of ADP/ATP exchange, respiratory enzymes and oxidative phosphorylation [4,20,31]. PSs targeting lysosomes could induce the release of cathepsins upon photodamage, which could cleave pro-apoptotic protein Bid and promote mitochondrial apoptosis, or cleave caspase-3 and inhibit apoptosis [31]. Necrosis is caused by high levels of cell damage and usually requires a higher dose than apoptosis. When PSs is predominantly present in the plasma membrane, this is the main form of cell death. In this type of injury, plasma membrane integrity is lost, cells dissolve, and tissue inflammation is triggered. PDT has been reported to induce autophagy, a mechanism for cell survival or adaptation in which injured cells attempt to repair or remove dysfunctional organelles to promote survival. If the initial response fails, autophagy turns into a cell death signal. PDT-induced autophagy is associated with subcellular sites damaged by ROS and can be triggered by light damage to key organelles such as endoplasmic reticulum, mitochondria and lysosome [32,33].

In addition, the fluorescence capability of PSs is widely used in clinical imaging, especially NIR fluorescence imaging technology, which can depict tumor tissue in real time, thus being used to provide highly sensitive images for surgery or to monitor drug therapy [34].

2. Nanotechniques to Improve Photodynamic Therapy

Poor water solubility is a common feature of PSs and limits their clinical application. Chemical coupling combining hydrophobic PS and hydrophilic substances could enhance the circulation time in the blood [24,35]. Physical binding is a more common approach. PSs are loaded into chitosan (CS) [23,36], cationic polymer liposome microcapsules [37–39] and other carriers, which can not only improve the physical and chemical properties but also avoid degradation in the physiological environment [40–42].

The use of targeted vectors helps reduce toxicity and allows the same therapeutic effect to be achieved with smaller doses of PS. This is mainly related to increasing the selectivity of PSs tissue distribution and improving drug bioavailability [4]. In addition to targeting specific tissues, simultaneous targeting of multiple organelles has also been reported to have a stronger therapeutic effect. This can be achieved by combining PSs with different subcellular localization or by using different nanocarriers [27,43,44].

Hypoxia at the treatment site [45,46], low ROS generation efficiency, and low light penetration are also limitations. Inorganic NPs such as AgNPs can mediate greater ROS production through Ag^+ ions released from the surface and have been reported to enhance the anticancer effect of PSs such as MB and Ce6 [47–49]. GO is also commonly used to enhance ROS production, and studies have found that the use of GO loaded with MB can raise the local tumor temperature to approximately 40 °C, effectively preventing tumor metastasis and regeneration [50]. The use of noncovalently bound graphene oxide dihydrogen porphyrin derivatives as long-wavelength absorbers of PS (λ_{max} of 707 nm) enables light to penetrate deeper into the tumor site, overcoming the limitations of low light penetration [51]. For some hypoxic tumors, oxygen or oxygen generators can be codelivered with the PS to enhance the PDT effect through a self-supply of oxygen. Common oxygen transport carriers include nanoscale artificial red blood cell tumors targeting human serum albumin, which can deliver oxygen-loaded hemoglobin and PSs to the tumor site [52,53]. Perfluorocarbon (PFC), an artificial blood substitute that can dissolve large amounts of oxygen, can also alleviate tumor hypoxia after cotargeted delivery with PS [54]. Another method is to use metal carriers to react with peroxide to generate oxygen at tumor sites [55,56]. For example, an activated system using linoleic acid peroxide (LAHP) and iron oxide NPs (IO NPs) can induce the apoptosis of cancer cells through tumor-specific $^1O_2$ generation and subsequent ROS-mediated mechanisms [46]. In addition, it is feasible to transform type II oxygen-sensitive photochemical reactions into Type I photochemical reactions [57]. Other approaches to overcome hypoxia include the use of siRNA to inhibit hypoxia-inducible factors.

The upregulation of vascular endothelial growth factor (VEGF) and heat shock protein 70 (HSP-70) are the main causes of PDT tolerance. To obtain a more ideal PDT treatment effect, PS can be delivered together with gene therapy drugs or small molecule inhibitors targeting VEGF or HSP-70 [58]. In addition, NO produced by photostressed tumor cells can induce anti-PDT effect and enhance tumor aggressiveness. This can be addressed by codelivery with iNOS inhibitors. These would be described in detail in the section on codelivery treatment [59–61].

3. Codelivery of PSs and Anticancer Drugs with Nanoparticles

There are many factors that contribute to decline in photodynamic therapy, including the metastatic tumor at unknown sites, inadequate light delivery, lack of sufficient oxygen and induction of an anti-PDT effect [1]. To overcome these limitations and to improve efficiency, the researchers have combined PDT with other treatments. Codelivery is one of the most common methods to achieve combination therapy and has been widely studied. Currently, common treatment schemes that are amenable to PS codelivery can be divided into the following types: chemotherapy, gene therapy, immunotherapy, photothermal therapy (PTT), hyperthermia (HT), radiotherapy, sonodynamic therapy and multiple drugs codelivery [62–71] (Figure 1). Here, we will mainly introduce the nanocarriers used for the codelivery of PSs and antitumor drugs and discuss how the drugs enhance each other.

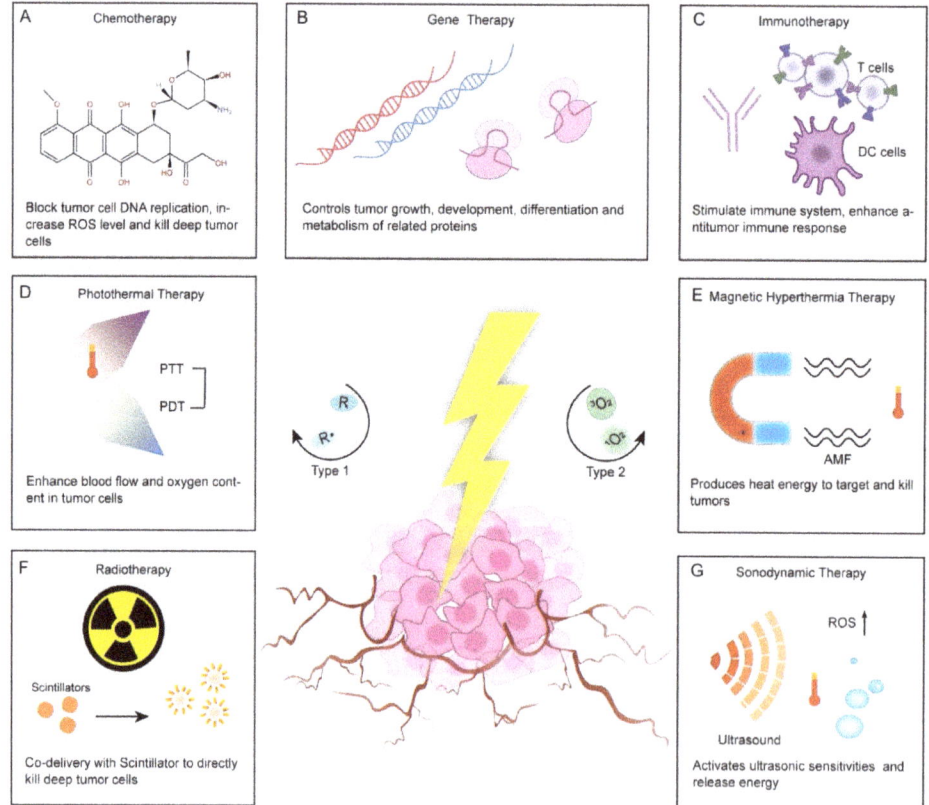

Figure 1. Combination of photodynamic therapy with various therapeutic regimens and possible synergistic antitumor mechanisms. (**A**) Chemotherapy, (**B**) Gene therapy, (**C**) Immunotherapy, (**D**) Photothermal therapy, (**E**) Hyperthermia therapy/Magnetic hyperthermia therapy, (**F**) Radiotherapy, and (**G**) Sonodynamic therapy.

3.1. Chemotherapy

Chemotherapy is a commonly used method for tumor treatment, but systemic toxicity and side effects cause patients to face great pain when receiving treatment, and the efficacy is limited by stability, targeting and multidrug resistance [72]. Many reports have proven that the application of targeted delivery vectors can improve the physical and chemical properties of chemotherapy drugs, while combination with PDT can help to improve multidrug resistance and other problems [73,74]. Mechanistically, chemotherapeutic drugs bind to the DNA of tumor cells and block DNA replication, which leads to suppressed cell division and ultimately death [75]. It has also been found that many chemotherapeutic drugs can increase intracellular ROS levels and oxidation-reduction homeostasis of cancer cells, thus enhancing the sensitivity of tumor cells to PDT [76]. On the other hand, light-independent chemotherapy can kill deep-level tumor cells that PDT cannot, while increased tumor vascular permeability induced by PDT can enhance the accumulation of nanomaterials in tumors, thus enhancing the efficacy of chemotherapy [77,78].

Cationic liposomes are widely used in the codelivery system of PSs and chemotherapeutic drugs due to their preferential accumulation in the vascular endothelium [79]. The introduction of porphyrin-phospholipid (PoP), which is a kind of PS-coupled lipid, enables photoprogrammed controlled release of cationic liposomes. ROS produced by irradiation can oxidize unsaturated lipids and accelerates the release of chemotherapeutic drugs [80,81] (Figure 2A). Doxorubicin (DOX) was loaded into PoP liposomes for intravenous injection. Tumor vascular permeability and drug accumulation were significantly increased under near-infrared light, while empty PoP liposomes without drug loading also showed antitumor effects, suggesting that conjugation with phospholipids did not affect the photodynamic effect of PS [82,83]. In the synthesis of PoP liposomes, the selection of PoP and the proportion of other raw materials are crucial to the morphology and serum stability of the liposomes. Generally, a lower content of PoP in the lipid bilayer leads to higher serum stability [84]. Moreover, the dosage needs to be considered. When DOX is loaded in excess, the bilayer of PoP liposomes becomes elliptical due to instability, while loading irinotecan (a camptothecin-derived anticancer drug) does not affect the morphology of the liposomes [62]. In addition, carrier modification can achieve multiple functions; for example, ^{64}Cu-labeled POP liposomes can be used for imaging simultaneously with treatment and have been shown to not cause drug leakage [85]. The timing of illumination after POP liposome administration is also important, and studies have shown that the drug accumulates more in tumors at short drug–light intervals [86].

Hypoxia is the cause of drug resistance in both chemotherapy and PDT. The effect of photochemotherapy can be enhanced by codelivery of oxygen carriers [87] or oxygen generators [88] loaded with therapeutic drugs. There are also substances that can serve as both chemotherapeutic agents and oxygen donors. For example, nanoplatinum (Pt), when encapsulated in liposomes with PSs, can provide oxygen as a catalase-like nanoenzyme, while Pt ions leached separately can also exert cytotoxic effects [89]. Although the application of nanocarriers can reduce the toxicity and side effects of chemotherapy drugs, it cannot improve the antitumor tolerance caused by the upregulation of heat shock protein HSP-70 after PDT. Hailong Tian [90] combined quercetin (Qu), a chemotherapy drug with the dual effects of anticancer and heat shock protein inhibition, with IR780. IR780 modified with hydrophilic biotin and Qu were assembled into a delivery carrier in solution, which successfully enhanced the therapeutic effect of PDT by inhibiting the expression of HSP-70. PDT and some chemotherapeutic agents, such as DOX and Pt, can mediate ICD. For example, the combined action of oxaliplatin and PDT was shown to expose calreticulin (CRT) on tumor cells, successfully activating host immunity and creating a suitable microenvironment for subsequent immunotherapy combination [91]. More examples of recently published studies on the codelivery of photosensitizers and chemotherapy drugs based on nanocarriers are illustrated in Table 1.

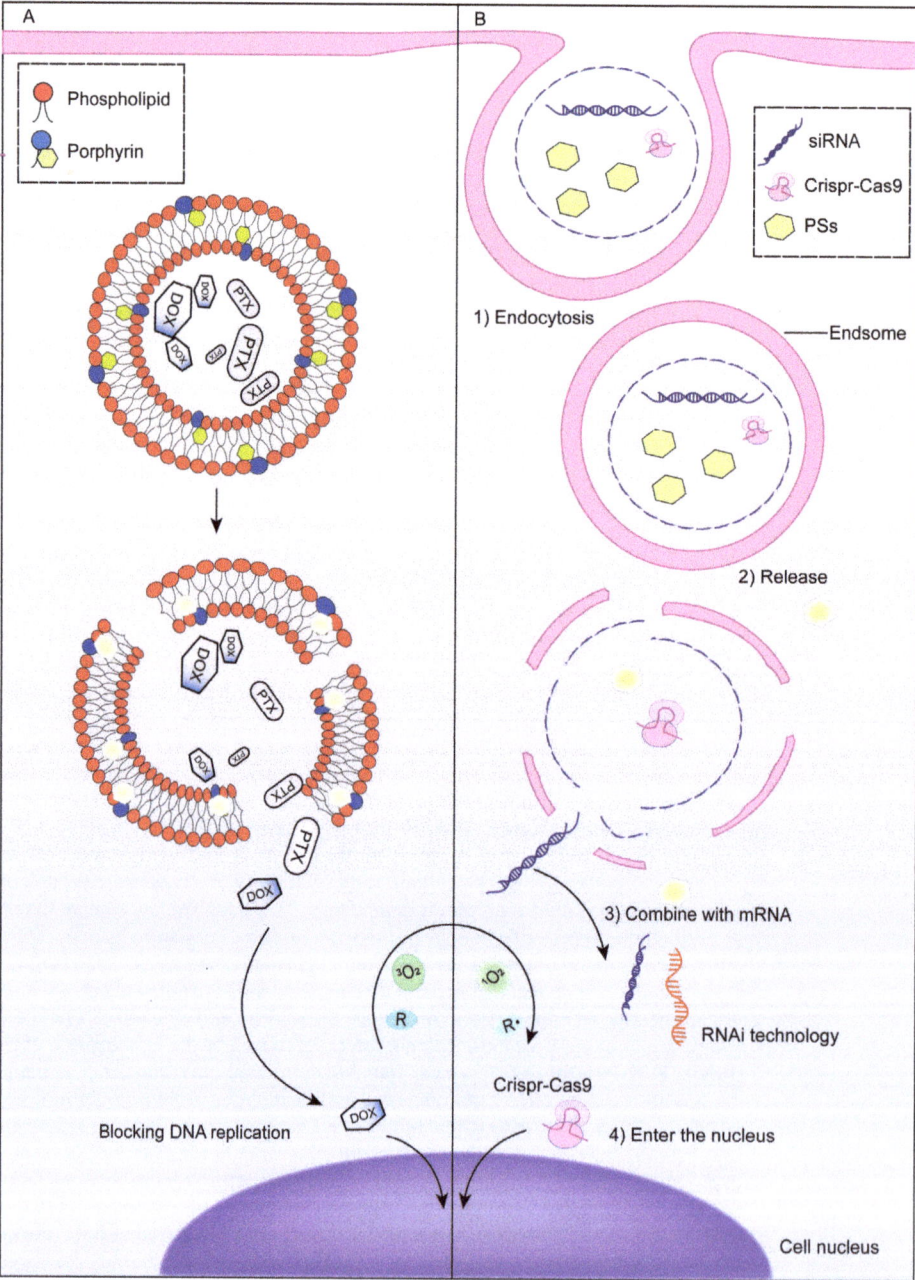

Figure 2. Mechanism of chemotherapy or gene therapy synergistic with PDT to enhance the antitumor effect. (**A**) Diagrammatic illustration of the mechanism of PDT-mediated controlled release of chemotherapy drugs. ROS produced by irradiation can oxidize unsaturated lipids and accelerate the release of chemotherapeutic drugs from porphyrin-phospholipid liposomes. (**B**) Diagrammatic illustration of the mechanism of photochemical internalization (PCI)-mediated endosome escape of nucleic acid drugs. When a photosensitizer is activated by an exogenous light, ROS can be produced rapidly in a short time, destroy the membrane of the intracellular body and release therapeutic genes in the cytoplasm.

Table 1. Codelivery of photosensitizers and chemotherapy drugs based on nanocarriers.

Nanoparticle	Photosensitizers	Chemotherapy Drugs	Tumor	Data Sources	Findings	Ref
Azobenzene-containing conjugated polymers-camptothecin-chlorin e6 NPs (CPs-CPT-Ce6)	Chlorin e6 (Ce6)	Camptothecin (CPT)	HeLa	In vitro, Animals	• The –N=N– functional groups in azobenzene could be reduced and cleaved by AZO reductase in tumor hypoxia, promoting ROS production. • Controlled release of CPT through the reduction of CPs by AZO reductase.	[92] 2018
Cyclic pentapeptide cRGDfk and Chlorin e6 conjugated silk fibroin (SF)-based NPs	Chlorin e6 (Ce6)	5-Fluorouracil (5-FU)	MGC-803	In vitro, Animals	• cRGDfk specifically targets and binds overexpressed $\alpha_v\beta_3$ integrin receptors on MGC-803 cells to increase tumor aggregation of the drug. • Induced high reactive oxygen species generation and produced a good antitumor effect.	[93] 2018
DOX- and perfluorocarbon (PFC)- loaded fluorinated aza-boron-dipyrromethene (NBF) NPs	Fluorinated aza-boron-dipyrromethene (NBF)	DOX	4T1	In vitro, Animals	• High doxorubicin loading efficiency (25%). • PDNBF NPs could be effectively enriched at the tumor site, and DOX could be explosively released by laser irradiation. • Significantly inhibited tumor growth and mediated in vivo ultrasound and photoacoustic imaging.	[94] 2020
Pluronic F127 encapsulated halogenated boron-dipyrromethene NPs (LBBr$_2$ NPs and LBCl$_2$ NPs)	Halogenated boron-dipyrromethene (BDPBr$_2$ and BDPCl$_2$)	Lenvatinib	Hep3B, Huh7	In vitro	• Improved the water solubility of drugs • Controlled release through pH response and enhanced the targeting of chemotherapy drugs. • Significantly inhibited tumor growth by chemotherapy/photodynamic cotherapy.	[95] 2021
Lactobionic acid-catalase-cis-aconitic anhydride-linked doxorubicin @ chlorin e6 (LA-CAT-CAD@Ce6)	Chlorin e6 (Ce6)	cis-Aconitic anhydride-linked doxorubicin (DOX precursor)	EMT6	In vitro, Animals	• Lactobionic acid acted as an active targeting ligand to increase cellular internalization. • Controlled release through pH response. • Decreased the expression of hypoxia-inducible factor-1α and improved the therapeutic effect.	[96] 2020
Pyropheophorbide a-polyethylene glycol 2000 (Ppa-PEG2k)	Pyropheophorbide a (Ppa)	ROS-responsive oleate prodrug of paclitaxel (PTX)	A549, 4T1	In vitro, Animals	• Enhanced the loading efficiency and avoided the quenching effect (ACQ) of PSs. • ROS produced by PDT controlled the release of chemotherapy drug PTX.	[97] 2019

Table 1. Cont.

Nanoparticle	Photosensitizers	Chemotherapy Drugs	Tumor	Data Sources	Findings	Ref
Poly (oligo (ethylene glycol) methacrylate)-Paclitaxel @Chlorin e6 NPs	Chlorin e6 (Ce6)	B-sensitive polymer-paclitaxel (PTX)	T24	In vitro, Animals	• Photointernalization (PCI) accelerated the uptake of NPs by tumor cells. • Tumor growth was significantly inhibited in a PDX model, and the inhibition rate was more than 98%.	[98] 2021
Polyethylene glycol-peptide-poly(ω-pentadecalactone-co-N-methyldiethyleneamine-co-3,3′-thiodipropionate) (PEG-M-PPMT) nanoparticles (NPs)	Chlorin e6 (Ce6)	Sorafenib (SRF)	A549	In vitro, Animals	• Increased serum stability of Ce6 and SRF and enhanced drug aggregation in tumors by EPR. • Overexpressed MMP-2 in tumor extracellular matrix could partially shed PEG from NPs and form smaller particles that penetrate into tumor tissue. • Acidic pH and high intracellular ROS levels accelerated drug release and rapidly killed tumor cells.	[99] 2020
(Phenylboronic acid$_4$-E$_2$E)$_2$-Protoporphyrin IX-(Lipoic acid)$_2$	Protoporphyrin IX (PpIX)	Paclitaxel (PTX)	A549	In vitro, Animals	• PTX blocks mitosis and makes cells stay at G2/M, prolonging the destruction time of nuclear membrane and promoting the accumulation of photosensitizer in the nucleus. • PDT enhanced the internalization and release rate of PTX by destroying lysosomes.	[100] 2020
Poly(ethylene glycol)-b-PMPMC-g-paclitaxel-g-PyTPE micelles (PMPT)	PyTPE, TB	Paclitaxel-SS-N$_3$ (PTX-SS-N$_3$)	HeLa	In vitro, Animals	• Increased uptake of drugs by cells through photochemical internalization (PCI). • The high expression of intracellular glutathione was used to break disulfide bonds and induce the release and aggregation of PTX to induce the change in aggregation state of luminescence.	[101] 2021

3.2. Gene Therapy

The rapid development of nanodelivery systems has improved the penetration ability of cells and tissues and stability of exogenous genes under physiological conditions, allowing gene therapy technology to break through previous bottlenecks and enable clinical application [102,103]. The combination of gene therapy and PDT offers a high degree of precision based on complementary base pairs, which most other therapeutic combinations lack. Exogenous genes are required to efficiently enter cells and successfully escape intracellular bodies before they can play a therapeutic role, which poses great challenges to the material properties of delivery vectors [104]. Programmable vectors have been proposed to solve this problem to some extent and are commonly released under internal stimuli such as enzymes under special pH conditions. Photochemical internalization (PCI) is an intracellular delivery technique using an exogenous light as a stimulus. After activation of PS, ROS can be rapidly produced within a short time to destroy the membrane of the intracellular body and release therapeutic agents such as nucleic acid drugs in the cytoplasm [105,106] (Figure 2B). This external light-dependent regulation is more controllable and stable than the internal response-dependent system and can achieve higher spatially controlled and targeted gene delivery [107]. Another type of photoprogrammed gene regulation uses PDT active nanomaterials as gene delivery vectors, such as PPBP, the black phosphorus (BP) nanosheets prepared with PEG and PEI modification, a black scale nanomaterial that shows PDT activity under light and then specifically degrades to release siRNA in a high ROS and acidic tumor environment to achieve targeted delivery [108].

Hypoxia influences PDT, while upregulation of VEGF and HSP-70 leads to PDT tolerance. Changing the expression of these proteins by gene therapy can help resolve these challenges to some extent and enhance the sensitivity of tumor cells to PDT. HIF1α is a hypoxia-inducible factor that plays a key role in tumor cell proliferation and angiogenesis [109]. Zheng WH [110] used anisamide-targeted lipid-calcium-phosphate (LCP) nanoparticles to achieve codelivery of protoporphyrin IX (PpIX) and HIF-1α siRNA. The results showed that HIF1α downregulation not only directly inhibited tumor cell generation but also promoted ROS production in the tumor environment, thereby enhancing PDT-mediated apoptosis. Nrf2 is a key antioxidation regulator that prevents ROS accumulation and promotes angiogenesis. Deng S [111] codelivered CRISPR–Cas9 ribonucleoprotein (RNP) with Ce6, ROS generated by the latter caused release of Cas9/sgRNA into cytoplasm, resulting in Nrf2 interference and preventing tumor cells escaping from ROS-mediated killing. In terms of improving PDT-induced tolerance, Jang Y [112] prepared a DOX-siVEGF-NPS/Ce6-MBS complex coloaded with VEGF siRNA and Ce6 for the treatment of squamous cell carcinoma. Under the action of VEGF siRNA, tumor angiogenesis was significantly reduced, and the antitumor effect was improved. Similar results were reported in Cao Y [113], the MnO_2 nanosheet was first surface decorated with $Cu_{2-x}S$ and then loaded with HSP-70 siRNA to form $MnO_2/Cu_{2-x}S$-HSP-70-siRNA, which mediated the heat shock response and showed superior synergistic antitumor ability. In addition, the use of therapeutic genes to regulate the expression of proteins related to the growth, development, differentiation and metabolism of tumor cells can enhance the effect of PDT or supplement the limitations of PDT. For example, gene therapy can activate the body's immune system to treat metastatic cancer [114] and inhibit epithelial-mesenchymal transition (EMT) to avoid tumor recurrence [115]. Overall, the diversity of cancer-causing genes and the complexity of pathogenesis, as well as the innate differences of individuals, give gene therapy and PDT to infinite possibilities in combination. More examples of recently published studies on the codelivery of photosensitizers and gene therapy drugs based on nanocarriers are illustrated in Table 2.

Table 2. Codelivery of photosensitizers and gene therapy drugs based on nanocarriers.

Nanoparticle	Photosensitizers	Gene Therapy Drugs	Tumor	Data Sources	Findings	Ref
Chlorin e6-DNAzyme/Cu(I)1,2,4-triazolate nanoscale coordination polymers (Ce6-DNAzyme/[Cu(tz)] CPs)	Chlorin e6 (Ce6)	Early Growth Response Factor-1 (EGR-1) targeted DNAzyme	MCF-7	In vitro, Animals	• [Cu(TZ)] CPs and Ce6 induced type 1 and type 2 PDT at 808 nm and 660 nm, respectively, enhancing the therapeutic effect in hypoxia environment (tumor regression rate was 88.0%). • Ce6-DNAzyme was degraded by glutathione overexpressed in tumors, resulting in DNAzyme targeted release and catalytic cleavage of EGR-1 mRNA.	[116] 2021
Cationic guanidylated porphyrin/siRNA complexes (H2-PG/siRNA)	Porphyrin	Inhibitor of apoptosis siRNA (siIAP)	MDA-MB-231	In vitro	• The H2-PG/siRNA complex promoted siRNA internalization. • Cationic guanidylated modification did not affect the PDT activity of porphyrin.	[117] 2019
CaCO$_3$ layer modified MnO$_2$ NPs (Mn@CaCO$_3$)	Indocyanine green (ICG)	Programmed death ligand 1 siRNA (siPD-L1)	Lewis	In vitro, Animals	• Increased oxygen production mediated by MnO$_2$ and reduced H$^+$ consumption mediated by CaCO$_3$ jointly enhanced the PDT effect. • siPD-L1 silencing and PDT together activated the immune system, mediating a powerful antitumor immune response.	[118] 2019
(PGL-NH2)2 and fluorocarbon inert gas of C3F8 grafted cationic porphyrin microbubbles (CpMBs)/siRNA	Porphyrin	Pioneer transcription factor 1 siRNA (siFOXA1)	MCF-7	In vitro, Animals	• Enhanced drug loading of photosensitizer and siRNA. • Under the guidance of contrast-enhanced ultrasound, the accumulation of local microbubbles in tumors was significantly increased through the ultrasound-induced superpore effect. • The codelivery system showed superior breast cancer inhibition.	[119] 2018
(NaYF$_4$:Yb, Er) upconversion NPs (UCNPs)	5,10,15,20-tetrakis (1-methyl pyridinium-4-yl) porphyrin (TMPyP$_4$)	ssDNA with chitosan aptamer (AS1411) and chitosan-targeted DNAzyme	MCF-7	In vitro, Animals	• The multivalence of the ssDNA endowed the UCNPs with high recognition and loading capacity of TMPyP4 and DNAzymes.	[120] 2020
Versatile function of cationic phosphonium-conjugated polythiophenes	Polythiophenes	Luciferase gene siRNA	MDA-MB-231	In vitro	• The vector effectively self-assembled with siRNA and mediated effective gene silencing (35% and 52% gene silencing efficiencies, respectively). • After successful delivery of siRNA, the photoactivity of the vector was restored, which could mediate further PDT.	[121] 2020

Table 2. Cont.

Nanoparticle	Photosensitizers	Gene Therapy Drugs	Tumor	Data Sources	Findings	Ref
Cationic polyporphyrin vectors	Porphyrin	Hypoxia-inducible factor-1α siRNA (siHIF-1α)	H22	In vitro, Animals	• Cationic photosensitive drugs were polymerized by an ROS splitting linker to achieve separation in space and avoid ACQ effects and could be used as a carrier to deliver siRNA. • Mediated effective intracellular internalization and gene silencing efficiency (60%), synergistic enhancement of phototoxicity.	[122] 2021
Periodic mesoporous ionosilica NPs (PMINPs)	Tetrasilylated porphyrin precursor	Luciferase gene siRNA	MDA-MB-231-Luc-RFP	In vitro	• PDT effectively induced cell death with 95% mortality. • As a delivery carrier of siRNA, it can successfully escape from endosomes and play a therapeutic role, with gene silencing efficiency up to 83%. • It presented triple functions, namely, imaging, PDT and PCI.	[123] 2021
Dendritic arginine-rich peptide conjugated with cystamine-modified stearic acid (ALS)	HPPH	Vascular endothelial growth factor (VEGF) siVEGF	HeLa	In vitro, Animals	• Alternating low and high doses of light drove siRNA internalization and PDT, respectively. • The liver and lung metastasis of HeLa cells were successfully inhibited, and the therapeutic effect was superior.	[58] 2021

3.3. Immunotherapy

PDT can activate the body's immune response in two ways: one is to induce an acute inflammatory response of the host and release various proinflammatory signals; the other is to trigger ICD by injured or dead tumor cells to release damage-associated molecular patterns (DAMPs) and neoantigens as danger signals [3,124]. Although the immune response mediated by PDT is not enough to kill tumor cells, it can create a reconstructed immune microenvironment for further antitumor immunotherapy [63].

Immune adjuvants are a class of immune-stimulating molecules that activate tumor-specific immune responses by interacting with Toll-like receptors (TLRs) on antigen-presenting cells (APCs) [125]. The combination of immune adjuvant and PDT has the dual ability to activate the immune system. A nanometal organic framework (nMOF) formed by direct self-assembly of metal ions and PSs is often used as a codelivery carrier and is characterized by a high loading efficiency and good biocompatibility [126]. Cai Z [127] prepared PCN-ACF-CpG@HA NPs loaded with the immune adjuvant CPG by combining PS tetrakis (4-carboxyphenyl) porphyrin (H_2TCPP) with zirconium ions to target tumors with high expression of the CD44 receptor. CPG and PDT together mediated a strong antitumor immune response, with significantly higher CD8+ and CD4+ T cell infiltration at the tumor site than that in the control group. Similarly, the cationic W-TBP designed by Ni K [128] based on nMOF can directly adsorb negatively charged CPG through electrostatic action, promote its internalization and DC maturation, and enhance antigen presentation in coordination with PDT-induced CRT exposure. In addition to treating tumors in situ, this codelivery combination kills distant metastatic cancer cells. Xia Y [129] evaluated the efficacy of CPG combined with the PS verteporfin in the treatment of 4T1 metastatic breast cancer; the results showed that the activation of DC cells was significantly increased, and the tumor volume of tumor-bearing mice was smaller than that of other control groups. Xu C [130] also achieved similar results in the treatment of local and metastatic B160F10 melanoma, which was enhanced by promoting DC recruitment and cytotoxic T cell infiltration at the tumor site. Exogenous antigens can also activate immune responses. Ovalbumin (OVA), a commonly used model antigen, can be used as a supplement to immune stimulation induced by PDT. The effect of such codelivery was evaluated in the studies of Huang R [131] and Ding B [132], both of which showed synergistic immune enhancement.

Immune checkpoint therapy has made significant breakthroughs in recent years and can effectively improve the immune system's response to tumors. At present, several immune checkpoint inhibitors have been approved by the FDA for clinical treatment [133]. Tumor vascular abnormalities and the immunosuppressive tumor microenvironment (TME) caused by indoleamine 2,3-dioxygenase 1 (IDO1) seriously affect the efficacy of PDT-mediated immunotherapy. Codelivery of PSs with IDO1 inhibitors is beneficial for amplifying the effects of photodynamic immunotherapy. Combinations that have been reported include ferritin and polyethylene glycol–PLGA (PEG–PLGA) coloaded with $ZnF_{16}Pc$ and IDO inhibitor NLG919 [134] or Ce6, tyrosinase inhibitor axitinib (AXT), IDO1 inhibitor dextro-1-methyltryptophan (1MT) and human serum albumin self-assembled NPs [135]. These combinations can improve the tumor microenvironment by normalizing tumor blood vessels, improving hypoxia levels, promoting the invasion of immune effector CD8+ T cells in tumors, and reducing the immunosuppressive properties of tumors, which represents a promising tumor treatment strategy. Cytotoxic T-lymphocyte-associated antigen 4 (CTLA-4) and programmed death-ligand 1 (PD-L1) are the most common immune checkpoints and are closely related to the immune function of T cells. Xu J [136] used the self-assembly property of Ce6 and immunoglobulin G (IgG) in the nanoscale affinity range to bind Ce6 to αPD-L1 or double bind to αPD-L1 and αCTLA-4 in the immunocheckpoint blocking treatment of glioma in situ and colon cancer. This combination therapy successfully prolonged the survival of tumor-bearing mice and produced a long-term memory response, avoiding tumor recurrence. In addition, zinc phthalocyanine and aCTLA4 have been coadded into microneedles prepared by hyaluronic acid and dextran for skin cancer delivery. This minimally invasive percutaneous drug delivery platform can also effectively induce an antitumor immune response and avoid the systemic distribution of drugs to reduce toxicity and side effects [137]. Without affecting coloaded drugs, nanodelivery systems targeting important organelles such as mitochondria [138] and the endoplasmic reticulum [139] can be designed to enhance PDT-triggered ICD, thereby enhancing immune activation (Figure 3).

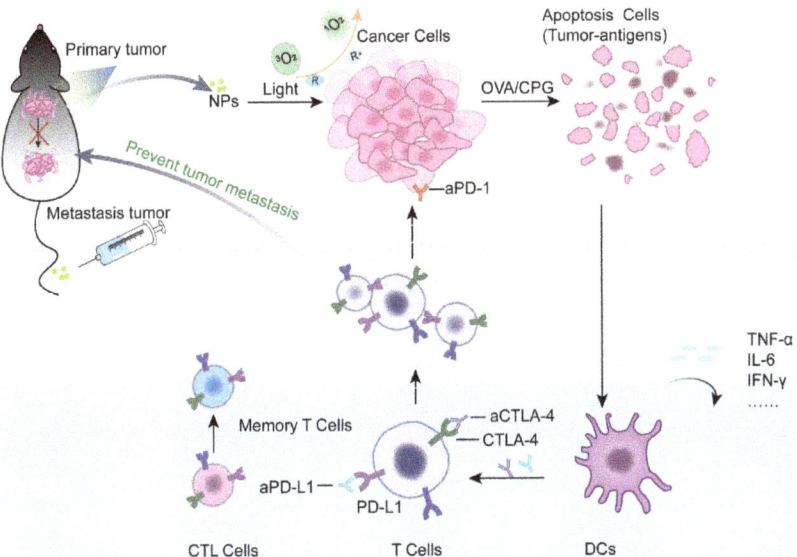

Figure 3. Mechanism by which photodynamic therapy and immunotherapy synergistically enhance antitumor effects. When photosensitizers in tumor sites are activated, they can cause acute inflammation and induce cell apoptosis or necrosis. Dendritic cells mature when stimulated by cytokines released at the site of inflammation and provide antigens to T lymphocytes in regional lymph nodes. Activated T lymphocytes become effector T cells, which are attracted to chemokines, migrate to the tumor and kill tumor cells. Different types of immunotherapy drugs play a role in different steps of the complete antitumor immune cycle. Codelivery of a photosensitizer with an immune adjuvant or tumor antigen can synergistically enhance the activation of the host immune system and improve the immunosuppressive microenvironment. The codelivery of a photosensitizer with CTLA-4 and PD-L1 monoclonal antibodies can enhance the antitumor immunity effect of T cells. The activation of these immune cells also plays a role in preventing metastasis and recurrence.

Photoimmunotherapy is a tumor-targeting therapy using specific antibodies to tumor-associated receptors chemically coupled with PSs, which is more accurate than conventional PDT and is suitable for tumors at sensitive anatomical sites. Hasan T [140] coupled epidermal growth factor receptor (EGFR) monoclonal antibody Cetuximab with benzoporphyrin derivative for pancreatic ductal adenocarcinoma treatment. The results showed that the photoimmune nanoconjugate (PIN) had a high binding specificity and could rapidly penetrate heteromorphic organoids, providing approximately 16-fold enhancement in molecular targeted NIR photodestruction. Nevertheless, single-receptor targeted therapy may cause tumor subsets with low receptor expression to evade treatment and thus fail to completely ablate tumors. Hasan T [141] further constructs a triple receptor-targeted PIN (TR-PIN), cetuximab, holo-transferrin, and trastuzumab conferred specificity for EGFR, transferrin receptor (TfR), and human epidermal growth factor receptor 2 (HER-2). Researchers compared the binding ability of TR-PIN to tumor cells with different levels of receptor expression (EGFR, TfR or HER-2), and found that TR-PIN has the ability to recognize multiple tumor targets, effectively photodynamically eradicating different tumor subsets and reducing escape. More examples of recently published studies on the codelivery of photosensitizers and immunotherapy drugs based on nanocarriers are illustrated in Table 3.

Table 3. Codelivery of photosensitizers and immunotherapy drugs based on nanocarriers.

Nanoparticle	Photosensitizers	Immunotherapy Drugs	Tumor	Data Sources	Findings	Ref
Ce6-Gold nanoclusters-PEG2000-CD3 antibody-cytokine-induced killer cell NPs	Chlorin e6 (Ce6)	CD3 antibody	MGC-803	In vitro, Animals	• The fluorescence intensity of GNCS-CE6 was approximately 4.5 times that of GNCs, thereby mediating a stronger PDT effect. • Increased drug aggregation at the tumor site by targeting CIK cells.	[142] 2018
Human-induced pluripotent stem cells loaded with MnO_2@Chlorin e6 NPs (iPS-MnO_2@Ce6)	Chlorin e6 (Ce6)	Tumor antigens of human-induced pluripotent stem cells	Lewis	In vitro, Animals	• iPS promoted the aggregation of nanoparticles at the tumor site and could be lysed by ROS produced by PDT to release tumor antigens. • MnO_2 interacted with H_2O_2 to release oxygen and alleviated tumor hypoxia.	[143] 2020
Chlorin e6- and imiquimod-loaded upconversion NPs (UCNPs-Ce6-R837 NPs)	Chlorin e6 (Ce6)	Imiquimod (R837)	CT26	In vitro, Animals	• Lanthanide ions in UCNP nanoparticles could transform long near-infrared light into shorter wave light, improving tissue permeability. • Toll-like receptor 7 agonist R837 was used as an adjuvant for enhanced antitumor immune response.	[144] 2017
Diblock copolymer azide-modified polyethylene glycol block polyaspartic acid(benzylamine) (Azide PEG-Pasp(Bz) micelles	Zinc phthalocyanine (ZnPc)	Mal-GGPLGVRG-Pra peptide modified aPD-L1	B16-F10	In vitro, Animals	• Dual corresponding functions of pH and MMP-2 responses enhanced the aggregation of NPs in tumor cells. • The blood circulation of NPs was prolonged, and their antitumor ability was enhanced.	[145] 2021
Serum albumin-coated boehmite B NPs	Chlorin e6 (Ce6)	Bee Venom Melittin (MLT)	4T1	In vitro, Animals	• Significantly reduced the hemolysis caused by MLT and decreased the toxic side effects. • MLT enhanced immunogenic cell death and dendritic cell activation, coactivating antitumor immunity with PDT.	[5] 2019

3.4. Photothermal Therapy (PTT)

Additionally, as a minimally invasive treatment, PTT has certain similarities with PDT. Photothermal agents concentrated at the tumor site absorb laser radiation energy and convert light energy into hyperthermia, resulting in the thermal ablation of adjacent cells. PTT enhances the effect of PDT, mainly by improving blood flow and increasing oxygen content in tumors [146] (Figure 4A).

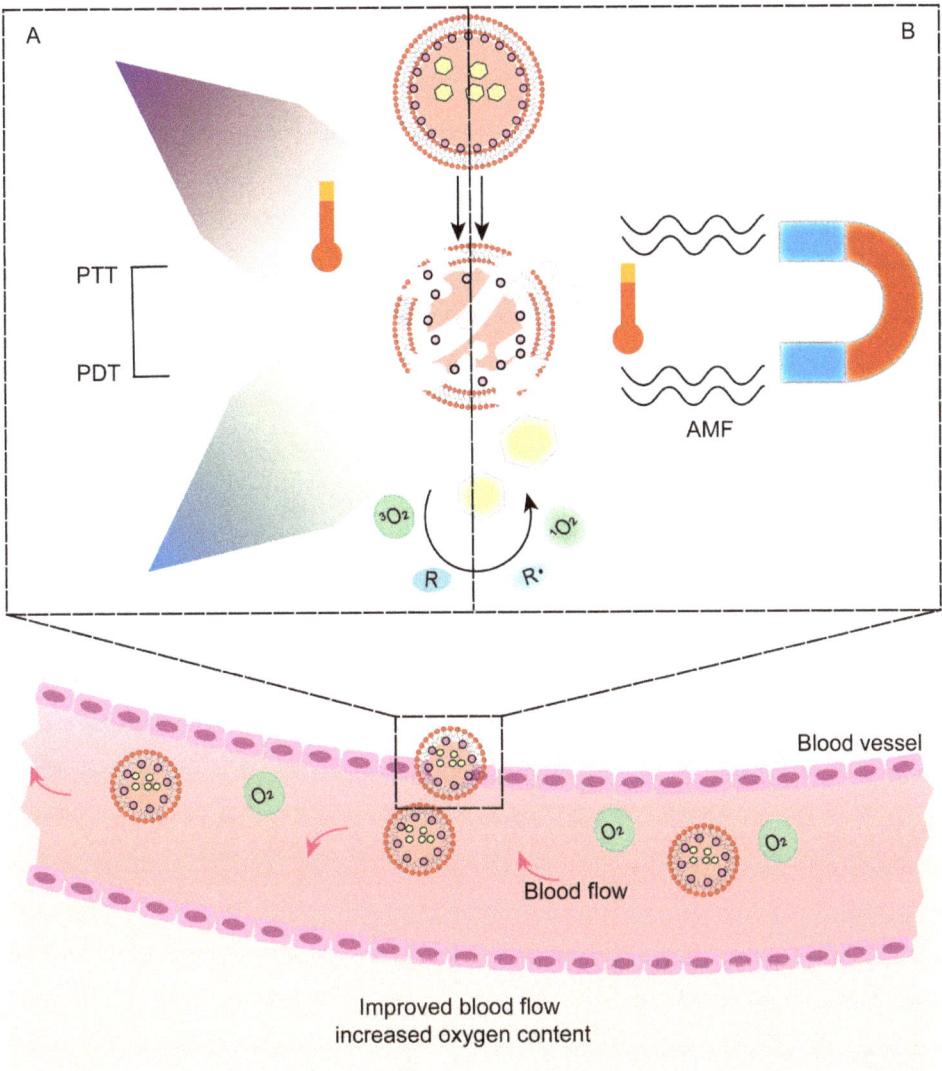

Figure 4. Mechanism of photodynamic therapy combined with photothermal therapy, hyperthermia and magnetic hyperthermia in synergistic enhancement of the antitumor effect based on codelivery systems. (**A**) When light-activated photothermal agents, (**B**) or alternating magnetic fields are applied to magnetic nanoparticles, heat is generated at the tumor site, increasing blood flow and synergistically enhancing PDTSome photothermal agents of inorganic materials themselves can be used as nanocarriers, which makes the combination of PTT and PDT convenient. Gold nanorods have been used as carriers with photothermal conversion capability, and the joint delivery of DOX and PS ICG can simultaneously achieve

chemo-PTT-PDT triple therapy [69]. Gold nanocages [147] show strong absorption in the NIR region, and their empty interior and porous walls are suitable for encapsulating PSs. Bo Tian et al. [148] coupled Ce6 on PEG-functionalized GO (GO-PEG-CE6). The photothermal effect of GO promoted the transfer of Ce6, and its destruction effect on cancer cells was significantly better than that of free Ce6. The photothermal agent plasma copper sulfide (Cu_2-XS) has also been reported to have photodynamic properties [149], allowing the combination of PTT and PDT to be achieved simultaneously, and has been verified in in vitro cultured melanoma cells and mouse melanoma models. The poor photostability and potential long-term toxicity of inorganic nanomaterials limit their clinical application, so more materials with good biocompatibility and high stability have been developed as alternatives. The conductive polymer polypyrrole is a material with relatively high biocompatible photostability and photothermal conversion efficiency, using polyacrylamide (PAH), polyacrylic acid (PAA) and $AlPCS_4$. Further modification of polypyrrole resulted in a more stable $AlPCS_4$@PPyCONH-PAH-PAA nanoneedle complex in a physiological environment. The results showed an enhanced synergistic effect, with tumor ablation in mice 14 days after treatment and no recurrence within 30 days [150].

Another more conventional codelivery method is to simultaneously load the photothermal agent and PS or prodrug of PS in nanodelivery systems such as micelles, vesicles, and liposomes. Gang Chen et al. [151] developed CS NPs as codelivery carriers of photothermal agents (IR780) and prodrug of protoporphyrin IX (5-aminolevulinic acid, 5-ALA) for oral administration in the treatment of subcutaneous colon cancer in mice. CS keeps the drug stable even under acidic conditions in the stomach, allowing the drug to successfully accumulate at the tumor site. Mechanistic studies have shown that the oxidative stress response at the tumor site is enhanced, producing more ROS, superoxide and $^1O_2$. The enhanced effect of this synergistic administration of light and heat on cancer treatment was also reported in the research of Xiaodong Liu [65]. The high singlet oxygen generation capacity and photothermal conversion efficiency make this treatment strategy more severely phototoxic to both superficial and deep tumor cells.

When the excitation wavelengths of the PS and photothermal agent were different, the complexity of the treatment was greatly increased. To solve this problem, Jing Lin [152] designed a gold vesicle with a strong plasma coupling effect. This gold vesicle was densely packed with monolayer gold NPs, and Ce6 was encapsulated inside. The enhancement of plasma coupling between gold NPs in close proximity lead to a redshift in extinction spectra. Therefore, the photothermal and photodynamic effects could be stimulated simultaneously by a single 671 nm laser irradiation. Some special materials, such as nano GO, themselves have the dual nature of promoting both PDT and PTT, and their development for PTT can reduce the complexity of material preparation [153]. More examples of recently published studies on the codelivery of photosensitizers and photothermal agents based on nanocarriers are illustrated in Table 4.

Table 4. Codelivery of photosensitizers and photothermal agents based on nanocarriers.

Nanoparticle	Photosensitizers	Photothermal Agents	Tumor	Data Sources	Findings	Ref
Boron dipyrromethene conjugated hyaluronic acid polymer NPs (BODIPY-HA NPs)	Boron dipyrromethene (BODIPY)	Boron dipyrromethene (BODIPY)	4T1	In vitro	• BODIPY showed only PTT activity due to P-P stacking after self-assembly to form NPs. • BODIPY-HA NPs were decomposed into BODIPY-HA molecules, restoring PDT activity and producing ROS after internalization by tumor cells.	[154] 2021
1,2-Distearoyl-sn-glycero-3-phosphoethanolamine-N-[carboxy(polyethylene glycol)-2000]-coated nanographene oxide-copper sulfide NPs (pGO-CuS NPs)	GO, CuS	Indocyanine green (ICG), CuS	MCF-7	In vitro	• Photosensitizer-assembled NPs improved the drug loading efficiency and stability.	[155] 2015
Polypyrrole NPs	Phycocyanin (Pc)	Phycocyanin (Pc)	MDA-MB-231	In vitro	• Pc produced PDT and PTT activity under 600 nm and 900 nm laser activation, respectively. • It had good synergistic antitumor effects and cell imaging ability of PDT and PTT.	[156] 2017
Indocyanine green-coated single-walled carbon nanohorn NPs (SWNH-ICGs)	Indocyanine green (ICG)	Indocyanine green (ICG)	4T1	In vitro, Animals	• The stability of ICG was improved, and ICG was protected from photodegradation. • Under 808 nm laser irradiation, local hyperthermia and a large number of ROS were produced simultaneously, effectively inhibiting the growth of 4T1 tumors.	[157] 2018
Iridium oxide-manganese dioxide mineralized Chlorin e6 conjugated bovine serum albumin NPs (BSA-Ce6@IrO$_2$/MnO$_2$)	Chlorin e6 (Ce6)	Iridium oxide (IrO$_2$)	MDA-MB-231, 4T1, PC3	In vitro, Animals	• IrO$_2$ and MnO$_2$ decomposed endogenous H$_2$O$_2$ to alleviate tumor hypoxia and improve PDT. • IrO$_2$ presented excellent photothermal conversion efficiency (65.3%) and high X-ray absorption coefficient, enabling NPs to be used in computer CT and PA imaging.	[158] 2020
Lipid-purpurin 18 and pure lipid self-assembled NPs (Pp18-lipos)	Lipid-purpurin 18 (Pp18-lipids)	Lipid-purpurin 18 (Pp18-lipids)	4T1	In vitro, Animals	• The Pp18-lipos with 2 mol% Pp18-lipids can perform PDT while with 65mol% can perform potent PTT. • PTT/PDT synergistically inhibited tumor growth and enhanced tumor T cell immune response.	[159] 2020

Table 4. Cont.

Nanoparticle	Photosensitizers	Photothermal Agents	Tumor	Data Sources	Findings	Ref
Folic acid-polyethylene glycol-coated black phosphorus nanosheets conjugated with copper sulfide (BP-CuS-FA)	Black phosphorus (BP)	Copper sulfide (CuS), Black phosphorus (BP)	4T1	In vitro, Animals	• FA could target tumor cells with FA receptor overexpression and enhance drug aggregation at tumor site. • BP nanosheets could be degraded by ROS through oxidation processes to reduce toxic and side effects. • BP-CuS-FA simultaneously mediated synergically enhanced the PDT-PTT antitumor effect and photoacoustic imaging.	[160] 2020
Poly(lactic-co-glycolic acid) (PLGA) NPs	IR780 iodide	Perfluorocarbon (PFC)	4T1	In vitro, Animals	• PFC could be used as an artificial blood substitute to effectively increase hypoxia in the tumor microenvironment and enhance PTT and PDT. • IR780 could simultaneously act as a PS and mediate mitochondrial targeting, disrupt the balance of mitochondrial ROS and induce irreversible apoptosis of tumor cells.	[161] 2020
Amino-modified nanomaterial based on MoS2 quantum-dot-doped disulfide-based SiO$_2$ NPs coated with hyaluronic acid and chlorin e6 (MoS$_2$@ss- SiO$_2$-Ce6/HA)	Chlorin e6 (Ce6)	MoS$_2$ quantum dots	4T1	In vitro, Animals	• Effectively prolonged the blood circulation time of MoS$_2$ quantum dots and increased the uptake of tumor cells. • It could also be used for fluorescence/CT/MSOT image-guided PDT and PTT combination therapy.	[162] 2019
Isoindigo/triphenylamine donor-acceptor-donor conjugated small molecule NPs (IID-ThTPA NPs)	IID-ThTPA	IID-ThTPA	4T1	In vitro, Animals	• The photothermal conversion efficiency reached 35.4%, and the singlet oxygen yield was 84%. • The ultrahigh singlet oxygen quantum yield of IID-ThTPA NPs originated from the narrow singlet–triplet energy gap of IID-ThTPA.	[163] 2020
MoSe$_2$/Bi$_2$Se$_3$ nanoheterostructure	MoSe$_2$/Bi$_2$Se$_3$	MoSe$_2$/Bi$_2$Se$_3$	HepG$_2$	In vitro, Animals	• ROS generation was promoted through photoinduced effective separation of electron-hole pairs. • The photothermal conversion efficiency was increased to 59.3% by the nanoheterostructure. • Displayed acid/photothermal sensitive drug release behavior.	[164] 2019
Polyethylene glycolated triphenylphosphine modified chitosan/iron oxide NPs (PEG-CS/Fe$_2$O$_3$ NPs)	Methylene blue (MB)	Iron oxide	HeLa, A549, MCF-7	In vitro, Animals	• Improved the aggregation in the tumor site, reduce the toxic and side effects on normal tissues. • Under low-power near-infrared light, NPs produced singlet oxygen, which can damage tumor cells.	[165] 2020

Table 4. Cont.

Nanoparticle	Photosensitizers	Photothermal Agents	Tumor	Data Sources	Findings	Ref
Indocyanine green-grafted gold nanobipyramids covalently conjugated with folic acid (AuBPs@FLA@ICG@FA NPs)	Indocyanine green (ICG)	Gold nanobipyramids (AuBPs)	B16-F10	In vitro	• Enhanced the overall PTT-PDT efficiency by increasing the temperature by 2 °C and doubling $^1O_2$ species generation.	[166] 2020
Pardaxin peptide-modified, indocyanine green-conjugated hollow gold nanospheres (FAL-ICG-HAuNS)	Indocyanine green (ICG)	Gold nanospheres	CT26	In vitro, Animals	• FAL modification imparted endoplasmic reticulum targeting capability to NPs • NIR irradiation induced strong ER stress and calcium reticulin (CRT) exposure, facilitating ICD-mediated immunotherapy. • The antigen presentation function of dendritic cells was enhanced, and CD8+T cell proliferation and secretion of cytotoxic factors were activated.	[139] 2019
Gd^{3+} and chlorin e6 loaded single-walled carbon nanohorns (Gd-Ce6@SWNHs)	Chlorin e6 (Ce6)	Gd^{3+}	4T1	In vitro, Animals	• NPs could migrate from targeted tumors to tumors-draining lymph nodes, continuously activating DCs, and ultimately eliminating metastases.	[167] 2020

3.5. Hyperthermia Therapy (HT) and Magnetic Hyperthermia Therapy (MH)

As one of the emerging noninvasive treatment options, HT may enhance PDT by alleviating hypoxia [168,169]. The mechanism is that as temperature increases, blood flow at the tumor site increases and microcirculation improves, thereby increasing tumor oxygenation [170]. MH, also known as magnetic therapy, is based on the heat generated by magnetic NPs (MNPs) under the action of an alternating magnetic field (AMF) to target and kill tumors without harming surrounding healthy tissue [171]. The emergence of MH has made the combination of HT and PDT a possibility, and the generated heat affects deeper tumors, which is beneficial for enhancing PDT [172] (Figure 4B). In terms of codelivery, magnetic nanomaterials can be directly used as carriers or loaded with PS in other carriers. Hongwei Gu [66] conjugated magnetite Fe_3O_4 with porphyrin derivatives, which is highly efficient and has a low systemic toxicity. Huang WC [173] used monocytes derived from bone marrow as carriers to jointly transport Ce6 and oxygen superparamagnetic iron oxide NPs for combined therapy. This is an interesting combination strategy, but the relevant literature is still limited, and researchers need to conduct more in-depth research and discussions. More examples of recently published studies on the codelivery of photosensitizers and hyperthermia agents based on nanocarriers are illustrated in Table 5.

Table 5. Codelivery of photosensitizer and hyperthermia agent drugs based on nanocarriers.

Nanoparticle	Photosensitizers	Hyperthermia Agents	Tumor	Data Sources	Findings	Ref
Cancer cell membrane-cloaked Ce6-loaded Janus magnetic mesoporous organosilica NPs (CM@M-MON@Ce6)	Chlorin e6 (Ce6)	Magnetic mesoporous silica nanoparticles (M-MSNs)	4T1	In vitro, Animals	• It exhibited the function of REDOX/PH double stimulation to induce PS release and matrix degradation. • Increased the ability of targeted tumor aggregation and prolonged blood circulation time. • Enhanced anticancer activity, simultaneously triggering a series of immunogenic cell death, resulting in a synergistic tumor-specific immune response.	[174] 2019
Ultramagnetic photosensitive liposomes	Foscan	Iron oxide NPs	SKOV-3	In vitro, Animals	• The combination of photodynamic and magnetothermal therapy triggered the synergistic action of apoptotic signaling pathways, leading to complete eradication of tumor cells.	[175] 2015
Magneto low-density nanoemulsion (MLDE)	Chlorin e6 (Ce6)	Iron oxide NPs	MCF-7	In vitro	• Improved the stability and biocompatibility of drugs. • Identified the low-density lipoprotein receptor on the surface of tumor cells and improved the targeting selectivity of drugs.	[176] 2018

3.6. Radiotherapy

Band gap materials convert X-rays into light photons in the UV-vis region, which can be used to activate PSs. This is the basis of a combination of PDT and radiation therapy known as X-ray PDT (XPDT) [177,178]. The use of light is one of the limitations of PDT, and the strong tissue penetration of X-rays can compensate for this shortcoming. The method of operation delivers scintillators and PSs together to the tumor site. Under the action of X-rays, scintillators emit persistent light to activate PSs. This strategy can also produce good therapeutic effects for deep tumors [179], and the therapeutic effect depends to some extent on the energy transfer efficiency of the scintillator. The primary choices of scintillators are rare earth materials [180–182] with high photon conversion rates and some metallic materials [183], in addition to a few nonmetallic materials [184] and even quantum dots [185].

Another factor affecting the therapeutic effect is the distance between the PS and the scintillator. One approach is to physically package PS in a coating bound to the scintillator by electrostatic or hydrophobic means or to load both the scintillator and PS into NPs [186,187]; for example, the combination of protoporphyrin IX (PpIX) and scintillator $LaF_3:Ce^{3+}$ coloaded in PEG-PLGA was shown to exhibit highly efficient loading and high stability under physiological conditions [188]. Physical combination has a certain risk of missing the target, whereas chemical bonding based on covalent bonds or conjugation is complex but more stable. K. K. Popovich [67] coated $CeF_3:Tb^{3+}$ with PpIX-coupled SiO_2. The monodisperse SiO_2 coating had high energy transfer efficiency and protected the scintillator encapsulated within it [189].

The combination of a scintillator and PS solves the problem of light sources, but it is still subject to the strong oxygen dependence of PDT. Zhang C [190] was inspired to integrate scintillators and semiconductor quantum dots with unique optical properties into ionizing radiation-induced PDT synchronous radiotherapy. The addition of a PS without traditional effects reduces the oxygen dependence of the complex, which can subsequently produce a process similar to type I PDT under ionizing radiation. Chuang YC [191] introduced the annealing process to achieve PS-free PDT. The yttrium oxide nanoscintillation complex coated with a silica shell ($Y_2O_3:Eu@SiO_2$) was subjected to X-ray irradiation and subsequent annealing, and then, photodynamic effects were promoted to mediate tumor cell damage in conjunction with radiotherapy.

Radionuclide-mediated Cerenkov luminescence is a phenomenon produced by the interaction of high-speed charged particles with the surrounding medium. The codelivery of radionuclides with PSs has been reported in several studies to have antitumor effects and prolong the survival of tumor-bearing mice. In addition to mediating Cerenkov luminescence, radionuclides can directly kill tumor cells [192,193]. Although this combination has achieved some success in the treatment of deep tumors, there are still many shortcomings to be overcome, such as the blueshift of the low-energy radiation emission spectrum to the ultraviolet region. More examples of recently published studies on the codelivery of photosensitizers and scintillators/radionuclides based on nanocarriers are illustrated in Table 6.

Table 6. Codelivery of photosensitizers and scintillators/radionuclides based on nanocarriers.

Nanoparticle	Photosensitizers	Scintillators/Radionuclides	Tumor	Data Sources	Findings	Ref
Hollow mesoporous silica NPs (HMSNs)	Chlorin e6 (Ce6)	Zirconium-89 (^{89}Zr)	4T1	In vitro, Animals	• ^{89}Zr activated Ce6 in the codelivery system and inhibited tumor growth. • It did not rely on external light source and instead used internal radiation to achieve deep tumor treatment.	[194] 2016
Dextran modified TiO$_2$ NPs (D-TiO$_2$ NPs)	TiO$_2$	Gallium-68 (Ga-68)	4T1	In vitro, Animals	• The Cerenkov productivity of GA-68 was 30 times that of 18F-fluorodeoxyglucose. • Ga-68 is an effective radionuclide for PDT, which can enhance DNA damage of tumor cells by codelivery.	[195] 2018
Magetic NPs with ^{89}Zr radiolabeling and porphyrin molecules surface modification (^{89}Zr-MNFs/TCPP)	Meso-tetrakis(4-carboxyphenyl)porphyrin (TCPP)	Zirconium-89 (^{89}Zr)	4T1	In vitro, Animals	• Under an external magnetic field, the NPs were highly concentrated in the tumor. • Multimodal imaging of fluorescence, Cerenkov luminescence and Cerenkov resonance energy transfer could be implemented to detect the treatment process.	[196] 2018
Titanocene-modified, transferrin-coated TiO$_2$ NPs (TiO$_2$-Tf-Tc)	TiO$_2$	Radiolabeled 2′-deoxy-2′-(18F)fluoro-D-glucose (FDG)	HT1080	In vitro, Animals	• Low radiation induced radionuclide Cerenkov luminescence and activation of oxygen-independent photosensitizer TiO$_2$, overcoming the limitation of the tumor hypoxia environment. • Selectively destroyed a large number of tumor cells and induced lymphocyte infiltration.	[192] 2015
Folic acid-poly(lactide-co-glycolide) polymeric nanoparticles-verteporfin (VP), (FA-PLGA-VP NPs)	Verteporfin (VP)	Verteporfin (VP)	HCT116	In vitro	• The NPs effectively killed HCT116 cells in the presence 6 MeV X-ray radiation. • The 6 MeV X-ray radiation from LINAC produced energetic secondary electrons and Cerenkov radiation in the samples, which in turn excited the VP molecules.	[197] 2018
^{131}I-labeled zinc tetra(4-carboxyphenoxy) phthalocyaninate conjugated Cr^{3+}-doped zinc gallate NPs (^{131}I-ZGCs-ZnPcC4)	Zinc tetra(4-carboxyphenoxy) phthalocyaninate (ZnPcC4)	Cr^{3+}-doped zinc gallate (ZnGa$_2$O$_4$:Cr^{3+})	4T1	In vitro, Animals	• ^{131}I could not only achieve long-term activation of PDT through Cerenkov luminescence and ionizing radiation but also directly kill tumor cells.	[193] 2021
LiLuF$_4$:Ce@SiO$_2$@Ag$_3$PO$_4$@cisplatin prodrug (Pt(IV)) NPs (LAPNP NPs)	Ag$_3$PO$_4$	LiLuF$_4$:Ce	HeLa	In vitro, Animals	• Pt(IV) acted as a sacrificial electrical receptor to enhance the yield of hydroxyl radicals by increasing the separation of electrons and holes in the photosensitizer. • Pt(IV) generated cisplatin after receiving electrons, further enhancing the damage to tumor cells.	[198] 2018
NaGdF$_4$:Tb,Ce@NaGdF$_4$ core/shell structure NPs	Rose Bengal (RB)	NaGdF$_4$:Tb,Ce	PC3	In vitro, Animals	• The combination of X-ray guided photodynamic therapy and anaerobic oncolytic bacteria killed hypoxic and aerobic tumor tissue.	[199] 2020

3.7. Sonodynamic Therapy (SDT)

Sonodynamic therapy (SDT) uses ultrasound and acoustic sensitizers to treat cancer. Ultrasound, on the one hand, activates ultrasonic-sensitive species gathered in tumor cells through transient sonoluminescence to produce ROS. Hot spots from ultrasonic radiation, on the other hand, release energy high enough to cause bubbles to form and oscillate, resulting in permanent cell damage. The latter phenomenon is also defined as sonography-induced cavitation effects that together lead to tumor cell apoptosis or necrosis [200–203]. The extent of tumor cell death depends on the intensity and frequency of ultrasound and the duration of exposure, so it is controllable, safe and noninvasive, similar to PDT.

The strong penetration ability and low tissue attenuation of ultrasound make sonophotodynamic therapy (SPDT) have a wider range of indications. PDT is suitable for superficial cancer types such as skin cancer [204] and esophageal cancer [205], but the treatment effect for melanoma skin cancer has not been ideal, which is caused by the absorption of visible light by melanin to remove ROS [206]. In contrast, SDT was significantly more effective for melanoma than PDT, although there was no differences between the two treatments for common skin cancer [207].

The ultrasonic activation ability of PSs has also been verified to some extent. Some PSs have both SPDT activity, which are referred to as photoacoustic agents. We only need to use a specific wavelength of light and a specific frequency of sound to activate the photoacoustic agent so that the photoacoustic combination can be achieved without considering the coordination of physical and chemical properties in the process of multidrug combination. Currently, porphyrins as well as Ce6, Photolon™/Fotolon™, and Sonoflora 1 Sonnelux-1 have been verified [208–210]; several studies have reported their therapeutic efficacy and safety, and there are many potential PSs whose ultrasonic activation ability is being verified, which will also find applications in photoacoustic combination in the near future [211].

The modification of codelivery vectors helps to achieve multifunctional and integrated photoacoustic therapy with high spatial activation and preferential treatment of deep penetration. Hong L et al. [68] prepared Ce6 and the high oxygen carrying capacity carrier perfluoropolyether into a nanoemulsion and tested the ROS generation ability at different tissue depths after the application of ultrasound or light. The results showed that PDT had a high degree of spatial selectivity for surface and endoscopically accessible areas, which made it more suitable for the treatment of tumors in vital organs, such as brain cancer. SDT, on the other hand, had the same ROS production efficiency for tissues at different depths. SPDT was conducive to targeting different depths and meeting specific spatial accuracy requirements. Accordingly, sensitive drugs can be combined with tissue-engineered scaffolds to kill tumor cells after surgery. The results showed that SPDT had fewer toxic side effects than conventional chemotherapy, so it has great potential [212]. More examples of recently published studies on the codelivery of photosensitizers and sonophotosensitizers based on nanocarriers are illustrated in Table 7.

Table 7. Codelivery of photosensitizers and sonophotosensitizers based on nanocarriers.

Nanoparticle	Photosensitizers	Sonophotosensitizers	Tumor	Data Sources	Findings	Ref
Glypican-3-targeted, curcumin-loaded microbubbles (GPC3-CUR-MBs)	Curcumin (CUR)	Curcumin (CUR)	HepG2	In vitro, Animals	• The combined therapy sonophotodynamic therapy (SPDT) had more obvious antitumor effects than SDT or PDT alone.	[213] 2020
Curcumin-loaded poly(L-lactic-co-glycolic acid) microbubbles (CUR-PLGA-MBs)	Curcumin (CUR)	Curcumin (CUR)	HepG2	In vitro	• Mitochondrial membrane potential loss was induced by increased reactive oxygen species (ROS) generation, leading to tumor cell apoptosis and thermal decay.	[214] 2020
5-Aminolevulinic acid/titanium dioxide NPs (5-ALA/TiO$_2$)	5-Aminolevulinic acid (5-ALA)	Titanium dioxide (TiO$_2$)	SCC	In vitro, Animals	• Using countercurrent chromatography to obtain regular size nanoparticles enhanced the efficacy of codelivery of PDT and SDT for tumor treatment.	[215] 2016

3.8. Multidrug Codelivery

Cumbersome drug delivery processes, limited efficiency, slow release and low efficacy are common characteristics of multidrug codelivery. Therefore, the main research direction is still focused on solving the problem of coloading and controlled release.

Chen Y [70] designed an NIR-sensitive nanocomposite DLA-UCNPs@SiO$_2$-C/HA@ mSiO$_2$-DOX@NB. This complex breaks the chemical bond and releases paclitaxel (PTX) when irradiated by NIR light at 980 nm, which is then activated by visible light at 450–480 nm to exert synergistic photodynamic and photothermal therapeutic effects. Similarly, the Fe$_3$O$_4$/g-C$_3$N$_4$@Ppy-DOX nanocomposite prepared by Cheng HL [4] and graphite-like carbon oxide (G-C$_3$N$_4$) can not only generate O$_2$ through photocatalytic degradation to improve the hypoxic state of solid tumors but also enable the loading of PTX into its mesoporous structure. Polypyrrole, as a photothermal agent, was shown to enhance the antitumor effect of chemo-PDT.

CuS NPs with both PTT and PDT activities were used to achieve the triple combination of PTT-PDT-HT [216]. Curcio A [217] prepared a maghemite (γ-Fe$_2$O$_3$) nanoflower-like multicore nanoparticle conceived for MH and coated it with a spiky copper sulfide shell (IONF@CuS) for PTT and PDT. This combination showed a good therapeutic effect and reduced the dose of maghemite, which meant lower toxicity. Simultaneous activation of PDT and PTT by X-ray radiation-induced scintillator luminescence can be triply magnified when combined with radiotherapy. Luo L [218] conjugated a scintillator complex and a gold nanorod nanosensitizer. Lanthanide complexes can provide excellent luminescence under X-ray excitation, while gold nanorods can be used not only as PSs for PTT but also as radiosensitizers for enhanced radiotherapy due to their strong near-infrared light and X-ray absorption capacity. As expected, the group treated with both laser and X-ray irradiation showed the best synergistic effect, with significantly more effective tumor ablation than that in the other monotherapy groups.

Low-dose docetaxel has been reported to mediate ICD-activated immune effects [219], and this function of PDT is also mentioned above. Therefore, folic acid-modified mesoporous CuS NPs coloaded with DOX, polyethylenimide-PpIX (PEI-PpIX) and CPG for the treatment of cold tumor breast cancer can effectively rebuild the tumor microenvironment and promote the invasion of cytotoxic T lymphocytes (CTLs) [220]. In addition, it was reported that a MOF was used to integrate chemotherapy-phototherapy-photothermo-immunotherapy. Cus PpIX and DOX were loaded into the core and shell of the metal-organic skeleton ZIF-8, respectively, while CPG was adsorbed outside the shell. This design effectively realized the organic unification of antitumor and antirecurrence/metastasis [221]. More examples of recently published studies on the codelivery of multidrugs based on nanocarriers are illustrated in Table 8.

Table 8. Codelivery of multidrugs based on nanocarriers.

Nanoparticle	Type of Combination Therapy	Tumor	Data Sources	Findings	Ref
Human serum albumin-paclitaxel-sinoporphyrin sodium nanotheranostics (HAS-PTX-DVDMS)	Photodynamic therapy/Chemotherapy/Sonodynamic therapy	4T1	In vitro, Animals	• As a cosolvent, HAS improved the water solubility of the photosensitizer and dispersed it sufficiently to reduce the aggregation quenching effect. • It could be used as fluorescent probe, with stronger fluorescence imaging ability and $^1O_2$ generation ability than that of DVDMS alone. • The addition of ultrasound increased the tumor cell mortality rate from 70% to 90%, and the effect of triple therapy was superior.	[222] 2020
ZrO_2-coated, doxorubicin hydrochloride-, chlorin e6- and tetradecanol-loaded upconversion NPs ($UCNPs@ZrO_2$-Ce6/DOX/PCM)	Photodynamic therapy/Chemotherapy/Hyperthermia	U14	In vitro, Animals	• It could be used to realize multimodal imaging guidance (MRI, CT and UCL) in conjunction with tumor therapy. • Under near-infrared light, the heat generated by UCNPs helped to kill cancer cells and dissolve PCM, triggering the release of drugs and the production of ROS, resulting in an effective integration of photothermal/photodynamic therapy with chemotherapy.	[223] 2017
Iron-dependent artesunate-loaded, transferrin-modified, hollow mesoporous CuS NPs (AS/Tf-HMCuS NPs)	Photodynamic therapy/Photothermal therapy/Chemotherapy	MCF-7	In vitro, Animals	• Tf-mediated endocytosis enhanced accumulation and retention in tumor cells. • Effective near-infrared light was converted to heat while producing high levels of ROS for PDT.	[224] 2017
1-Tetradecanol-, doxorubicin- and chlorin e6-loaded hollow mesoporous copper sulfide NPs (H-CuS@PCM/DOX/Ce6 (HPDC) NPs)	Photodynamic therapy/Photothermal therapy/Chemotherapy	4T1	In vitro, Animals	• Under near-infrared laser radiation, the NPs produced a strong photothermal effect, which induced controlled release of DOX and Ce6. • The NPs presented low systemic toxicity and good blood compatibility and were able to eradicate breast cancer in 4T1 mice.	[225] 2019
(Enaminitrile molecule gel encapsulating doxorubicin core/Mesoporous silica-coated, CuS-loaded, lanthanide ion-doped upconversion shell) NPs wrapped with a cancer cell membrane	Photodynamic therapy/Photothermal therapy/Chemotherapy	MCF-7, 4T1	In vitro, Animals	• Wrapping NPs in cancer cell membranes imparted unique advantages such as immune escape and homologous binding ability. • Through the transformation of near-infrared energy into ultraviolet light from the UCNP nucleus, enaminitrile molecule phase transition was stimulated to generate ROS for PDT, thus avoiding the limited penetration of ultraviolet light to tissues.	[226] 2021

Table 8. Cont.

Nanoparticle	Type of Combination Therapy	Tumor	Data Sources	Findings	Ref
(Upconversion core/chlorin e6, doxorubicin hydrochloride coloaded mesoporous silica shell) NPs conjugated with polyethylene glycol-modified graphene (DOX-UMCG)	Photodynamic therapy/Photothermal therapy/Chemotherapy	HeLa	In vitro, Animals	• Only low-intensity near-infrared light was required to produce a domino effect, avoiding the phototoxicity of high-intensity exposure to nearby healthy cells. • Synergistic Chemo/PTT/PDT anticancer effect with low systemic toxicity.	[227] 2020
Thiol-terminated monomethoxyl poly(ethylene glycol) and mercaptoropionylhydrazide-modified gold nanorods covalently conjugated with 5-aminolevulinic acid and doxorubicin (GNRs-MPH-$^{ALA/DOX}$-PEG)	Photodynamic therapy/Photothermal therapy/Chemotherapy	MCF-7	In vitro, Animals	• Combined CT/PDT/PTT therapy killed McF-7 cells more effectively, with superadditive antitumor effects and no obvious systemic toxicity. • The circulating half-life of GNRs-MPH-$^{ALA/DOX}$-PEG in blood was approximately 52 min, and the tumor aggregation rate was 3.3%.	[228] 2018
Folic acid-functionalized, paclitaxel-loaded MgAl layered double hydroxide gated mesoporous silica NPs (MT@L-PTX@FA)	Photodynamic therapy/Photothermal therapy/Chemotherapy	HepG2	In vitro	• Under near-infrared irradiation, the NPs effectively converted photon energy into ROS and heat, enhancing toxicity to tumor cells. • It presented obvious slow-release characteristics and was sensitive to pH. It could dissolve MgAl LDHs into Mg^{2+} and Al^{3+} under the low pH of the tumor site, selectively releasing PTX for chemotherapy.	[229] 2019
Folic acid-CuS/docetaxel@polyethylenimine-protoporphyrin IX-CPG (FA-CuS/DTX@PEI-PpXCpG)	Photodynamic therapy/Photothermal therapy/Chemotherapy/Immunotherapy	4T1	In vitro, Animals	• FA-CD@PP-CpG medium and low-dose DTX promoted CTL infiltration, improved the efficacy of anti-PD-L1 antibody (APD-L1), inhibited MDSCs, and effectively polarized MDSCs to the M1 phenotype.	[220] 2019

4. Outlook and Discussion

Complex microenvironments, abnormal growth rates and drug resistance during treatment make cancer treatment difficult. PDT, as a new treatment scheme, has the advantages of simple operation, noninvasiveness, safety and few side effects. The emergence of nano-carriers has made great contributions to the development of photodynamic therapy, and the limitation of physical and chemical properties of PS in PDT was solved. In addition to therapeutic effects, PS-mediated fluorescence can also be used for optical imaging to detect tumors, or as image guidance for surgery [230]. The major issues contributing to the failure of PDT are metastatic tumor at unknown sites, inadequate light delivery and lack of sufficient oxygen. This limitation can be addressed by multidrug combination. The combination of PDT and other treatment schemes, such as chemotherapy and radiotherapy, immunotherapy, gene therapy and PTT, has obvious advantages over the single application of one treatment scheme. With the development of nanodelivery vectors, codelivery has become a common method of multidrug combination. In this paper, we review the research progress of PDT combined with other therapies to improve the therapeutic effect on tumors based on the codelivery of nanodelivery carriers.

The combination of PDT and chemotherapy can significantly reduce the dose of chemotherapy drugs, overcome the deep-seated tumors that PDT cannot kill by multidrug resistant chemotherapy, and increase the level of ROS in the tumor microenvironment to enhance the sensitivity of cancer cells to PDT. In combination with immunotherapy, the PDT-mediated inflammatory response and ICD activate the body's immune response, which can be further enhanced by codelivering an immune adjuvant CPG or tumor antigen, providing a reconstructed immune microenvironment for tumor immunotherapy. PDT can be codelivered with therapeutic genes that target the regulation of hypoxia, angiogenesis, and heat shock proteins, alleviating the tolerance of long-term PDT therapy. Combined with therapeutic genes that target the regulation of other key proteins in tumor growth and metabolism, multimechanism antitumor effects can be achieved. The combination of PDT and PTT can synergistically increase the oxidative stress response at the tumor site, and the PTT-mediated increase in reactive oxygen species levels at the tumor site enhances the sensitivity of tumor cells to PDT. Studies on the combination of PDT and HT are still scarce. Although the discovery of MH is of great help to this codelivery strategy, more studies are still needed to confirm any synergistic effects. PDT combined with radiotherapy can overcome the limitation of PDT in light and can significantly improve the therapeutic effect of PDT on deep tumors. Combined sonodynamic therapy is beneficial to achieve accurate treatment, while satisfying different depths and is suitable for tumor treatment of fine organs. Multidrug codelivery can realize the organic unity of antitumor and antimetastatic effects, as well as recurrence through different antitumor mechanisms.

Although these different antitumor combinations have shown good results, they have their own limitations. PDT has been reported many times to induce sustained systemic immunosuppression, but the current mechanism has not been clarified. The speculated reasons are as follows: (1) ROS produced during PDT inactivate DAMPs released by apoptotic tumor cells, thus failing to stimulate immunity; and (2) apoptotic tumor cells release IL-10, TGF-beta and other immunosuppressive cytokines that affect the generation of CD8+ T cells [231]. This immunosuppression will affect not only the subsequent treatment effect of PDT but also the combination of PDT and immunotherapy. The combination of PDT and PTT is dependent on laser irradiation, which has a poor effect on deep tumors. The combination of PDT and radiotherapy is also subject to the strong oxygen dependence of PDT. Multidrug combination delivery is limited by the development of delivery vectors, drug loading and release. These problems are one of the reasons why codelivery systems based on nanocarriers have not been applied in clinical applications, while other reasons include incomplete safety assessment of the preparation protocol and difficulty in large-scale clinical applications of the preparation.

In summary, this paper focuses on the synergistic enhancement of antitumor therapeutic effects by codelivery combinations of PDT and different treatment regimens. This type of approach is definitely a potential therapeutic strategy, and the existing problems mentioned above need more research to resolve.

Author Contributions: Y.-L.Y. and K.L. conceived the concept of the review article, and prepared the content outline. Y.-L.Y. and K.L. contributed to the review writing for different sections. L.Y. supervised the writing and final revision of the manuscript. All authors have read and agreed to the published version of the manuscript.

Funding: This research received no external funding.

Institutional Review Board Statement: Not applicable.

Informed Consent Statement: Not applicable.

Data Availability Statement: Not applicable.

Conflicts of Interest: The authors declare no conflict of interest.

Abbreviations

PDT	photodynamic therapy
PTT	photothermal therapy
HT	hyperthermia therapy
MT	magnetic hyperthermia therapy
MNPs	magnetic nanoparticles
AMF	alternating magnetic field
ROS	reactive oxygen
ICD	immunogenic cell death
PFC	perfluorocarbon
CS	chitosan
NPs	nanoparticles
OVA	ovalbumin
DOX	doxorubicin
PS	photosensitisers
PoP	Porphyrin-phospholipid
Qu	quercetin
Pt	platinum
CRT	calreticulin
DAMPs	damage-associated molecular patterns
TLR	toll-like receptor
APC	antigen-presenting cell
nMOF	nano-metal organic framework
TME	tumor microenvironment
PEG	polyethylene glycol
PLGA	poly(lactide-co-glycolic)
GO	graphene oxide
PpIX	protoporphyrin IX
PTX	paclitaxel
SDT	sonodynamic therapy
SPDT	sono-photodynamic therapy
IgG	immunoglobulin G
HIF1α	hypoxia-inducible factor α
VEGF	vascular growth factor
PCI	photochemical Internalization
IDO1	indoleamine 2, 3-dioxygenase 1
CLTA-4	cytotoxic T-lymphocyte-associated antigen 4
PD-L1	programmed death-ligand 1
Ce6	chlorin e6

PEI	polythylenimide
ERP	enhanced permeability and retention effects
XPDT	X-ray photodynamic therapy
LDL	low-density lipoprotein
1MT	dextro-1-methyltryptophan
LCP	lipid-calcium-phosphate
EMT	epithelial mesenchymal transition
HPD	hematoporphyrin
MB	methylene blue
NIR	near infrared
ZnPc	zinc phthalocyanine
$ZnF_{16}Pc$	zinc hexadecafluorophthalocyanine
ClAlPc	aluminum chloride phthalocyanine
HYP	hypericin
LAHP	linoleic acid peroxide
CRT	calreticulin
AXT	axitinib
5-ALA	5-aminolevulinic acid
PAH	polyacrylamide
PAA	polyacrylic acid
H_2TCPP	tetrakis (4-carboxyphenyl) porphyrin
RNP	ribonucleoprotein
EGFR	epidermal growth factor receptor
HER-2	human epidermal growth factor receptor 2
TfR	transferrin receptor
PIN	photoimmune nanoconjugated platform

References

1. Kumar, A.; Moralès, O.; Mordon, S.; Delhem, N.; Boleslawski, E. Could Photodynamic Therapy Be a Promising Therapeutic Modality in Hepatocellular Carcinoma Patients? A Critical Review of Experimental and Clinical Studies. *Cancers* **2021**, *13*, 5176. [CrossRef]
2. Donohoe, C.; Senge, M.O.; Arnaut, L.G.; Gomes-da-Silva, L.C. Cell death in photodynamic therapy: From oxidative stress to anti-tumor immunity. *Biochim. Biophys. Acta Rev. Cancer* **2019**, *1872*, 188308. [CrossRef]
3. Wachowska, M.; Muchowicz, A.; Demkow, U. Immunological aspects of antitumor photodynamic therapy outcome. *Central-Eur. J. Immunol.* **2015**, *40*, 481–485. [CrossRef]
4. Kwiatkowski, S.; Knap, B.; Przystupski, D.; Saczko, J.; Kedzierska, E.; Knap-Czop, K.; Kotlinska, J.; Michel, O.; Kotowski, K.; Kulbacka, J. Photodynamic therapy-mechanisms, photosensitizers and combinations. *Biomed. Pharmacother.* **2018**, *106*, 1098–1107. [CrossRef] [PubMed]
5. Liu, H.; Hu, Y.; Sun, Y.; Wan, C.; Zhang, Z.; Dai, X.; Lin, Z.; He, Q.; Yang, Z.; Huang, P.; et al. Co-delivery of Bee Venom Melittin and a Photosensitizer with an Organic-Inorganic Hybrid Nanocarrier for Photodynamic Therapy and Immunotherapy. *ACS Nano* **2019**, *13*, 12638–12652. [CrossRef]
6. Tardivo, J.P.; Del Giglio, A.; de Oliveira, C.S.; Gabrielli, D.S.; Junqueira, H.C.; Tada, D.B.; Severino, D.; de Fatima Turchiello, R.; Baptista, M.S. Methylene blue in photodynamic therapy: From basic mechanisms to clinical applications. *Photodiagn. Photodyn. Ther.* **2005**, *2*, 175–191. [CrossRef]
7. Junqueira, H.C.; Severino, D.; Dias, L.G.; Gugliotti, M.S.; Baptista, M.S. Modulation of methylene blue photochemical properties based on adsorption at aqueous micelle interfaces. *Phys. Chem. Chem. Phys.* **2002**, *4*, 2320–2328. [CrossRef]
8. Ma, M.; Cheng, L.; Zhao, A.; Zhang, H.; Zhang, A. Pluronic-based graphene oxide-methylene blue nanocomposite for photodynamic/photothermal combined therapy of cancer cells. *Photodiagn. Photodyn. Ther.* **2020**, *29*, 101640. [CrossRef]
9. Vallejo, M.C.S.; Moura, N.M.M.; Ferreira Faustino, M.A.; Almeida, A.; Gonçalves, I.; Serra, V.V.; Neves, M.G.P.M.S. An Insight into the Role of Non-Porphyrinoid Photosensitizers for Skin Wound Healing. *Int. J. Mol. Sci.* **2020**, *22*, 234. [CrossRef] [PubMed]
10. Vallejo, M.C.S.; Moura, N.M.M.; Gomes, A.T.P.C.; Joaquinito, A.S.M.; Faustino, M.A.F.; Almeida, A.; Goncalves, I.; Serra, V.V.; Neves, M.G.P.M.S. The Role of Porphyrinoid Photosensitizers for Skin Wound Healing. *Int. J. Mol. Sci.* **2021**, *22*, 4121. [CrossRef] [PubMed]
11. Rahmanian, N.; Eskandani, M.; Barar, J.; Omidi, Y. Recent trends in targeted therapy of cancer using graphene oxide-modified multifunctional nanomedicines. *J. Drug Target.* **2017**, *25*, 202–215. [CrossRef] [PubMed]
12. Kang, M.S.; Lee, S.Y.; Kim, K.S.; Han, D.W. State of the Art Biocompatible Gold Nanoparticles for Cancer Theragnosis. *Pharmaceutics* **2020**, *12*, 701. [CrossRef]

13. Bekmukhametova, A.; Ruprai, H.; Hook, J.M.; Mawad, D.; Houang, J.; Lauto, A. Photodynamic therapy with nanoparticles to combat microbial infection and resistance. *Nanoscale* **2020**, *12*, 21034–21059. [CrossRef] [PubMed]
14. Qin, L.; Jiang, S.; He, H.; Ling, G.; Zhang, P. Functional black phosphorus nanosheets for cancer therapy. *J. Control Release* **2020**, *318*, 50–66. [CrossRef] [PubMed]
15. Huang, Y.Y.; Sharma, S.K.; Yin, R.; Agrawal, T.; Chiang, L.Y.; Hamblin, M.R. Functionalized fullerenes in photodynamic therapy. *J. Biomed. Nanotechnol.* **2014**, *10*, 1918–1936. [CrossRef]
16. Liu, C.; Qin, H.; Kang, L.; Chen, Z.; Wang, H.; Qiu, H.; Ren, J.; Qu, X. Graphitic carbon nitride nanosheets as a multifunctional nanoplatform for photochemical internalization-enhanced photodynamic therapy. *J. Mater. Chem. B* **2018**, *6*, 7908–7915. [CrossRef]
17. Kessel, D. Photodynamic Therapy: A Brief History. *J. Clin. Med.* **2019**, *8*, 1581. [CrossRef]
18. Lin, C.; Zhang, Y.; Wang, J.; Sui, A.; Xiu, L.; Zhu, X. The study of effect and mechanism of 630-nm laser on human lung adenocarcinoma cell xenograft model in nude mice mediated by hematoporphyrin derivatives. *Lasers Med. Sci.* **2020**, *35*, 1085–1094. [CrossRef]
19. Dougherty, T.J.; Lawrence, G.; Kaufman, J.H.; Boyle, D.; Weishaupt, K.R.; Goldfarb, A. Photoradiation in the treatment of recurrent breast carcinoma. *J. Natl. Cancer Inst.* **1979**, *62*, 231–237. [PubMed]
20. Gunaydin, G.; Gedik, M.E.; Ayan, S. Photodynamic Therapy-Current Limitations and Novel Approaches. *Front. Chem.* **2021**, *9*, 691697. [CrossRef] [PubMed]
21. Liang, H.; Zhou, Z.; Luo, R.; Sang, M.; Liu, B.; Sun, M.; Qu, W.; Feng, F.; Liu, W. Tumor-specific activated photodynamic therapy with an oxidation-regulated strategy for enhancing anti-tumor efficacy. *Theranostics* **2018**, *8*, 5059–5071. [CrossRef]
22. Ormond, A.B.; Freeman, H.S. Dye Sensitizers for Photodynamic Therapy. *Materials* **2013**, *6*, 817–840. [CrossRef] [PubMed]
23. Jeong, Y.I.; Cha, B.; Lee, H.L.; Song, Y.H.; Jung, Y.H.; Kwak, T.W.; Choi, C.; Jeong, G.W.; Nah, J.W.; Kang, D.H. Simple nanophotosensitizer fabrication using water-soluble chitosan for photodynamic therapy in gastrointestinal cancer cells. *Int. J. Pharm.* **2017**, *532*, 194–203. [CrossRef] [PubMed]
24. Son, J.; Yi, G.; Kwak, M.H.; Yang, S.M.; Park, J.M.; Lee, B.I.; Choi, M.G.; Koo, H. Gelatin-chlorin e6 conjugate for in vivo photodynamic therapy. *J. Nanobiotechnol.* **2019**, *17*, 50. [CrossRef]
25. Petrovic, L.Z.; Xavierselvan, M.; Kuriakose, M.; Kennedy, M.D.; Nguyen, C.D.; Batt, J.J.; Detels, K.B.; Mallidi, S. Mutual impact of clinically translatable near-infrared dyes on photoacoustic image contrast and in vitro photodynamic therapy efficacy. *J. Biomed. Opt.* **2020**, *25*, 063808.
26. Yan, L.; Luo, L.; Amirshaghaghi, A.; Miller, J.; Meng, C.; You, T.; Busch, T.M.; Tsourkas, A.; Cheng, Z. Dextran-Benzoporphyrin Derivative (BPD) Coated Superparamagnetic Iron Oxide Nanoparticle (SPION) Micelles for T2-Weighted Magnetic Resonance Imaging and Photodynamic Therapy. *Bioconjug. Chem.* **2019**, *30*, 2974–2981. [CrossRef]
27. Rizvi, I.; Nath, S.; Obaid, G.; Ruhi, M.K.; Moore, K.; Bano, S.; Kessel, D.; Hasan, T. A Combination of Visudyne and a Lipid-anchored Liposomal Formulation of Benzoporphyrin Derivative Enhances Photodynamic Therapy Efficacy in a 3D Model for Ovarian Cancer. *Photochem. Photobiol.* **2019**, *95*, 419–429. [CrossRef]
28. Roguin, L.P.; Chiarante, N.; García Vior, M.C.; Marino, J. Zinc(II) phthalocyanines as photosensitizers for antitumor photodynamic therapy. *Int. J. Biochem. Cell Biol.* **2019**, *114*, 105575. [CrossRef]
29. Santos, K.L.M.; Barros, R.M.; da Silva Lima, D.P.; Nunes, A.M.A.; Sato, M.R.; Faccio, R.; de Lima Damasceno, B.P.G.; Oshiro-Junior, J.A. Prospective application of phthalocyanines in the photodynamic therapy against microorganisms and tumor cells: A mini-review. *Photodiagn. Photodyn. Ther.* **2020**, *32*, 102032. [CrossRef]
30. Lo, P.C.; Rodríguez-Morgade, M.S.; Pandey, R.K.; Ng, D.; Torres, T.; Dumoulin, F. The unique features and promises of phthalocyanines as advanced photosensitisers for photodynamic therapy of cancer. *Chem. Soc. Rev.* **2020**, *49*, 1041–1056. [CrossRef]
31. Oleinick, N.L.; Morris, R.L.; Belichenko, I. The role of apoptosis in response to photodynamic therapy: What, where, why, and how. *Photochem. Photobiol. Sci.* **2002**, *1*, 1–21.
32. Buytaert, E.; Dewaele, M.; Agostinis, P. Molecular effectors of multiple cell death pathways initiated by photodynamic therapy. *Biochim. Biophys. Acta* **2007**, *1776*, 86–107. [CrossRef] [PubMed]
33. Buytaert, E.; Callewaert, G.; Hendrickx, N.; Scorrano, L.; Hartmann, D.; Missiaen, L.; Vandenheede, J.R.; Heirman, I.; Grooten, J.; Agostinis, P. Role of endoplasmic reticulum depletion and multidomain proapoptotic BAX and BAK proteins in shaping cell death after hypericin-mediated photodynamic therapy. *FASEB J.* **2006**, *20*, 756–758. [CrossRef] [PubMed]
34. Owens, E.A.; Henary, M.; El Fakhri, G.; Choi, H.S. Tissue-Specific Near-Infrared Fluorescence Imaging. *Acc. Chem. Res.* **2016**, *49*, 1731–1740. [CrossRef]
35. Duse, L.; Agel, M.R.; Pinnapireddy, S.R.; Schafer, J.; Selo, M.A.; Ehrhardt, C.; Bakowsky, U. Photodynamic Therapy of Ovarian Carcinoma Cells with Curcumin-Loaded Biodegradable Polymeric Nanoparticles. *Pharmaceutics* **2019**, *11*, 282. [CrossRef]
36. Machado, F.C.; Adum de Matos, R.P.; Primo, F.L.; Tedesco, A.C.; Rahal, P.; Calmon, M.F. Effect of curcumin-nanoemulsion associated with photodynamic therapy in breast adenocarcinoma cell line. *Bioorg. Med. Chem.* **2019**, *27*, 1882–1890. [CrossRef]
37. de Morais, F.A.P.; Goncalves, R.S.; Vilsinski, B.H.; Lazarin-Bidoia, D.; Balbinot, R.B.; Tsubone, T.M.; Brunaldi, K.; Nakamura, C.V.; Hioka, N.; Caetano, W. Hypericin photodynamic activity in DPPC liposomes-part II: Stability and application in melanoma B16-F10 cancer cells. *Photochem. Photobiol. Sci.* **2020**, *19*, 620–630. [CrossRef]

38. Liu, Y.; Ma, K.; Jiao, T.; Xing, R.; Shen, G.; Yan, X. Water-Insoluble Photosensitizer Nanocolloids Stabilized by Supramolecular Interfacial Assembly towards Photodynamic Therapy. *Sci. Rep.* **2017**, *7*, 42978. [CrossRef] [PubMed]
39. Amanda Pedroso de Morais, F.; Sonchini Goncalves, R.; Souza Campanholi, K.; Martins de Franca, B.; Augusto Capeloto, O.; Lazarin-Bidoia, D.; Bento Balbinot, R.; Vataru Nakamura, C.; Carlos Malacarne, L.; Caetano, W.; et al. Photophysical characterization of Hypericin-loaded in micellar, liposomal and copolymer-lipid nanostructures based F127 and DPPC liposomes. *Spectrochim. Acta A Mol. Biomol. Spectrosc.* **2021**, *248*, 119173. [CrossRef]
40. Wu, P.T.; Lin, C.L.; Lin, C.W.; Chang, N.C.; Tsai, W.B.; Yu, J. Methylene-Blue-Encapsulated Liposomes as Photodynamic Therapy Nano Agents for Breast Cancer Cells. *Nanomaterials* **2018**, *9*, 14. [CrossRef]
41. Khanal, A.; Bui, M.P.; Seo, S.S. Microgel-encapsulated methylene blue for the treatment of breast cancer cells by photodynamic therapy. *J. Breast Cancer* **2014**, *17*, 18–24. [CrossRef]
42. Zheng, Y.; Li, Z.; Chen, H.; Gao, Y. Nanoparticle-based drug delivery systems for controllable photodynamic cancer therapy. *Eur. J. Pharm. Sci.* **2020**, *144*, 105213. [CrossRef]
43. Huang, Y.; Wang, T.; Tan, Q.; He, D.; Wu, M.; Fan, J.; Yang, J.; Zhong, C.; Li, K.; Zhang, J. Smart Stimuli-Responsive and Mitochondria Targeting Delivery in Cancer Therapy. *Int. J. Nanomed.* **2021**, *16*, 4117–4146. [CrossRef] [PubMed]
44. Biswas, S.; Torchilin, V.P. Nanopreparations for organelle-specific delivery in cancer. *Adv. Drug Deliv. Rev.* **2014**, *66*, 26–41. [CrossRef]
45. Liu, C.; Li, Y.; Li, Y.; Duan, Q. Preparation of a star-shaped copolymer with porphyrin core and four PNIPAM-b-POEGMA arms for photodynamic therapy. *Mater. Sci. Eng. C Mater. Biol. Appl.* **2019**, *98*, 74–82. [CrossRef]
46. Weishaupt, K.R.; Gomer, C.J.; Dougherty, T.J. Identification of singlet oxygen as the cytotoxic agent in photoinactivation of a murine tumor. *Cancer Res.* **1976**, *36*, 2326–2329. [PubMed]
47. Dabrzalska, M.; Janaszewska, A.; Zablocka, M.; Mignani, S.; Majoral, J.P.; Klajnert-Maculewicz, B. Complexing Methylene Blue with Phosphorus Dendrimers to Increase Photodynamic Activity. *Molecules* **2017**, *22*, 345. [CrossRef] [PubMed]
48. Wang, P.; Tang, H.; Zhang, P. Plasmonic Nanoparticle-based Hybrid Photosensitizers with Broadened Excitation Profile for Photodynamic Therapy of Cancer Cells. *Sci. Rep.* **2016**, *6*, 34981. [CrossRef]
49. Liang, R.; Liu, L.; He, H.; Chen, Z.; Han, Z.; Luo, Z.; Wu, Z.; Zheng, M.; Ma, Y.; Cai, L. Oxygen-boosted immunogenic photodynamic therapy with gold nanocages@manganese dioxide to inhibit tumor growth and metastases. *Biomaterials* **2018**, *177*, 149–160. [CrossRef] [PubMed]
50. Zhang, C.; Cheng, X.; Chen, M.; Sheng, J.; Ren, J.; Jiang, Z.; Cai, J.; Hu, Y. Fluorescence guided photothermal/photodynamic ablation of tumours using pH-responsive chlorin e6-conjugated gold nanorods. *Colloids Surf. B Biointerfaces* **2017**, *160*, 345–354. [CrossRef]
51. Amanda Pedroso de Morais, F.; Sonchini Gonçalves, R.; Souza Campanholi, K.; Martins de França, B.; Augusto Capeloto, O.; Lazarin-Bidoia, D.; Bento Balbinot, R.; Vataru Nakamura, C.; Carlos Malacarne, L.; Caetano, W.; et al. Nanographene oxide-methylene blue as phototherapies platform for breast tumor ablation and metastasis prevention in a syngeneic orthotopic murine model. *J. Nanobiotechnol.* **2018**, *16*, 9.
52. Shi, X.; Zhan, Q.; Yan, X.; Zhou, J.; Zhou, L.; Wei, S. Oxyhemoglobin nano-recruiter preparation and its application in biomimetic red blood cells to relieve tumor hypoxia and enhance photodynamic therapy activity. *J. Mater. Chem. B* **2020**, *8*, 534–545. [CrossRef]
53. Luo, Z.; Tian, H.; Liu, L.; Chen, Z.; Liang, R.; Chen, Z.; Wu, Z.; Ma, A.; Zheng, M.; Cai, L. Tumor-targeted hybrid protein oxygen carrier to simultaneously enhance hypoxia-dampened chemotherapy and photodynamic therapy at a single dose. *Theranostics* **2018**, *8*, 3584–3596. [CrossRef] [PubMed]
54. Fang, H.; Gai, Y.; Wang, S.; Liu, Q.; Zhang, X.; Ye, M.; Tan, J.; Long, Y.; Wang, K.; Zhang, Y.; et al. Biomimetic oxygen delivery nanoparticles for enhancing photodynamic therapy in triple-negative breast cancer. *J. Nanobiotechnol.* **2021**, *19*, 81. [CrossRef]
55. Zhou, Z.; Song, J.; Tian, R.; Yang, Z.; Yu, G.; Lin, L.; Zhang, G.; Fan, W.; Zhang, F.; Niu, G.; et al. Activatable Singlet Oxygen Generation from Lipid Hydroperoxide Nanoparticles for Cancer Therapy. *Angew. Chem. Int. Ed. Engl.* **2017**, *56*, 6492–6496. [CrossRef]
56. Hu, D.; Chen, L.; Qu, Y.; Peng, J.; Chu, B.; Shi, K.; Hao, Y.; Zhong, L.; Wang, M.; Qian, Z. Oxygen-generating Hybrid Polymeric Nanoparticles with Encapsulated Doxorubicin and Chlorin e6 for Trimodal Imaging-Guided Combined Chemo-Photodynamic Therapy. *Theranostics* **2018**, *8*, 1558–1574. [CrossRef] [PubMed]
57. Usacheva, M.; Swaminathan, S.K.; Kirtane, A.R.; Panyam, J. Enhanced photodynamic therapy and effective elimination of cancer stem cells using surfactant-polymer nanoparticles. *Mol. Pharm.* **2014**, *11*, 3186–3195. [CrossRef]
58. Yue, D.; Cai, X.; Fan, M.; Zhu, J.; Tian, J.; Wu, L.; Jiang, Q.; Gu, Z. An Alternating Irradiation Strategy-Driven Combination Therapy of PDT and RNAi for Highly Efficient Inhibition of Tumor Growth and Metastasis. *Adv. Healthc. Mater.* **2021**, *10*, e2001850. [CrossRef] [PubMed]
59. Girotti, A.W.; Fahey, J.M.; Korytowski, W. Multiple Means by Which Nitric Oxide can Antagonize Photodynamic Therapy. *Curr. Med. Chem.* **2016**, *23*, 2754–2769. [CrossRef]
60. Girotti, A.W.; Fahey, J.M.; Korytowski, W. Upregulation of nitric oxide in tumor cells as a negative adaptation to photodynamic therapy. *Lasers Surg. Med.* **2018**, *50*, 590–598. [CrossRef]
61. Fahey, J.M.; Girotti, A.W. Nitric oxide-mediated resistance to photodynamic therapy in a human breast tumor xenograft model: Improved outcome with NOS_2 inhibitors. *Nitric Oxide* **2017**, *62*, 52–61. [CrossRef]

62. Carter, K.A.; Luo, D.; Razi, A.; Geng, J.; Shao, S.; Ortega, J.; Lovell, J.F. Sphingomyelin Liposomes Containing Porphyrin-phospholipid for Irinotecan Chemophototherapy. *Theranostics* **2016**, *6*, 2329–2336. [CrossRef]
63. Cramer, G.M.; Moon, E.K.; Cengel, K.A.; Busch, T.M. Photodynamic Therapy and Immune Checkpoint Blockade†. *Photochem. Photobiol.* **2020**, *96*, 954–961. [CrossRef]
64. El-Daly, S.M.; Abba, M.L.; Gamal-Eldeen, A.M. The role of microRNAs in photodynamic therapy of cancer. *Eur. J. Med. Chem.* **2017**, *142*, 550–555. [CrossRef]
65. Liu, X.; Yang, G.; Zhang, L.; Liu, Z.; Cheng, Z.; Zhu, X. Photosensitizer cross-linked nano-micelle platform for multimodal imaging guided synergistic photothermal/photodynamic therapy. *Nanoscale* **2016**, *8*, 15323–15339. [CrossRef] [PubMed]
66. Gu, H.; Xu, K.; Yang, Z.; Chang, C.K.; Xu, B. Synthesis and cellular uptake of porphyrin decorated iron oxide nanoparticles-a potential candidate for bimodal anticancer therapy. *Chem. Commun.* **2005**, 4270–4272. [CrossRef] [PubMed]
67. Popovich, K.; Procházková, L.; Pelikánová, I.T.; Vlk, M.; Palkovský, M.; Jarý, V.; Nikl, M.; Múčka, V.; Mihóková, E.; Čuba, V. Preliminary study on singlet oxygen production using CeF$_3$:Tb$_3$+@SiO$_2$-PpIX. *Radiat. Meas.* **2016**, *90*, 325–328. [CrossRef]
68. Hong, L.; Pliss, A.M.; Zhan, Y.; Zheng, W.; Xia, J.; Liu, L.; Qu, J.; Prasad, P.N. Perfluoropolyether Nanoemulsion Encapsulating Chlorin e6 for Sonodynamic and Photodynamic Therapy of Hypoxic Tumor. *Nanomaterials* **2020**, *10*, 2058. [CrossRef]
69. Yu, Y.; Zhang, Z.; Wang, Y.; Zhu, H.; Li, F.; Shen, Y.; Guo, S. A new NIR-triggered doxorubicin and photosensitizer indocyanine green co-delivery system for enhanced multidrug resistant cancer treatment through simultaneous chemo/photothermal/photodynamic therapy. *Acta Biomater.* **2017**, *59*, 170–180. [CrossRef]
70. Chen, Y.; Zhang, F.; Wang, Q.; Tong, R.; Lin, H.; Qu, F. Near-infrared light-mediated LA-UCNPs@SiO$_2$-C/HA@mSiO$_2$-DOX@NB nanocomposite for chemotherapy/PDT/PTT and imaging. *Dalton Trans.* **2017**, *46*, 14293–14300. [CrossRef] [PubMed]
71. Cheng, H.L.; Guo, H.L.; Xie, A.J.; Shen, Y.H.; Zhu, M.Z. 4-in-1 Fe$_3$O$_4$/g-C$_3$N$_4$@PPy-DOX nanocomposites: Magnetic targeting guided trimode combinatorial chemotherapy/PDT/PTT for cancer. *J. Inorg. Biochem.* **2021**, *215*, 111329. [CrossRef]
72. Bukowski, K.; Kciuk, M.; Kontek, R. Mechanisms of Multidrug Resistance in Cancer Chemotherapy. *Int. J. Mol. Sci.* **2020**, *21*, 3233. [CrossRef] [PubMed]
73. Qin, S.Y.; Cheng, Y.J.; Lei, Q.; Zhang, A.Q.; Zhang, X.Z. Combinational strategy for high-performance cancer chemotherapy. *Biomaterials* **2018**, *171*, 178–197. [CrossRef]
74. Chistiakov, D.A.; Myasoedova, V.A.; Orekhov, A.N.; Bobryshev, Y.V. Nanocarriers in Improving Chemotherapy of Multidrug Resistant Tumors: Key Developments and Perspectives. *Curr. Pharm. Des.* **2017**, *23*, 3301–3308. [CrossRef] [PubMed]
75. Srinivas, U.S.; Tan, B.W.Q.; Vellayappan, B.A.; Jeyasekharan, A.D. ROS and the DNA damage response in cancer. *Redox Biol.* **2019**, *25*, 101084. [CrossRef] [PubMed]
76. Yang, H.; Villani, R.M.; Wang, H.; Simpson, M.J.; Roberts, M.S.; Tang, M.; Liang, X. The role of cellular reactive oxygen species in cancer chemotherapy. *J. Exp. Clin. Cancer Res.* **2018**, *37*, 266. [CrossRef]
77. Schreiber, S.; Gross, S.; Brandis, A.; Harmelin, A.; Rosenbach-Belkin, V.; Scherz, A.; Salomon, Y. Local photodynamic therapy (PDT) of rat C6 glioma xenografts with Pd-bacteriopheophorbide leads to decreased metastases and increase of animal cure compared with surgery. *Int. J. Cancer* **2002**, *99*, 279–285. [CrossRef]
78. Luo, D.; Carter, K.A.; Miranda, D.; Lovell, J.F. Chemophototherapy: An Emerging Treatment Option for Solid Tumors. *Adv. Sci.* **2017**, *4*, 1600106. [CrossRef]
79. Lila, A.S.; Ishida, T.; Kiwada, H. Targeting anticancer drugs to tumor vasculature using cationic liposomes. *Pharm. Res.* **2010**, *27*, 1171–1183. [CrossRef]
80. Luo, D.; Li, N.; Carter, K.A.; Lin, C.; Geng, J.; Shao, S.; Huang, W.C.; Qin, Y.; Atilla-Gokcumen, G.E.; Lovell, J.F. Rapid Light-Triggered Drug Release in Liposomes Containing Small Amounts of Unsaturated and Porphyrin-Phospholipids. *Small* **2016**, *12*, 3039–3047. [CrossRef]
81. Miranda, D.; Lovell, J.F. Mechanisms of Light-induced Liposome Permeabilization. *Bioeng. Transl. Med.* **2016**, *1*, 267–276. [CrossRef]
82. Luo, D.; Geng, J.; Li, N.; Carter, K.A.; Shao, S.; Atilla-Gokcumen, G.E.; Lovell, J.F. Vessel-Targeted Chemophototherapy with Cationic Porphyrin-Phospholipid Liposomes. *Mol. Cancer Ther.* **2017**, *16*, 2452–2461. [CrossRef]
83. Luo, D.; Carter, K.A.; Molins, E.A.G.; Straubinger, N.L.; Geng, J.; Shao, S.; Jusko, W.J.; Straubinger, R.M.; Lovell, J.F. Pharmacokinetics and pharmacodynamics of liposomal chemophototherapy with short drug-light intervals. *J. Control Release* **2019**, *297*, 39–47. [CrossRef]
84. Luo, D.; Carter, K.A.; Razi, A.; Geng, J.; Shao, S.; Giraldo, D.; Sunar, U.; Ortega, J.; Lovell, J.F. Doxorubicin encapsulated in stealth liposomes conferred with light-triggered drug release. *Biomaterials* **2016**, *75*, 193–202. [CrossRef]
85. Luo, D.; Goel, S.; Liu, H.J.; Carter, K.A.; Jiang, D.; Geng, J.; Kutyreff, C.J.; Engle, J.W.; Huang, W.C.; Shao, S.; et al. Intrabilayer (64)Cu Labeling of Photoactivatable, Doxorubicin-Loaded Stealth Liposomes. *ACS Nano* **2017**, *11*, 12482–12491. [CrossRef] [PubMed]
86. Luo, D.; Carter, K.A.; Geng, J.; He, X.; Lovell, J.F. Short Drug-Light Intervals Improve Liposomal Chemophototherapy in Mice Bearing MIA PaCa-2 Xenografts. *Mol. Pharm.* **2018**, *15*, 3682–3689. [CrossRef]
87. Jiang, W.; Delahunty, I.M.; Xie, J. Oxygenating the way for enhanced chemophototherapy. *Theranostics* **2018**, *8*, 3870–3871. [CrossRef] [PubMed]
88. Sunil, V.; Mozhi, A.; Zhan, W.; Teoh, J.H.; Wang, C.H. Convection enhanced delivery of light responsive antigen capturing oxygen generators for chemo-phototherapy triggered adaptive immunity. *Biomaterials* **2021**, *275*, 120974. [CrossRef]

89. Liu, X.L.; Dong, X.; Yang, S.C.; Lai, X.; Liu, H.J.; Gao, Y.; Feng, H.Y.; Zhu, M.H.; Yuan, Y.; Lu, Q.; et al. Biomimetic Liposomal Nanoplatinum for Targeted Cancer Chemophototherapy. *Adv. Sci.* **2021**, *8*, 2003679. [CrossRef] [PubMed]
90. Tian, H.; Zhang, J.; Zhang, H.; Jiang, Y.; Song, A.; Luan, Y. Low side-effect and heat-shock protein-inhibited chemo-phototherapy nanoplatform via co-assembling strategy of biotin-tailored IR780 and quercetin. *Chem. Eng. J.* **2020**, *382*, 123043. [CrossRef]
91. He, C.; Duan, X.; Guo, N.; Chan, C.; Poon, C.; Weichselbaum, R.R.; Lin, W. Core-shell nanoscale coordination polymers combine chemotherapy and photodynamic therapy to potentiate checkpoint blockade cancer immunotherapy. *Nat. Commun.* **2016**, *7*, 12499. [CrossRef]
92. Zhang, X.; Wu, M.; Li, J.; Lan, S.; Zeng, Y.; Liu, X.; Liu, J. Light-Enhanced Hypoxia-Response of Conjugated Polymer Nanocarrier for Successive Synergistic Photodynamic and Chemo-Therapy. *ACS Appl. Mater. Interfaces* **2018**, *10*, 21909–21919. [CrossRef] [PubMed]
93. Mao, B.; Liu, C.; Zheng, W.; Li, X.; Ge, R.; Shen, H.; Guo, X.; Lian, Q.; Shen, X.; Li, C. Cyclic cRGDfk peptide and Chlorin e6 functionalized silk fibroin nanoparticles for targeted drug delivery and photodynamic therapy. *Biomaterials* **2018**, *161*, 306–320. [CrossRef]
94. Zhang, J.; Huang, H.; Xue, L.; Zhong, L.; Ge, W.; Song, X.; Zhao, Y.; Wang, W.; Dong, X. On-demand drug release nanoplatform based on fluorinated aza-BODIPY for imaging-guided chemo-phototherapy. *Biomaterials* **2020**, *256*, 120211. [CrossRef] [PubMed]
95. Zong, J.; Peng, H.; Qing, X.; Fan, Z.; Xu, W.; Du, X.; Shi, R.; Zhang, Y. pH-Responsive Pluronic F127-Lenvatinib-Encapsulated Halogenated Boron-Dipyrromethene Nanoparticles for Combined Photodynamic Therapy and Chemotherapy of Liver Cancer. *ACS Omega* **2021**, *6*, 12331–12342. [CrossRef]
96. Cheng, X.; He, L.; Xu, J.; Fang, Q.; Yang, L.; Xue, Y.; Wang, X.; Tang, R. Oxygen-producing catalase-based prodrug nanoparticles overcoming resistance in hypoxia-mediated chemo-photodynamic therapy. *Acta Biomater.* **2020**, *112*, 234–249. [CrossRef]
97. Sun, B.; Chen, Y.; Yu, H.; Wang, C.; Zhang, X.; Zhao, H.; Chen, Q.; He, Z.; Luo, C.; Sun, J. Photodynamic PEG-coated ROS-sensitive prodrug nanoassemblies for core-shell synergistic chemo-photodynamic therapy. *Acta Biomater.* **2019**, *92*, 219–228. [CrossRef] [PubMed]
98. Tan, P.; Cai, H.; Wei, Q.; Tang, X.; Zhang, Q.; Kopytynski, M.; Yang, J.; Yi, Y.; Zhang, H.; Gong, Q.; et al. Enhanced chemo-photodynamic therapy of an enzyme-responsive prodrug in bladder cancer patient-derived xenograft models. *Biomaterials* **2021**, *277*, 121061. [CrossRef]
99. Shu, M.; Tang, J.; Chen, L.; Zeng, Q.; Li, C.; Xiao, S.; Jiang, Z.; Liu, J. Tumor microenvironment triple-responsive nanoparticles enable enhanced tumor penetration and synergetic chemo-photodynamic therapy. *Biomaterials* **2021**, *268*, 120574. [CrossRef] [PubMed]
100. Zhong, D.; Wu, H.; Wu, Y.; Li, Y.; Yang, J.; Gong, Q.; Luo, K.; Gu, Z. Redox dual-responsive dendrimeric nanoparticles for mutually synergistic chemo-photodynamic therapy to overcome drug resistance. *J. Control Release* **2021**, *329*, 1210–1221. [CrossRef] [PubMed]
101. Yi, X.; Hu, J.J.; Dai, J.; Lou, X.; Zhao, Z.; Xia, F.; Tang, B.Z. Self-Guiding Polymeric Prodrug Micelles with Two Aggregation-Induced Emission Photosensitizers for Enhanced Chemo-Photodynamic Therapy. *ACS Nano* **2021**, *15*, 3026–3037. [CrossRef] [PubMed]
102. Naldini, L. Gene therapy returns to centre stage. *Nature* **2015**, *526*, 351–360. [CrossRef]
103. Xin, Y.; Huang, M.; Guo, W.W.; Huang, Q.; Zhang, L.Z.; Jiang, G. Nano-based delivery of RNAi in cancer therapy. *Mol. Cancer* **2017**, *16*, 134. [CrossRef]
104. Vaughan, H.J.; Green, J.J.; Tzeng, S.Y. Cancer-Targeting Nanoparticles for Combinatorial Nucleic Acid Delivery. *Adv. Mater.* **2020**, *32*, e1901081. [CrossRef] [PubMed]
105. Goodman, A.M.; Hogan, N.J.; Gottheim, S.; Li, C.; Clare, S.E.; Halas, N.J. Understanding Resonant Light-Triggered DNA Release from Plasmonic Nanoparticles. *ACS Nano* **2017**, *11*, 171–179. [CrossRef]
106. Matsushita-Ishiodori, Y.; Ohtsuki, T. Photoinduced RNA interference. *Acc. Chem. Res.* **2012**, *45*, 1039–1047. [CrossRef] [PubMed]
107. Wang, Y.; He, H.; Xu, X.; Wang, X.; Chen, Y.; Yin, L. Far-red light-mediated programmable anti-cancer gene delivery in cooperation with photodynamic therapy. *Biomaterials* **2018**, *171*, 72–82. [CrossRef]
108. Chen, L.; Chen, C.; Chen, W.; Li, K.; Chen, X.; Tang, X.; Xie, G.; Luo, X.; Wang, X.; Liang, H.; et al. Biodegradable Black Phosphorus Nanosheets Mediate Specific Delivery of hTERT siRNA for Synergistic Cancer Therapy. *ACS Appl. Mater. Interfaces* **2018**, *10*, 21137–21148. [CrossRef]
109. Vaupel, P.; Kallinowski, F.; Okunieff, P. Blood flow, oxygen and nutrient supply, and metabolic microenvironment of human tumors: A review. *Cancer Res.* **1989**, *49*, 6449–6465.
110. Chen, W.H.; Lecaros, R.L.; Tseng, Y.C.; Huang, L.; Hsu, Y.C. Nanoparticle delivery of HIF1α siRNA combined with photodynamic therapy as a potential treatment strategy for head-and-neck cancer. *Cancer Lett.* **2015**, *359*, 65–74. [CrossRef]
111. Deng, S.; Li, X.; Liu, S.; Chen, J.; Li, M.; Chew, S.Y.; Leong, K.W.; Cheng, D. Codelivery of CRISPR-Cas9 and chlorin e6 for spatially controlled tumor-specific gene editing with synergistic drug effects. *Sci. Adv.* **2020**, *6*, eabb4005. [CrossRef]
112. Jang, Y.; Kim, D.; Lee, H.; Jang, H.; Park, S.; Kim, G.E.; Lee, H.J.; Kim, H.J.; Kim, H. Development of an ultrasound triggered nanomedicine-microbubble complex for chemo-photodynamic-gene therapy. *Nanomedicine* **2020**, *27*, 102194. [CrossRef] [PubMed]
113. Cao, Y.; Meng, X.; Wang, D.; Zhang, K.; Dai, W.; Dong, H.; Zhang, X. Intelligent $MnO_2/Cu_{2-x}S$ for Multimode Imaging Diagnostic and Advanced Single-Laser Irradiated Photothermal/Photodynamic Therapy. *ACS Appl. Mater. Interfaces* **2018**, *10*, 17732–17741. [CrossRef] [PubMed]

114. Yang, C.; Fu, Y.; Huang, C.; Hu, D.; Zhou, K.; Hao, Y.; Chu, B.; Yang, Y.; Qian, Z. Chlorin e6 and CRISPR-Cas9 dual-loading system with deep penetration for a synergistic tumoral photodynamic-immunotherapy. *Biomaterials* **2020**, *255*, 120194. [CrossRef] [PubMed]
115. Ma, C.; Shi, L.; Huang, Y.; Shen, L.; Peng, H.; Zhu, X.; Zhou, G. Nanoparticle delivery of Wnt-1 siRNA enhances photodynamic therapy by inhibiting epithelial-mesenchymal transition for oral cancer. *Biomater. Sci.* **2017**, *28*, 494–501. [CrossRef]
116. Liu, S.Y.; Xu, Y.; Yang, H.; Liu, L.; Zhao, M.; Yin, W.; Xu, Y.T.; Huang, Y.; Tan, C.; Dai, Z.; et al. Ultrathin 2D Copper(I) 1,2,4-Triazolate Coordination Polymer Nanosheets for Efficient and Selective Gene Silencing and Photodynamic Therapy. *Adv. Mater.* **2021**, *33*, e2100849. [CrossRef]
117. Laroui, N.; Coste, M.; Lichon, L.; Bessin, Y.; Gary-Bobo, M.; Pratviel, G.; Bonduelle, C.; Bettache, N.; Ulrich, S. Combination of photodynamic therapy and gene silencing achieved through the hierarchical self-assembly of porphyrin-siRNA complexes. *Int. J. Pharm.* **2019**, *659*, 118585. [CrossRef]
118. Liu, Y.; Pan, Y.; Cao, W.; Xia, F.; Liu, B.; Niu, J.; Alfranca, G.; Sun, X.; Ma, L.; de la Fuente, J.M.; et al. A tumor microenvironment responsive biodegradable CaCO$_3$/MnO$_2$-based nanoplatform for the enhanced photodynamic therapy and improved PD-L1 immunotherapy. *Theranostics* **2019**, *9*, 6867–6884. [CrossRef]
119. Zhao, R.; Liang, X.; Zhao, B.; Chen, M.; Liu, R.; Sun, S.; Yue, X.; Wang, S. Ultrasound assisted gene and photodynamic synergistic therapy with multifunctional FOXA1-siRNA loaded porphyrin microbubbles for enhancing therapeutic efficacy for breast cancer. *Biomaterials* **2018**, *173*, 58–70. [CrossRef]
120. Jin, Y.; Wang, H.; Li, X.; Zhu, H.; Sun, D.; Sun, X.; Liu, H.; Zhang, Z.; Cao, L.; Gao, C.; et al. Multifunctional DNA Polymer-Assisted Upconversion Therapeutic Nanoplatform for Enhanced Photodynamic Therapy. *ACS Appl. Mater. Interfaces* **2020**, *12*, 26832–26841. [CrossRef]
121. Lichon, L.; Kotras, C.; Myrzakhmetov, B.; Arnoux, P.; Daurat, M.; Nguyen, C.; Durand, D.; Bouchmella, K.; Ali, L.M.A.; Durand, J.O.; et al. Polythiophenes with Cationic Phosphonium Groups as Vectors for Imaging, siRNA Delivery, and Photodynamic Therapy. *Nanomaterials* **2020**, *10*, 1432. [CrossRef] [PubMed]
122. Zheng, N.; Luo, X.; Zhang, Z.; Wang, A.; Song, W. Cationic Polyporphyrins as siRNA Delivery Vectors for Photodynamic and Gene Synergistic Anticancer Therapy. *ACS Appl. Mater. Interfaces* **2021**, *13*, 27513–27521. [CrossRef] [PubMed]
123. Mezghrani, B.; Ali, L.M.A.; Richeter, S.; Durand, J.O.; Hesemann, P.; Bettache, N. Periodic Mesoporous Ionosilica Nanoparticles for Green Light Photodynamic Therapy and Photochemical Internalization of siRNA. *ACS Appl. Mater. Interfaces* **2021**, *13*, 29325–29339. [CrossRef]
124. Nath, S.; Obaid, G.; Hasan, T. The Course of Immune Stimulation by Photodynamic Therapy: Bridging Fundamentals of Photochemically Induced Immunogenic Cell Death to the Enrichment of T-Cell Repertoire. *Photochem. Photobiol.* **2019**, *95*, 1288–1305. [CrossRef]
125. Banstola, A.; Jeong, J.H.; Yook, S. Immunoadjuvants for cancer immunotherapy: A review of recent developments. *Acta Biomater.* **2020**, *114*, 16–30. [CrossRef]
126. Lu, K.; Aung, T.; Guo, N.; Weichselbaum, R.; Lin, W. Nanoscale Metal-Organic Frameworks for Therapeutic, Imaging, and Sensing Applications. *Adv. Mater.* **2018**, *30*, e1707634. [CrossRef]
127. Cai, Z.; Xin, F.; Wei, Z.; Wu, M.; Lin, X.; Du, X.; Chen, G.; Zhang, D.; Zhang, Z.; Liu, X.; et al. Photodynamic Therapy Combined with Antihypoxic Signaling and CpG Adjuvant as an In Situ Tumor Vaccine Based on Metal-Organic Framework Nanoparticles to Boost Cancer Immunotherapy. *Adv. Healthc. Mater.* **2020**, *9*, e1900996. [CrossRef] [PubMed]
128. Ni, K.; Luo, T.; Lan, G.; Culbert, A.; Song, Y.; Wu, T.; Jiang, X.; Lin, W. A Nanoscale Metal-Organic Framework to Mediate Photodynamic Therapy and Deliver CpG Oligodeoxynucleotides to Enhance Antigen Presentation and Cancer Immunotherapy. *Angew. Chem. Int. Ed. Engl.* **2020**, *59*, 1108–1112. [CrossRef]
129. Xia, Y.; Gupta, G.K.; Castano, A.P.; Mroz, P.; Avci, P.; Hamblin, M.R. CpG oligodeoxynucleotide as immune adjuvant enhances photodynamic therapy response in murine metastatic breast cancer. *J. Biophotonics* **2014**, *7*, 897–905. [CrossRef]
130. Huang, Y.; Ding, Z.; Jiang, B.P.; Luo, Z.; Chen, T.; Guo, Z.; Ji, S.C.; Liang, H.; Shen, X.C. Artificial Metalloprotein Nanoanalogues: In Situ Catalytic Production of Oxygen to Enhance Photoimmunotherapeutic Inhibition of Primary and Abscopal Tumor Growth. *Small* **2020**, *16*, e2004345. [CrossRef]
131. Ding, B.; Shao, S.; Yu, C.; Teng, B.; Wang, M.; Cheng, Z.; Wong, K.L.; Ma, P.; Lin, J. Large-Pore Mesoporous-Silica-Coated Upconversion Nanoparticles as Multifunctional Immunoadjuvants with Ultrahigh Photosensitizer and Antigen Loading Efficiency for Improved Cancer Photodynamic Immunotherapy. *Adv. Mater.* **2018**, *30*, e1802479. [CrossRef]
132. Xu, C.; Nam, J.; Hong, H.; Xu, Y.; Moon, J.J. Positron Emission Tomography-Guided Photodynamic Therapy with Biodegradable Mesoporous Silica Nanoparticles for Personalized Cancer Immunotherapy. *ACS Nano* **2019**, *13*, 12148–12161. [CrossRef]
133. Pardoll, D.M. The blockade of immune checkpoints in cancer immunotherapy. *Nat. Rev. Cancer* **2012**, *12*, 252–264. [CrossRef]
134. Yang, X.; Zhang, W.; Jiang, W.; Kumar, A.; Zhou, S.; Cao, Z.; Zhan, S.; Yang, W.; Liu, R.; Teng, Y.; et al. Nanoconjugates to enhance PDT-mediated cancer immunotherapy by targeting the indoleamine-2,3-dioxygenase pathway. *J. Nanobiotechnol.* **2021**, *19*, 182. [CrossRef]
135. Zhou, Y.; Ren, X.; Hou, Z.; Wang, N.; Jiang, Y.; Luan, Y. Engineering a photosensitizer nanoplatform for amplified photodynamic immunotherapy via tumor microenvironment modulation. *Nanoscale Horiz.* **2021**, *6*, 120–131. [CrossRef] [PubMed]

136. Xu, J.; Yu, S.; Wang, X.; Qian, Y.; Wu, W.; Zhang, S.; Zheng, B.; Wei, G.; Gao, S.; Cao, Z.; et al. High Affinity of Chlorin e6 to Immunoglobulin G for Intraoperative Fluorescence Image-Guided Cancer Photodynamic and Checkpoint Blockade Therapy. *ACS Nano* **2019**, *13*, 10242–10260. [CrossRef] [PubMed]
137. Chen, S.X.; Ma, M.; Xue, F.; Shen, S.; Chen, Q.; Kuang, Y.; Liang, K.; Wang, X.; Chen, H. Construction of microneedle-assisted co-delivery platform and its combining photodynamic/immunotherapy. *J. Control Release* **2020**, *324*, 218–227. [CrossRef] [PubMed]
138. Wu, C.; Wang, L.; Tian, Y.; Guan, X.; Liu, Q.; Li, S.; Qin, X.; Yang, H.; Liu, Y. "Triple-Punch" Anticancer Strategy Mediated by Near-Infrared Photosensitizer/CpG Oligonucleotides Dual-Dressed and Mitochondria-Targeted Nanographene. *ACS Appl. Mater. Interfaces* **2018**, *10*, 6942–6955. [CrossRef]
139. Li, W.; Yang, J.; Luo, L.; Jiang, M.; Qin, B.; Yin, H.; Zhu, C.; Yuan, X.; Zhang, J.; Luo, Z.; et al. Targeting photodynamic and photothermal therapy to the endoplasmic reticulum enhances immunogenic cancer cell death. *Nat. Commun.* **2019**, *10*, 3349. [CrossRef]
140. Obaid, G.; Bano, S.; Mallidi, S.; Broekgaarden, M.; Kuriakose, J.; Silber, Z.; Bulin, A.L.; Wang, Y.; Mai, Z.; Jin, W.; et al. Impacting Pancreatic Cancer Therapy in Heterotypic in Vitro Organoids and in Vivo Tumors with Specificity-Tuned, NIR-Activable Photoimmunonanoconjugates: Towards Conquering Desmoplasia? *Nano Lett.* **2019**, *19*, 7573–7587. [CrossRef]
141. Bano, S.; Obaid, G.; Swain, J.W.R.; Yamada, M.; Pogue, B.W.; Wang, K.; Hasan, T. NIR Photodynamic Destruction of PDAC and HNSCC Nodules Using Triple-Receptor-Targeted Photoimmuno-Nanoconjugates: Targeting Heterogeneity in Cancer. *J. Clin. Med.* **2020**, *9*, 2390. [CrossRef]
142. Xia, F.; Hou, W.; Liu, Y.; Wang, W.; Han, Y.; Yang, M.; Zhi, X.; Li, C.; Qi, D.; Li, T.; et al. Cytokine induced killer cells-assisted delivery of chlorin e6 mediated self-assembled gold nanoclusters to tumors for imaging and immuno-photodynamic therapy. *Biomaterials* **2018**, *170*, 1–11. [CrossRef] [PubMed]
143. Liu, Y.; Yang, J.; Liu, B.; Cao, W.; Zhang, J.; Yang, Y.; Ma, L.; de la Fuente, J.M.; Song, J.; Ni, J.; et al. Human iPS Cells Loaded with MnO$_2$-Based Nanoprobes for Photodynamic and Simultaneous Enhanced Immunotherapy Against Cancer. *Nano-Micro Lett.* **2020**, *12*, 127. [CrossRef] [PubMed]
144. Xu, J.; Xu, L.; Wang, C.; Yang, R.; Zhuang, Q.; Han, X.; Dong, Z.; Zhu, W.; Peng, R.; Liu, Z. Near-Infrared-Triggered Photodynamic Therapy with Multitasking Upconversion Nanoparticles in Combination with Checkpoint Blockade for Immunotherapy of Colorectal Cancer. *ACS Nano* **2017**, *11*, 4463–4474. [CrossRef]
145. Su, Z.; Xiao, Z.; Huang, J.; Wang, Y.; An, Y.; Xiao, H.; Peng, Y.; Pang, P.; Han, S.; Zhu, K.; et al. Dual-Sensitive PEG-Sheddable Nanodrug Hierarchically Incorporating PD-L1 Antibody and Zinc Phthalocyanine for Improved Immuno-Photodynamic Therapy. *ACS Appl. Mater. Interfaces* **2021**, *13*, 12845–12856. [CrossRef] [PubMed]
146. Li, X.; Kwon, N.; Guo, T.; Liu, Z.; Yoon, J. Innovative Strategies for Hypoxic-Tumor Photodynamic Therapy. *Angew. Chem. Int. Ed. Engl.* **2018**, *57*, 11522–11531. [CrossRef]
147. Gao, L.; Fei, J.; Zhao, J.; Li, H.; Cui, Y.; Li, J. Hypocrellin-loaded gold nanocages with high two-photon efficiency for photothermal/photodynamic cancer therapy in vitro. *ACS Nano* **2012**, *6*, 8030–8040. [CrossRef]
148. Tian, B.; Wang, C.; Zhang, S.; Feng, L.; Liu, Z. Photothermally enhanced photodynamic therapy delivered by nano-graphene oxide. *ACS Nano* **2011**, *5*, 7000–7009. [CrossRef]
149. Wang, S.; Riedinger, A.; Li, H.; Fu, C.; Liu, H.; Li, L.; Liu, T.; Tan, L.; Barthel, M.J.; Pugliese, G.; et al. Plasmonic copper sulfide nanocrystals exhibiting near-infrared photothermal and photodynamic therapeutic effects. *ACS Nano* **2015**, *9*, 1788–1800. [CrossRef]
150. Liu, X.; Su, H.; Shi, W.; Liu, Y.; Sun, Y.; Ge, D. Functionalized poly(pyrrole-3-carboxylic acid) nanoneedles for dual-imaging guided PDT/PTT combination therapy. *Biomaterials* **2018**, *167*, 177–190. [CrossRef]
151. Paszko, E.; Ehrhardt, C.; Senge, M.O.; Kelleher, D.P.; Reynolds, J.V. Nanodrug applications in photodynamic therapy. *Photodiagn. Photodyn. Ther.* **2011**, *8*, 14–29. [CrossRef]
152. Lin, J.; Wang, S.; Huang, P.; Wang, Z.; Chen, S.; Niu, G.; Li, W.; He, J.; Cui, D.; Lu, G.; et al. Photosensitizer-loaded gold vesicles with strong plasmonic coupling effect for imaging-guided photothermal/photodynamic therapy. *ACS Nano* **2013**, *7*, 5320–5329. [CrossRef]
153. Kalluru, P.; Vankayala, R.; Chiang, C.S.; Hwang, K.C. Nano-graphene oxide-mediated In vivo fluorescence imaging and bimodal photodynamic and photothermal destruction of tumors. *Biomaterials* **2016**, *95*, 1–10. [CrossRef] [PubMed]
154. Chen, B.; Cao, J.; Zhang, K.; Zhang, Y.N.; Lu, J.; Zubair Iqbal, M.; Zhang, Q.; Kong, X. Synergistic photodynamic and photothermal therapy of BODIPY-conjugated hyaluronic acid nanoparticles. *J. Biomater. Sci. Polym. Ed.* **2021**, *32*, 2028–2045. [CrossRef]
155. Wu, C.; Zhu, A.; Li, D.; Wang, L.; Yang, H.; Zeng, H.; Liu, Y. Photosensitizer-assembled PEGylated graphene-copper sulfide nanohybrids as a synergistic near-infrared phototherapeutic agent. *Expert Opin. Drug Deliv.* **2016**, *13*, 155–165. [CrossRef] [PubMed]
156. Bharathiraja, S.; Manivasagan, P.; Santha Moorthy, M.; Bui, N.Q.; Jang, B.; Phan, T.; Jung, W.K.; Kim, Y.M.; Lee, K.D.; Oh, J. Photo-based PDT/PTT dual model killing and imaging of cancer cells using phycocyanin-polypyrrole nanoparticles. *Eur. J. Pharm. Biopharm.* **2018**, *123*, 20–30. [CrossRef] [PubMed]

157. Gao, C.; Dong, P.; Lin, Z.; Guo, X.; Jiang, B.P.; Ji, S.; Liang, H.; Shen, X.C. Near-Infrared Light Responsive Imaging-Guided Photothermal and Photodynamic Synergistic Therapy Nanoplatform Based on Carbon Nanohorns for Efficient Cancer Treatment. *Chemistry* **2018**, *24*, 12827–12837. [CrossRef]
158. Wu, J.; Williams, G.R.; Niu, S.; Yang, Y.; Li, Y.; Zhang, X.; Zhu, L.M. Biomineralized Bimetallic Oxide Nanotheranostics for Multimodal Imaging-Guided Combination Therapy. *Theranostics* **2020**, *10*, 841–855. [CrossRef]
159. Sun, Y.; Zhang, Y.; Gao, Y.; Wang, P.; He, G.; Blum, N.T.; Lin, J.; Liu, Q.; Wang, X.; Huang, P. Six Birds with One Stone: Versatile Nanoporphyrin for Single-Laser-Triggered Synergistic Phototheranostics and Robust Immune Activation. *Adv. Mater.* **2020**, *32*, e2004481. [CrossRef] [PubMed]
160. Jana, D.; Jia, S.; Bindra, A.K.; Xing, P.; Ding, D.; Zhao, Y. Clearable Black Phosphorus Nanoconjugate for Targeted Cancer Phototheranostics. *ACS Appl. Mater. Interfaces* **2020**, *12*, 18342–18351. [CrossRef]
161. Chen, S.; Huang, B.; Pei, W.; Wang, L.; Xu, Y.; Niu, C. Mitochondria-Targeting Oxygen-Sufficient Perfluorocarbon Nanoparticles for Imaging-Guided Tumor Phototherapy. *Int. J. Nanomed.* **2020**, *15*, 8641–8658. [CrossRef]
162. Li, P.; Liu, L.; Lu, Q.; Yang, S.; Yang, L.; Cheng, Y.; Wang, Y.; Wang, S.; Song, Y.; Tan, F.; et al. Ultrasmall MoS$_2$ Nanodots-Doped Biodegradable SiO$_2$ Nanoparticles for Clearable FL/CT/MSOT Imaging-Guided PTT/PDT Combination Tumor Therapy. *ACS Appl. Mater. Interfaces* **2019**, *11*, 5771–5781. [CrossRef]
163. Shao, W.; Yang, C.; Li, F.; Wu, J.; Wang, N.; Ding, Q.; Gao, J.; Ling, D. Molecular Design of Conjugated Small Molecule Nanoparticles for Synergistically Enhanced PTT/PDT. *Nano-Micro Lett.* **2020**, *12*, 147. [CrossRef] [PubMed]
164. Wang, Y.; Zhao, J.; Chen, Z.; Zhang, F.; Wang, Q.; Guo, W.; Wang, K.; Lin, H.; Qu, F. Construct of MoSe$_2$/Bi$_2$Se$_3$ nanoheterostructure: Multimodal CT/PT imaging-guided PTT/PDT/chemotherapy for cancer treating. *Biomaterials* **2019**, *217*, 119282. [CrossRef] [PubMed]
165. Zhang, G.; Gou, H.; Liu, Y.; Xi, K.; Jiang, D.; Jia, X. pH-responsive PEG-chitosan/iron oxide hybrid nanoassemblies for low-power assisted PDT/PTT combination therapy. *Nanomedicine* **2020**, *15*, 1097–1112. [CrossRef]
166. Campu, A.; Focsan, M.; Lerouge, F.; Borlan, R.; Tie, L.; Rugina, D.; Astilean, S. ICG-loaded gold nano-bipyramids with NIR activatable dual PTT-PDT therapeutic potential in melanoma cells. *Colloids Surf. B Biointerfaces* **2020**, *194*, 111213. [CrossRef] [PubMed]
167. Yang, J.; Hou, M.; Sun, W.; Wu, Q.; Xu, J.; Xiong, L.; Chai, Y.; Liu, Y.; Yu, M.; Wang, H.; et al. Sequential PDT and PTT Using Dual-Modal Single-Walled Carbon Nanohorns Synergistically Promote Systemic Immune Responses against Tumor Metastasis and Relapse. *Adv. Sci.* **2020**, *7*, 2001088. [CrossRef]
168. Detty, M.R.; Gibson, S.L.; Wagner, S.J. Current clinical and preclinical photosensitizers for use in photodynamic therapy. *J. Med. Chem.* **2004**, *47*, 3897–3915. [CrossRef]
169. Streffer, C. Biological Basis of Thermotherapy (With Special Reference to Oncology). In *Biological Basis of Oncologic Thermotherapy*; Gauthrie, M., Ed.; Springer: Berlin/Heidelberg, Germany, 1990; pp. 1–71.
170. Van Rhoon, G.C.; Franckena, M.; Ten Hagen, T.L. A moderate thermal dose is sufficient for effective free and TSL based thermochemotherapy. *Adv. Drug Deliv. Rev.* **2020**, *163–164*, 145–156. [CrossRef] [PubMed]
171. Jordan, A.; Scholz, R.; Wust, P.; Fahling, H.; Felix, R. Magnetic fluid hyperthermia (MFH): Cancer treatment with AC magnetic field induced excitation of biocompatible superparamagnetic nanoparticles. *J. Magn. Magn. Mater.* **1999**, *201*, 413–419. [CrossRef]
172. Huang, W.C.; Shen, M.Y.; Chen, H.H.; Lin, S.C.; Chiang, W.H.; Wu, P.H.; Chang, C.W.; Chiang, C.S.; Chiu, H.C. Monocytic delivery of therapeutic oxygen bubbles for dual-modality treatment of tumor hypoxia. *J. Control Release* **2015**, *220*, 738–750. [CrossRef]
173. Yanase, S.; Nomura, J.; Matsumura, Y.; Nagata, T.; Fujii, T.; Tagawa, T. Synergistic interaction of 5-aminolevulinic acid-based photodynamic therapy with simultaneous hyperthermia in an osteosarcoma tumor model. *Int. J. Oncol.* **2006**, *29*, 365–373. [CrossRef]
174. Wang, Z.; Zhang, F.; Shao, D.; Chang, Z.; Wang, L.; Hu, H.; Zheng, X.; Li, X.; Chen, F.; Tu, Z.; et al. Janus Nanobullets Combine Photodynamic Therapy and Magnetic Hyperthermia to Potentiate Synergetic Anti-Metastatic Immunotherapy. *Adv. Sci.* **2019**, *6*, 1901690. [CrossRef] [PubMed]
175. Di Corato, R.; Bealle, G.; Kolosnjaj-Tabi, J.; Espinosa, A.; Clement, O.; Silva, A.K.; Menager, C.; Wilhelm, C. Combining magnetic hyperthermia and photodynamic therapy for tumor ablation with photoresponsive magnetic liposomes. *ACS Nano* **2015**, *9*, 2904–2916. [CrossRef]
176. Pellosi, D.S.; Macaroff, P.P.; Morais, P.C.; Tedesco, A.C. Magneto low-density nanoemulsion (MLDE): A potential vehicle for combined hyperthermia and photodynamic therapy to treat cancer selectively. *Mater. Sci. Eng. C* **2018**, *92*, 103–111. [CrossRef] [PubMed]
177. Chen, W.; Zhang, J. Using nanoparticles to enable simultaneous radiation and photodynamic therapies for cancer treatment. *J. Nanosci. Nanotechnol.* **2006**, *6*, 1159–1166. [CrossRef]
178. Gadzhimagomedova, Z.; Zolotukhin, P.; Kit, O.; Kirsanova, D.; Soldatov, A. Nanocomposites for X-Ray Photodynamic Therapy. *Int. J. Mol. Sci.* **2020**, *21*, 4004. [CrossRef]
179. Hu, J.; Tang, Y.; Elmenoufy, A.H.; Xu, H.; Cheng, Z.; Yang, X. Nanocomposite-Based Photodynamic Therapy Strategies for Deep Tumor Treatment. *Small* **2015**, *11*, 5860–5887. [CrossRef]
180. Rimoldi, T.; Orsi, D.; Lagonegro, P.; Ghezzi, B.; Galli, C.; Rossi, F.; Salviati, G.; Cristofolini, L. CeF$_3$-ZnO scintillating nanocomposite for self-lighted photodynamic therapy of cancer. *J. Mater. Sci. Mater. Med.* **2016**, *27*, 159. [CrossRef] [PubMed]

181. Chen, M.H.; Jenh, Y.J.; Wu, S.K.; Chen, Y.S.; Hanagata, N.; Lin, F.H. Non-invasive Photodynamic Therapy in Brain Cancer by Use of Tb^{3+}-Doped LaF$_3$ Nanoparticles in Combination with Photosensitizer Through X-ray Irradiation: A Proof-of-Concept Study. *Nanoscale Res. Lett.* **2017**, *12*, 62. [CrossRef]
182. Yu, X.; Liu, X.; Wu, W.; Yang, K.; Mao, R.; Ahmad, F.; Chen, X.; Li, W. CT/MRI-Guided Synergistic Radiotherapy and X-ray Inducible Photodynamic Therapy Using Tb-Doped Gd-W-Nanoscintillators. *Angew. Chem. Int. Ed. Engl.* **2019**, *58*, 2017–2022. [CrossRef] [PubMed]
183. Kirakci, K.; Zelenka, J.; Rumlová, M.; Martinčík, J.; Nikl, M.; Ruml, T.; Lang, K. Octahedral molybdenum clusters as radiosensitizers for X-ray induced photodynamic therapy. *J. Mater. Chem. B* **2018**, *6*, 4301–4307. [CrossRef]
184. Rossi, F.; Bedogni, E.; Bigi, F.; Rimoldi, T.; Cristofolini, L.; Pinelli, S.; Alinovi, R.; Negri, M.; Dhanabalan, S.C.; Attolini, G.; et al. Porphyrin conjugated SiC/SiO$_x$ nanowires for X-ray-excited photodynamic therapy. *Sci. Rep.* **2015**, *5*, 7606. [CrossRef]
185. Juzenas, P.; Chen, W.; Sun, Y.P.; Coelho, M.A.; Generalov, R.; Generalova, N.; Christensen, I.L. Quantum dots and nanoparticles for photodynamic and radiation therapies of cancer. *Adv. Drug Deliv. Rev.* **2008**, *60*, 1600–1614. [CrossRef]
186. Yuan, Q.; Wu, Y.; Wang, J.; Lu, D.; Zhao, Z.; Liu, T.; Zhang, X.; Tan, W. Targeted bioimaging and photodynamic therapy nanoplatform using an aptamer-guided G-quadruplex DNA carrier and near-infrared light. *Angew. Chem. Int. Ed. Engl.* **2013**, *52*, 13965–13969. [CrossRef]
187. Yu, Z.; Sun, Q.; Pan, W.; Li, N.; Tang, B. A Near-Infrared Triggered Nanophotosensitizer Inducing Domino Effect on Mitochondrial Reactive Oxygen Species Burst for Cancer Therapy. *ACS Nano* **2015**, *9*, 11064–11074. [CrossRef]
188. Dinakaran, D.; Sengupta, J.; Pink, D.; Raturi, A.; Chen, H.; Usmani, N.; Kumar, P.; Lewis, J.D.; Narain, R.; Moore, R.B. PEG-PLGA nanospheres loaded with nanoscintillators and photosensitizers for radiation-activated photodynamic therapy. *Acta Biomater.* **2020**, *117*, 335–348. [CrossRef] [PubMed]
189. Chen, H.; Wang, G.D.; Chuang, Y.J.; Zhen, Z.; Chen, X.; Biddinger, P.; Hao, Z.; Liu, F.; Shen, B.; Pan, Z.; et al. Nanoscintillator-mediated X-ray inducible photodynamic therapy for in vivo cancer treatment. *Nano Lett.* **2015**, *15*, 2249–2256. [CrossRef]
190. Zhang, C.; Zhao, K.; Bu, W.; Ni, D.; Liu, Y.; Feng, J.; Shi, J. Marriage of scintillator and semiconductor for synchronous radiotherapy and deep photodynamic therapy with diminished oxygen dependence. *Angew. Chem. Int. Ed. Engl.* **2015**, *54*, 1770–1774. [CrossRef]
191. Chuang, Y.C.; Chu, C.H.; Cheng, S.H.; Liao, L.D.; Chu, T.S.; Chen, N.T.; Paldino, A.; Hsia, Y.; Chen, C.T.; Lo, L.W. Annealing-modulated nanoscintillators for nonconventional X-ray activation of comprehensive photodynamic effects in deep cancer theranostics. *Theranostics* **2020**, *10*, 6758–6773. [CrossRef]
192. Kotagiri, N.; Sudlow, G.P.; Akers, W.J.; Achilefu, S. Breaking the depth dependency of phototherapy with Cerenkov radiation and low-radiance-responsive nanophotosensitizers. *Nat. Nanotechnol.* **2015**, *10*, 370–379. [CrossRef]
193. Wang, Q.; Liu, N.; Hou, Z.; Shi, J.; Su, X.; Sun, X. Radioiodinated Persistent Luminescence Nanoplatform for Radiation-Induced Photodynamic Therapy and Radiotherapy. *Adv. Healthc. Mater.* **2021**, *10*, e2000802. [CrossRef]
194. Kamkaew, A.; Cheng, L.; Goel, S.; Valdovinos, H.F.; Barnhart, T.E.; Liu, Z.; Cai, W. Cerenkov Radiation Induced Photodynamic Therapy Using Chlorin e6-Loaded Hollow Mesoporous Silica Nanoparticles. *ACS Appl. Mater. Interfaces* **2016**, *8*, 26630–26637. [CrossRef]
195. Duan, D.; Liu, H.; Xu, Y.; Han, Y.; Xu, M.; Zhang, Z.; Liu, Z. Activating TiO$_2$ Nanoparticles: Gallium-68 Serves as a High-Yield Photon Emitter for Cerenkov-Induced Photodynamic Therapy. *ACS Appl. Mater. Interfaces* **2018**, *10*, 5278–5286. [CrossRef]
196. Ni, D.; Ferreira, C.A.; Barnhart, T.E.; Quach, V.; Yu, B.; Jiang, D.; Wei, W.; Liu, H.; Engle, J.W.; Hu, P.; et al. Magnetic Targeting of Nanotheranostics Enhances Cerenkov Radiation-Induced Photodynamic Therapy. *J. Am. Chem. Soc.* **2018**, *140*, 14971–14979. [CrossRef]
197. Clement, S.; Chen, W.; Deng, W.; Goldys, E.M. X-ray radiation-induced and targeted photodynamic therapy with folic acid-conjugated biodegradable nanoconstructs. *Int. J. Nanomed.* **2018**, *13*, 3553–3570. [CrossRef]
198. Wang, H.; Lv, B.; Tang, Z.; Zhang, M.; Ge, W.; Liu, Y.; He, X.; Zhao, K.; Zheng, X.; He, M.; et al. Scintillator-Based Nanohybrids with Sacrificial Electron Prodrug for Enhanced X-ray-Induced Photodynamic Therapy. *Nano Lett.* **2018**, *18*, 5768–5774. [CrossRef]
199. Park, W.; Cho, S.; Kang, D.; Han, J.H.; Park, J.H.; Lee, B.; Lee, J.; Kim, D.H. Tumor Microenvironment Targeting Nano-Bio Emulsion for Synergistic Combinational X-Ray PDT with Oncolytic Bacteria Therap. *Adv. Healthc. Mater.* **2020**, *9*, e1901812. [CrossRef]
200. McHale, A.P.; Callan, J.F.; Nomikou, N.; Fowley, C.; Callan, B. Sonodynamic Therapy: Concept, Mechanism and Application to Cancer Treatment. *Adv. Exp. Med. Biol.* **2016**, *880*, 429–450.
201. Ashush, H.; Rozenszajn, L.A.; Blass, M.; Barda-Saad, M.; Azimov, D.; Radnay, J.; Zipori, D.; Rosenschein, U. Apoptosis induction of human myeloid leukemic cells by ultrasound exposure. *Cancer Res.* **2000**, *60*, 1014–1020.
202. Umemura, S.; Yumita, N.; Nishigaki, R.; Umemura, K. Mechanism of cell damage by ultrasound in combination with hematoporphyrin. *Jpn. J. Cancer Res.* **1990**, *81*, 962–966. [CrossRef]
203. Ma, A.; Chen, H.; Cui, Y.; Luo, Z.; Liang, R.; Wu, Z.; Chen, Z.; Yin, T.; Ni, J.; Zheng, M.; et al. Metalloporphyrin Complex-Based Nanosonosensitizers for Deep-Tissue Tumor Theranostics by Noninvasive Sonodynamic Therapy. *Small* **2019**, *15*, e1804028. [CrossRef] [PubMed]
204. Lu, Y.G.; Wang, Y.Y.; Yang, Y.D.; Zhang, X.C.; Gao, Y.; Yang, Y.; Zhang, J.B.; Li, G.L. Efficacy of topical ALA-PDT combined with excision in the treatment of skin malignant tumor. *Photodiagn. Photodyn. Ther.* **2014**, *11*, 122–126. [CrossRef]

205. Yano, T.; Muto, M.; Minashi, K.; Iwasaki, J.; Kojima, T.; Fuse, N.; Doi, T.; Kaneko, K.; Ohtsu, A. Photodynamic therapy as salvage treatment for local failure after chemoradiotherapy in patients with esophageal squamous cell carcinoma: A phase II study. *Int. J. Cancer* **2012**, *131*, 1228–1234. [CrossRef] [PubMed]
206. Li, X.Y.; Tan, L.C.; Dong, L.W.; Zhang, W.Q.; Shen, X.X.; Lu, X.; Zheng, H.; Lu, Y.G. Susceptibility and Resistance Mechanisms During Photodynamic Therapy of Melanoma. *Front. Oncol.* **2020**, *10*, 597. [CrossRef]
207. McEwan, C.; Nesbitt, H.; Nicholas, D.; Kavanagh, O.N.; McKenna, K.; Loan, P.; Jack, I.G.; McHale, A.P.; Callan, J.F. Comparing the efficacy of photodynamic and sonodynamic therapy in non-melanoma and melanoma skin cancer. *Bioorg. Med. Chem.* **2016**, *24*, 3023–3028. [CrossRef]
208. An, Y.W.; Liu, H.Q.; Zhou, Z.Q.; Wang, J.C.; Jiang, G.Y.; Li, Z.W.; Wang, F.; Jin, H.T. Sinoporphyrin sodium is a promising sensitizer for photodynamic and sonodynamic therapy in glioma. *Oncol. Rep.* **2020**, *44*, 1596–1604. [CrossRef] [PubMed]
209. Xiong, W.; Wang, P.; Hu, J.; Jia, Y.; Wu, L.; Chen, X.; Liu, Q.; Wang, X. A new sensitizer DVDMS combined with multiple focused ultrasound treatments: An effective antitumor strategy. *Sci. Rep.* **2015**, *5*, 17485. [CrossRef]
210. Sadanala, K.C.; Chaturvedi, P.K.; Seo, Y.M.; Kim, J.M.; Jo, Y.S.; Lee, Y.K.; Ahn, W.S. Sono-photodynamic combination therapy: A review on sensitizers. *Anticancer Res.* **2014**, *34*, 4657–4664.
211. Chen, H.J.; Zhou, X.B.; Wang, A.L.; Zheng, B.Y.; Yeh, C.K.; Huang, J.D. Synthesis and biological characterization of novel rose bengal derivatives with improved amphiphilicity for sono-photodynamic therapy. *Eur. J. Med. Chem.* **2018**, *145*, 86–95. [CrossRef]
212. Sun, D.; Zhang, Z.; Chen, M.; Zhang, Y.; Amagat, J.; Kang, S.; Zheng, Y.; Hu, B.; Chen, M. Co-Immobilization of Ce6 Sono/Photosensitizer and Protonated Graphitic Carbon Nitride on PCL/Gelation Fibrous Scaffolds for Combined Sono-Photodynamic Cancer Therapy. *ACS Appl. Mater. Interfaces* **2020**, *12*, 40728–40739. [CrossRef]
213. Zhu, J.; Wang, Y.; Yang, P.; Liu, Q.; Hu, J.; Yang, W.; Liu, P.; He, F.; Bai, Y.; Gai, S.; et al. GPC3-targeted and curcumin-loaded phospholipid microbubbles for sono-photodynamic therapy in liver cancer cells. *Colloids Surf. B Biointerfaces* **2021**, *197*, 111358. [CrossRef] [PubMed]
214. Zhu, J.X.; Zhu, W.T.; Hu, J.H.; Yang, W.; Liu, P.; Liu, Q.H.; Bai, Y.X.; Xie, R. Curcumin-Loaded Poly(L-lactide-co-glycolide) Microbubble-Mediated Sono-photodynamic Therapy in Liver Cancer Cells. *Ultrasound Med. Biol.* **2020**, *46*, 2030–2043. [CrossRef]
215. Miyoshi, N.; Kundu, S.K.; Tuziuti, T.; Yasui, K.; Shimada, I.; Ito, Y. Combination of Sonodynamic and Photodynamic Therapy against Cancer Would Be Effective through Using a Regulated Size of Nanoparticles. *Nanosci. Nanoeng.* **2016**, *4*, 1–11. [CrossRef]
216. Li, L.; Rashidi, L.H.; Yao, M.; Ma, L.; Chen, L.; Zhang, J.; Zhang, Y.; Chen, W. CuS nanoagents for photodynamic and photothermal therapies: Phenomena and possible mechanisms. *Photodiagn. Photodyn. Ther.* **2017**, *19*, 5–14. [CrossRef]
217. Curcio, A.; Silva, A.K.A.; Cabana, S.; Espinosa, A.; Baptiste, B.; Menguy, N.; Wilhelm, C.; Abou-Hassan, A. Iron Oxide Nanoflowers @ CuS Hybrids for Cancer Tri-Therapy: Interplay of Photothermal Therapy, Magnetic Hyperthermia and Photodynamic Therapy. *Theranostics* **2019**, *9*, 1288–1302. [CrossRef]
218. Luo, L.; Sun, W.; Feng, Y.; Qin, R.; Zhang, J.; Ding, D.; Shi, T.; Liu, X.; Chen, X.; Chen, H. Conjugation of a Scintillator Complex and Gold Nanorods for Dual-Modal Image-Guided Photothermal and X-ray-Induced Photodynamic Therapy of Tumors. *ACS Appl. Mater. Interfaces* **2020**, *12*, 12591–12599. [CrossRef] [PubMed]
219. Kodumudi, K.N.; Woan, K.; Gilvary, D.L.; Sahakian, E.; Wei, S.; Djeu, J.Y. A novel chemoimmunomodulating property of docetaxel: Suppression of myeloid-derived suppressor cells in tumor bearers. *Clin. Cancer Res.* **2010**, *16*, 4583–4594. [CrossRef] [PubMed]
220. Chen, L.; Zhou, L.; Wang, C.; Han, Y.; Lu, Y.; Liu, J.; Hu, X.; Yao, T.; Lin, Y.; Liang, S.; et al. Tumor-Targeted Drug and CpG Delivery System for Phototherapy and Docetaxel-Enhanced Immunotherapy with Polarization toward M1-Type Macrophages on Triple Negative Breast Cancers. *Adv. Mater.* **2019**, *31*, e1904997. [CrossRef]
221. Yang, J.C.; Shang, Y.; Li, Y.H.; Cui, Y.; Yin, X.B. An "all-in-one" antitumor and anti-recurrence/metastasis nanomedicine with multi-drug co-loading and burst drug release for multi-modality therapy. *Chem. Sci.* **2018**, *9*, 7210–7217. [CrossRef]
222. Zhang, Y.; Wan, Y.; Chen, Y.; Blum, N.T.; Lin, J.; Huang, P. Ultrasound-Enhanced Chemo-Photodynamic Combination Therapy by Using Albumin "Nanoglue"-Based Nanotheranostics. *ACS Nano* **2020**, *14*, 5560–5569. [CrossRef]
223. Feng, L.; Gai, S.; He, F.; Dai, Y.; Zhong, C.; Yang, P.; Lin, J. Multifunctional mesoporous ZrO_2 encapsulated upconversion nanoparticles for mild NIR light activated synergistic cancer therapy. *Biomaterials* **2017**, *147*, 39–52. [CrossRef]
224. Hou, L.; Shan, X.; Hao, L.; Feng, Q.; Zhang, Z. Copper sulfide nanoparticle-based localized drug delivery system as an effective cancer synergistic treatment and theranostic platform. *Acta Biomater.* **2017**, *54*, 307–320. [CrossRef]
225. Li, Q.; Sun, L.; Hou, M.; Chen, Q.; Yang, R.; Zhang, L.; Xu, Z.; Kang, Y.; Xue, P. Phase-Change Material Packaged within Hollow Copper Sulfide Nanoparticles Carrying Doxorubicin and Chlorin e6 for Fluorescence-Guided Trimodal Therapy of Cancer. *ACS Appl. Mater. Interfaces* **2019**, *11*, 417–429. [CrossRef]
226. Xu, X.; Han, C.; Zhang, C.; Yan, D.; Ren, C.; Kong, L. Intelligent phototriggered nanoparticles induce a domino effect for multimodal tumor therapy. *Theranostics* **2021**, *11*, 6477–6490. [CrossRef] [PubMed]
227. Han, R.; Tang, K.; Hou, Y.; Yu, J.; Wang, C.; Wang, Y. Ultralow-intensity near infrared light synchronously activated collaborative chemo/photothermal/photodynamic therapy. *Biomater. Sci.* **2020**, *8*, 607–618. [CrossRef] [PubMed]
228. Xu, W.; Qian, J.; Hou, G.; Wang, Y.; Wang, J.; Sun, T.; Ji, L.; Suo, A.; Yao, Y. PEGylated hydrazided gold nanorods for pH-triggered chemo/photodynamic/photothermal triple therapy of breast cancer. *Acta Biomater.* **2018**, *82*, 171–183. [CrossRef]

229. Wen, J.; Yang, K.; Ding, X.; Li, H.; Xu, Y.; Liu, F.; Sun, S. In Situ Formation of Homogeneous Tellurium Nanodots in Paclitaxel-Loaded MgAl Layered Double Hydroxide Gated Mesoporous Silica Nanoparticles for Synergistic Chemo/PDT/PTT Trimode Combinatorial Therapy. *Inorg. Chem.* **2019**, *58*, 2987–2996. [CrossRef]
230. Obaid, G.; Broekgaarden, M.; Bulin, A.L.; Huang, H.C.; Kuriakose, J.; Liu, J.; Hasan, T. Photonanomedicine: A convergence of photodynamic therapy and nanotechnology. *Nanoscale* **2016**, *8*, 12471–12503. [CrossRef]
231. Mroz, P.; Hamblin, M.R. The immunosuppressive side of PDT. *Photochem. Photobiol. Sci.* **2011**, *10*, 751–758. [CrossRef] [PubMed]

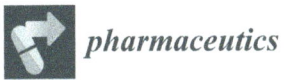

Review

Phthalocyanine and Its Formulations: A Promising Photosensitizer for Cervical Cancer Phototherapy

Lucimara R. Carobeli [1], Lyvia E. de F. Meirelles [1], Gabrielle M. Z. F. Damke [1], Edilson Damke [1], Maria V. F. de Souza [1], Natália L. Mari [1], Kayane H. Mashiba [1], Cristiane S. Shinobu-Mesquita [1], Raquel P. Souza [1], Vânia R. S. da Silva [1], Renato S. Gonçalves [2], Wilker Caetano [2] and Márcia E. L. Consolaro [1,*]

[1] Department of Clinical Analysis and Biomedicine, Universidade Estadual de Maringá, Maringá 87020-900, PR, Brazil; lucimaracarobeli@gmail.com (L.R.C.); lyvia.fmeirelles@gmail.com (L.E.d.F.M.); gabizago@gmail.com (G.M.Z.F.D.); edilsondamke@gmail.com (E.D.); mariavitoriafesouza@gmail.com (M.V.F.d.S.); nlmari95@gmail.com (N.L.M.); kayanehmashiba@gmail.com (K.H.M.); cristianeshinobu@gmail.com (C.S.S.-M.); raquelpantarotto@gmail.com (R.P.S.); vaniasela@gmail.com (V.R.S.d.S.)

[2] Department of Chemistry, Universidade Estadual de Maringá, Maringá 87020-900, PR, Brazil; rsonchini@gmail.com (R.S.G.); wcaetano@uem.br (W.C.)

* Correspondence: melconsolaro@gmail.com; Tel.: +55-44-3011-5455

Abstract: Cervical cancer is one of the most common causes of cancer-related deaths in women worldwide. Despite advances in current therapies, women with advanced or recurrent disease present poor prognosis. Photodynamic therapy (PDT) has emerged as an effective therapeutic alternative to treat oncological diseases such as cervical cancer. Phthalocyanines (Pcs) are considered good photosensitizers (PS) for PDT, although most of them present high levels of aggregation and are lipophilic. Despite many investigations and encouraging results, Pcs have not been approved as PS for PDT of invasive cervical cancer yet. This review presents an overview on the pathophysiology of cervical cancer and summarizes the most recent developments on the physicochemical properties of Pcs and biological results obtained both in vitro in tumor-bearing mice and in clinical tests reported in the last five years. Current evidence indicates that Pcs have potential as pharmaceutical agents for anti-cervical cancer therapy. The authors firmly believe that Pc-based formulations could emerge as a privileged scaffold for the establishment of lead compounds for PDT against different types of cervical cancer.

Keywords: phthalocyanine; uterine cervical neoplasms; photochemotherapy; in vitro; in vivo

1. Introduction

Cervical cancer is one of the most common types of cancer in women worldwide with an estimated 604,000 cases and 342,000 deaths worldwide in 2020 [1,2]. Globally, it represents the fourth most frequent type of cancer and the fourth leading cause of cancer death in women despite being considered nearly completely preventable because of the highly effective primary (human *Papillomavirus*-HPV vaccine) and secondary (screening) prevention measures available [1–4]. Specifically, since 2006 HPV vaccination has been available for the prevention of cervical cancer. However, even if high coverage vaccination can be quickly implemented, a substantial effect on disease burden will be seen after three to four decades and the short-term impact will require cervical screenings for older cohorts not covered by the HPV vaccine [3,4]. These preventable measures have not been equitably implemented across and within countries [2,5]. This is evidenced by the data that around 90% of cervical cancer cases occur in low- and medium-income countries (LMICs), where the incidence and disease-specific mortality continue to increase [2,6]. Indeed, the data show that rates remain disproportionately high in developing versus developed countries (18.8 vs. 11.3 per 100,000 for incidence; 12.4 vs. 5.2 per 100,000 for mortality) [2]. Additionally, analyzing data from different countries, cervical cancer is the most common type of cancer in 23 countries and the leading cause of cancer death in 36 countries, especially in sub-Saharan Africa, Melanesia, South America, and South-Eastern Asia [2]. All these data highlight that cervical cancer is a striking example of a global health disparity [6].

Surgery and radiation therapy are the most common options for the treatment of invasive cervical cancer. The type of treatment will depend on factors such as the stage of the disease; the size of the tumor; and personal factors, such as age and desire to have children [7]. The clinical staging of cervical cancer follows the guidelines of the International Federation of Gynecology and Obstetrics (FIGO) [8], and for treatment, patients can be grouped in early-stage disease; locally advanced disease; and advanced disease, which includes persistent, recurrent, or metastatic disease [9]. For early-stage disease, surgery is the primary treatment modality with high cure rates and overall 5-year survival up to 92% [10]. Surgery or radiation associated with chemotherapy can be used [11,12]. In advanced cervical cancer, the main therapeutic option is chemoradiation with a platinum-based agent [13], and chemotherapy before surgery or chemoradiation that is associated with inferior outcomes compared to concurrent chemoradiation [14]. Specifically, chemotherapy can work as an adjuvant when used immediately after the primary treatment of the tumor by surgery or radiation therapy. It can also be a neoadjuvant when performed before local treatment with the aim of reducing the tumor size and providing adequate conditions for the subsequent surgical and/or radiotherapy treatment. In addition, there is concomitant chemo-radiotherapy that is administered simultaneously with radiotherapy to enhance the treatment effect and increase the patient's survival; however, the side effects tend to be worse [11]. The most commonly used chemotherapeutics for the treatment of cervical cancer include cisplatin, carboplatin, paclitaxel, topotecan, and gemcitabine. Cisplatin is the most effective cytotoxic agent against metastatic cervical cancer; in addition, it increases sensitivity to radiotherapy [15]. The side effects of chemotherapy depend on the type of drug, the dose administered, and the duration of treatment. These effects are temporary and can include nausea and vomiting, loss of appetite, mouth sores, hair loss, inflammation in the mouth, infection, bleeding or bruising after minor cuts or injuries, and shortness of breath [11].

The use of concomitant chemoradiotherapy improves the 5-year survival rates of patients with advanced cervical cancer. Nevertheless, once post-treatment failure occurs, the 1-year survival rates are less than 20%. Therefore, the occurrence of local recurrence and distant metastasis is still very common in these patients, significantly decreasing survival rates [16]. Therefore, early-stage and locally advanced disease can be cured, but women with advanced or recurrent disease present a poor prognosis. Despite these alarming facts, efficient treatment methods are still lacking. This underscores the need for different treatment strategies, particularly for advanced cervical cancer, which is still the leading cause of death in developing nations with limited access to care [13].

In the last 20 years, little progress has been made on the development of novel therapeutic modalities for preinvasive (cervical intraepithelial neoplasia-CIN) or invasive cervical cancer [17]. Since the first use of a hematoporphyrin derivative in conjunction with red light irradiation to kill tumor cells in 1975, photodynamic therapy (PDT) has attracted attention as a promising strategy for cancer treatment [18]. The main elements of PDT are a photoactive drug (PS), light at an appropriate wavelength, and molecular oxygen [9,10]. Light excites the PS to its triplet state, interacting with the oxygen present in the tissue to produce reactive oxygen species (ROS) via a type I or type II mechanism. This interaction results in the production of free radicals [11] or singlet oxygen ($^1O_2$) [12], respectively. PDT is an attractive treatment modality for cancer because the PS, light, and oxygen separately do not present any toxic effects on the body, unlike chemotherapy, which induces systemic toxicity and radiotherapy that damage neighboring normal tissues [19]. PDT is currently applied against numerous cancers, and it is clinically approved in the United States for esophageal and non-small cell lung cancers. Additionally, PDT is being tested in clinical trials for several other types of cancers, including glioma, pediatric brain cancer, prostate cancer, head and neck cancer, cervical cancer, pancreatic cancer, breast cancer, and oral cancer [18]. For cervical cancer, the Photocure system (Cevira®), a multinational Phase III trial, was developed to treat persistent oncogenic HPV and cervical precancerous lesions. This technology is based on the hexylaminolevulinate (prodrug of protoporphyrin IX) that is administered locally to the cervix by a drug and light delivery device. Cevira has been shown in patients to be efficient and safe [20]. Overall, PDT has the following advantages in the treatment of CIN and invasive cervical cancer: localized treatment through light application, HPV inactivation if properly applied, selectivity of action in dysplastic and neoplastic cells, the possibility of repeated use without leading to cumulative toxicity, the possibility of combination with chemotherapy and radiotherapy to obtain better results, and the improvement of antitumor immunity helping in tumor elimination as well as tumor control in the medium and long term [21]. Moreover, PDT does not induce systemic side effects and can be repeated several times without tumor resistance, with a short delay between consecutive therapies [22]. Finally, PDT does not require anesthesia in many patients and generally does not cause bleeding, which makes its use applicable to the outpatient setting [17].

A PS should ideally have the following key features: (1) be a pure compound; (2) present a long life of the triplet reactive excited species generated by the photoactive pathways (greater than 500 ns), enough to react with molecular oxygen and induce ROS production; (3) present a strong absorption peak in the red to near-infrared spectral region (NIR) (between 650 and 800 nm) because the absorption of single photons with wavelengths longer than 800 nm does not provide enough energy to excite oxygen to its singlet state. Additionally, the NIR is used because most tissues transmit light reasonably well in this spectral domain; (4) present a substantial triplet quantum yield leading to good production of ROS upon irradiation; (5) no dark toxicity and relatively rapid clearance from normal tissues, thereby minimizing the side effects of PDT; and (6) present good solubility and biocompatibility [23–29]. Since the discovery of PDT, continuous efforts have been made to identify new ideal PS with this set of characteristics.

Historically, the first approaches to PDT are found in ancient texts such as the Egyptian medical treatise Ebers Papyrus and the Atharvaveda from the Hinduism. Despite this background, the observation of photochemical sensitization of tissues was first performed in detail by Raab (1900) in Germany and shortly afterwards by Von Tappeiner (1900), who coined the term "photodynamic action" to describe the treatment of skin tumors by using topical administration of eosin combined with sunlight [30]. The majority of PS currently in use for PDT are cyclic tetrapyrrolic structures: porphyrins and their analogs; chlorins; bacteriochlorins; and phthalocyanines (Pcs). Among them, Pcs include a variety of substances considered good PS for cancer PDT, with activation in the range from 670 to 690 nm and well-defined tissue penetration in the target cells. Since Pcs absorb long-wavelength light strongly; localization is in their cells; and they have triplet yield, among other features, they can be used in small doses [31]. Despite their interesting optical properties in the NIR, the applications of these hydrophobic planar molecules were not fully performed because of poor solubility, which is crucial in order to reach the therapeutic target and also a tendency to form aggregates. Aggregation causes the formation of exiplexes upon light absorption, quenches excited state lifetimes, and diminishes photophysical properties. More specifically, the formation of aggregates in solution decreases the capacity to produce singlet oxygen because the photochemical activity is exclusively related to monomer species. Thus, aggregates decrease not only the photoactivity of the Pc but also limit the access to the neoplastic cells, affecting its bioavailability [32–34]. Additionally, depending on the dose, some Pcs such as ZnPc can cause skin phototoxicity in patients [32]. As result, several studies sought for structural variations in Pcs molecules, such as incorporation of appropriate aromatic substitutions or an element in the molecule's core structure to reduce the degree of hydrophobicity. These attempts led to the development of easy synthetic routes for a new generation of Pcs with improved solubility and reduced aggregation [34,35]. Another option to increase the solubility and bioavailability of hydrophobic Pcs and their derivatives is a formulation using various drug delivery systems (DDSs) such as nanoemulsions and liposomal, among others [36], which present themselves as feasible approaches to increase Pcs' biocompatibility. Despite these advances and encouraging results, Pcs are not yet approved as PS for invasive cervical cancer PDT.

This review presents an overview of the pathophysiology of cervical cancer that may influence the interpretation of results from studies with different formulations using Pcs for PDT against cancer. We also review the photophysical properties of Pcs, the in vitro effects and antitumor mechanism of action in cell cultures, and the in vivo effectiveness as anticancer agents in a tumor-bearing mice model and clinical trials reported in the last five years. There is also an emphasis on various strategies to enhance the functions of Pcs, showing the great promise of this class of functional dyes as advanced PS for PDT of CIN and cervical cancer.

2. Cervical Cancer

2.1. Basic Concepts

The endocervical canal is lined with the stratified squamous epithelium and columnar epithelium, which cover the ectocervix and endocervix, respectively. The transition zone between these cells is called the squamocolumnar junction. Any premalignant cellular transformation occurs mostly at the squamocolumnar junction and is closely associated with high-risk HPV types. The premalignant changes or dysplasia of squamous cells in the cervical epithelium are collectively known as CIN [6,8]. CIN grade 3 (CIN 3) precedes the development of invasive cervical cancer by 10–20 years, making cervical cancer preventable if these lesions are detected and effectively treated [37]. Most of the therapeutic methods for the treatment of CIN3 can be divided into two basic groups: (a) destructive methods (diathermocoagulation, cryodestruction, and laser evaporation) and (b) removal of the pathologic tissue (surgical, laser, or electrosurgical excision). Different treatment modalities, including cold-knife excision, electrocautery, cryosurgery, laser ablation, and large-loop excision of the transformation zone (LLETZ), have shown high success rates [12]. However, the most common adverse effects of such treatment are hemorrhage, traumatization of subjacent tissues with a formation of rough scraps, stenosis, and stricture of the cervical canal. Changes in the anatomic structure of the cervix uteri lead to the loss of functionality; specifically, a reduction of cervical secretions results in a decrease in the probability of conception, an increase in spontaneous abortion, an increase in the level of perinatal mortality, and impairment to normal delivery [38]. Indeed, the optimal management of CIN3 requires development and introduction of novel therapeutic approaches. On the other hand, mild and moderate lesions (CIN1 and CIN2), which may precede CIN3, are generally not treated but require periodic long-term screening to monitor its development or disappearance [39]. However, considering that the accuracy of Papanicolaou (Pap) smear in diagnosing cervical precancerous lesions is low, sometimes contradictory results between biopsy and Pap smear are reported, which hinders the clinical decision concerning whether or not to adopt treatment as well as the type of treatment.

The main types of invasive cervical cancer are squamous cell carcinoma (SCC) (around 70% of cases), adenocarcinoma (AC) (around 25% of cases), adenosquamous cell carcinoma (ASC), neuroendocrine-endocrine cancer, glassy cell carcinoma, and undifferentiated cancer [40]. It is common knowledge that the most important cause of cervical cancer is persistent HPV infection. HPV is detected in 99% of cervical tumors [41], with HPV-16 being the most prevalent type, followed by HPV-18; together, these types account for around 70% of SCC and over 80% of AC cases [42,43]. However, oncogenic or high-risk HPV types (hrHPV) are virtually necessary but not sufficient causes for cervical cancer development [41]. Most hrHPV infections are eventually cleared, but some cases progress to high-grade squamous intraepithelial lesions (HSIL) (10% of HPV infections) and invasive cervical cancer (<1% of HPV infections) [44–47]. The reasons for this variable natural history are poorly understood [48], but it is generally assumed that other causes or cofactors are important for the development of neoplasia in HPV-infected women [44,46,49]. Other important cofactors to cervical cancer development include immunosuppression (particularly human immunodeficiency virus), smoking, parenthood (a higher number of full-term pregnancies increases risk), use of oral contraceptive [50], and sexually transmitted infections (such as chronic infection by *Chlamydia trachomatis* [48]).

HPVs are small, non-enveloped, double-stranded DNA viruses that exhibit a strict tropism for cutaneous and mucosal (e.g., oropharynx, anogenital tract) epithelium [51,52]. At present, more than 200 different types of HPV have been identified [53] and approximately 54 are able to infect the reproductive tract mucosa [54], with 12 oncogenic types classified as group 1 carcinogens [55]. The most common hrHPV types include HPV-16, 18, 31, 33, 35, 39, and 45 [54]. HPV infects the actively proliferating, undifferentiated basal keratinocytes of the stratified squamous cervical epithelium that are thought to become exposed through a microlesion [56]. Two viral promoters, early (E) and late (L), regulate viral gene expression and are active at different stages in the life cycle [57]. The establishment and maintenance of HPV genomes in infected cells are associated with the expression of early genes E5, E6, and E7, which encode their respective oncoproteins, as well as the replication proteins E1 and E2. In the basal undifferentiated cells, viral genomes are subsequently maintained at low copy number by replicating along with cellular DNA [52,58]. During cell division, basal cells leave the basal layer, migrate to the suprabasal region and begin to differentiate. At this stage, the viral genome is divided among the daughter cells, which, when migrating to the upper layers of the epithelium during the differentiation process, continue with the active cell cycle. In differentiated layers of the epithelium, the viral DNA is packaged into new capsids and virus progeny is released from the upper layer of the epithelium [57,59–63].

The development of cervical cancer is associated with loss of regulation of the HPV production cycle, an event observed in persistent hrHPV infections, which tend to integrate their genome to the host cell [46,49]. During the integration process, the viral genome may lose the E4 gene and part of the E2 gene, which play roles in controlling the transcription of other viral genes. The consequence of the loss of E2 function is an increase in the expression of the E6 and E7 genes. In this scenario, there is no maturation of host cells and no production of new viral particles [46,64,65]. Thus, HPV oncogenic potential depends on the expression of E6/E7 genes whose products, the E6 and E7 proteins, have as their main target the p53 and pRb proteins of the host genome, inducing lack of control of the cell cycle [66–72].

In face of the complexity of cervical carcinogenesis and the different types of hrHPV involved, it is important to correctly apply in vitro and in vivo models that represent this complexity for testing molecules or biologics for anti cervical cancer drug development.

2.2. Human Cervical Cancer-Derived Cell Lines to In Vitro and In Vivo (Tumor-Bearing Mice) Studies

Human tumor-derived cell lines present a historically important role in the discovery and development of new therapeutic agents against cancer. In vitro studies using immortalized human cancer cell lines provide controlled conditions to assess the effectiveness of drugs and provide unrestricted availability of human-derived material [73]. For the discovery of new anti cervical cancer drugs, human tumor-derived cell lines are even more important, since no animal model of HPV infection exists [74]. This is due to the fact that Papillomaviruses are strictly species-specific and even in experimental conditions do not infect any other host than their natural one. There is only one known case of cross infection between horses and other equidae by bovine papillomavirus (BPV) types 1 and 2. Additionally, HPV is strictly tissue-restricted and cannot be propagated in vitro. Consequently, to evaluate tumors triggered by HPV on in vivo animal studies, an experimental model of tumor induction could be performed where researchers would inoculate the human cervical cancer-derived cell lines through subcutaneous injection in mice, for example, tumor-bearing mice. Therefore, major knowledge regarding the HPV life cycle, the oncogenicity, and the synergy with cofactors was first established in vitro or by animal papillomaviruses in vivo. However, DNA sequences of HPV-16, -18, -45, and -68 have been found in cell lines established from human cervical carcinomas [75–77]. Since animal models for cellular transformation by HPV are not available, cervical cancer cell lines are unique tools for understanding the biology and tumor response as well for testing small molecules or biologics for anti-cancer drug development.

At present, immortalized cervical cancer cell lines available in major cell repositories, including American Type Culture Collection (ATCC) and European Collection of Authenticated Cell Cultures (ECACC), represent six cervical cancers (not considering HeLa-derived cell lines) [78], reflecting the two main types of cervical cancer (SCC and AD) and the two main types of hrHPV involved in cervical carcinogenesis (HPV-16 and 18) as well as HPV-45 and HPV-68. Still, the availability of a series of HPV-positive (Hela, SiHa, Caski, MS751, ME-180, and C-4I) and HPV-negative (C-33A) human cervical carcinoma cell lines provides the opportunity to evaluate whether a new drug candidate is effective or not in both scenarios. Table 1 summarizes the main human immortalized cervical cancer cell lines and their characteristics.

Table 1. Main human immortalized cervical cancer cell lines available for in vitro studies from uterine cervix tissues.

Cell Line	Histologic Type	Donor Age	HPV	p53	pRb
HeLa (ATCC® CCL-2™)	Adenocarcinoma	31	HPV-18	Positive (low)	Positive (normal)
SiHa (ATCC® HTB-35™)	Squamous cell carcinoma	55	HPV-16, 1 to 2 copies per cell	Positive	Positive
CasKi (ATCC® CRM-CRL-1550™)	Squamous cell carcinoma	40	HPV-16, about 600 copies per cell, and HPV-18	NA	NA
C-33A (ATCC® HTB-31™)	Squamous cell carcinoma	66	Negative	Positive	Positive
MS751 (ATCC® HTB-34™)	Squamous cell carcinoma	47	HPV-18 HPV-45	NA	NA
ME-180 (ATCC® HTB-33™)	Squamous cell carcinoma	66	HPV DNA with higher homology to HPV-68 than HPV-18	Positive	Positive
C-4 I (ATCC® CRL-1594™)	Squamous cell carcinoma	41	HPV-18	NA	NA

NA: not applicable; pRb, retinoblastoma protein; p53, protein 53; and HPV, human papillomavirus.

3. Photodynamic Therapy (PDT)

3.1. Principles and Applications

PDT is a promising treatment modality. The light is absorbed by the PS either systemically, locally, or topically for the treatment of a variety of pathologies such as oncological [79], cardiovascular [80], dermatological [81], ophthalmic [82], bacterial, viral, and parasitic infections [83]. Possibly the main use of PDT in the world up until now has been its use in ophthalmology, i.e., in the treatment of wet age-related macular degeneration and PVC [82]. Photoactivation of the PS in the presence of oxygen and a target cell or tissue are necessary for PDT. Specifically, the PS is excited by light inducing two photochemical mechanisms (type I and type II). In Type I, the PS in its excited triplet state interacts with a biomolecule transferring or acquiring one electron/hydrogen via the radical mechanism, leading to the generation of ROS, including superoxide anions ($O_2^{-\bullet}$), singlet oxygen ($^1O_2$), hydroxyl radicals ($HO^\bullet$), and hydrogen peroxide (H_2O_2), that attack cellular targets and damage cellular components. However, original free radicals can cause cellular damage directly [19,36,83,84]. In Type II, the direct energy transfer occurs from the PS in the triplet excited state to the oxygen in the fundamental triplet state, producing cytotoxic singlet oxygen [19,83,84]. Singlet oxygen presents a short lifetime in a time-scale of microseconds, but a sufficient concentration of highly cytotoxic singlet oxygen can induce irreversible cell damage [36]. Furthermore, the location of the PS changes over time, and therefore, soon after the application, it is located in the vasculature and PDT can mainly result in the closure of blood vessels. Although both types of reactions (Type I and II) take place at the same time, most PS used for anti-cancer PDT are believed to operate via the Type II rather than the Type I mechanism [84–88], possibly due to ROS generation via Type

II chemistry being mechanistically much simpler than via Type I. After photochemical reaction, light-mediated destruction of the PS can occur [89] or the PS can return to its ground state without modifications and can be prepared to repeat the excitation-energy transfer process multiple times [23,90–92] (Scheme 1).

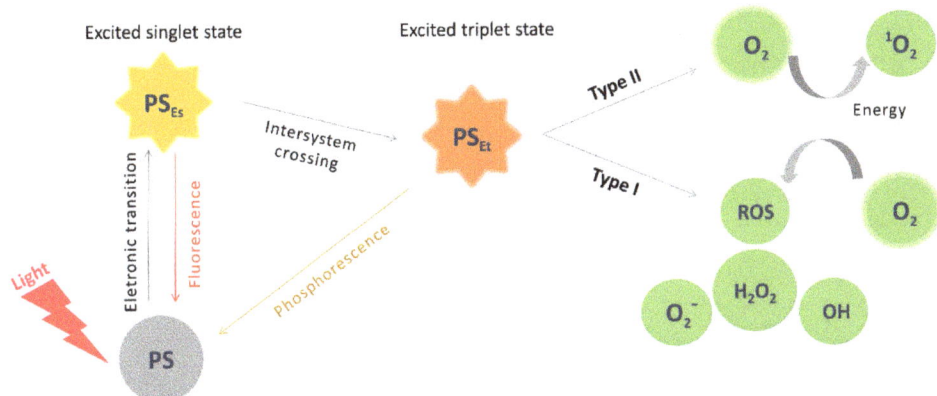

Scheme 1. Photodynamic reaction mechanism.

As mentioned earlier, in order to ensure high effectiveness in PDT, is important that the PS present some outstanding characteristics, such as low (or no) toxicity to normal tissue, high therapeutic selectivity, non-prolonged photosensitivity, long circulation time in plasma, and enhanced accumulation in target tissue [93].

Several types of fiber tip or light applicator, e.g., lens, cylindrical diffuser, and spherical diffuser, have been developed to facilitate the light delivery and to optimize the light transmission and distribution in the lesion site. Lens-based fiber-optic light distributors are very useful for the frontal irradiation of superficial lesions as the optical lens can offer better light uniformity and beam expansion. The thin flexible fiber with microlens tip is particularly suitable for endoscopic applications. Recently, macrobendings (two perpendicular mode scramblers) have been used in PDT fibers to improve the uniformity of light beam [94]. The aforementioned Cevira technology clearly emphasizes the importance of developing light distribution devices specifically dedicated to the cervix [20].

3.2. PDT on Cancer

PDT effectiveness on cancer treatment is closely related to the high selectivity of PS accumulation rate in the cancer tissue. The high selectivity in PDT comes from a partially selective accumulation of the drug combined with the selective application of light. Consequently, the short lifetime of ROS especies can be enough to generate the photodynamic activity and oxidative damage to endogenous biomolecules (e.g., proteins and DNAs), leading to cell death via apoptosis, necrosis, or autophagy-associated mechanisms [95–99]. ROS can also be indirectly related to stimulation of the transcription and release of inflammation mediators [100]. In addition, an elevated ROS level leads to cellular oxidation process by damaging plasma membranes and cell organelles and subsequent alteration in permeability and transport function between intra and extracellular media [101]. PDT targets include tumor cells, tissue microvasculature, and the host's inflammatory and immune systems. The combination of all these components is necessary for the long-term control of the tumor [36,102,103] (Figure 1).

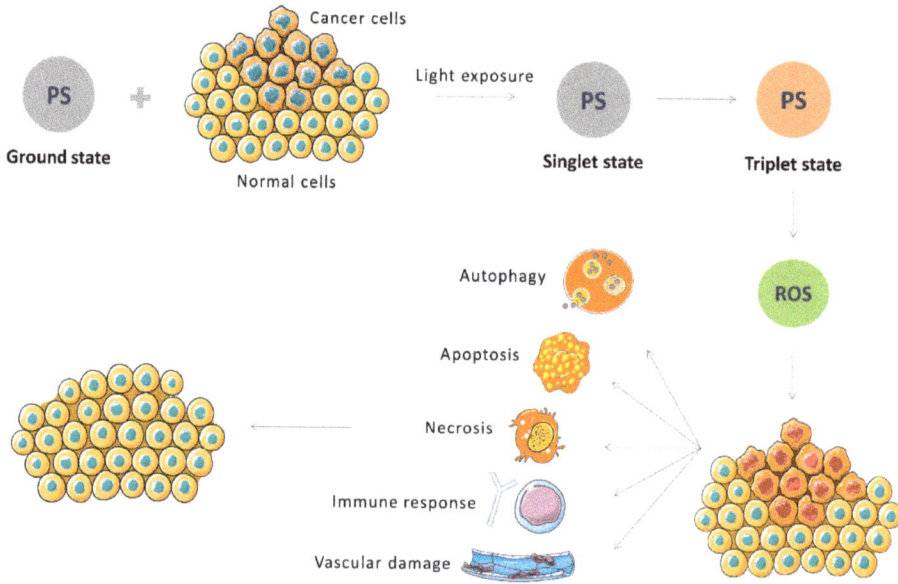

Figure 1. Photodynamic therapy (PDT) for cancer treatment.

The extent of damage and the cell death pathways involved depend on the type and concentration of the PS, its subcellular location, the energy applied, and the type of tumor [104]. The uptake of the PS by cancer cells as well as the localization within or on the cell surface depend on its chemical characteristics [105–107]. Hydrophobic PS tend to diffuse rapidly into plasma membranes and gather in intracellular membrane structures such as mitochondria and endoplasmic reticulum (ER). Hydrophilic PS tend to be internalized by endocytosis or transport by lipids and serum proteins [79,84]. After internalization, the intracellular location of the PS can be highly specific or quite broad [79,84] and has been reported to include the ER, mitochondria, Golgi complex, lysosomes, and plasma membrane [79,84]. Furthermore, it is very important that the PS does not accumulate in cell nuclei in order to limit DNA damage and prevent the appearance of genetically resistant cells [79]. Importantly, the location of the PS in cells is critical to determine the cell death pathway resulting from PDT and consequently the cell response to photodamage [105–107]. In this sense, it is very important to understand the preferential subcellular location of the PS in order to predict its cytotoxic potential [105–108]. The best described cytotoxic effects of organelle-specific PDT are in mitochondria, lysosomes, and ER [104].

As discussed above, PDT induces cell death via necrosis, apoptosis, or autophagy. The predominant mechanism depends on the PS and light dose, cell type, and subcellular localization [109,110]. The production of ROS at the mitochondrial, lysosomal, or ER location of the PS can directly initiate apoptotic cell death [111], which can be defined as a type of programmed cell death. Apoptosis is an induced and regulated process that activates a family of proteins (known as caspase) as well as precise cellular events, which degrade nucleic and polypeptide materials [103]. Necrosis is a non-programmed cell death and is more often observed when the PS site of action is in the plasma membrane and/or when it is activated with high-energy doses [79]. In order to suppress undesired damage to normal tissues, this effect should in general be avoided [112]. On the other hand, necrosis is an unscheduled cell death and is most often observed when the PS localizes in the plasma membrane and/or when it is activated by high doses of energy [79]. In the latter case, it is called accidental necrosis, and in order to prevent damage to normal cells, it must be avoided [112] with the use of appropriate doses of energy. Some reports have suggested that a pronounced inflammatory response resulting from necrotic cell death after PDT is important because it aids the immune-stimulating function of PDT [113]. Finally, the autophagic pathway is an evolutionarily old cytoprotective mechanism that aims to reestablish homeostasis [105,114,115]. This is a death pathway that appears not to be limited to the subcellular compartment in which PS accumulates [105,114]. The induction of autophagy appears to be a common response in PDT protocols [114], despite the role of autophagy as a factor in PDT-induced cell death is not yet clear. Despite this, PDT-induced autophagy appears to play a prosurvival role in apoptosis-competent cells and possibly a prodeath role in apoptosis-defective cells [105,114]. Additionally, when impaired or insufficient autophagy is triggered, induction of cell death is the most common result observed [105,114,115].

Although PDT has been proven as an effective broad-spectrum therapeutic, and it has been used with relative success in the field of oncology specially for the treatment of superficial oncologic lesions [116,117]. Recent advances in fiber optic technology have enabled the use of PDT far beyond its dermatological applications. Light sources such as lasers can be coupled with fiber optic systems to allow deep or difficult-to-treat tumors to be treated with PDT, such as urinary bladder, digestive tract, and brain and breast tumors [118]. Moreover, PDT can be used in association with other therapeutic techniques such as surgery or chemotherapy. In the case of surgery for tumor resection, PDT can help to destroy any remaining cancer cells after surgery. Several trials have demonstrated synergistic effects by combining PDT with low-dose chemotherapeutics [118–120]. For example, the PS can overcome the multi-drug resistance of the chemotherapeutic, whereas the chemotherapeutic can address the limitations of light penetration and hypoxia-related resistance in PDT [120].

Regarding the light power, it was previously established that the fluence rate affects the PDT tumor response. A high fluence rate decreases or even totally inhibits tumor control. The influence of fluence rate is not restricted to cytocidal effects, but it can also be seen in sublethal conditions such as vascular permeability. This has been shown to be true in pre-clinical and clinical settings. Therefore, this is an extremely important parameter in PDT in vitro and in vivo studies [121].

Several PS are in clinical use or undergoing clinical trials to treat cancer. Among them, the hematoporphyrin derivative (Photofrin), a first-generation PS with prolonged cutaneous phototoxicity can be highlighted. Photofrin is a HPLC-purified form of hematoporphyrin and has already been approved by the Food and Drug Administration (FDA) for the palliative treatment of obstructive diseases such as lung and esophageal cancers. Other PS can still be mentioned. Among them, a second generation have improved pharmacokinetics and reduced skin photosensitivity, such as benzoporphyrin derivative (BPD), 5-ethylamino-9-diethyl-aminobenzo [a] phenothiazine chloride (EtNBS), silicon phthalocyanine (Pc4), m-tetrahydroxyphenylchlorine (mTHPC), mesochlorin e6 (Mce6), and mono-L-aspartylchlorin e6 (NPe6). Additionally, there are several other PS at different stages of development [122].

3.3. Pcs as Photosensitizers for Cancer PDT

Pcs are referred to as tetrabenzotetraazaporphyrins and belong to the group of 2nd generation PS. Pcs are synthetic macromolecules related to tetra-aza porphyrins (porphyrazines) and have a benzene ring fused to each of four pyrrole subunits, which are linked by four nitrogen atoms (like porphyrazines macrocycle) instead of four bridging carbon atoms in porphyrin macrocycle [123]. Pcs are usually prepared in the form of complexes with metal cations such as zinc, aluminum, and gallium, co-ordinated to the centre of the macrocycle. This is due to the fact that during synthesis transition, metal cation helps to close the ring to easily form a macrocycle. The photophysical properties of Pcs are strongly influenced by the presence and nature of the central metal ion and result in metallophthalocyanines (MPcs) with high singlet oxygen quantum yields [31,124–129].

Considering that Pcs are flexible and stable compounds that improved light absorption capabilities, they have been used but not limited to chemical sensors and semiconductors, in nonlinear optics and as PS [130,131]. The first metal-free Pcs were discovered by Braun and Tcherniac in 1907 as a product during the preparation of ortho-cyanobenzamide from phthalamide in acetone (Scheme 2) [103,132,133]. Pcs can be obtained by the classic template reactions starting from diverse precursors, such as phthalonitrile (PN), o-cyanobenzamide, 1,3-diiminoisoindoline (1,3-D), phthalimide (PM), and phthalic acid, generally in high-boiling non-aqueous solvents at elevated temperatures or electrochemically from phthalonitrile [103,133]. No characterization studies were performed until 1929, when Linstead and co-workers synthesized and elucidated their structure as tetraazabenzoporphyrin [134–137]. Therefore, Pcs evolved from porphyrins and share some features with their precursors. Moreover, it is a highly efficient PS with a high fluorescence quantum yield and improved spectroscopic properties that are within the therapeutic window for PDT applications in relation to its precursor [138,139]. Overall, most Pcs have been extensively studied as a PS in PDT of cancer due several characteristics, including chemical stability under physiological conditions, optimal selectivity in tumor cells, quick clearance from the body, low cytotoxicity in the dark with high phototoxicity, absorption in the optical transmission window of biological tissues, and high quantum yield of singlet oxygen production [121,140,141].

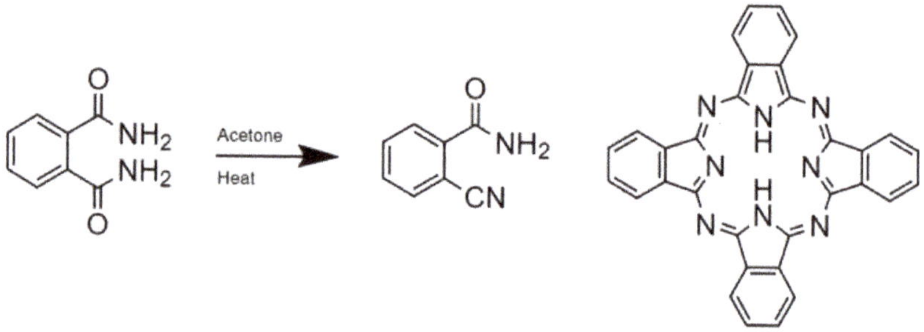

Scheme 2. Synthesis of the first metal-free phthalocyanine as a product during the preparation of ortho-cyanobenzamide from phthalamide in acetone.

Among the Pcs, MPcs have been identified as strong inducers of cyto damage and preferentially accumulate in tumor cells, where they stimulate photo damages in various in vitro and in vivo tumor models [142,143]. In vitro, MPcs family members were used to investigate their phototherapeutic activities in various cancer cell lines, including lung, colon, esophageal, cervical, and breast cancer cells [144–147]. Still, several MPc-based photosensitizers have been used in clinical trials against cancer such as CGP55847 (liposomal formulation of unsubstituted ZnPc), photosens (Pc derivative containing aluminum as the central metal), and photocyanine (isomeric mixture of di-(potassium sulfonate)-di-phthalimidomethyl ZnPc) [148,149]. Finally, among the Pcs evaluated so far in the clinic, Pc4, a silicon-based MPc developed by Vitex/USA, presented the greatest potential against breast, human colon, and ovarian cancers [150,151].

3.4. Pcs Optimization of Photophysical Properties and Biocompatibility

Pcs are large planar aromatic systems composed of four isoindole units linked by nitrogen atoms. Therefore, Pcs present the ability to form stable chelates with at least sixty metal and metalloid ions inserted into the central ring replacing two hydrogens originating the MPcs [36] (Figure 2). Whereas the properties of MPcs vary according to the nature of the central ion, the selection of this ion as well as the synthetic modifications offer numerous options to control their physical properties. Therefore, closed-shell diamagnetic Pcs present higher yields, longer lifetimes of triplet states, and greater tumor retention compared to paramagnetic Pcs, being more suitable for PDT [90,124,152–155].

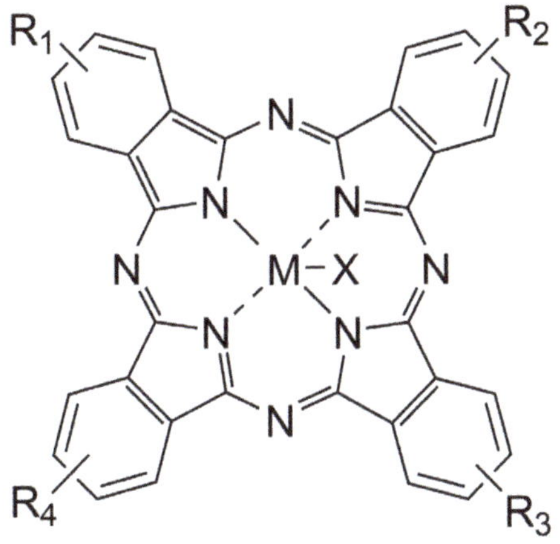

Figure 2. General chemical structure of metallated phthalocyanines (MPcs).

As discussed above, unsubstituted Pcs and their metal complexes suffer poor solubility in water and aggregation tendency, limiting their clinical application [32–34]. However, due to the chemical structure of PCs, it is possible to introduce various peripheral (macrocycle) and axial (coordination to the central metal ion) substitutions that modulate the tendency for aggregation, pharmacokinetics, biodistribution, and solubility, as well as fine-tuning of NIR absorbance [90,156–159]. The advantage of increasing solubility through appropriate replacement is that it allows for direct biological administration without the need for an additional vehicle [36].

Typical substitutions to the periphery of the Pcs macrocycle are sulfonation, phosphonation [127,160], glycosylation [161], or carboxylation, or addition of other soluble substituents such as glucose, quaternary amino, hydroxyl, or nitro groups [162]. These peripheral substitutions generate Pcs with increased solubility and reduced tendency to aggregate [90,162]. Suitable ions for axial substitution of the Pcs central ion are Al^{3+} with one or Si^{4+} and Ge^{4+}, with two coordination sites. MPcs not substituted with central ions, such as silicon or iron, tend to bond through oxo-bridges. Typical organic substitutes are soluble polymers such as poly(ethylene glycol) or poly(vinyl alcohol). Shorter polymers tend to shorten plasma half-life, but polymers with longer chains significantly prolong plasma half-life compared to unsubstituted MPcs. Axial substitution generally decreases the MPcs aggregation tendency and modulates solubility among other properties [36,163,164]. Additionally, exocyclically metallated Pcs are also an option to improve the properties of Pcs [165].

The solubility and bioavailability of hydrophobic Pcs can be further improved with the use of DDSs. Furthermore, DDSs also have the advantages of improving efficacy and/or reduced toxicity of a PS and delivering them to targeted tissues [36]. Some examples of DDSs used in PCs are liposomes, micelles, nanocapsules, microemulsion, polymeric nanoparticles, solid lipid particles, niosomes, and carbon nanotubes. The use of formulations with DDSs has currently been considered as a very promising strategy to control Pcs' biological properties [166]. Finally, mitochondria are important regulators of apoptosis. In general, they are responsible from most of the ATP in a cell. Therefore, it is reasonable to design and develop PS that target the mitochondria. PS can be chemically modified (e.g., with triphenylphosphonium derivatives, which insert to the inner membrane of mitochondria) so that they can be actively targeted to mitochondria. Several PS can accumulate in mitochondria owing to their charge in case of positively charged agents. On the other hand, negatively charged agents accumulate in the mitochondria as a result of their hydrophobicity. Furthermore, mitochondrial targeting can also be achieved by synthesizing

PS that are attached to mitochondria targeting sequences, which can direct molecules to the mitochondrial matrix [167].

4. Pcs as a PS for Cervical Cancer PDT

In this section, we cover the main studies reported in the last five years focusing new Pcs approaches being developed and tested in vitro and/or in tumor-bearing mice and in clinical tests against cervical cancer. More specifically, a review was conducted following a systematic search to identify studies reported between January 2016 and April 2021 focused on "Phthalocyanine" and "Uterine Cervical Neoplasms" in PubMed, Embase, Scopus, and Web of Science databases. To expand the search, references of the original selected articles were evaluated to find papers that could complement this review.

4.1. In Vitro Studies Evaluating Pcs on Hela Cells

In the last 5 years, several in vitro studies have been performed using Pcs as a PDT agent against the HeLa cell line. These studies are presented in detail in Table 2. HeLa cells are immortalised cells and the oldest and most commonly used human cell line [168]. The HeLa cell line is derived from cervical cancer cells (adenocarcinoma) taken on 8 February 1951, from Henrietta Lacks, a 31-year-old African-American mother of five, who died of cancer on 4 October 1951 [169]. The cell line is remarkably durable and prolific, which allows it to be used extensively in scientific study [170]. Therefore, in many of the studies that tested different Pcs formulations in HeLa, the main objective was not to evaluate its effectiveness against cervical cancer but against cancer as a whole. However, indirectly, these studies evaluated the activity of these PCs against cervical adenocarcinoma.

Table 2. Main recent (2016–2021) in vitro studies evaluating different formulations of phthalocyanines in HeLa cells.

Title	Reference	PS/Concentration/ Time of Exposure to PS	Light Source/ Wavelength/Fluence/ Power-Density/ Time of Exposure	Main Outcomes
Exocyclically metallated tetrapyridinoporphyrazine as a potential photosensitizer for photodynamic therapy	[165]	Exocyclically metallated tetrapyridinoporphyrazine [tetrakis-(trans-Pt(NH3)2Cl)-tetra(3,4-pyrido)porphyrazine-zinc(II)](NO3)4, 1.6 µM, and 4 h	600 nm, 5.8 mW/cm^{-2}, 6.96 J/cm^{-2}, and 20 min	Single digit micromolar concentrations are able to induce photocytotoxicity while maintaining low toxicity in the dark. The compound mainly accumulates in the nucleus, suggesting that interacts with DNA, leading to subsequent DNA damage and resulting in photocytotoxicity.
Peripherally crowded cationic phthalocyanines as efficient photosensitizers for photodynamic therapy	[171]	Zinc phthalocyanine bearing four or eight bulky 2,6-di(pyridin-3-yl)phenoxy substituents, 0–10 µM, and 12 h	570 nm, 12.4 mW/cm^2, 11.2 J/cm^2, and 15 min	High photodynamic activity against cancer cells while maintaining low toxicity in the dark. Localization in the lysosomes, inducing an apoptotic cell death pathway with secondary necrosis.
Facile synthesis of cyclic peptide–phthalocyanine conjugates for epidermal growth factor receptor-targeted photodynamic therapy	[172]	Cyclic peptide-conjugated zinc(II) phthalocyanine, 0–60 nM, and 2 h	610 nm, 23 mW/cm^2, 28 J/cm^2, and 20 min	The intensity of cell uptake in EGFR-positive HT29 and HCT116 cells is up to 25 times higher than against EGFR-negative HeLa and HEK293 cells. This conjugate also shows high photo cytotoxicity for HT29 and HCT116 cells.
Synthesis and photodynamic activities of novel silicon(IV) phthalocyanines axially substituted	[173]	Quaternized cationic silicon(IV) phthalocyanine (SiPc) derivatives, 0–10 µM, and 24 h	680 ± 10 nm, 2/J cm^2, and NR	High photodynamic activity against cancer cells while maintaining low toxicity in the dark.

Table 2. Cont.

Title	Reference	PS/Concentration/ Time of Exposure to PS	Light Source/ Wavelength/Fluence/ Power-Density/ Time of Exposure	Main Outcomes
Effects of zinc porphyrin and zinc phthalocyanine derivatives in photodynamic anticancer therapy under different partial pressures of oxygen in vitro	[174]	Disulphonated zinc phthalocyanine (ZnPcS$_2$) and tetrasulphonated zinc tetraphenylporphyrin (ZnTPPS$_4$), 0–10 µM, and 24 h	ZnTPPS$_4$: 415 ± 10 nm ZnPcS$_2$: 660 ± 15 nm; 7 mW/cm^2, 4.2 J/cm^2, and 10 min	ZnTPPS$_4$ was internalized in the cytosol and lysosomes, whereas ZnPcS$_2$ was attached to membrane structures and was photodynamically effective at a minimal level of oxygen, with a higher effect on mitochondrial respiration.
Assessing amphiphilic ABAB Zn(II) phthalocyanines with enhanced photosensitization abilities in in vitro photodynamic therapy studies against cancer	[175]	Triethylene glycol (TEG)-containing Zn(II)Pcs, namely, ABAB-1, A3B-1, and A4-1	ABAB-1, A3B-1, and A4-1; 637 nm ± 17 nm; different red light doses (3, 6 and 9 J/cm^2), NR	ABAB-1 and A3B-1 presented high photodynamic activity on cancer cells while maintaining low toxicity in the dark.
In vitro bioeffects of polyelectrolyte multilayer microcapsules post-loaded with water-soluble cationic photosensitizer	[176]	Dextran sulfate (DS) and poly-L-arginine (PArg) PMC ([DS/PAgr]4) capsules loaded with zinc phthalocyanine choline derivative (cholosens), NR	-	High drug release rate, internalization, light toxicities, and low dark effects.
Improved targeting for photodynamic therapy via a biotin–phthalocyanine conjugate: synthesis, photophysical and photochemical measurements, and in vitro cytotoxicity assay	[177]	Peripherally biotin-substituted zinc(II) phthalocyanine (Pc$_2$), 0.25–5 µM, and 24 h	690 ± 10 nm, 1/J cm^2 and 2/J cm^2, and NR	The biotin-conjugated zinc(II) phthalocyanine derivative presented a higher cytotoxic effect than the amino functionalized zinc(II) phthalocyanine derivative. Pcs were located in the cytoplasm, leading to cell death by apoptosis and reduction of colony capacity after PDT.
Cationic versus anionic phthalocyanines for photodynamic therapy: what a difference the charge makes	[178]	Anionic and cationic zinc(II) phthalocyanines, 1–10 mM, and 12 h	570 nm, 12.4 mW/cm^2, 11.2 J/cm^2, and 15 min	Hydrophilic compounds were localized into lysosomes and amphiphilic compounds were also detected in the cellular membrane. Hydrophilic cationic Pcs were relocalized into the cytoplasm upon irradiation and damaged the nuclear membrane. A high dose of Pcs induced morphological changes and phototoxicity.
Multiple functions integrated inside a single molecule for amplification of photodynamic therapy activity	[179]	Arg and Lys zinc phthalocyanines, 0–10 µM, and 48 h	665 nm, 5 W, 0.4 W/cm^2, and 4 min	The phototoxic effects were more accentuated and the percentage of apoptotic cells was higher in the cells treated with Arg-ZnPc.
Apomyoglobin is an efficient carrier for zinc phthalocyanine in photodynamic therapy of tumors	[180]	Zinc phthalocyanine carried by apomyoglobin, 500 nM, and NR	647 nm, 2.5 mW, 130 mW/cm^2, 40 J/cm^2, and 5 min	The uptake of ZnPc by cells was efficient, with no dark toxicity. When illuminated, a moderate fluence and low concentrations were sufficient to induce extensive cell death.
Novel theranostic zinc phthalocyanine–phospholipid complex self-assembled nanoparticles for imaging-guided targeted photodynamic treatment with controllable ROS production and shape-assisted enhanced cellular uptake	[181]	Zinc phthalocyanine-soybean phosphatidylcholine (ZnPc-SPC) complex, 0.3–10 µg/mL, and 12 or 24 h	630 nm, NR, and 5 min	Pcs could target folate receptors-overexpressed cancer cells while internalized in the cytoplasm. Apoptosis rate increased after PDT.

Table 2. Cont.

Title	Reference	PS/Concentration/ Time of Exposure to PS	Light Source/ Wavelength/Fluence/ Power-Density/ Time of Exposure	Main Outcomes
Zinc phthalocyanine-soybean phospholipid complex based drug carrier for switchable photoacoustic/fluorescence image, multiphase photothermal/photodynamic treatment and synergetic therapy	[182]	Zinc phthalocyanine-soybean phospholipid complex with doxorubicin (DZSM), 0.3–10 µg/mL, and 12 h	638 nm, 1 W/cm^2, NR, and 5 min	ZnPc was distributed in the cytoplasm. Dox was almost located in the nucleus. DZSM presented high selectivity for FRα over-expressed tumor cells as HeLa, excellent switchable image, significant multiphase photothermal therapy (PTT)/PDT effect, and great synergetic therapy potential, leading to notable inhibition of tumor growth.
Novel core-interlayer-shell DOX/ZnPc Co-loaded MSNs@ pH-sensitive CaP@PEGylated liposome for enhanced synergetic chemo-photodynamic therapy	[183]	DOX/ZnPc co-loaded MSNs@CaP@PEGylated liposome, NR, and 24 h	630 nm, 0.05 W/cm^2, NR, and 5 min	ZnPc in the nanoparticles successfully produced the intracellular singlet oxygen under the light that could eventually induce the cytotoxicity of PDT in the cells and could be a promising candidate for PDT besides serving as a chemotherapeutic agent.
Silicon(IV) phthalocyanine-biotin conjugates: synthesis, photo physicochemical properties and in vitro biological activity for photodynamic therapy	[184]	Axially biotin substituted silicon(IV) phthalocyanine, 0–10 µM, and 24 h	NR, 1 J/cm^2 or 2 J/cm^2, and NR	Both axially mono- and bis-biotin substituted silicon(IV) phthalocyanines presented high photo cytotoxicity against HeLa cancer cells with the cell survival degree ranging from 13% to 50%. The photosensitivity and the intensity of damage were found to be directly related to the concentration of the used photosensitizers.
Positively charged phthalocyanine-arginine conjugates as efficient photosensitizer for photodynamic therapy	[185]	Arginine substituted zinc phthalocyanines (ArgEZnPc and ArgZnPc), 0–4 µM, and 4 h	665 nm, 96 mW/cm^2, 28.8 J/cm^2, 5 min, and NR	ArgEZnPc presented higher cellular uptake, high water solubility and ROSs generation ability. HeLa cells showed shrinkage and cell scatter, membrane deformation, and chromatin damage. ArgEZnPc can target the lysosomes and exhibited high cytotoxicity.
Intracellular uptake and fluorescence imaging potential in tumor cell of zinc phthalocyanine	[186]	Zinc phthalocyanine (ZnPc), 10–90 mM, and 24 h	NR	The IC$_{50}$ values were observed to be 35 mM in HeLa cells, maximum uptake was determined at 6 h, and the uptake was decreased at 24 h.
In vitro effects of photodynamic therapy induced by chloro aluminum phthalocyanine nanoemulsion	[187]	Chloroaluminum phthalocyanine nanoemulsion (ClAlPc/NE) or MX+ ClAlPc/NE (methoxyamine), NR, and 3 h	670 nm, 0.1, 0.5 and 1.0 J/cm^2, and NR	A dose-dependent cell death reduced clonogenic survival rates, and sub-G1 accumulation and apoptosis induction were observed in HeLa cells. MX increased PDT effects.
Synthesis of asymmetric zinc(II) phthalocyanines with two different functional groups and spectroscopic properties and photodynamic activity for photodynamic therapy	[188]	Zinc(II) phthalocyanine functionalized, 0–10 µM, and 24 h	690 ± 10 nm, 2 J/cm^2, and NR	The photodynamic efficiency is micromolar. Biotin conjugated zinc(II) phthalocyanine displayed a higher photo cytotoxicity relative to amino phthalocyanine, probably attributed to its high triplet quantum yield of $^1O_2$.

Table 2. Cont.

Title	Reference	PS/Concentration/ Time of Exposure to PS	Light Source/ Wavelength/Fluence/ Power-Density/ Time of Exposure	Main Outcomes
Triblock copolymers encapsulated poly (aryl benzyl ether) dendrimer zinc(II) phthalocyanine nanoparticles for enhancement in vitro photodynamic efficacy	[189]	Zinc (II) phthalocyanines nanoparticles with triblock copolymer (G2-DPcZn), 0.02–10 µM, and 24 h	670 nm, 25, 50, and 100 mW/cm^2, 0–6 J/cm^2, and 2 min	The nanocarriers enhanced intracellular uptake, phototoxicity, and ROS production. The nanoparticle surface with positive charge seems to localize G2-DPcZn in mitochondria.
Cyclodextrin type dependent host-guest interaction mode with phthalocyanine and their influence on photodynamic activity against cancer	[190]	Phthalocyanines (Pc) with cyclodextrins (CDs), 5 µM, and 4 h	665 nm, NR, and 5 min.	The aggregation degree of Pcs was decreased, the water solubility and photodynamic activity were increased. The cellular uptake and ROS generation efficiency of (-CD)4-ZnPc was higher. PDT induced morphology changes, such as chromatin condensation, shrinkage, and fragmentation.
Drug delivery function of carboxymethyl-β-cyclodextrin modified upconversion nanoparticles for adamantine phthalocyanine and their NIR-triggered cancer treatment	[191]	UCNP/COOH-β-CD/Ad-ZnPc, 2–8 µM, and 4 h	980 nm, NR, and 1–4 sessions of 2 min	The complex was mainly located in the cytoplasm and after irradiation induced morphology changes, such as chromatin condensation, shrinkage, and fragmentation. The UCNPs and Ad-ZnPc and UCNP/COOH-β-CD/Ad-ZnPc treated cell survival percent sharply decreased with the increasing of drug concentration and light dose.
Phototoxicity of liposomal Zn- and Al-phthalocyanine against cervical and oral squamous cell carcinoma cells in vitro	[192]	Liposomal Zn- and Al-phthalocyanine, 0.1–1 µM, and 24 h	ZnPc: 350–800 nm, 43.2 J/cm^2; AlPc: 690 nm, 3.6 J/cm^2; 20 min	Liposome-embedded ZnPc and AlPc were more effective than free ZnPc and AlPc in reducing cell viability. HeLa cervical adenocarcinoma cells were more sensitive to AlPc.
Photodynamic therapy and nuclear imaging activities of zinc phthalocyanine-integrated TiO$_2$ nanoparticles in breast and cervical tumors	[193]	Zinc phthalocyanine integrated to the TiO$_2$ nanoparticle (ZnPc-TiO$_2$), 1–6.25 µM, and 3h	LED light source, 10 mW/cm^2, 30, 60, and 90 J/cm^2, and NR	TiO$_2$ nanoparticles increased the cytotoxicity of ZnPc in the HeLa cell line. Phototoxic effects increased depending on the dose of light. Cellular localization of the Pcs was found especially in cytoplasm but not nuclei.
Cervical cancer cells (HeLa) response to photodynamic therapy using a zinc phthalocyanine photosensitizer	[194]	Sulphonated zinc phthalocyanine PS (ZnPcSmix), 0.25–1 µM, and 24 h	673 nm diode laser, 96 mW, 2, 4 and 8 J/cm^2, and NR	The PS was located in the cytoplasm and perinuclear region of HeLa cells. PDT induced dose-dependent structural changes, with decreased cell viability and proliferation, as well as membrane damage.

PS, photosensitizer; NR, not reported.

4.1.1. MPcs

In general, MPcs were the most studied Pcs against HeLa cells and mostly presented the main objective to increase the solubility and bioavailability of hydrophobic Pcs and their derivatives using various DDSs. It was possible to observe that MPcs formulations demonstrated high photodynamic activity against HeLa cells upon light activation [165,171,175–183,185–190,192–194] while presenting low or absent toxicity in the dark [165,175,176,178,179,181,183,185,188,190,192,193]. Overall, these results show that Pcs formulations were effective in subtoxic doses and had a dose- and time-dependent cytotoxic effect against HeLa cells, highlighting their potential for PDT against cervical cancer.

MPcs formulations successfully entered cells and localized mainly in the cytoplasm of tumor cells [174,177,178,181,182,191,193,194] rather than in cellular membrane [180]. Taken together, these data demonstrate that the Pcs formulations tested exhibited a higher capacity to permeate the cytoplasmic membrane and to internalize in the cytoplasm of HeLa cells. The uptake of the PS by cancer cells is crucial for PDT to be effective since ROS present a short half-life and can only act close to the generation site [104,195]. Hydrophobic molecules can rapidly diffuse into plasmatic membranes, while more polar drugs tend to be internalized via endocytosis or assisted transport by serum lipids and proteins. However, the exact mechanisms of MPcs cellular uptake against HeLa cells are still unclear and require further investigation.

The PDT efficiency depends on the illumination conditions, the chemical properties, and the intra-tumoral localization of the PS. Still, the type of photodamage in cells loaded with a PS and illuminated depends on the precise subcellular location of the PS. Thus, understanding the location of the PS is an important principle to consider the most effective PS for each application [104,195]. The subcellular localization of MPcs in Hela cells included mitochondria [174,193] and lysosomes [171,172,174,175,177,178,194] but rarely at the nucleus [165]. This evidence highlights the potential of MPcs as a PS for PDT against cervical adenocarcinoma, since most potent PS are usually localized in mitochondria and/or lysosomes [196].

It is well known that the production of ROS at mitochondrial, lysosomal, or ER loci can directly initiate apoptotic cell death [111]. Accordingly, the HeLa cells death pathway induced by MPcs was apoptosis [171,177,180,185,187,192], compatible with its sub-localization in the mitochondria and lysosomes. These results are very promising as overall apoptosis is considered the most desired mechanism of programmed cell death in PDT due to the absence of side effects compared to necrosis. High doses of PDT and/or uncontrolled photodamage lead to the uncontrolled release of biomolecules of unscheduled cell death into the extracellular space, initiating an inflammatory response in the surrounding tissue. For this reason, necrosis is generally seen as an undesirable mechanism. On the other hand, specific photodamage at adequate doses of PDT can be lethal to cells without harming surrounding healthy cells [196].

MPcs also exerted long-term dose-dependent phototoxic effects against HeLa cells according to the study of Balçik-Erçi et al. 2020 [177]. This effect was obtained with a peripherally biotin substituted zinc(II) Pc that reduced the cell colony capacity, which reflects the decrease in long-term cell proliferation. In general, the results of in vitro studies were promising and suggested that different formulations of MPcs are among the best currently-used PS of cervical adenocarcinoma PDT and their use in clinical studies should be encouraged for prospective means of managing this cancer.

Additionally, the combination of PDT and chemotherapy can induce synergistic therapeutic effects: the PS can overcome multidrug resistance, while the chemotherapeutic drugs can address the limitations of light penetration and hypoxia-related resistance in PDT and enhance the sensitivity of cancer cells to ROS [197]. Recently, Ma et al. 2018 [182] developed a ZnPC-soybean phospholipid complex based on DDSs with doxorubicin (Dox). In vitro evaluations indicated that MTX-decorated self-assembled ZnPc-SPC complex nanoparticles (NPs), referred as DZSM, presented high selectivity for FRα over-expressed tumor cells as HeLa cells; significant multiphase PDT effect; significant cytotoxicity; and great synergetic therapy potential. Additionally, Ma et al. 2018 [183] developed novel DOX/ZnPc co-loaded mesoporous silica (MSNs)@ calcium phosphate (CaP)@PEGylated liposome NPs. In vitro assays with HeLa cells indicated that CaP could not only achieve the controllable release of PS triggered by pH but also promote its cellular uptake and induce apoptosis. According to the authors, the MSNs@CaP@PEGylated liposomes could serve as a promising nanoplatform for cancer treatment by synergic chemo-PDT and superior tumor-targeting ability.

The results of both studies highlight that MPcs could serve as a promising multifunctional platform in anticancer treatment by synergic chemo-PDT and superior tumor-targeting ability.

4.1.2. Silicon Pcs (SiPcs)

Two recent studies investigated the in vitro activity of silicon Pcs (SiPcs) formulations against HeLa cells. Unlike most other Pcs, SiPcs possess two additional axial bonds that reduce aggregation in solution and can be synthetically tailored, thereby creating further scope for modulation of optical, chemical, and electronic properties [198]. The results of both studies [173,184] were very promising as they showed that SiPcs presented high photo cytotoxicity against HeLa cells and were non-cytotoxic/low-cytotoxic in the dark.

Finally, as far as we know, little has been studied about photobleaching in metal-free Pc and MPC formulations against HeLa cells or other cervical cancer cell lineages.

Although the results presented in Table 2 are promising, some important points should be highlighted:

1. Considering that the different studies included in Table 2 used different concentrations of MPCs, different light exposure times, and different light sources, it is very difficult to compare the results obtained between these studies.
2. Still, for the same reasons, it is very difficult to assess which formulation presented the best therapeutic efficacy.
3. The number of recent studies evaluating the combination of PDT and chemotherapy is very small and restricted to doxorubicin, limiting interpretations of its real benefit.

4.2. Both In Vitro and In Tumor-Bearing Mice Pcs Studies Based on HeLa Cells

A small number of studies evaluated Pcs effects against HeLa cells in vitro and in vivo. Regarding in vivo data, these were performed in tumor-bearing mice with HeLa cells [29,199–201] (Table 3). Briefly, Wang et al. 2019 [201] proposed that the therapeutic activity of the MPc (sulfonated Al-phthalocyanine-AlPcS) can be efficiently excited via plasmonic-resonance energy transfer from the two-photon excited gold nanobipyramids (GBPs) and further generates cytotoxic singlet oxygen for cancer eradication. In vitro, after incubation with GBP-AlPcS and exposure to laser irradiation, approximately 80% of HeLa-cell mortality rate was achieved at GBP-AlPcS. In comparison, the compound presented low dark cytotoxicity. In the study conducted by Li et al. 2019 [29], other MPc (zinc II Pc) derivative entrapped mesoporous silica NPs (MSNs) and a wrapping DNA (O1) (PcC4-MSN-514 O1) displayed in vitro selective phototoxicity against HeLa cells. In vivo, with systemic administration of PcC4-MSN-O1, there was accumulation in HeLa tumors of xenograft-bearing mice. After laser irradiation, tumor growth was inhibited and apoptosis was induced. Moreover, the time-modulated activation process in tumors and the relatively fast excretion of PcC4-MSN-O1 indicated its advantages in reducing potential side effects. Li et al. 2019 [199] introduced two polyethylene glycol (PEG) linkers on SiPc to synthesize a new water-soluble and tumor-targeting photosensitizer compound. In vitro, this compound accumulated in biotin receptor (BR)-positive Hela cells through BR-mediated internalization. In vivo, SiPc preferentially accumulated in the tumor tissue of the tumor-bearing mice. Furthermore, SiPc significantly depressed tumor progression after irradiation. Finally, Liang et al. 2021 [200] tested FA-TiO2-Pc in conjunction with folic acid (FA), a tumor-targeting agent. In vitro, FA-TiO2-Pc presented high therapeutic efficiency at low concentration and with a short incubation time, under one-photon excitation. In mice with HeLa xenograft tumors, FA-TiO2-Pc led to decreased tumor growth with minimal side effects, even at low concentrations and low light irradiation.

Therefore, the results of these studies highlight that the tested MPcs formulations are very promising for cervical cancer PDT, including in vivo and presented great potential for future use in clinical studies. However, the limitations highlighted above for the studies included in Table 2 can be applied to the studies shown in Table 3. Therefore, additional interpretations of these studies are greatly impaired.

Table 3. Recent (2016–2021) in vitro and in vivo studies evaluating different formulations of phthalocyanines on HeLa cells.

Title	Reference	Animal Model	PS/Concentration/ Time of Exposure to PS	Light Source/Wavelength/ Fluence/Power/Density/Time of Exposure	Main In Vitro Outcomes	Main In Vivo Outcomes
Functional titanium dioxide nanoparticle conjugated with phthalocyanine and folic acid as a promising photosensitizer for targeted photodynamic therapy in vitro and in vivo	[200]	Female BALB/c nude mice inoculated subcutaneously on the right armpit with 100 μL HeLa cells (1×10^7 cells) in PBS.	TiO_2 nanoparticle conjugated with folic acid (FA), and Al (III) phthalocyanine chloride tetrasulfonic acid (FA-TiO_2-Pc), 0.52 μmol/kg, 6 h	420–800 nm, 0.75 W/cm^2, 10 min.	FA-TiO_2-Pc presented high therapeutic drug efficiency at a low concentration dose and short incubation time under one-photon excitation.	Tumor growth of the FA-TiO_2-Pc treated mice was significantly inhibited. The survival rates were 100%, and no significant physiological morphology changes were observed in heart, liver, spleen, lungs, and kidney, indicating no toxic effects after treatment.
A biotin receptor-targeted silicon(IV) phthalocyanine for in vivo tumor imaging and photodynamic therapy	[199]	Female BALB/c nude mice inoculated subcutaneously on the right foreleg armpit with 100 μL of PBS containing HeLa cells (1×10^7)	Biotin receptor-targeted silicon(IV) phthalocyanine, 2 μmol/kg, 2 h	670 nm, 10 mW/cm^2, 30 min	High photodynamic activity on cancer cells while maintaining low toxicity in the dark.	The compound specifically accumulated in tumor tissue through the biotin receptor-mediated process, allowing for the targeted imaging of the tumor tissue in vivo. Moreover, under-irradiation induced clear necrosis of the tumor tissues and the tumor's growth was inhibited.
Sequential protein-responsive nanophotosensitizer complex for enhancing tumor-specific therapy	[29]	Male NOD-SCID mice injected subcutaneously with HeLa cells (2×10^7 cells)	zinc(II) phthalocyanine derivative entrapped mesoporous silica nanoparticles (MSNs) and a wrapping DNA (O1) (PcC4-MSN-O1), 200 μM, 24 h	670 nm, 0.5 W/cm^2, 20 min	PcC4-MSN-O1 displayed selective phototoxicity against HeLa over normal cells (HEK-293).	There was an accumulation in HeLa tumors of xenograft-bearing mice, and irradiation induced the inhibition of tumor growth and apoptosis. The time-modulated activation process in tumors and the relatively fast excretion of PcC4-MSN-O1 indicated its advantages in reducing potential side effects.
AlPcS-loaded gold nanobipyramids with high two-photon efficiency for photodynamic therapy in vivo	[201]	Nude mice inoculated subcutaneously with HeLa cells	Sulfonated Al-phthalocyanine (AlPcS)-loaded by gold nanobipyramids, 5 nM, 2 h	800 nm 2.8 W/cm^2, 30 min	High photodynamic activity against cancer cells.	An evident inhibition in tumor growth and extensive necrosis was observed in mice after PDT treatment with GBP-AlPcS. Moreover, no side effect or toxicity to normal tissues was observed.

PS, photosensitizer.

4.3. Studies Evaluating Pcs in Other Cervical Cancer Cells than Hela

In the last 5 years, only one study evaluated Pcs in other cervical cancer cell lines in addition to HeLa [17]. This study evaluated the effectiveness of PDT using Silicon phthalocyanine 4 (Pc4) in vitro and in vivo against human cervical cancer cells CaSki (squamous cell carcinoma drive cell line, HPV-16 about 600 copies per cell, and HPV-18) and ME-180 (squamous cell carcinoma drive cell line, HPV DNA with greater homology to HPV-68 than HPV-18). Specifically, cell growth and cytotoxicity were measured in vitro using a methyl thiazole tetrazolium assay. Pc4 cellular uptake and intracellular distribution were determined. For in vitro Pc4 PDT, cells were irradiated at 670 nm at a fluence of 2.5 J/cm^2. SCID mice (female C.B-17 mice) were implanted with CaSki and ME-180 cells both subcutaneously and intracervical. Forty-eight hours after Pc4 administration, the tumors were irradiated at 75 and 150 J/cm^2, for 4 min. In vitro, Pc4 itself was relatively non-toxic and Pc4 PDT was effective in killing cervical cancer cells grown as either spheroids or monolayers. Additionally, in both cervical cancer cell lines, the subcellular distribution of Pc4 occurred in the cytoplasm, lysosomes, RE, and mitochondria. In vivo, intracervical tumors became necrotic after Pc4 PDT. In general, this study highlighted the in vitro and in vivo potential of PDT with Pcs against invasive cervical cancer due to HPV-16, the most prevalent HPV type in cervical cancer. Furthermore, these results occurred more specifically in squamous cell carcinoma, which is the most common type of cervical cancer worldwide (approximately 70% of total) [40].

4.4. Clinical Studies

As far as we know, only a recent study performed the clinical treatment of CIN with Pcs [24]. PDT was performed using a chitosan NP containing chlorocyan-aluminum Pc in patients with CIN1 and CIN2. The compound was applied on the surface of the cervix of each selected patient with CIN1 (n = 11) or CIN2 (n = 1), which was then illuminated after 30 min with a red laser lighting (minimum dose of 200 J, power of 1.20 W, irradiance of 0.30 W·cm^{-2}, and fluency of 50 J·cm^{-2}). Among the 12 patients treated primarily, 11 (91.7%) presented negative cervical cytology in the first evaluation after treatment, but 1 (8.3%) presented no therapeutic benefit, even after reapplication. Two of the patients who presented a good initial therapeutic response had relapse, but evolved to cytological remission after a new round of PDT, remaining negative until the last follow-up. No important side effects were observed in any of the patients. According to the authors, the trial demonstrated that the treatment of CIN1 and CIN2 lesions using PDT with CNP-AlClPc is feasible and safe. However, they suggested large randomized clinical trials to establish efficacy.

To date, Pcs have not been used in clinical studies for the PDT of invasive cervical cancer. According to clinicaltrials.gov, there is only one published study of a clinical trial involving cervical cancer and PDT [202].

5. Conclusions

Throughout this review, we highlighted that the main topics in Pcs as agents for PDT against cervical cancer are solubility, targeting capacity, and therapeutic efficiency. At a chemical level, it is concluded that Pcs amphiphilic character leads to higher efficiency in vitro and in vivo. Furthermore, the phototoxic potential as well as its cellular uptake and internalization seem to be improved, making it difficult to stack it via axial ligation and inclusion of positive charge(s). Additionally, the latest in vitro and in vivo studies of Pcs against cervical cancer reported in this review strongly suggest that the application of nanotechnologies as DDSs allowed for increased PDT efficacy and reduced side-effects associated with the Pcs administration, which shows promise for cervical cancer treatment.

Hence, only considering their chemistry, Pcs exhibit this flexibility, enabling further screening and investigations, which raises hope for cervical cancer treatment. However, we highlight some important considerations as follows:

- Current evidence indicates that despite the increasing number of studies with a growing number of different Pcs formulations and their generally increased number of favorable aspects as mainly related to in vitro low effective concentration (mainly against the tumour cell line), low dark toxicity, increased photo cytotoxicity, and cellular uptake in a dose-dependent manner for cervical cancer, only a few Pcs were evaluated in cervical cancer cell lines other than HeLa. As a result, most studies assessed the activity of different Pcs formulations against cervical adenocarcinoma and not against squamous cervical cancer, which is the most common type of cervical cancer worldwide (approximately 70% of total) [40]. Additionally, few preclinical animal studies and no clinical studies with Pcs in invasive cervical cancer have been performed to date.
- Regarding pre-clinical animal models [203], there are only a few studies in tumor-bearing mice xenograft tumors based on HeLa cells. Therefore, there is an urgent need for more in vivo studies in tumor-bearing mice and primates based on HeLa cells and in other cervical cancer lineages to continue studies on the effectiveness of different Pc formulations against cervical cancer.
- Indeed, our review showed that in the field of Pcs in cervical cancer, the photophysical and photochemical properties, subcellular localization, phototoxic activity, mechanisms of cell death, and improved targeting to tumor tissues have been the main topics explored. However, up to this moment, there is an immediate need to increase the number of clinical trials evaluating Pcs in CIN and invasive cervical cancer. As a result, it would be possible to confirm preclinical studies and orient future research.
- Additionally, we showed that the combination of PDT with MPcs and chemotherapy using Dox can induce synergistic therapeutic effects, highlighting that MPcs could serve as a promising multifunctional platform in anticancer treatment by synergic chemo-PDT and superior tumor-targeting ability. However, the number of studies with this approach is still limited, so we strongly suggest implementing research in this area.
- Finally, the search for new possible mechanisms of action in different cervical cancer cells may consequently contribute to novel applications for single or combined Pcs treatments to CIN and invasive cervical cancer.

In conclusion, Pcs are promising as pharmaceutical entities for anti-cervical cancer agents. Major research requirements are needed to encourage studies evaluating Pcs in cervical cancer cell lines other than HeLa and in squamous cervical cancer type; increase preclinical animal studies and clinical trials evaluating Pcs in CIN and invasive cervical cancer to confirm preclinical in vitro studies and orientate future research; implement research in by combining PDT with Pcs and chemotherapy; and understand the new exact mode of actions of Pcs in different cervical cancer cells. Despite all the drawbacks and limitations mentioned above, the authors firmly believe that Pc-based formulations could emerge as a privileged scaffold for the establishment of lead compounds for PDT against cervical cancer. A deeper understanding of the effects of PDT with Pcs could enable the future improvement of currently used protocols and the treatment of different cervical cancer types.

Author Contributions: Conceptualization, L.R.C. and M.E.L.C.; methodology, L.R.C., L.E.d.F.M., G.M.Z.F.D., E.D., M.V.F.d.S., K.H.M., C.S.S.-M. and R.P.S.; validation, V.R.S.d.S., R.S.G. and W.C.; formal analysis, M.E.L.C.; writing—original draft preparation, L.R.C., L.E.d.F.M., G.M.Z.F.D., E.D., M.V.F.d.S., N.L.M., K.H.M., C.S.S.-M. and R.P.S.; validation, V.R.S.d.S., R.S.G. and W.C.; writing—review and editing, M.E.L.C.; supervision, M.E.L.C.; project administration, M.E.L.C.; funding acquisition, M.E.L.C. All authors have read and agreed to the published version of the manuscript.

Funding: This research was funded by Conselho Nacional de Desenvolvimento Científico e Tecnológico (CNPq) (grants 409382/2018-3 and 304037/2019-2) and Coordenação de Aperfeiçoamento de Pessoal de Nível Superior (CAPES) (PROAP), Brazilian Government.

Institutional Review Board Statement: Not applicable.

Informed Consent Statement: Not applicable.

Conflicts of Interest: The authors declare no conflict of interest.

References

1. Tian, T.; Gong, X.; Gao, X.; Li, Y.; Ju, W.; Ai, Y. Comparison of survival outcomes of locally advanced cervical cancer by histopathological types in the surveillance, epidemiology, and end results (SEER) database: A propensity score matching study. *Infect. Agent. Cancer* **2020**, *15*, 33. [CrossRef]
2. Sung, H.; Ferlay, J.; Siegel, R.L.; Laversanne, M.; Soerjomataram, I.; Jemal, A.; Bray, F. Global Cancer Statistics 2020: GLOBOCAN estimates of incidence and mortality worldwide for 36 cancers in 185 countries. *CA Cancer J. Clin.* **2021**, *71*, 209–249. [CrossRef]
3. Schiffman, M.; Doorbar, J.; Wentzensen, N.; De Sanjosé, S.; Fakhry, C.; Monk, B.J.; Stanley, M.A.; Franceschi, S. Carcinogenic human papillomavirus infection. *Nat. Rev. Dis. Prim.* **2016**, *2*, 16086. [CrossRef]
4. Zhao, F.; Qiao, Y. Cervical cancer prevention in China: A key to cancer control. *Lancet* **2019**, *393*, 969–970. [CrossRef]
5. Ogilvie, G.S.; Krajden, M.; van Niekerk, D.; Smith, L.W.; Cook, D.; Ceballos, K.; Lee, M.; Gentile, L.; Gondara, L.; Elwood-Martin, R.; et al. HPV for cervical cancer screening (HPV FOCAL): Complete Round 1 results of a randomized trial comparing HPV-based primary screening to liquid-based cytology for cervical cancer. *Int. J. Cancer* **2017**, *15*, 440–448. [CrossRef]
6. Cohen, P.A.; Jhingran, A.; Oaknin, A.; Denny, L. Cervical cancer. *Lancet* **2019**, *393*, 169–182. [CrossRef]
7. American Cancer Society Cervical Cancer Early Detection, Diagnosis, and Staging. Available online: https://www.cancer.org/content/dam/CRC/PDF/Public/8601.00.pdf (accessed on 7 July 2021).
8. Salvo, G.; Odetto, D.; Pareja, R.; Frumovitz, M.; Ramirez, P.T. Revised 2018 International Federation of Gynecology and Obstetrics (FIGO) cervical cancer staging: A review of gaps and questions that remain. *Int. J. Gynecol. Cancer* **2020**, *30*, 873–878. [CrossRef]
9. Serrano-Olvera, A.; Cetina, L.; Coronel, J.; Dueñas-González, A. Emerging drugs for the treatment of cervical cancer. *Expert Opin. Emerg. Drugs* **2015**, *20*, 165–182. [CrossRef]
10. American Cancer Society Cancer Facts & Figures. 2018. Available online: https://www.cancer.org/content/dam/cancer-org/research/cancer-facts-and-statistics/annual-cancer-facts-and-figures/2018/cancer-facts-and-figures-2018.pdf (accessed on 7 July 2021).
11. American Cancer Society Treating Cervical Cancer. Available online: https://www.cancer.org/content/dam/CRC/PDF/Public/8602.00.pdf (accessed on 7 July 2021).
12. Tao, X.H.; Guan, Y.; Shao, D.; Xue, W.; Ye, F.S.; Wang, M.; He, M.H. Efficacy and safety of photodynamic therapy for cervical intraepithelial neoplasia: A systemic review. *Photodiagn. Photodyn. Ther.* **2014**, *11*, 104–112. [CrossRef]
13. Wolford, J.E.; Tewari, K.S. Rational design for cervical cancer therapeutics: Cellular and non-cellular based strategies on the horizon for recurrent, metastatic or refractory cervical cancer. *Expert Opin. Drug Discov.* **2018**, *13*, 445–457. [CrossRef]
14. Gupta, S.; Maheshwari, A.; Parab, P.; Mahantshetty, U.; Hawaldar, R.; Sastri Chopra, S.; Kerkar, R.; Engineer, R.; Tongaonkar, H.; Ghosh, J.; et al. Neoadjuvant chemotherapy followed by radical surgery versus concomitant chemotherapy and radiotherapy in patients with stage IB2, IIA, or IIB squamous cervical cancer: A randomized controlled trial. *J. Clin. Oncol.* **2018**, *36*, 1548–1555. [CrossRef]
15. Yang, H.; Wu, X.L.; Wu, K.H.; Zhang, R.; Ju, L.L.; Ji, Y.; Zhang, Y.W.; Xue, S.L.; Zhang, Y.X.; Yang, Y.F.; et al. MicroRNA-497 regulates cisplatin chemosensitivity of cervical cancer by targeting transketolase. *Am. J. Cancer Res.* **2016**, *6*, 2690–2699.
16. Gadducci, A.; Sartori, E.; Maggino, T.; Landoni, F.; Zola, P.; Cosio, S.; Pasinetti, B.; Alessi, C.; Maneo, A.; Ferrero, A. The clinical outcome of patients with stage Ia1 and Ia2 squamous cell carcinoma of the uterine cervix: A Cooperation Task Force (CTF) study. *Eur. J. Gynaecol. Oncol.* **2003**, *24*, 513–516.
17. Gadzinski, J.A.; Guo, J.; Philips, B.J.; Basse, P.; Craig, E.K.; Bailey, L.; Latoche, J.; Comerci, J.T.; Eiseman, J.L. Evaluation of silicon phthalocyanine 4 photodynamic therapy against human cervical cancer cells in vitro and in mice. *Adv. Biol. Chem.* **2016**, *6*, 193–215. [CrossRef]
18. Dougherty, T.J.; Grindey, G.B.; Fiel, R.; Weishaupt, K.R.; Boyle, D.G. Photoradiation therapy. II. Cure of animal tumors with hematoporphyrin and light. *J. Natl. Cancer Inst.* **1975**, *55*, 115–121. [CrossRef]
19. Agostinis, P.; Berg, K.; Cengel, K.A.; Foster, T.H.; Girotti, A.W.; Gollnick, S.O.; Hahn, S.M.; Hamblin, M.R.; Juzeniene, A.; Kessel, D.; et al. Photodynamic therapy of cancer: An update. *CA Cancer J. Clin.* **2011**, *61*, 250–281. [CrossRef]
20. Photocure-The Bladder Cancer Company. Available online: https://https://photocure.com/about/about-us/ (accessed on 10 October 2021).
21. Shishkova, N.; Kuznetsova, O.; Berezov, T. Photodynamic therapy for gynecological diseases and breast cancer. *Cancer Biol. Med.* **2012**, *9*, 9–17. [CrossRef]
22. Castano, A.P.; Mroz, P.; Hamblin, M.R. Photodynamic therapy and anti-tumour immunity. *Nat. Rev. Cancer* **2006**, *6*, 535–545. [CrossRef]
23. Ochsner, M. Photophysical and photobiological processes in the photodynamic therapy of tumours. *J. Photochem. Photobiol. B* **1997**, *39*, 1–18. [CrossRef]
24. Vendette, A.C.F.; Piva, H.L.; Muehlmann, L.A.; de Souza, D.A.; Tedesco, A.C.; Azevedo, R.B. Clinical treatment of intra-epithelia cervical neoplasia with photodynamic therapy. *Int. J. Hyperth.* **2020**, *37*, 50–58. [CrossRef]
25. Mroz, P.; Yaroslavsky, A.; Kharkwal, G.B.; Hamblin, M.R. Cell death pathways in photodynamic therapy of cancer. *Cancers* **2011**, *3*, 2516–2539. [CrossRef]
26. Lucky, S.S.; Soo, K.C.; Zhang, Y. Nanoparticles in photodynamic therapy. *Chem. Rev.* **2015**, *115*, 1990–2042. [CrossRef]

27. Fan, W.; Huang, P.; Chen, X. Overcoming the Achilles' heel of photodynamic therapy. *Chem. Soc. Rev.* **2016**, *45*, 6488–6519. [CrossRef]
28. Hu, F.; Xu, S.; Liu, B. Photosensitizers with aggregation-induced emission: Materials and biomedical applications. *Adv. Mater.* **2018**, *30*, 1801350. [CrossRef]
29. Li, X.; Fan, H.; Guo, T.; Bai, H.; Kwon, N.; Kim, K.H.; Yu, S.; Cho, Y.; Kim, H.; Nam, K.T.; et al. Sequential protein-responsive nanophotosensitizer complex for enhancing tumor-specific therapy. *ACS Nano* **2019**, *13*, 6702–6710. [CrossRef]
30. Kou, J.; Dou, D.; Yang, L. Porphyrin photosensitizers in photodynamic therapy and its applications. *Oncotarget* **2017**, *8*, 81591–81603. [CrossRef]
31. Reddi, E.; Lo Castro, G.; Biolo, R.; Jori, G. Pharmacokinetic studies with zinc(II)-phthalocyanine in tumour-bearing mice. *Br. J. Cancer* **1987**, *56*, 597–600. [CrossRef]
32. Chen, J.; Wang, Y.; Fang, Y.; Jiang, Z.; Wang, A.; Xue, J. Improved photodynamic anticancer activity and mechanisms of a promising zinc(II) phthalocyanine-quinoline conjugate photosensitizer in vitro and in vivo. *Biomed. Opt. Express.* **2020**, *11*, 3900–3912. [CrossRef]
33. Wasielewski, M.R. Self-assembly strategies for integrating light harvesting and charge separation in artificial photosynthetic systems. *Acc. Chem. Res.* **2009**, *42*, 1910–1921. [CrossRef]
34. Revuelta-Maza, M.A.; Hally, C.; Nonell, S.; de la Torre, G.; Torres, T. Crosswise phthalocyanines with collinear functionalization: New paradigmatic derivatives for efficient singlet oxygen photosensitization. *ChemPlusChem* **2019**, *84*, 673–679. [CrossRef]
35. Dumoulin, F.; Durmuş, M.; Ahsen, V.; Nyokong, T. Synthetic pathways to water-soluble phthalocyanines and close analogs. *Coord. Chem. Rev.* **2010**, *254*, 2792–2847. [CrossRef]
36. Rak, J.; Pouckova, P.; Benes, J.; Vetvicka, D. Drug delivery systems for phthalocyanines for photodynamic therapy. *Anticancer Res.* **2019**, *39*, 3323–3339. [CrossRef]
37. Castle, P.; Murokora, D.; Perez, C.; Alvarez, M.; Quek, S.; Campbell, C. Treatment of cervical intraepithelial lesions. *Int. J. Gynaecol. Obstet.* **2017**, *138*, 20–25. [CrossRef]
38. Nene, B.M.; Hiremath, P.S.; Kane, S.; Fayette, J.M.; Shastri, S.S.; Sankaranarayanan, R. Effectiveness, safety, and acceptability of cryotherapy by midwives for cervical intraepithelial neoplasia in Maharashtra, India. *Int. J. Gynaecol. Obstet.* **2008**, *103*, 232–236. [CrossRef]
39. Mizuno, M.; Mitsui, H.; Kajiyama, H.; Teshigawara, T.; Inoue, K.; Takahashi, K.; Ishii, T.; Ishizuka, M.; Nakajima, M.; Kikkawa, F. Efficacy of 5-aminolevulinic acid and LED photodynamic therapy in cervical intraepithelial neoplasia: A clinical trial. *Photodiagn. Photodyn. Ther.* **2020**, *32*, 102004. [CrossRef]
40. Hu, K.; Wang, W.; Liu, X.; Meng, Q.; Zhang, F. Comparison of treatment outcomes between squamous cell carcinoma and adenocarcinoma of cervix after definitive radiotherapy or concurrent chemoradiotherapy. *Radiat. Oncol.* **2018**, *13*, 1–7. [CrossRef]
41. Walboomers, J.M.M.; Jacobs, M.V.; Manos, M.M.; Bosch, F.X.; Kummer, J.A.; Shah, K.V.; Snijders, P.J.F.; Peto, J.; Meijer, C.J.L.M.; Muñoz, N.J.M.M. Human papillomavirus is a necessary cause of invasive cervical cancer worldwide. *J. Pathol.* **1999**, *189*, 12–19. [CrossRef]
42. Castellsagué, X.; Diaz, M.; de Sanjosé, S.; Muñoz, N.; Herrero, R.; Franceschi, S.; Peeling, R.W.; Ashley, R.; Smith, J.S.; Snijders, P.J.F.; et al. Worldwide human papillomavirus etiology of cervical adenocarcinoma and its cofactors: Implications for screening and prevention. *J. Natl. Cancer Inst.* **2006**, *98*, 303–315. [CrossRef]
43. De Sanjose, S.; Quint, W.G.V.; Alemany, L.; Geraets, D.T.; Klaustermeier, J.E.; Lloveras, B.; Tous, S.; Felix, A.; Bravo, L.E.; Shin, H.R.; et al. Human papillomavirus genotype attribution in invasive cervical cancer: A retrospective cross-sectional worldwide study. *Lancet Oncol.* **2010**, *11*, 1048–1056. [CrossRef]
44. Ho, G.Y.F.; Bierman, R.; Beardsley, L.; Chang, C.J.; Burk, R.D. Natural History of cervicovaginal papillomavirus infection in young women. *N. Engl. J. Med.* **1998**, *338*, 423–428. [CrossRef]
45. Koh, W.J.; Greer, B.E.; Abu-Rustum, N.R.; Apte, S.M.; Campos, S.M.; Cho, K.R.; Chu, C.; Cohn, D.; Crispens, M.A.; Dorigo, O.; et al. Cervical cancer, version 2.2015: Featured updates to the NCCN guidelines featured updates to the NCCN guidelines. *J. Natl. Compr. Cancer Netw.* **2015**, *13*, 395–404. [CrossRef]
46. Tota, J.E.; Chevarie-Davis, M.; Richardson, L.A.; DeVries, M.; Franco, E.L. Epidemiology and burden of HPV infection and related diseases: Implications for prevention strategies. *Prev. Med.* **2011**, *53*, S12–S21. [CrossRef]
47. Monsonego, J.; Cox, J.T.; Behrens, C.; Sandri, M.; Franco, E.L.; Yap, P.S.; Huh, W. Prevalence of high-risk human papilloma virus genotypes and associated risk of cervical precancerous lesions in a large U.S. screening population: Data from the ATHENA trial. *Gynecol. Oncol.* **2015**, *137*, 47–54. [CrossRef]
48. De Abreu, A.L.P.; Malaguti, N.; Souza, R.P.; Uchimura, N.S.; Ferreira, É.C.; Pereira, M.W.; Carvalho, M.D.B.; Pelloso, S.M.; Bonini, M.G.; Gimenes, F.; et al. Association of human papillomavirus, *Neisseria gonorrhoeae* and *Chlamydia trachomatis* co-infections on the risk of high-grade squamous intraepithelial cervical lesion. *Am. J. Cancer Res.* **2016**, *6*, 1371–1383.
49. Bodily, J.; Laimins, L.A. Persistence of human papillomavirus infection: Keys to malignant progression. *Trends Microbiol.* **2011**, *19*, 33–39. [CrossRef]
50. Herrero, R.; Murillo, R. Cervical Cancer. In *Cancer Epidemiology and Prevention*; Thun, M., Linet, M.S., Cerhan, J.R., Haiman, C.A., Schottenfeld, D., Eds.; Oxford University Press: New York, NY, USA, 2018; pp. 925–946. ISBN 13:9780190238667.
51. Egawa, N.; Egawa, K.; Griffin, H.; Doorbar, J. Human papillomaviruses; Epithelial tropisms, and the development of neoplasia. *Viruses* **2015**, *7*, 3863–3890. [CrossRef]

52. Mac, M.; Moody, C.A. Epigenetic regulation of the human papillomavirus life cycle. *Pathogens* **2020**, *9*, 483. [CrossRef]
53. PaVE: Papilloma Virus Genome Database. Available online: https://pave.niaid.nih.gov/ (accessed on 6 January 2020).
54. Huh, W.K.; Joura, E.A.; Giuliano, A.R.; Iversen, O.E.; de Andrade, R.P.; Ault, K.A.; Bartholomew, D.; Cestero, R.M.; Fedrizzi, E.N.; Hirschberg, A.L.; et al. Final efficacy, immunogenicity, and safety analyses of a nine-valent human papillomavirus vaccine in women aged 16–26 years: A randomised, double-blind trial. *Lancet* **2017**, *390*, 2143–2159. [CrossRef]
55. WHO. *IARC Monographs on the Evaluation of Carcinogenic Risks to Humans Human Papillomaviruses*; WHO: Lyon, France, 2007; Volume 90, ISBN 9789283212904.
56. Pyeon, D.; Pearce, S.M.; Lank, S.M.; Ahlquist, P.; Lambert, P.F. Establishment of human papillomavirus infection requires cell cycle progression. *PLoS Pathog.* **2009**, *5*, e1000318. [CrossRef]
57. Ozbun, M.A.; Meyers, C. Temporal usage of multiple promoters during the life cycle of human papillomavirus type 31b. *J. Virol.* **1998**, *72*, 2715–2722. [CrossRef]
58. Moody, C.A. Mechanisms by which HPV induces a replication competent environment in differentiating keratinocytes. *Viruses* **2017**, *9*, 261. [CrossRef]
59. Hummel, M.; Hudson, J.B.; Laimins, L.A. Differentiation-induced and constitutive transcription of human papillomavirus type 31b in cell lines containing viral episomes. *J. Virol.* **1992**, *66*, 6070–6080. [CrossRef]
60. Klumpp, D.; Laimins, L. Differentiation-induced changes in promoter usage for transcripts encoding the human papillomavirus type 31 replication protein E1. *Virology* **1999**, *25*, 239–246. [CrossRef]
61. Bedell, M.A.; Hudson, J.B.; Golub, T.R.; Turyk, M.E.; Hosken, M.; Wilbanks, G.D.; Laimins, L.A. Amplification of human papillomavirus genomes in vitro is dependent on epithelial differentiation. *J. Virol.* **1991**, *65*, 2254–2260. [CrossRef]
62. Hummel, M.; Lim, H.B.; Laimins, L.A. Human papillomavirus type 31b late gene expression is regulated through protein kinase C-mediated changes in RNA processing. *J. Virol.* **1995**, *69*, 3381–3388. [CrossRef]
63. Ozbun, M.A.; Meyers, C. Characterization of late gene transcripts expressed during vegetative replication of human papillomavirus type 31b. *J. Virol.* **1997**, *71*, 5161–5172. [CrossRef]
64. Verteramo, R.; Pierangeli, A.; Calzolari, E.; Patella, A.; Recine, N.; Mancini, E.; Marcone, V.; Masciangelo, R.; Bucci, M.; Antonelli, G.; et al. Direct sequencing of HPV DNA detected in gynaecologic outpatients in Rome, Italy. *Microbes Infect.* **2006**, *8*, 2517–2521. [CrossRef]
65. Lehtinen, M.; Ault, K.; Lyytikainen, E.; Dillner, J.; Garland, S.; Ferris, D.; Koutsky, L.; Sings, H.; Lu, S.; Haupt, R.; et al. Chlamydia trachomatis infection and risk of cervical intraepithelial neoplasia. *Sex. Transm. Infect.* **2011**, *87*, 372–376. [CrossRef]
66. Longworth, M.S.; Wilson, R.; Laimins, L.A. HPV31 E7 facilitates replication by activating E2F2 transcription through its interaction with HDACs. *EMBO J.* **2005**, *24*, 1821–1830. [CrossRef]
67. Howie, H.L.; Katzenellenbogen, R.A.; Galloway, D.A. Papillomavirus E6 proteins. *Virology* **2009**, *384*, 324–334. [CrossRef]
68. Munger, K.; Werness, B.A.; Dyson, N.; Phelps, W.C.; Harlow, E.; Howley, P.M. Complex formation of c-myc papillomavirus E7 proteins with the retinoblastoma tumor suppressor gene product. *EMBO J.* **1989**, *8*, 4099–4105. [CrossRef] [PubMed]
69. Dyson, N.; Howley, P.M.; Münger, K.; Harlow, E. The human papilloma virus-16 E7 oncoprotein is able to bind to the retinoblastoma gene product. *Science* **1989**, *243*, 934–937. [CrossRef] [PubMed]
70. Scheffner, M.; Werness, B.A.; Huibregtse, J.M.; Levine, A.J.; Howley, P.M. The E6 oncoprotein encoded by human papillomavirus types 16 and 18 promotes the degradation of p53. *Cell* **1990**, *63*, 1129–1136. [CrossRef]
71. Huibregtse, J.M.; Scheffner, M.; Howley, P.M. A cellular protein mediates association of p53 with the E6 oncoprotein of human papillomavirus types 16 or 18. *EMBO J.* **1991**, *10*, 4129–4135. [CrossRef] [PubMed]
72. Scheffner, M.; Huibregtse, J.M.; Vierstra, R.D.; Howley, P.M. The HPV-16 E6 and E6-AP complex functions as a ubiquitin-protein ligase in the ubiquitination of p53. *Cell* **1993**, *75*, 495–505. [CrossRef]
73. Sharma, S.V.; Haber, D.A.; Settleman, J. Cell line-based platforms to evaluate the therapeutic efficacy of candidate anticancer agents. *Nat. Rev. Cancer* **2010**, *10*, 241–253. [CrossRef]
74. Campo, M.S. Animal models of papillomavirus pathogenesis. *Virus Res.* **2002**, *89*, 249–261. [CrossRef]
75. Boshart, M.; Gissmann, L.; Ikenberg, H.; Kleinheinz, A.; Scheurlen, W.; zur Hausen, H. A new type of papillomavirus DNA, its presence in genital cancer biopsies and in cell lines derived from cervical cancer. *EMBO J.* **1984**, *3*, 1151–1157. [CrossRef] [PubMed]
76. Schwarz, E.; Freese, U.K.; Gissmann, L.; Mayer, W.; Roggenbuck, B.; Stremlau, A.; Zur Hausen, H. Structure and transcription of human papillomavirus sequences in cervical carcinoma cells. *Nature* **1985**, *314*, 111–114. [CrossRef] [PubMed]
77. Pater, M.M.; Pater, A. Human papillomavirus types 16 and 18 sequences in carcinoma cell lines of the cervix. *Virology* **1985**, *145*, 313–318. [CrossRef]
78. Rosa, M.N.; Evangelista, A.F.; Leal, L.F.; De Oliveira, C.M.; Silva, V.A.O.; Munari, C.C.; Munari, F.F.; Matsushita, G.D.M.; Dos Reis, R.; Andrade, C.E.; et al. Establishment, molecular and biological characterization of HCB-514: A novel human cervical cancer cell line. *Sci. Rep.* **2019**, *9*, 1913. [CrossRef] [PubMed]
79. Van Straten, D.; Mashayekhi, V.; de Bruijn, H.S.; Oliveira, S.; Robinson, D.J. Oncologic photodynamic therapy: Basic principles, current clinical status and future directions. *Cancers* **2017**, *9*, 19. [CrossRef]
80. Levy, J.G. Photodynamic therapy. *Trends Biotechnol.* **1995**, *13*, 14–18. [CrossRef]
81. Wolf, P. Photodynamic therapy in dermatology: State of the art. *J. Eur. Acad. Dermatol. Venereol.* **2001**, *15*, 508–509. [CrossRef] [PubMed]

82. Ghodasra, D.H.; Demirci, H. Photodynamic therapy for choroidal metastasis. *Am. J. Ophthalmol.* **2016**, *161*, 104–109. [CrossRef]
83. Kharkwal, G.B.; Sharma, S.K.; Huang, Y.Y.; Dai, T.; Hamblin, M.R. Photodynamic therapy for infections: Clinical applications. *Lasers Surg. Med.* **2011**, *43*, 755–767. [CrossRef] [PubMed]
84. Abrahamse, H.; Hamblin, M.R. New photosensitizers for photodynamic therapy. *Biochem. J.* **2016**, *473*, 347–364. [CrossRef] [PubMed]
85. Gannon, M.J.; Brown, S.B. Photodynamic therapy and its applications in gynaecology. *Br. J. Obstet. Gynaecol.* **1999**, *106*, 1246–1254. [CrossRef] [PubMed]
86. Konan, Y.N.; Gurny, R.; Allémann, E. State of the art in the delivery of photosensitizers for photodynamic therapy. *J. Photochem. Photobiol. B Biol.* **2002**, *66*, 89–106. [CrossRef]
87. Kalka, K.; Merk, H.; Mukhtar, H. Photodynamic therapy in dermatology. *J. Am. Acad. Dermatol.* **2000**, *42*, 389–413. [CrossRef]
88. Calixto, G.M.F.; Bernegossi, J.; De Freitas, L.M.; Fontana, C.R.; Chorilli, M.; Grumezescu, A.M. Nanotechnology-based drug delivery systems for photodynamic therapy of cancer: A review. *Molecules* **2016**, *21*, 342. [CrossRef]
89. Moan, J.; Streckyte, G.; Bagdonas, S.; Bech, O.; Berg, K. The pH dependency of protoporphyrin IX formation in cells incubated with 5-aminolevulinic acid. *Cancer Lett.* **1997**, *113*, 25–29. [CrossRef]
90. Tedesco, A.; Rotta, J.; Lunardi, C. Synthesis, photophysical and photochemical aspects of phthalocyanines for photodynamic therapy. *Curr. Org. Chem.* **2003**, *7*, 187–196. [CrossRef]
91. Tokumaru, K. Photochemical and photophysical behaviour of porphyrins and phthalocyanines irradiated with violet or ultraviolet light. *J. Porphyr. Phthalocyanines* **2001**, *5*, 77–86. [CrossRef]
92. Ahmad, N.; Mukhtar, H. Mechanism of photodynamic therapy-Induced cell death. *Methods Enzym.* **2000**, *319*, 342–358. [CrossRef]
93. Allison, R.R.; Downie, G.H.; Cuenca, R.; Hu, X.H.; Childs, C.J.H.; Sibata, C.H. Photosensitizers in clinical PDT. *Photodiagn. Photodyn. Ther.* **2004**, *1*, 27–42. [CrossRef]
94. Nagata, J.Y.; Hioka, N.; Kimura, E.; Batistela, V.R.; Terada, R.S.S.; Graciano, A.X.; Baesso, M.L.; Hayacibara, M.F. Antibacterial photodynamic therapy for dental caries: Evaluation of the photosensitizers used and light source properties. *Photodiagn. Photodyn. Ther.* **2012**, *9*, 122–131. [CrossRef] [PubMed]
95. Andrzejak, M.; Price, M.; Kessel, D.H. Apoptotic and autophagic responses to photodynamic therapy in 1c1c7 murine hepatoma cells. *Autophagy* **2011**, *7*, 979–984. [CrossRef] [PubMed]
96. Chiaviello, A.; Postiglione, I.; Palumbo, G. Targets and mechanisms of photodynamic therapy in lung cancer cells: A brief overview. *Cancers* **2011**, *3*, 1014–1041. [CrossRef] [PubMed]
97. Kim, J.; Lim, W.; Kim, S.; Jeon, S.; Hui, Z.; ni, K.; Kim, C.; Im, Y.; Choi, H.; Kim, O. Photodynamic therapy (PDT) resistance by PARP1 regulation on PDT-induced apoptosis with autophagy in head and neck cancer cells. *J. Oral Pathol. Med.* **2014**, *43*, 675–684. [CrossRef]
98. Buytaert, E.; Dewaele, M.; Agostinis, P. Molecular effectors of multiple cell death pathways initiated by photodynamic therapy. *Biochim. Biophys. Acta-Rev. Cancer* **2007**, *1776*, 86–107. [CrossRef]
99. Taylor, E.L.; Brown, S.B. The advantages of aminolevulinic acid photodynamic therapy in dermatology. *J. Dermatolog. Treat.* **2002**, *13*, s3–s11. [CrossRef]
100. Calzavara-Pinton, P.G.; Venturini, M.; Sala, R. Photodynamic therapy: Update 2006 Part 1: Photochemistry and photobiology. *J. Eur. Acad. Dermatol. Venereol.* **2007**, *21*, 293–302. [CrossRef] [PubMed]
101. Dougherty, T.J.; Gomer, C.J.; Henderson, B.W.; Jori, G.; Kessel, D.; Korbelik, M.; Moan, J.; Peng, Q. Photodynamic therapy. *J. Natl. Cancer Inst.* **1998**, *90*, 889–905. [CrossRef]
102. Issa, M.C.A.; Manela-Azulay, M. Photodynamic therapy: A review of the literature and image documentation. *An. Bras. Dermatol.* **2010**, *85*, 501–511. [CrossRef]
103. Tedesco, A.C.; Primo, F.L.; Beltrame, M. Phtalocyanines: Synthesis, characterization and biological applications of photodynamic therapy (PDT), nanobiotechnology, magnetohypertermia and photodiagnosis (theranostics). In *Reference Module in Materials Science and Materials Engineering*; Elsevier: Amsterdam, The Netherlands, 2016. [CrossRef]
104. Dos Santos, A.F.; De Almeida, D.R.Q.; Terra, L.F.; Baptista, M.S.; Labriola, L. Photodynamic therapy in cancer treatment—An update review. *J. Cancer Metastasis Treat.* **2019**, *5*, 25. [CrossRef]
105. Tsubone, T.M.; Martins, W.K.; Pavani, C.; Junqueira, H.C.; Itri, R.; Baptista, M.S. Enhanced efficiency of cell death by lysosome-specific photodamage. *Sci. Rep.* **2017**, *7*, 6734. [CrossRef] [PubMed]
106. Oliveira, C.S.; Turchiello, R.; Kowaltowski, A.J.; Indig, G.L.; Baptista, M.S. Major determinants of photoinduced cell death: Subcellular localization versus photosensitization efficiency. *Free Radic. Biol. Med.* **2011**, *51*, 824–833. [CrossRef] [PubMed]
107. Kessel, D.; Reiners, J.J. Promotion of proapoptotic signals by lysosomal photodamage. *Photochem. Photobiol.* **2015**, *91*, 931–936. [CrossRef] [PubMed]
108. Feng, X.; Shi, Y.; Xie, L.; Zhang, K.; Wang, X.; Liu, Q.; Wang, P. Synthesis, Characterization, and Biological Evaluation of a Porphyrin-Based Photosensitizer and Its Isomer for Effective Photodynamic Therapy against Breast Cancer. *J. Med. Chem.* **2018**, *61*, 7189–7201. [CrossRef]
109. Agarwal, M.L.; Clay, M.E.; Harvey, E.J.; Evans, H.H.; Antunez, A.R.; Oleinick, L.N. Photodynamic therapy induces rapid cell death by apoptosis in LSI78Y mouse lymphoma cells. *Cancer Res.* **1991**, *51*, 5993–5996. [PubMed]
110. Kessel, D. Death pathways associated with photodynamic therapy. *Med. Laser Appl.* **2006**, *15*, 219–224. [CrossRef] [PubMed]

111. Kessel, D.; Oleinick, N.L. Cell death pathways associated with photodynamic therapy: An update. *Photochem. Photobiol.* **2018**, *94*, 213–218. [CrossRef] [PubMed]
112. Kushibiki, T.; Hirasawa, T.; Okawa, S.; Ishihara, M. Responses of cancer cells induced by photodynamic therapy. *J. Healthc. Eng.* **2013**, *4*, 87–108. [CrossRef] [PubMed]
113. Garg, A.; Nowis, D.; Golab, J.; Vandenabeele, P.; Krysko, D.; Agostinis, P. Immunogenic cell death, DAMPs and anticancer therapeutics: An emerging amalgamation. *Biochim. Biophys. Acta* **2010**, *1805*, 53–71. [CrossRef]
114. Reiners, J.J.; Agostinis, P.; Berg, K.; Oleinick, N.L.; Kessel, D. Assessing autophagy in the context of photodynamic therapy. *Autophagy* **2010**, *6*, 7–18. [CrossRef]
115. Galluzzi, L.; Bravo-San Pedro, J.M.; Kroemer, G. Organelle-specific initiation of cell death. *Nat. Cell Biol.* **2014**, *16*, 728–736. [CrossRef]
116. Babilas, P.; Schreml, S.; Landthaler, M.; Szeimies, R.M. Photodynamic therapy in dermatology: State-of-the-art. *Photodermatol. Photoimmunol. Photomed.* **2010**, *26*, 118–132. [CrossRef]
117. Baldeia, I.; Filip, A. Photodynamic therapy in melanoma—an update. *J. Physiol. Pharmacol.* **2012**, *63*, 109–118.
118. Marmo Moreira, L.; Fábio Vieira dos Santos, B.; Juliana Pereira Lyon, A.; Maira Maftoum-Costa, A.; Cristina Pacheco-Soares, A.; Soares da Silva, N.A. Photodynamic therapy: Porphyrins and phthalocyanines as photosensitizers. *Aust. J. Chem.* **2008**, *61*, 741–754. [CrossRef]
119. Crescenzi, E.; Chiaviello, A.; Canti, G.; Reddi, E.; Veneziani, B.M.; Palumbo, G. Low doses of cisplatin or gemcitabine plus Photofrin/photodynamic therapy: Disjointed cell cycle phase-related activity accounts for synergistic outcome in metastatic non-small cell lung cancer cells (H1299). *Mol. Cancer Ther.* **2006**, *5*, 776–785. [CrossRef] [PubMed]
120. Aniogo, E.C.; George, B.P.A.; Abrahamse, H. Phthalocyanine induced phototherapy coupled with Doxorubicin; a promising novel treatment for breast cancer. *Expert Rev. Anticancer Ther.* **2017**, *17*, 693–702. [CrossRef] [PubMed]
121. Henderson, V.W.; Busch, T.M.; Snyder, J.W. Fluence rate as a modulator of PDT mechanisms. *Lasers Surg. Med.* **2006**, *38*, 489–493. [CrossRef] [PubMed]
122. Spring, B.Q.; Rizvi, I.; Xu, N.; Hasan, T. The role of photodynamic therapy in overcoming cancer drug resistance. *Photochem. Photobiol. Sci.* **2015**, *14*, 1476–1491. [CrossRef]
123. Cid, J.J.; Yum, J.H.; Jang, S.R.; Nazeeruddin, M.K.; Martínez-Ferrero, E.; Palomares, E.; Ko, J.; Grätzel, M.; Torres, T. Molecular cosensitization for efficient panchromatic dye-sensitized solar cells. *Angew. Chem.-Int. Ed.* **2007**, *46*, 8358–8362. [CrossRef] [PubMed]
124. Brasseur, N. Sensitizers for PDT: Phthalocyanines. In *Photodynamic Therapy*; Royal Society of Chemistry: London, UK, 2007; pp. 105–118. ISBN 978-1-84755-165-8.
125. Ogura, S.I.; Tabata, K.; Fukushima, K.; Kamachi, T.; Okura, I. Development of phthalocyanines for photodynamic therapy. *J. Porphyr. Phthalocyanines* **2006**, *10*, 1116–1124. [CrossRef]
126. Mantareva, V.; Kussovski, V.; Angelov, I.; Borisova, E.; Avramov, L.; Schnurpfeil, G.; Wöhrle, D. Photodynamic activity of water-soluble phthalocyanine zinc(II) complexes against pathogenic microorganisms. *Bioorg. Med. Chem.* **2007**, *15*, 4829–4835. [CrossRef]
127. Ali, H.; Van Lier, J.E. Metal complexes as photo- and radiosensitizers. *Chem. Rev.* **1999**, *99*, 2379–2450. [CrossRef]
128. Nyman, E.S.; Hynninen, P.H. Research advances in the use of tetrapyrrolic photosensitizers for photodynamic therapy. *J. Photochem. Photobiol. B Biol.* **2004**, *73*, 1–28. [CrossRef]
129. Ball, D.J.; Wood, S.R.; Vernon, D.I.; Griffiths, J.; Dubbelman, T.M.A.R.; Brown, S.B. The characterisation of three substituted zinc phthalocyanines of differing charge for use in photodynamic therapy. A comparative study of their aggregation and photosensitising ability in relation to mTHPC and polyhaematoporphyrin. *J. Photochem. Photobiol. B Biol.* **1998**, *45*, 28–35. [CrossRef]
130. Kadish, K.M.; Smith, K.M.; Guilard, R. *The Porphyrin Handbook*; Academic Press: San Diego, CA, USA, 2003.
131. Pinzón, J.R.; Plonska-Brzezinska, M.E.; Cardona, C.M.; Athans, A.J.; Gayathri, S.S.; Guldi, D.M.; Herranz, M.Á.; Martín, N.; Torres, T.; Echegoyen, L. Sc3N@C80-ferrocene electron-donor/acceptor conjugates as promising materials for photovoltaic applications. *Angew. Chemie-Int. Ed.* **2008**, *47*, 4173–4176. [CrossRef] [PubMed]
132. Braun, A.; Tcherniac, J. Über die produkte der einwirkung von acetanhydrid auf phthalamid. *Ber. Dtsch. Chem. Ges.* **1907**, *40*, 2709–2714. [CrossRef]
133. Kharisov, B.I.; Mendez, U.O.; Garza, J.L.A.; Rodrı´guez, J.R.A. Synthesis of non-substituted phthalocyanines by standard and non-standard techniques. Influence of solvent nature in phthalocyanine preparation at low temperature by UV-treatment of the reaction system. *New J. Chem.* **2005**, *29*, 686–692. [CrossRef]
134. De Diesbach, H.; von der Weid, E. Quelques sels complexes des o-dinitriles avec le cuivre et la pyridine. *Helv. Chim. Acta* **1927**, *10*, 886–888. [CrossRef]
135. Linstead, R.P. Phthalocyanines. Part I. A new type of synthetic colouring matters. *J. Chem. Soc.* **1934**, *95*, 1016–1017. [CrossRef]
136. Linstead, R.P.; Lowe, A.R. Phthalocyanines. Part III. Preliminary experiments on the preparation of phthalocyanines from phthalonitrile. *J. Chem. Soc.* **1934**, 1022–1027. [CrossRef]
137. Dent, C.E.; Linstead, R.P.; Lowe, A.R. Phthalocyanines. Part VI. The structure of the phthalocyanines. *J. Chem. Soc.* **1934**, *1033*, 184. [CrossRef]

138. Sharman, W.M.; Allen, C.M.; Van Lier, J.E. Photodynamic therapeutics: Basic principles and clinical applications. *Drug Discov. Today* **1999**, *4*, 507–517. [CrossRef]
139. Medina, W.S.G.; dos Santos, N.A.G.; Curti, C.; Tedesco, A.C.; dos Santos, A.C. Effects of zinc phthalocyanine tetrasulfonate-based photodynamic therapy on rat brain isolated mitochondria. *Chem. Biol. Interact.* **2009**, *179*, 402–406. [CrossRef]
140. Staicu, A.; Pascu, A.; Nuta, A.; Sorescu, A.; Raditoiu, V.; Pascu, M.L. Studies about phthalocyanine photosensitizers to be used in photodynamic therapy. *Rom. Rep. Phys.* **2013**, *65*, 1032–1051.
141. Spikes, J.D.; Jori, G. Photodynamic therapy of tumours and other diseases using porphyrins. *Laser Med. Sci.* **1987**, *2*, 3–15. [CrossRef]
142. Whitacre, C.M.; Feyes, D.K.; Satoh, T.; Grossmann, J.; Mulvihill, J.W.; Mukhtar, H.; Oleinick, N.L. Photodynamic therapy with the phthalocyanine photosensitizer Pc 4 of SW480 human colon cancer xenografts in athymic mice. *Clin. Cancer Res.* **2000**, *6*, 2021–2027. [PubMed]
143. Vieira Velloso, N.; Muehlmann, L.A.; Longo, P.F.; Rodrigues Da Silva, J.; Zancanela, D.C.; Tedesco, A.C.; Bentes De Azevedo, R. Aluminum-phthalocyanine chloride-based photodynamic therapy inhibits pi3k/akt/mtor pathway in oral squamous cell carcinoma cells in vitro. *Chemotherapy* **2012**, *2012*, 5. [CrossRef]
144. Abrahamse, H.; Kresfelder, T.; Horne, T.; Cronje, M.; Nyokong, T. Apoptotic inducing ability of a novel photosensitizing agent, Ge sulfophthalocyanine, on oesophageal and breast cancer cell lines. *Opt. Methods Tumor Treat. Detect. Mech. Tech. Photodyn. Ther. XV* **2006**, *6139*, 613904. [CrossRef]
145. Seotsanyana-Mokhosi, I.; Kresfelder, T.; Abrahamse, H.; Nyokong, T. The effect of Ge, Si and Sn phthalocyanine photosensitizers on cell proliferation and viability of human oesophageal carcinoma cells. *J. Photochem. Photobiol. B Biol.* **2006**, *83*, 55–62. [CrossRef] [PubMed]
146. Manoto, S.L.; Sekhejane, P.R.; Houreld, N.N.; Abrahamse, H. Localization and phototoxic effect of zinc sulfophthalocyanine photosensitizer in human colon (DLD-1) and lung (A549) carcinoma cells (in vitro). *Photodiagn. Photodyn. Ther.* **2012**, *9*, 52–59. [CrossRef]
147. Manoto, S.L.; Houreld, N.N.; Abrahamse, H. Phototoxic effect of photodynamic therapy on lung cancer cells grown as a monolayer and three dimensional multicellular spheroids. *Lasers Surg. Med.* **2013**, *45*, 186–194. [CrossRef]
148. Love, W.G.; Duk, S.; Biolo, R.; Jori, G.; Taylor, P.W. Liposome-mediated delivery of photosensitizers: Localization of zinc (II)-phthalocyanine within implanted tumors after intravenous administration. *Photochem. Photobiol.* **1996**, *63*, 656–661. [CrossRef]
149. Shao, J.; Xue, J.; Dai, Y.; Liu, H.; Chen, N.; Jia, L.; Huang, J. Inhibition of human hepatocellular carcinoma HepG2 by phthalocyanine photosensitiser photocyanine: ROS production, apoptosis, cell cycle arrest. *Eur. J. Cancer* **2012**, *48*, 2086–2096. [CrossRef] [PubMed]
150. Miller, J.D.; Baron, E.D.; Scull, H.; Hsia, A.; Berlin, J.C.; McCormick, T.; Colussi, V.; Kenney, M.E.; Cooper, K.D.; Oleinick, N.L. Photodynamic therapy with the phthalocyanine photosensitizer Pc 4: The case experience with preclinical mechanistic and early clinical-translational studies. *Toxicol. Appl. Pharmacol.* **2007**, *224*, 290–299. [CrossRef] [PubMed]
151. Baran, T.M.; Giesselman, B.R.; Hu, R.; Biel, M.A.; Foster, T.H. Factors influencing tumor response to photodynamic therapy sensitized by intratumor administration of methylene blue. *Lasers Surg. Med.* **2010**, *42*, 728–735. [CrossRef]
152. Spikes, J.D. Phthalocyanines as photosensitizers in biological systems and for the photodynamic therapy of tumors. *Photochem. Photobiol.* **1986**, *43*, 691–699. [CrossRef] [PubMed]
153. Zaidi, S.I.A.; Agarwal, R.; Eichler, G.; Rihter, B.D.; Kenney, M.E.; Mukhtar, H. Photodynamic effects of new silicon phthalocyanines: In vitro studies utilizing rat hepatic microsomes and human erythrocyte ghosts as model membrane sources. *Photochem. Photobiol.* **1993**, *58*, 204–210. [CrossRef] [PubMed]
154. Agarwal, R.; Athar, M.; Elmets, C.A.; Bickers, D.R.; Mukhtar, H. Photodynamic therapy of chemically- and ultraviolet B radiation-induced murine skin papillomas by chloroaluminum phthalocyanine tetrasulfonate. *Photochem. Photobiol.* **1992**, *56*, 43–50. [CrossRef] [PubMed]
155. Brasseur, N.; Ali, H.; Autenrieth, D.; Langlois, R.; van Lier, J.E. Biological activities of Phthalocyanines—iii. Photoinactivation of v-79 chinese hamster cells by tetrasulfophthalocyanines. *Photochem. Photobiol.* **1985**, *42*, 515–521. [CrossRef] [PubMed]
156. Cook, M.J.; Chambrier, I.; Cracknell, S.J.; Mayes, D.A.; Russell, D.A. Octa-alkyl zinc phthalocyanines: Potential photosensitizers for use in the photodynamic therapy of cancer. *Photochem. Photobiol.* **1995**, *62*, 542–545. [CrossRef] [PubMed]
157. Stilts, C.E.; Nelen, M.I.; Hilmey, D.G.; Davies, S.R.; Gollnick, S.O.; Oseroff, A.R.; Gibson, S.L.; Hilf, R.; Detty, M.R. Water-soluble, core-modified porphyrins as novel, longer-wavelength- absorbing sensitizers for photodynamic therapy. *J. Med. Chem.* **2000**, *43*, 2403–2410. [CrossRef] [PubMed]
158. Yates, N.C.; Moan, J.; Western, A. Water-soluble metal naphthalocyanines-near-IR photosensitizers: Cellular uptake, toxicity and photosensitizing properties in nhik 3025 human cancer cells. *J. Photochem. Photobiol. B Biol.* **1990**, *4*, 379–390. [CrossRef]
159. Cruse-Sawyer, J.E.; Griffiths, J.; Dixon, B.; Brown, S.B. The photodynamic response of two rodent tumour models to four zinc (II)-substituted phthalocyanines. *Br. J. Cancer* **1998**, *77*, 965–972. [CrossRef]
160. Sharman, W.M.; Kudrevich, S.V.; Van Lier, J.E. Novel water-soluble phthalocyanines substituted with phosphonate moieties on the benzo rings. *Tetrahedron Lett.* **1996**, *37*, 5831–5834. [CrossRef]
161. Wöhrle, D. Phthalocyanines: Properties and applications, volume 3. Edited by C. C. Leznoff and A. B. P. Lever, VCH, Weinheim 1993, 303 pp., hardcover, DM 198, ISBN3-527-89638-4. *Adv. Mater.* **1993**, *5*, 943–944. [CrossRef]

162. Lo, P.C.; Rodríguez-Morgade, M.S.; Pandey, R.K.; Ng, D.K.P.; Torres, T.; Dumoulin, F. The unique features and promises of phthalocyanines as advanced photosensitisers for photodynamic therapy of cancer. *Chem. Soc. Rev.* **2020**, *49*, 1041–1056. [CrossRef]
163. Brasseur, N.; Ouellet, R.; La Madeleine, C.; Van Lier, J. Water soluble aluminium phthalocyanine-polymer conjugates for PDT: Photodynamic activities and pharmacokinetics in tumour bearing mice. *Br. J. Cancer* **1999**, *80*, 1533–1541. [CrossRef] [PubMed]
164. Yamaoka, T.; Tabata, Y.; Ikada, Y. Distribution and tissue uptake of poly(ethylene glycol) with different molecular weights after intravenous administration to mice. *J. Pharm. Sci.* **1994**, *83*, 601–606. [CrossRef] [PubMed]
165. Schneider, L.; Larocca, M.; Wu, W.; Babu, V.; Padrutt, R.; Slyshkina, E.; König, C.; Ferrari, S.; Spingler, B. Exocyclically metallated tetrapyridinoporphyrazine as a potential photosensitizer for photodynamic therapy. *Photochem. Photobiol. Sci.* **2019**, *18*, 2792–2803. [CrossRef] [PubMed]
166. Md, S.; Haque, S.; Madheswaran, T.; Zeeshan, F.; Meka, V.S.; Radhakrishnan, A.K.; Kesharwani, P. Lipid based nanocarriers system for topical delivery of photosensitizers. *Drug Discov. Today* **2017**, *22*, 1274–1283. [CrossRef]
167. Gunaydin, G.; Gedik, M.E.; Ayan, S. Photodynamic Therapy—Current Limitations and Novel Approaches. *Front. Chem.* **2021**, *9*, 691697. [CrossRef] [PubMed]
168. Rahbari, R.; Sheahan, T.; Modes, V.; Collier, P.; Macfarlane, C.; Badge, R.M. A novel L1 retrotransposon marker for HeLa cell line identification. *Biotechniques* **2009**, *46*, 277–284. [CrossRef] [PubMed]
169. Scherer, W.F.; Syverton, J.T.; Gey, G.O. Studies on the propagation in vitro of poliomyelitis viruses: IV. Viral multiplication in a stable strain of human malignant epithelial cells (strain HeLa) derived from an epidermoid carcinoma of the cervix. *J. Exp. Med.* **1953**, *97*, 695–710. [CrossRef] [PubMed]
170. Capes-Davis, A.; Theodosopoulos, G.; Atkin, I.; Drexler, H.G.; Kohara, A.; MacLeod, R.A.F.; Masters, J.R.; Nakamura, Y.; Reid, Y.A.; Reddel, R.R.; et al. Check your cultures! A list of cross-contaminated or misidentified cell lines. *Int. J. Cancer* **2010**, *127*, 1–8. [CrossRef] [PubMed]
171. Halaskova, M.; Rahali, A.; Almeida-Marrero, V.; Machacek, M.; Kucera, R.; Jamoussi, B.; Torres, T.; Novakova, V.; de la Escosura, A.; Zimcik, P. Peripherally crowded cationic phthalocyanines as efficient photosensitizers for photodynamic therapy. *ACS Med. Chem. Lett.* **2021**, *12*, 502–507. [CrossRef]
172. Chu, J.C.H.; Fong, W.-P.; Wong, C.T.T.; Ng, D.K.P. Facile synthesis of cyclic peptide–phthalocyanine conjugates for epidermal growth factor receptor-targeted photodynamic therapy. *J. Med. Chem.* **2021**, *64*, 2064–2076. [CrossRef] [PubMed]
173. Göksel, M.; Durmuş, M.; Biyiklioglu, Z. Synthesis and photodynamic activities of novel silicon(IV) phthalocyanines axially substituted with water soluble groups against HeLa cancer cell line. *Dalt. Trans.* **2021**, *50*, 2570–2584. [CrossRef] [PubMed]
174. Pola, M.; Kolarova, H.; Ruzicka, J.; Zholobenko, A.; Modriansky, M.; Mosinger, J.; Bajgar, R. Effects of zinc porphyrin and zinc phthalocyanine derivatives in photodynamic anticancer therapy under different partial pressures of oxygen in vitro. *Investig. New Drugs* **2020**, *39*, 89–97. [CrossRef]
175. Revuelta-Maza, M.; Mascaraque, M.; González-Jiménez, P.; González-Camuñas, A.; Nonell, S.; Juarranz, Á.; de la Torre, G.; Torres, T. Assessing amphiphilic ABAB Zn(II) phthalocyanines with enhanced photosensitization abilities in in vitro photodynamic therapy studies against cancer. *Molecules* **2020**, *25*, 213. [CrossRef]
176. Ermakov, A.; Verkhovskii, R.; Babushkina, I.; Trushina, D.; Inozemtseva, O.; Lukyanets, E.; Ulyanov, V.; Gorin, D.; Belyakov, S.; Antipina, M. In vitro bioeffects of polyelectrolyte multilayer microcapsules post-loaded with water-soluble cationic photosensitizer. *Pharmaceutics* **2020**, *12*, 610. [CrossRef] [PubMed]
177. Balçik-Erçin, P.; Çetin, M.; Göksel, M.; Durmuş, M. Improved targeting for photodynamic therapy: Via a biotin-phthalocyanine conjugate: Synthesis, photophysical and photochemical measurements, and in vitro cytotoxicity assay. *New J. Chem.* **2020**, *44*, 3392–3401. [CrossRef]
178. Kollar, J.; Machacek, M.; Halaskova, M.; Lenco, J.; Kucera, R.; Demuth, J.; Rohlickova, M.; Hasonova, K.; Miletin, M.; Novakova, V.; et al. Cationic versus anionic phthalocyanines for photodynamic therapy: What a difference the charge makes. *J. Med. Chem.* **2020**, *63*, 7616–7632. [CrossRef] [PubMed]
179. Shi, Y.; Zhan, Q.; Li, Y.; Zhou, L.; Wei, S. Multiple functions integrated inside a single molecule for amplification of photodynamic therapy activity. *Mol. Pharm.* **2020**, *17*, 190–201. [CrossRef] [PubMed]
180. Cozzolino, M.; Pesce, L.; Pezzuoli, D.; Montali, C.; Brancaleon, L.; Cavanna, L.; Abbruzzetti, S.; Diaspro, A.; Bianchini, P.; Vlapplani, C. Apomyoglobin is an efficient carrier for zinc phthalocyanine in photodynamic therapy of tumors. *Biophys. Chem.* **2019**, *253*, 106228. [CrossRef]
181. Ma, J.; Li, Y.; Liu, G.; Li, A.; Chen, Y.; Zhou, X.; Chen, D.; Hou, Z.; Zhu, X. Novel theranostic zinc phthalocyanine–phospholipid complex self-assembled nanoparticles for imaging-guided targeted photodynamic treatment with controllable ROS production and shape-assisted enhanced cellular uptake. *Colloids Surf. B Biointerfaces* **2018**, *162*, 76–89. [CrossRef]
182. Ma, J.; Chen, D.; Li, Y.; Chen, Y.; Liu, Q.; Zhou, X.; Qian, K.; Li, Z.; Ruan, H.; Hou, Z.; et al. Zinc phthalocyanine-soybean phospholipid complex based drug carrier for switchable photoacoustic/fluorescence image, multiphase photothermal/photodynamic treatment and synergetic therapy. *J. Control. Release* **2018**, *284*, 1–14. [CrossRef]
183. Ma, J.; Wu, H.; Li, Y.; Liu, Z.; Liu, G.; Guo, Y.; Hou, Z.; Zhao, Q.; Chen, D.; Zhu, X. Novel core-interlayer-shell DOX/ZnPc co-loaded MSNs@ pH-sensitive CaP@PEGylated liposome for enhanced synergetic chemo-photodynamic therapy. *Pharm. Res.* **2018**, *35*, 57. [CrossRef] [PubMed]

184. Gülmez, A.D.; Göksel, M.; Durmuş, M. Silicon(IV) phthalocyanine-biotin conjugates: Synthesis, photophysicochemical properties and in vitro biological activity for photodynamic therapy. *J. Porphyr. Phthalocyanines* **2017**, *21*, 547–554. [CrossRef]
185. Wang, A.; Zhou, R.; Zhou, L.; Sun, K.; Jiang, J.; Wei, S. Positively charged phthalocyanine-arginine conjugates as efficient photosensitizer for photodynamic therapy. *Bioorg. Med. Chem.* **2017**, *25*, 1643–1651. [CrossRef]
186. Avşar, G.; Sari, F.A.; Yuzer, A.C.; Soylu, H.M.; Er, O.; Ince, M.; Lambrecht, F.Y. Intracellular uptake and fluorescence imaging potential in tumor cell of zinc phthalocyanine. *Int. J. Pharm.* **2016**, *505*, 369–375. [CrossRef] [PubMed]
187. Franchi, L.P.; Amantino, C.F.; Melo, M.T.; de Lima Montaldi, A.P.; Primo, F.L.; Tedesco, A.C. In vitro effects of photodynamic therapy induced by chloroaluminum phthalocyanine nanoemulsion. *Photodiagn. Photodyn. Ther.* **2016**, *16*, 100–105. [CrossRef]
188. Göksel, M. Synthesis of asymmetric zinc(II) phthalocyanines with two different functional groups & spectroscopic properties and photodynamic activity for photodynamic therapy. *Bioorg. Med. Chem.* **2016**, *24*, 4152–4164. [CrossRef] [PubMed]
189. Huang, Y.; Yu, H.; Lv, H.; Zhang, H.; Ma, D.; Yang, H.; Xie, S.; Peng, Y. Triblock copolymers encapsulated poly (aryl benzyl ether) dendrimer zinc(II) phthalocyanine nanoparticles for enhancement in vitro photodynamic efficacy. *Photodiagn. Photodyn. Ther.* **2016**, *16*, 124–131. [CrossRef]
190. Lu, S.; Wang, A.; Ma, Y.J.; Xuan, H.Y.; Zhao, B.; Li, X.D.; Zhou, J.H.; Zhou, L.; Wei, S.H. Cyclodextrin type dependent host-guest interaction mode with phthalocyanine and their influence on photodynamic activity to cancer. *Carbohydr. Polym.* **2016**, *148*, 236–242. [CrossRef] [PubMed]
191. Wang, A.; Jin, W.; Chen, E.; Zhou, J.; Zhou, L.; Wei, S. Drug delivery function of carboxymethyl-β-cyclodextrin modified upconversion nanoparticles for adamantine phthalocyanine and their NIR-triggered cancer treatment. *Dalt. Trans.* **2016**, *45*, 3853–3862. [CrossRef]
192. Young, J.; Yee, M.; Kim, H.; Cheung, J.; Chino, T.; Düzgüneş, N.; Konopka, K. Phototoxicity of liposomal Zn- and Al-phthalocyanine against cervical and oral squamous cell carcinoma cells in vitro. *Med. Sci. Monit. Basic Res.* **2016**, *22*, 156–164. [CrossRef] [PubMed]
193. Yurt, F.; Ocakoglu, K.; Ince, M.; Colak, S.G.; Er, O.; Soylu, H.M.; Gunduz, C.; Biray Avci, C.; Caliskan Kurt, C. Photodynamic therapy and nuclear imaging activities of zinc phthalocyanine-integrated TiO$_2$ nanoparticles in breast and cervical tumors. *Chem. Biol. Drug Des.* **2018**, *91*, 789–796. [CrossRef]
194. Hodgkinson, N.; Kruger, C.A.; Mokwena, M.; Abrahamse, H. Cervical cancer cells (HeLa) response to photodynamic therapy using a zinc phthalocyanine photosensitizer. *J. Photochem. Photobiol. B Biol.* **2017**, *177*, 32–38. [CrossRef] [PubMed]
195. Pazos, M.D.C.; Nader, H.B. Effect of photodynamic therapy on the extracellular matrix and associated components. *Braz. J. Med. Biol. Res.* **2007**, *40*, 1025–1035. [CrossRef] [PubMed]
196. Bacellar, I.; Tsubone, T.; Pavani, C.; Baptista, M. Photodynamic efficiency: From molecular photochemistry to cell death. *Int. J. Mol. Sci.* **2015**, *16*, 20523–20559. [CrossRef] [PubMed]
197. Hu, T.; Wang, Z.; Shen, W.; Liang, R.; Yan, D.; Wei, M. Recent advances in innovative strategies for enhanced cancer photodynamic therapy. *Theranostics* **2021**, *11*, 3278–3300. [CrossRef]
198. Mitra, K.; Hartman, M.C.T. Silicon phthalocyanines: Synthesis and resurgent applications. *Org. Biomol. Chem.* **2021**, *19*, 1168–1190. [CrossRef]
199. Li, K.; Dong, W.; Liu, Q.; Lv, G.; Xie, M.; Sun, X.; Qiu, L.; Lin, J. A biotin receptor-targeted silicon(IV) phthalocyanine for in vivo tumor imaging and photodynamic therapy. *J. Photochem. Photobiol. B Biol.* **2019**, *190*, 1–7. [CrossRef]
200. Liang, X.; Xie, Y.; Wu, J.; Wang, J.; Petković, M.; Stepić, M.; Zhao, J.; Ma, J.; Mi, L. Functional titanium dioxide nanoparticle conjugated with phthalocyanine and folic acid as a promising photosensitizer for targeted photodynamic therapy in vitro and in vivo. *J. Photochem. Photobiol. B Biol.* **2021**, *215*, 112122. [CrossRef]
201. Wang, J.; Zhuo, X.; Xiao, X.; Mao, R.; Wang, Y.; Wang, J.; Liu, J. AlPcS-loaded gold nanobipyramids with high two-photon efficiency for photodynamic therapy: In vivo. *Nanoscale* **2019**, *11*, 3397. [CrossRef]
202. Hillemanns, P.; Garcia, F.; Petry, K.U.; Dvorak, V.; Sadovsky, O.; Iversen, O.; Einstein, M.H. A randomized study of hexaminolevulinate photodynamic therapy in patients with cervical intraepithelial neoplasia 1/2. *Am. J. Obstet. Gynecol.* **2015**, *212*, 465.e1-7. [CrossRef]
203. Larmour, L.I.; Jobling, T.W.; Gargett, C.E. A review of current animal models for the study of cervical dysplasia and cervical carcinoma. *Int. J. Gynecol. Cancer* **2015**, *25*, 1345–1352. [CrossRef]

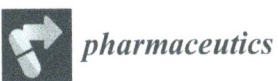

Review

Combining Nanocarrier-Assisted Delivery of Molecules and Radiotherapy

Eliza Rocha Gomes [1] and Marina Santiago Franco [2,*]

[1] Department of Pharmaceutical Products, Faculty of Pharmacy, Universidade Federal de Minas Gerais, Belo Horizonte 31270-901, Brazil; elizarochagomes@gmail.com
[2] Department of Radiation Sciences (DRS), Institute of Radiation Medicine (IRM), 85764 München, Germany
* Correspondence: marina.franco@helmholtz-muenchen.de; Tel.: +49-89-3187-48767

Abstract: Cancer is responsible for a significant proportion of death all over the world. Therefore, strategies to improve its treatment are highly desired. The use of nanocarriers to deliver anticancer treatments has been extensively investigated and improved since the approval of the first liposomal formulation for cancer treatment in 1995. Radiotherapy (RT) is present in the disease management strategy of around 50% of cancer patients. In the present review, we bring the state-of-the-art information on the combination of nanocarrier-assisted delivery of molecules and RT. We start with formulations designed to encapsulate single or multiple molecules that, once delivered to the tumor site, act directly on the cells to improve the effects of RT. Then, we describe formulations designed to modulate the tumor microenvironment by delivering oxygen or to boost the abscopal effect. Finally, we present how RT can be employed to trigger molecule delivery from nanocarriers or to modulate the EPR effect.

Keywords: nanocarriers; nanosystems; chemotherapy; radiotherapy; radiosensitizer; abscopal effect; hypoxia; synergism; cancer

---

Citation: Gomes, E.R.; Franco, M.S. Combining Nanocarrier-Assisted Delivery of Molecules and Radiotherapy. *Pharmaceutics* 2022, 14, 105. https://doi.org/10.3390/pharmaceutics14010105

Academic Editor: Carlos Alonso-Moreno

Received: 24 November 2021
Accepted: 29 December 2021
Published: 3 January 2022

Publisher's Note: MDPI stays neutral with regard to jurisdictional claims in published maps and institutional affiliations.

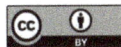

Copyright: © 2022 by the authors. Licensee MDPI, Basel, Switzerland. This article is an open access article distributed under the terms and conditions of the Creative Commons Attribution (CC BY) license (https://creativecommons.org/licenses/by/4.0/).

1. Introduction

Cancer is recognized as a leading cause of death all over the world. The disease is a barrier to increasing life expectancy, and its incidence and mortality keeps growing rapidly throughout the world. According to GLOBOCAN 2020, there were 19.3 million new cancer cases and around 10 million deaths from it in 2020 [1]. Currently, the main strategies used in cancer management are surgery, chemotherapy, and radiotherapy (RT). Chemotherapy acts not only in tumor cells but also in normal tissues, leading to systemic side effects that limit the doses that can be administered to the patients. One strategy to reduce the toxicity to normal tissues, thus enhancing the therapeutic index of chemotherapeutics, is the use of nanocarriers [2]. Nanosized formulations rely on their ability to passively accumulate in the tumor due to the enhanced permeability and retention (EPR) effect, discovered more than 30 years ago. Briefly, the EPR effect consists of nanocarriers taking advantage of the defective vascular architecture and poor lymphatic drainage in the tumoral area, to passively accumulate in this region [3,4]. This effect has been validated in both experimental animal models and different human tumors [3]. Since the approval of the first nanocarrier (Doxil®, liposomal doxorubicin) by the FDA in 1995, these formulations have been extensively researched and improved [5]. These improvements consist of different strategies. Active targeting to the tumor tissue is one of them. By decorating the surface of the nanocarriers with ligands directed to receptors known to be overexpressed in the tumor cells, it is possible to significantly increase drug delivery to the tumor as compared to passive targeting only [4,6]. Enhancing drug release kinetics at the tumor is also critical for the antitumoral effects. Therefore, nanocarriers designed to release their contents only when exposed to a trigger stimulus, either endogenous or exogenous, lead to superior anticancer effects [7]. The tumor microenvironment (TME) consists of different types of cells and many molecules released by tumor, stromal, and immune cells. It plays a role in tumor growth, differentiation, invasion, epigenetics, and immune evasion [8,9]. The complexity of the TME makes it an important target for cancer therapy with nanocarriers, which can carry and deliver multiple drugs with different targets [9,10]. The possibility to co-encapsulate molecules in nanocarriers allows for theranostic applications [11,12] as well as combination chemotherapy [13]. For combination chemotherapy, nanocarriers have been further finely designed to deliver specific synergistic ratios of drugs, significantly enhancing the antitumor activity [14,15].

The combination of different strategies to fight cancer will shape the future of cancer management. Understanding the mechanisms of strategies that can work together will lead to the greatest anticancer effects [2]. One strategy that is leading to good results is the combining nanocarrier-assisted delivery of molecules and RT. Commercialized nanocarriers such as Caelyx® (liposomal doxorubicin) and Abraxane® (albumin nanoparticles of paclitaxel) have already been combined to RT in clinical trials, showing to be a promising and safe treatment strategy [16–18]. These formulations, however, were not designed specifically with the purpose to be combined to RT.

RT deposits energy in the cells damaging their genetic material, thus hindering their ability to divide and proliferate. The damage to the cells occurs in a direct or indirect manner as illustrated in Figure 1. The direct action comprises approximately 50% of the damage to DNA. The direct-type effect consists of two different events. The first arises from energy deposited in the DNA itself, so that sites of electron loss (radical cations), electron gain (radical anions), and excitations (minor role) are created through ionizations. The second event consists of quasidirect effects, arising from the DNA solvation shell. When the solvation shell is ionized, radical cations and ejected electrons are rapidly transferred to DNA [19,20]. The indirect action consists of the radiolysis of water molecules present in the cells producing free radicals such as superoxide, hydrogen peroxide, and hydroxyl radical. These reactive oxygen species (ROS) interact with cellular molecules, such as DNA, lipids, and proteins [20,21]. ROS-mediated cell death is mainly caused by clustered DNA strand lesions, which are difficult to repair. The membranes and organelles of cells are also believed to be major targets of ROS. It acts by peroxidizing the membrane lipids, leading to structural and functional impairment, contributing to cell cycle arrest and apoptosis. Apoptosis can also arise from ROS-altered cellular homeostasis and ROS-modified signaling pathways [22]. Mitochondrial dysfunction due to ROS-mediated mitDNA damage leads to a sustained increase in endogenous ROS production, which culminates in more cell damage [23]. ROS are also related to early and late effects of RT, such as the bystander effect, field effect, inflammation, and fibrosis [24]. The direct and indirect disruption of the DNA molecular structure can lead to single-strand breaks (SSBs), base oxidation, apurinic, or apyrimidinic sites, and double-strand breaks (DSBs, the most important DNA damage) which culminate cell damage or death [25].

It is estimated that around 50% of cancer patients receive RT in their disease management. RT can be used as an isolated radical treatment or combined with surgery or systemic therapy in the curative setting. For patients with locally advanced or disseminated cancer, it is used to provide some symptom relief [27]. During RT, radiation doses that can be delivered to the patient are limited by normal tissue tolerance. Over the past few decades, thanks to engineering and computing, radiation instrumentation has strongly evolved. This allows an improved therapeutic ratio as radiation is delivered to the tumor with great precision, thereby minimizing normal tissue exposure, leading to higher cure rates. Additionally, radiobiology knowledge of tumor radiation sensitivity and resistance combined to normal tissue toxicity has improved RT outcome. The combined treatment of radiation and systemic drugs affects the radiobiological mechanisms in tumor and normal cells and is used in a large proportion of patients. Despite the good tumor control observed in many patients nowadays, some tumor types remain insensitive to RT or recur shortly after the treatment, indicating that there is still room for improvement [28–30]. The promising combination of nanocarriers and RT is the focus of the present review. Herein, we present how nanocarriers can be designed to modulate the effects of RT by delivering molecules that act either directly on the tumor cells or on TME. RT, in turn, can be used either as exogenous nanocarrier-trigger stimulus or to modulate the EPR effect. A summary of these strategies is depicted in Figure 2.

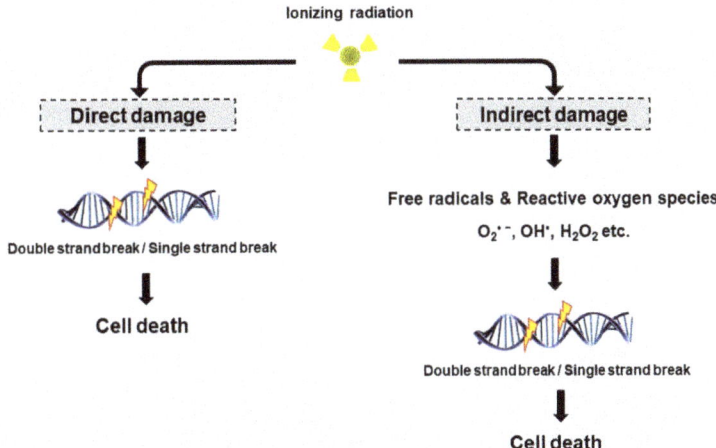

Figure 1. Ionizing radiation damages the DNA by direct and indirect effects. Direct damages arises from direct interaction between radiation and cellular DNA. Indirect DNA damage is caused by free radicals prevenient of the radiolysis of water molecules present in the cells. Reproduced from Hur and Yoon, MDPI, 2017 [26].

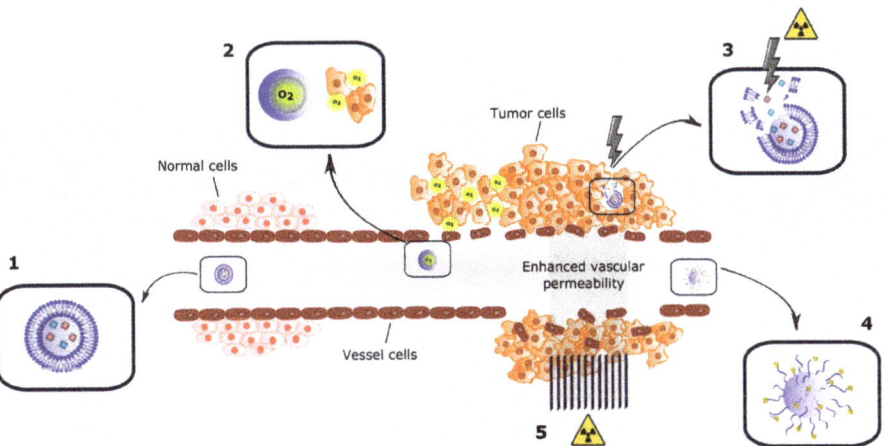

Figure 2. Strategies for combining nanocarrier-assisted delivery of molecules and radiotherapy. Encapsulation of single or multiple radiosensitizing agents in a nanocarrier (**1**); delivery of oxygen to diminish tumor hypoxia (**2**); radiation as exogenous triggering stimulus for in situ compound release (**3**); antigen-capturing nanocarriers to boost the abscopal effect; and (**4**) induction of transient enhanced vascular permeability by micro- and mini-beam irradiation modulating the EPR effect (**5**).

2. Nanocarriers Encapsulating Radiosensitizers

A range of compounds that influence, for example, DNA repair (especially double-strand break repair), act as radiosensitizers by increasing damage to the irradiated cells, leading to increased cell death [30]. However, these compounds present side effects that sometimes hamper their use [31]. Effective radiosensitizers should have less effect on normal tissues [21]. In this scenario, nanocarriers play an important role in directing the radiosensitizer to the tumor cells, sparing the normal tissue of the additional damage caused by irradiation.

2.1. Chemotherapeutic Drugs That Act as Radiosensitizers

Combinations of conventional chemotherapeutic drugs with RT led to most of the significant advances in cancer treatment in the last decades. Therefore, combinations of chemotherapy and RT are today the standard of care for many patients with solid tumors [32,33].

2.1.1. Cisplatin

Platinum analogs such as cisplatin (CDDP) are well-known radiosensitizers that have been widely used clinically in combination with RT for cancer treatment. Different potential mechanisms associated with radiation potentiation have been reported. Some of these mechanisms consist of adduct formation and DNA damage repair inhibition, an increase in cellular platinum uptake induced by radiation, synergistic effect due to cell cycle disruption, and enhanced formation of platinum intermediates when radiation-induced free radicals are present [32,33]. However, the use of CDDP is limited due to its severe nephrotoxicity [34], which can be overcome by its encapsulation in nanocarriers. Zhang et al. developed liposomes encapsulating CDDP (L-CDDP) and evaluated its antitumor efficacy in combination with RT (6 Gy) in a mouse model with human lung adenocarcinoma A549 tumor. L-CDDP plus irradiation led to a higher tumor growth suppression compared to CDDP plus irradiation and irradiation alone. The tumor growth delay (TGD) values were 11.95, 3.27, and 1.83 days, respectively. Sensitizer enhancement ratio (SER) values, when drugs were administrated 72 h before radiation, were 3.21 for CDDP and 4.92 for L-CDDP, confirming the effective role of L-CDDP in directing the radiosensitizer to the tumor [35]. More details about all formulations presented in this review can be found on Table 1.

Jung et al. [36] prepared liposomes modified with epidermal growth factor receptor (EGFR) antibodies encapsulating CDDP (EGFR:L-CDDP). A colony formation assay (CFA) was performed on A549 cells treated with the free drug, actively and nonactively targeted formulations combined to irradiation (0, 2, 5, or 10 Gy) 2 h later. This assay consists of an in vitro cell survival assay which assesses the ability of a single cell to grow into a colony, defined as a group of at least 50 cells. It is the gold-standard method in radiobiology to determine cell reproductive death after exposure to ionizing radiation [37]. This preliminary study indicated that both liposomes lead to enhanced radiosensitivity, with the actively targeted formulation being slightly more potent. The antitumor efficacy was evaluated in animals bearing A549 tumors. On the final date of the experiment, the change of tumor growth was compared between treated group and control group (T/C). The percentual changes of tumor growth were calculated as: T/C (%) = [(change in tumor growth for treated group)/(change in tumor growth for control group)] × 100. The T/C (%) were 53.1 for free CDDP, 61.3 for L-CDDP, and 46.8 for EGFR:L-CDDP. After the combination of drugs with irradiation (5 Gy), these values were 40.7, 32.2, and 20.7, for free CDDP, L-CDDP, and EGFR:L-CDDP, respectively, while it was 51.8, for the group treated with irradiation alone (5 Gy). These results reveal a higher efficacy of EGFR:L-CDDP either alone or combined to irradiation [36].

Table 1. Nanocarriers designed to be used in combination with radiotherapy.

Formulation	Composition	Encapsulated Agent	Mean Diameter	Irradiation Dose (Gy) *	Reference
Nanocarriers Encapsulating Radiosensitizers					
Liposome	HSPC:CHOL:DSPE-PEG2000	Cisplatin	~100 nm	6 Gy	[35]
Liposome	(DPPC):CHOL:ganglioside:DCP:DPPE) (35:40:15:5:5 molar ratio) and anti-EGFR antibodies	Cisplatin	247.9 nm	5 Gy	[36]
Liposome (Promitil®)	HSPC:CHOL:DSPE-PEG2000:MLP (60:30:5:5 molar ratio) HSPC:CHOL:DSPE-PEG2000:MLP (55:30:5:10 molar ratio)	Mitomycin C	98.61 nm	5 Gy	[38–41]
Liposome (Myocet®)	EPC:CHOL (55:34 molar ratio)	Doxorubicin	~160 nm	2 Gy	[42,43]
Liposome	DSPE-PEG2000:MDH:CHOL	Doxorubicin	169.4 nm	2 Gy	[44]
Micelles	PEG-PCL/P105	Doxorubicin	~20 nm	6 Gy	[45]
Nanoparticle	Precirol ATO, Pluronic F68, dimethyldioctadecyl-ammonium bromide	Curcumin	~300 nm	2 Gy to 9 Gy	[46]
Liposome	lecithin:CHOL:CUR (18:1:1 weight ratio)	Curcumin	114.9 nm	5 Gy	[47]
Liposome	DOPC:CHOL:DSPE-PEG2000	Cupric tirapazamine complex	160–180 nm	7 Gy or 10 Gy	[48]
Liposome	DPPC:MSPC:DSPE-PEG2000 (86:10:4 molar ratio)	Pimonidazole	~100 nm	4 Gy	[49]
Nanoparticle	H1 nanopolymer:Dbait	Dbait	170 nm	9 Gy	[50]
Co-delivery of Molecules: The Search for Synergism					
Nanoparticle	PLGA-PEG	Cisplatin and Paclitaxel	82.9 nm	5 Gy	[51]
Nanoparticle	PLGA-PEG	Wortmannin and Cisplatin	80–200 nm	5 Gy	[52]
Nanoparticle	PLGA-PEG	Cisplatin and Etoposide	100 nm	5 Gy	[53]
Nanoparticle	PLGA-PEG:transferrin at a molar ratio of 1:3	Tetrahydrocurcumin and Doxorubicin	255.8 nm	3 Gy	[54]
Nanoparticle	angiopep-2:DSPE-PEG2000:DOTAP:PLGA	Temozolomide and Dbait	99.9 nm	3 Gy	[55]
Nanoparticle	H1 nanopolymer:Docetaxel:Dbait	Docetaxel and Dbait	117 nm	3 Gy	[56]
Nanoparticle	magnetic graphene oxide:FePt nanoparticles	Metronidazol and 5-fluorouracil	243 nm	2 Gy	[57]
Nanoparticle	(Poly-metronidazole)n:DSPE-PEG2000: lecitina:angiopep-2-DSPE-PEG-2000	Metronidazol and Doxorubicin	~80 nm	2 Gy	[58]
Liposome	DSPE-PEG2000: MDH: CHOL	Metronidazole and Dbait	127 nm	2 Gy	[59]
Nanoparticle	1,4-dicarboxybenzene (BDC): Hafnium (Hf):PEG	Talazoparib and Buparlisib	112 nm	4 Gy or 8 Gy	[60]

Table 1. Cont.

Formulation	Composition	Encapsulated Agent	Mean Diameter	Irradiation Dose (Gy) *	Reference
\multicolumn{6}{c}{Nanocarriers Encapsulating Oxygen: Targeting Hypoxia}					
Nanoparticle	perfluorotributylamine (PFTBA)@albumin	Oxygen	150 nm	5 Gy	[61]
Nanodroplets	perfluoro-15-crown-5-ether (PFCE)@cisPt(IV) Lip cisPt(IV)-Lip is prepared by mixing 2.5 mg cisPt(IV)-DSPE, 5 mg DPPC, 1.5 mg cholesterol and 4 mg DSPE-mPEG5k	Oxygen Cisplatin	~200 nm	6 Gy	[62]
Nanoparticle	PEG-Bi_2Se_3 @perfluorohexane	Oxygen	~35 nm	6 Gy	[63]
Nanoparticle decorated nanodroplets	TaOx@PFC-PEG	Oxygen	~150	6 Gy	[64]
Liposome	PFH@DSPE-PEG2000:CHOL:lecithin (3.79:4.28:24.65 weight ratio)	Oxygen	~100 nm	10 Gy	[65]
\multicolumn{6}{c}{Nanocarriers Designed to Boost the Abscopal Effect}					
Nanoparticle	PLGA based NP coated with either amine polyethylene glycol; DOTAP or PEG-maleimide	-	<200 nm	-	[66]
Nanoparticle	Mesoporous silica nanoparticles functionalized with APTES	-	~100 nm	8 Gy	[67]
Nanoparticle	PEG-maleimide-mPEG-functionalized hollow mesoporous titanium dioxide ($HTiO_2$)	IDOi (Indole-amine-2,3-dioxygenase inhibitor)	~50 nm	4 Gy	[68]
\multicolumn{6}{c}{Radiation-Triggered Delivery Systems}					
Nanoparticle	DNA:AuNP	Doxorubicin	NA	5 Gy	[69]
Nanoparticle	bismuth nanoparticles functionalized with S-nitrosothiol	-	36 nm	5 Gy	[70]
Nanoparticle	Pegylated thioether-hybridized hollow mesoporous organosilica nanoparticles	tert-butyl hydroperoxide (TBHP) and iron pentacarbonyl (Fe(CO)5)	~50 nm	8 Gy	[71]
Liposome	DOTAP:DOPC (~1:1 weight ratio)	Doxorubicin	NA	4 Gy	[72]
Liposome	egg lecithin-80: DSPE-PEG2000 (60:9 w/w)	Hemoglobin and Doxorubicin	~140 nm	8 Gy	[73]

* Photon irradiation was used in all experiments. Abbreviations: (3-aminopropyl) triethoxysilane (APTES); cholesterol (CHOL); diacetyl phosphate (DCP); 1,2-dioleoyl-sn-glycero-3-phosphocholine (DOPC); 1,2-di-(9Z-octadecenoyl)-3-tri- methylammonium-propane (DOTAP); dipalmitoylphosphatidylcholine (DPPC); dipalmitoylphosphatidylethanolamine (DPPE); 1,2-distearoyl-sn-glycero-3-phosphoethanolamine-N-[amino(polyethylene glycol)-2000 (DSPE-PEG2000); folate–polyethylenimine600–cyclodextrin (H1 nanopolymer); hydrogenated Soy Phosphatidylcholine (HSPC); malate dehydrogenase (MDH); mitomycin and glycerol lipid (MMC lipid prodrug) (MLP); 1-stearoyl-2-hydroxy-sn-glycero-3-phosphocholine (MSPC); polyethylene glycol (PEG); polyethylene glycol-polycaprolactone/pluronic (PEG-PCL/P105); and poly(lactic-co-glycolic acid) (PLGA).

2.1.2. Mitomycin

Mitomycin C (MMC) is a DNA crosslinking agent considered to be a potent chemotherapeutic drug and radiosensitizer. It forms DNA adducts compromising the repair of radiation-induced DNA breaks by cells. MMC is attractive as a radiosensitizer as it may target hypoxic cell populations in detriment to oxygenated cells; however, its use is still associate with significant toxicity such as pulmonary fibrosis, hemolytic uremic syndrome, and damage to bone marrow and other tissues [38–40]. Thus, Gabizon et al. developed a lipidic prodrug consisting of MMC linked to 2,3-distearoyloxy-propane-1-dithio-4′-benzyloxycarbonyl, abbreviate as MLP and formulated into liposomes, known as Promitil® [40,41]. A phase 1A clinical study with Promitil® showed that toxicity was substantially reduced. Currently, Promitil® is in a phase 1B clinical study [38]. In vitro cytotoxicity of free MMC and Promitil® against colorectal cancer cell lines HT-29 and SW480 was evaluated, and both cell lines showed a dose-dependent response to the treatments. When HT-29 and SW480 cells were irradiated (doses ranging from 0 to 8 Gy) after drug treatments (10 nM MMC), radiation survival curves demonstrated that both Promitil® and MMC produced significant radiosensitization in HT-29 cells, with SER values of 1.4 and 1.3, respectively. However, there was no significant sensitization in SW480 cells. The antitumor efficacy was evaluated in human HT-29 and SW480 xenograft models. Animals treated with Promitil® and RT (5 Gy) had significantly prolonged TGD in both tumor models compared to free MMC plus RT, demonstrating the efficacy of Promitil® as a cancer therapy [38]. Promitil® has finally reached clinical testing as palliative therapy for two patients with oligometastases from colorectal cancer. Both patients presented durable clinical responses to the combination of Promitil® and RT, suggesting the combination as a chemoradiotherapy approach [39].

2.1.3. Doxorubicin

Doxorubicin (DXR) is a tetracycline antibiotic that induces DNA damage by inhibiting topoisomerase II and generating free radicals. Another mechanism of action consists of the formation of DXR-DNA adducts and interstrand crosslinks from DXR covalently binding to DNA. This makes DXR promising to be used in combination with RT, by increasing sublethal radiation-induced damage. DXR low solubility in water and severe dose-dependent cardiotoxicity are important reasons to support its delivery in nanocarriers [45,74].

Liu et al. developed liposomes composed of 1,2-distearoyl-sn-glycero-3-phosphoethanolamine-N-[amino(polyethylene glycol)-2000] (DSPE-PEG2000), cholesterol (CHOL), and malate dehydrogenase (MDH) to encapsulate DXR (MLP-DXR). The hypoxic radiosensitizer 2-methyl-5-nitroimidazole-1-ethanol (metronidazole) was conjugated to hexadecanedioic acid (HA), in order to form (16-(2-(2-methyl-5-nitro-1H-imidazol-1-yl) ethoxy)-16-oxohexadecanoic acid (MHA). The MHA was then coupled with 3-dimethylaminopropane-1,2-diol (DA) to form ester-linked MDH. The MDH lipid was used for obtaining hypoxia radiosensitizer liposomes. Liposomes without MDH were prepared as control (DLP-DXR). When tested in a xenograft glioma model obtained by intracranial injection of human glioblastoma U87 cells, MLP-DXR plus RT clearly demonstrated the strongest inhibition of glioma growth. Fourteen days after treatment, animals treated with MLP-DXR plus RT presented tumors with ~580 mm³, while those receiving RT alone and DLP-DXR plus RT presented tumors with ~4000 and ~1000 mm³, respectively [44].

DXR has been shown to be an effective therapeutic agent against malignant glioma cells. However, DXR has not been used for the treatment of brain tumors as its poor penetration across the blood–brain barrier hinders its efficacy. Liposomes encapsulating DXR have been studied to circumvent this poor penetration [42]. Labussière et al. evaluated the commercialized nonpegylated liposome of DXR (Myocet®) on two subcutaneous U87 and TCG4 and one intracranial U87 malignant glioma models xenografted on nude mice. After the treatment with RT alone (2 Gy), the median survival was 30.5 and 81.0 days, for U87 and TCG4 subcutaneous models, respectively. The combination of Myocet® plus RT (2 Gy), increased the median survival up to 36.5 days in U87 and 93.0 days in TCG4 subcutaneous models. However, in intracranial U87 model, the median survival was 39.5 days for the RT alone and 32.0 days for the Myocet® plus RT [43]. Chastagner et al. evaluated Myocet® and the commercialized pegylated liposome (Caelyx®, DXR) on U87 xenograft model. The overall survival was 22, 47, and 48 days when mice received RT alone (2 Gy), Myocet® plus RT (2 Gy) and Caelyx® plus RT (2 Gy), respectively. These results showed that both Myocet® and Caelyx® have a synergistic interaction with RT [42]. Han et al. showed that micelles composed of polyethylene glycol (PEG), polycaprolactone (PCL), and Pluronic P105, loading DXR inhibited the drug resistance of human myelogenous leukemia (K562/ADR) cells [75]. Lung adenocarcinoma is the most common primary lung cancer, and it is often detected at the metastastic stage [76]. Therefore, Xu et al. selected the A549 cell line to evaluate micelles consisting of PEG-PCL/P105 loading DXR. CFA using A549 lung cancer cells was performed to determine the effects of the treatment with DXR-micelles plus irradiation (at 0–6 Gy). The cell survival fraction was ~0.05% and ~0.005% after treatment with irradiation alone (6 Gy) and the DXR-micelles plus RT, respectively. Moreover, SER of cells treated with DXR-micelles was 1.44 [45].

2.2. Natural Products as Radiosensitizers

Natural products play a role as radiosensitizers, presenting different effects on irradiated normal and tumor cells. Despite promising effects in cancer treatment, their clinical applications in RT are few. This is possibly related to their low bioavailability, which can be overcome with the use of nanocarriers [77–79].

Curcumin

Curcumin (CUR) is a phenylpropanoid isolated from the roots of the herbaceous perennial plant *Curcuma longa*. It is a natural antioxidant and nuclear factor (NF-κB) inhibitor, used on the treatment of inflammatory conditions and cancer and as a radiosensitizer. The radiosensitizing role of CUR arises from its interference with many different pathways. It has been shown that CUR inhibits transcription factors (NF-KB, AP-1, and STAT3) highly expressed in cancer cells, and genes involved in processes such as proliferation (COX-2, c-Myc, and cyclin D1), survival (Bcl-2, Bcl-XL), invasion (MM9), and metastasis (ICAM-1, ELAM-1, VCAM-1). It has also been reported to interfere with the cell cycle, arresting cells in the most radiosensitive G2/M phase. In this phase, cells passing the G2 checkpoint are unable to repair DNA damage. CUR has also been found to increase the intrinsic and extrinsic apoptosis pathways induced by RT [46].

Minafra et al. prepared solid lipid nanoparticles loaded with CUR and evaluated its sensitizing effects in breast cancer cells. CUR nanoparticles (10 μM) were combined to different doses of irradiation (2, 4, 6, and 9 Gy) in order to obtain dose-response curves. The radiosensitizing effect was determined by the dose-modifying factor (DMF) obtained from the curves and calculated at the surviving fraction of 50%. DMFs of 1.78 and 1.38 were obtained for the MCF7 cell line and the triple-negative MDA-MB-231 cell line, respectively. Shi et al. prepared liposomes encapsulating CUR (L-CUR) and evaluated its sensitizing effects in a mouse model with LL2 (murine Lewis lung carcinoma) tumor. There was a significant inhibition of tumor growth in mice treated with L-CUR plus RT (5 Gy), in relation to the animals treated with either L-CUR or RT alone (5 Gy). Twenty-two days after treatment, animals treated with L-CUR plus RT presented a tumor volume of ~300 mm^3, while those receiving irradiation alone (6 Gy) presented a tumor volume of ~600 mm^3 [47].

2.3. Hypoxic Cell Radiosensitizers

Hypoxia plays an important role in RT as tumor cells have been reported to be 2–3 times more radioresistant when in a hypoxic environment as compared to tumor cells under normal oxygen level [80]. This cellular response dependency on oxygen after irradiation is known as the "oxygen fixation hypothesis". As previously mentioned, in the indirect action of ionizing radiation, ion pairs created in water react with molecules yielding free radicals (R•). These radicals cause a type of DNA base damage that can be easily repaired by antioxidants. However, peroxides (RO$_2$•) formed by the reaction of molecular oxygen with the R• in DNA lead to damage that is difficult or even impossible for the cell to repair. Thus, as the hypothesis postulates, molecular oxygen can permanently fix the DNA damage caused by radicals [81,82]. Oxygen deficiency is present in the majority of solid human tumors, due to inadequate and heterogeneous vascular network. For this reason, strategies to overcome hypoxia-induced radioresistance are of clinical importance [83,84].

2.3.1. Tirapazamine

Tirapazamine (TPZ) is a hypoxic cytotoxin, i.e., a type of radiosensitizer that is only activated under a hypoxia condition. In such a condition, TPZ is reduced into a radical intermediate (TPZ•−) which in sequence becomes protonated (TPZH•). The bioactive radicals which are precursors for DNA damage are formed in further reaction steps, still under debate. What is known is that they lead to the inactivation of the enzyme topoisomerase II, and then, DNA DSB arise. In the presence of O2, the TPZ•− radical is back-oxidized to the parent neutral state, hence the hypoxia selectivity [85,86].

Silva et al. synthetized a cupric-TPZ complex [Cu(TPZ)$_2$] that improved TPZ's hypoxia selectivity in prostate cancer, exhibited slower metabolism, and higher DNA binding, compared to TPZ [87]. Then, Silva et al. [48] developed liposomes of different lipidic compositions to load Cu(TPZ)$_2$. A formulation composed of 1,2-dioleoyl-*sn*-glycero-3-phosphocholine (DOPC):CHOL:DSPE-PEG2000, when tested in C4-2B (human prostatic carcinoma cells) spheroids presented an IC50 of ~22.0 µM, significantly reduced compared to that of the free complex (~42 µM). The combination of Cu(TPZ)$_2$-loaded liposomes with RT was evaluated in C4-2B spheroids, treated with 10 µM of total TPZ either as free Cu (TPZ)2 or liposomal-Cu(TPZ)$_2$ for 24 h followed by X-ray irradiation at a single dose of 7 or 10 Gray. The changes in spheroids diameter were monitored for 22 days. At the end of the experiment, liposomes significantly reduced spheroid growth rate compared to RT alone or in combination with the free complex [48].

2.3.2. Nitroimidazoles

Nitroimidazoles have also been studied as hypoxic cell radiosensitizers. They mimic the oxygen reacting with DNA radicals to "fix" radiation damage in hypoxic cells. The adducts formed lead to DNA strand breaks and, consequently, cell death [88]. So far, the toxicity of these compounds has limited its clinical translation making its encapsulation in nanocarriers a promising strategy [89]. Sadeghi et al. developed temperature-sensitive liposomes loaded with pimonidazole (PMZ) (TSL-PMZ). Cell survival was measured by CFA in FaDu (human hypopharyngeal carcinoma) cell line under hypoxic conditions. TSL-PMZ enhanced the effect of RT (4 Gy) in a concentration-dependent way. The SER of TSL-PMZ in concentrations of 0.25, 0.50, and 0.75 mM in FaDu cells were 1.7, 2.3, and 2.9, respectively [49].

2.4. DNA Repair Inhibitors

Tumor cells respond to the DNA damage caused by irradiation by activating the DNA signaling response, which upregulates DNA repair. The DNA repair pathways are promising targets for therapeutic intervention such as radiosensitization [90].

Dbait

Dbait (DNA strand break bait) are innovative molecules composed of 32 base-pair deoxyribonucleotides. They form intramolecular DNA double helix mimicking DNA damages, acting as a bait for DNA damage signaling enzymes. This "false" DNA damage signal prevents the recruitment of repair enzymes (DNA-PK and PARP) that would act on DSB and SSB. These molecules have given promising results as radiosensitizer in several types of tumors as they inhibit several repair pathways of DNA damage induced by RT [91,92]. Yao et al. 2016 developed a polycation nanoparticle to delivery Dbait (NP-Dbait). The therapeutic efficacy of NP-Dbait was evaluated in xenograft mouse models bearing PC-3 or 22Rv1 prostate cancer. The combination of NP-Dbait and RT (9 Gy) led to significantly longer TGD and prolonged the survival time of tumor-bearing mice when compared with controls groups. When tumor volumes of control group reached 3000 mm^3, animals treated with NP-Dbait plus RT presented tumor volumes of ~1300 mm^3 (PC-3 model) and ~700 mm^3 (22Rv1 model). Those receiving irradiation alone (9 Gy) presented tumor volume of ~2500 mm^3 (PC-3 model) and ~2000 mm^3 (22Rv1 model) [50].

3. Co-Delivery of Molecules: The Search for Synergism

The efficacy of chemotherapeutic agents is often hindered by the rapid development of drug resistance. Combination therapy based on the understanding of tumor biology, tumor environment, and molecular pathways is a successful strategy to overcome multidrug resistance [93,94]. The use of nanotechnology for cancer treatment keeps on evolving, particularly in combinatorial treatments [95,96]. The co-encapsulation of molecules in nanocarriers is a technical challenge that comes with advantages. Some of those consist of lower costs of constituents and manufacturing process as compared to two single formulations, as well as a lower adjuvant load to the patient. Another point is the uncertainty about the biodistribution when two different formulations are administered. Ultimately, established synergistic ratios can be encapsulated, guaranteeing a higher efficacy [14,15]. Nanocarriers co-encapsulating molecules are a promising strategy to increase the effectiveness of RT [95].

Tian et al. developed nanoparticles composed of poly(lactic-co-glycolic acid) (PLGA) coated with PEG to co-deliver paclitaxel (PTX, a chemotherapeutic drug that can cause myelosuppression and peripheral neuropathy [97]) and CDDP at a molar ratio of 1:1 (NP-PTX:CDDP 1:1). The efficacy was evaluated in murine models using both the human lung cancer 344SQ allograft and H460 xenograft models. NP-PTX:CDDP 1:1 plus RT (5 Gy) greatly retarded tumor growth rates compared to RT alone (5 Gy). Twenty-three days after treatment of mice bearing 344SQ tumors, a tumor volume variation of ~10 was observed in the animals treated with RT alone, while those receiving NP-PTX:CDDP 1:1 plus RT presented a tumor volume variation of ~5. For mice bearing H460 tumors, at the end of eighteen days, a change in tumor volume of ~12 was observed after treatment with RT alone and of ~5 after treatment with NP-PTX:CDDP 1:1 plus RT. These results showed the potential of NP-PTX:CDDP 1:1 as a promising chemoradiotherapy strategy [51]. Zhang et al. developed nanoparticles to co-encapsulate wortmannin (WTMN) and CDDP (NP-WTMN:CDDP), to enhance chemoradiotherapy and reverse platinum resistance in ovarian cancer models. These nanoparticles were evaluated in murine xenograft models of platinum-sensitive ovarian cancer (A2780 cell line) and CDDP-resistant ovarian cancer (A2780cis cell line). After treatment with NP-WTMN:CDDP followed by irradiation (5 Gy), the TGD was ~8 days in A2780 model. Moreover, the TGD was ~10 days in A2780cis model. For both models, the TGD was ~2 days, in animals treated with RT alone (5 Gy). These results showed that co-delivering WTMN:CDDP in nanoparticles is a strategy to reverse CDDP resistance and improve chemoradiotherapy efficacy [1]. In another study, Zhang et al. developed PLGA-PEG-based nanoparticles to co-deliver etoposide (ET) and CDDP at a molar ratio of 1:1.8 (NP-ET:CDDP). The efficacy of these nanoparticles in combination with RT was evaluated using both 344SQ and H460 murine lung cancer models. The TGD was ~8 days, after treatment with NP-ET:CDDP followed by 5 Gy irradiation, while for animals treated with RT alone (5 Gy), the TGD was ~2 days, for both 344SQ and H460 models [53].

Nanoparticles composed of PLGA-PEG conjugated to transferrin (Tf) were developed by Zhang et al. to co-deliver tetrahydrocurcumin (THC) and DXR (NP-Tf-THC:DXR) into glioma [54]. The overexpression of Tf receptors (TfR) in glioma cells is well known. Nanocarriers targeting TfR have been investigated for the effective delivery of drugs to brain tumors [98]. When tested in a xenograft glioma model obtained by subcutaneous injection of rat C6 glioma cell line, NP-Tf-THC:DXR combined with irradiation (3 Gy) showed a tumor inhibition rate of 94.49%, while that for treatment with irradiation alone (3 Gy) was ~40% [54].

Li et al. developed nanoparticles to co-deliver temozolomide (TMZ) and Dbait (NP-TMZ-Dbait). CFA using C6 mouse glioma cells was performed to determine the effects of the different treatments. The survival fractions of cells treated with radiation alone (3 Gy),

NP-TMZ-Dbait or NP-TMZ-Dbait plus RT (3 Gy), were −0.8, ~0.60, and ~0.20, respectively, confirming the synergistic potential of the combination [55].

Liu et al. developed a Dbait nanoparticle to deliver docetaxel (DTX, a chemotherapeutic drug that can lead to infusion reactions, febrile neutropenia, pneumonitis, and neuropathies [99]). The combination of RT (3 Gy) and nanoparticles was evaluated in mice bearing PC-3 tumor. Thirty days after treatment, animals receiving the formulation plus RT presented a tumor volume of ~850 mm^3. Those treated with irradiation alone (3 Gy) presented a tumor volume of ~1500 mm^3. This was reflected on longer survival time for animals receiving both the nanoparticles and RT compared to RT alone [56].

Magnetic graphene oxide nanoparticles were developed by Yang et al. to encapsulate 5-fluorouracil (5-FU, a chemotherapeutic drug that can lead to mucositis, leukopenia, neutropenia, and thrombocytopenia [100]). Firstly, magnetic graphene oxide (MGO) was conjugated with PEG2000 and covalently bonded with metronidazol. These nanocomposites (NCs) were mixed with FePt magnetic nanoparticles, and 5-FU was added. CFA under 2 Gy irradiation was conducted in H1975 and A549 human lung adenocarcinoma cells, to evaluate the radiation enhancement ratio (RER) of MGO-FU:MI NCs. Survival fractions of H1975 cells changed from 0.58 with radiation alone (2 Gy) to 0.36 with combined therapy, an RER of 1.6. For A549 cells, the RER was 1.5 with survival fractions of 0.79–0.52 after treatments with radiation alone and combined therapy, respectively. The dose enhancement factor (DEF) was calculated to evaluate the effect of MGO-FU:MI NCs [57]. DEF is defined as the ratio between the dose deposited in tumor with NCs and the dose deposited in control group [101]. The DEF values were 1.68 for H1975 cells at 15 µg/mL and 1.68 for A549 cells at 10 µg/mL. These results showed the radioprotective and dose enhancement effects of MGO-FU:MI NCs. In addition, the SER values of MGO-FU:MI NCs were 1.15 for H1975 cells at 15 µg/mL and 1.99 for A549 cells at 10 µg/mL, confirming the effective role of MGO-FU:MI NCs as a radiosensitizer [57].

Hua et al. synthetized metronidazole polymers to develop nanoparticles encapsulating DXR for glioma therapy. The nanoparticles obtained [ALP-(MIs)n:DXR] were evaluated in mice bearing C6 tumor, and ALP-(MIs)n:DXR plus RT (2 Gy) had significant effects on inhibiting glioma growth compared to other treatments. Nanoparticles composed of a nonradiosensitizer polymer (PLGA) were compared to ALP-(MIs)n:DXR to further investigate the radiosensitization effect of (P-MIs)n. Both the glioma inhibition rates of ALP-(MIs)25:DXR (19.6) and ALP-(MIs)48:DXR (13.7) presented a remarkably higher inhibition efficacy toward glioma growth than the AL-PLGA:DXR (68.3), which suggests that (P-MIs)n has a radiosensitizing effect [58].

Liu et al. developed liposomes to deliver Dbait (MLP-Dbait) for glioma therapy. To evaluate the antitumoral efficacy of MLP-Dbait, a xenograft glioma model was obtained by intracranial injection of C6 cells to mice. Liposomes containing the green fluorescent protein (GFP) gene were used as a control group. For the combination of RT (2 Gy) with free Dbait or MLP/GFP or MLP/Dbait, the tumor growth rates were 37.9%, 39.9%, and 21.1%. This higher effectivity of the combination of Dbait, MLP, and RT was also translated to a longest median survival rate, compared to the other treatments [59].

Neufeld et al. developed a formulation of talazoparib and buparlisib in Hafnium and 1,4-dicarboxybenzene (Hf-BDC) nanoscale metal organic frameworks (nMOFs) coated with DSPE-PEG (TB@Hf-BDC-PEG) [60]. Hf is a high atomic metallic ion, which interacts with ionizing radiation, to generate ROS for cancer treatment [102]. The results of CFA indicated that the growth rates and colony formation abilities of 4T1 cells were significantly inhibited by RT plus TB@Hf-BDC-PEG. The RER of TB@Hf-BDC-PEG combined with irradiation (8 Gy) was 12.68. The therapeutic efficacy of TB@Hf-BDC-PEG was evaluated on Balb/C mice bearing subcutaneous 4T1 murine breast tumors. Fourteen days after treatment, there was a change in tumor volume ~6 in the animals treated with RT alone (4 Gy), while those treated with TB@Hf-BDC-PEG plus RT (4 Gy) presented a change in tumor volume of ~4.5 [60].

It is important to highlight that some nanocarriers themselves, such as high atomic number nanoparticles (mainly gold nanoparticles), act as radiosensitizers by enhancing radiation energy deposition in the cells. This strategy has been recently reviewed elsewhere [103,104] and is not the focus of the present review. Herein, we describe nanocarriers designed to encapsulate and deliver radiosensitizing molecules.

4. Nanocarriers Encapsulating Oxygen: Targeting Hypoxia

On item 2.3, we describe how hypoxia plays an important role in radioresistance and the encapsulation of hypoxic cell radiosensitizers as one strategy to overcome it. Another strategy consists of the delivery of oxygen itself using agents such as fluorocarbons (FC). FC can dissolve oxygen and then deliver it in hypoxia regions by passive diffusion [84]. Perfluorocarbons (PFCs) are chemically inert and present excellent biocompatibility. They have been extensively studied as oxygen suppliers to improve RT outcome [61].

Zhou et al. used perfluorotributylamine (PFTBA), a PFC with strong platelet inhibition effect to obtain PFTBA:albumin nanoparticles. These nanoparticles were stored in an oxygen chamber for PFC oxygenation. These nanoparticles were designed to function as a two-stage oxygen delivery system. Once administered, the PFTBA:albumin nanoparticles take advantage of the EPR effect to passively accumulate at the tumor and release the bound O_2. At the same time, the PFTBA inhibits platelet activation in the tumor blood vessels disrupting the vessel barriers. This leads to higher red blood cell infiltration and consequently higher oxygen delivery to the tumor. The efficacy of combining PFTBA:albumin nanoparticles to radiation was evaluated in vivo. Balb/C mice bearing the highly hypoxic subcutaneous CT26 colon cancer tumors (~50 mm^3) were divided in groups to receive different treatments. Fourteen days after treatment, animals treated with PFTBA:albumin nanoparticles presented tumors >700 mm^3, while those receiving irradiation alone (5 Gy) presented tumors between 300 and 600 mm^3. Animals receiving PFTBA:albumin nanoparticles followed 10 h later by irradiation (5 Gy) presented tumors <150 mm^3. These results showed that PFTBA:albumin nanoparticles were able to sensitize the tumors to RT, effectively inhibiting tumor growth [61].

Yao et al. designed nanoparticles composed of commercial lipids and perfluoro-15-crown-5-ether (PFCE) loading CDDP prodrug (cisPt(IV)) for enhanced chemoradiotherapy efficacy. An in vivo study in mice bearing 4T1 murine breast tumor (~150 mm^3 at day 0) was performed to show the hypoxic relief enhanced chemoradiotherapy. At the end of fourteen days, animals treated with PFCE@cisPt(IV)-Lip nanoparticles (at days 0 and 3) presented tumors with ~800 mm^3. Animals receiving irradiation alone (6 Gy at days 1 and 4) presented tumors with ~600 mm^3, and animals receiving PFCE@cisPt(IV)-Lip nanoparticles (at days 0 and 3) followed by irradiation (6 Gy at days 1 and 4) presented tumors with ~200 mm^3. Tumor slices were stained with a hypoxia-probe (pimonidazole) to confirm the potency of the formulation on tumor oxygenation, as compared to a control. The semiquantitative analysis of positive hypoxia areas revealed positive area percentages of only ~2.5% for animals receiving the formulation, as compared to ~42.4% for control animals [62].

Song et al. prepared pegylated hollow Bi_2Se_3 nanoparticles which could be filled with perfluorohexane (a liquid PFC). This PEG-Bi_2Se_3@perfluorohexane functioned as an oxygen reservoir targeting hypoxia combined with the ability of the high Z element Bi to locally concentrate the radiation energy, further sensitizing the tumor. First, it was verified in vivo that the exposure of the oxygen-loaded PEG-Bi_2Se_3@perfluorohexane nanoparticles to NIR light (808 nm laser for 10 min) led to the burst release of oxygen from the nanoparticles, instantly increasing tumor oxygenation. Tumor slices stained with a hypoxia probe (pimonidazole) showed enhanced oxygenation level for tumors injected with PEG-Bi2Se3@perfluorohexane nanoparticles and exposed to NIR light (~35%) as compared to the control (~75%). Following that, the antitumor efficacy was evaluated in Balb/c mice bearing subcutaneous 4T1 murine breast cancer tumors. Therefore, the relative tumor volume (RTV) was calculated by using the formula: RTV = Tx × 100/T0, where Tx refers to the tumor volume of the respective tumor on day x, and T0 refers to the tumor volume of the same tumor when the treatment started. Sixteen days after treatment, animals treated with oxygen-loaded PEG-Bi_2Se_3 @perfluorohexane nanoparticles plus NIR presented RTV of ~11. Those receiving irradiation alone (6 Gy) presented RTV of ~7.5. Animals exposed to oxygen loaded PEG-Bi_2Se_3 @perfluorohexane nanoparticles plus NIR plus irradiation (6 Gy) presented RTV of ~1.5. This confirmed the synergistic effect of the combination of the nanoparticles with NIR and irradiation on tumor growth suppression [63]. In another study, Song et al. prepared another multifunctional RT sensitizer. The formulation consisted of pegylated PFC nanodroplets decorated with TaOx nanoparticles (TaOx@PFC-PEG). Similarly to the previously described formulation, this is also able to deliver oxygen loaded on PFC and to concentrate radiation energy at the tumor site due to the TaOx. Again, they evaluated the antitumor efficacy in Balb/c mice bearing subcutaneous 4T1 tumors. Twelve days after treatment, animals treated with oxygen-loaded TaOx@PFC-PEG presented RTV of ~9. Those receiving irradiation alone (6 Gy) presented RTV of ~6. Treatment with oxygen-loaded TaOx@PFC-PEG plus irradiation (6 Gy) presented the highest efficacy with an RTV of ~2, confirming the radiosensitizing potential of the formulation [64].

Xu et al. prepared a liposomal formulation encapsulating perfluorohexane (lip-PFH). Balb/c mice bearing CT26 (mice colon cancer) tumors with ~80 mm^3 were used in in vivo experiments. First, the accumulation of lip-PFH at the tumor site was verified 24 h after intravenous administration. Subsequently the antitumor efficacy was evaluated. When animals received the injection of lip(PFH) followed 24 h later by 10 Gy irradiation, the TGD was ~17.5 days. This was not that notable but significantly improved compared to the TGD (~14 days) for animals treated with irradiation only (10 Gy) [65].

5. Nanocarriers Designed to Boost the Abscopal Effect

The abscopal effect consists of a systemic anticancer response that can result from RT. It occurs in addition to the local effect of radiation. An antitumor response throughout the body is induced, reaching distant sites, which were not irradiated [105]. The mechanisms for the abscopal effect are not fully understood, but the immunological hypothesis supports that it occurs due to immunogenic responses initiated by RT-induced DNA breaks. This antitumor immune response, mediated by T-cell activation, leads to the regression of off-site, nonirradiated tumors [105,106]. Although considered promising, the practical efficacy of the abscopal effect is unsatisfactory. Therefore, new strategies as means to enhance it are highly desired [68]. One of these strategies consist of the development of antigen-capturing nanoparticles (AC-NPs). These nanoparticles bind to tumor antigens, released after RT-induced immunogenic cell death and improve their delivery to antigen presenting cells, enhancing cancer immunity. Antigens are then presented to T-cells, and the effector T-cells are directed to both primary and distant tumor sites boosting the abscopal effect [107,108].

Min et al. developed different poly(lactic-co-glycolic acid) (PLGA)-based AC-NPs, and showed that the set of captured antibodies is dependent on the surface properties of the NP. AC-NPs composed of unmodified PLGA bind to proteins through noncovalent hydrophobic–hydrophobic interactions. When coated with either amine polyethylene glycol or 1,2-dioleoyloxy-3-(trimethylammonium)propane (DOTAP), the AC-NPs bind to proteins via ionic interactions. When coated with PEG-maleimide, they bind to proteins through stable thioether bonds [66].

Yang et al. developed mesoporous silica nanoparticles (MSNs) functionalized with (3-aminopropyl) triethoxysilane (APTES) and investigated its potential to enhance the abscopal effect in the treatment of hepatocellular carcinoma. MSNs have a large surface area and porous structure that can absorb biomaterials such as antigens and deliver them to target cells. An in vivo experiment was performed in mice with bilateral Hepa1-6 (Murine hepatoma) tumors. The primary tumors received RT alone (8 Gy); MSN alone (injected into the tumor) or RT + MSN (same scheme) and the distant tumors (nonirradiated/non-treated) had their volumes evaluated. At the end of 40 days, the tumor volumes were ~1100 and

~1300 mm^3 for animals treated with RT alone and MSN alone, respectively. By comparison, when RT and MSN were combined, the tumor volume was reduced to ~550 mm^3 [67].

Chen et al. developed AC-NPs based on PEG-maleimide-mPEG-functionalized hollow mesoporous titanium dioxide (HTiO$_2$) aimed at eradicating metastatic breast tumor. In this formulation, the PEG-maleimide is responsible for capturing the tumor-associated antigens. To further boost the abscopal effect, this formulation was used to encapsulate an indole-amine-2,3-dioxygenase inhibitor (IDOi). IDO is an immunosupressive cytosolic enzyme often overexpressed in the tumor. The potential of the formulation on activating the abscopal effect was investigated in mice with bilateral 4T1 (murine mammary carcinoma) tumors. Animals received different formulations and irradiation (4 Gy) on the primary tumor, and the RTV of distant tumors (non-irradiated) was evaluated. At the end of 20 days, the RTV was ~4.5 and ~3.0 for animals treated with RT alone and HTiO$_2$-mPEG, respectively. By comparison, adding PEG-maleimide to the formulation (HTiO$_2$- mal-mPEG) allowed for an RTV of ~1.0 and combining PEG-maleimide and an IDOi to the formulation (IDOi@HTiO$_2$- mal-mPEG) led to an RTV of ~0.5. This study made it clear that the combination of RT with immunotherapy provided by the formulation was highly effective on tumor suppression [68].

6. Radiation-Triggered Delivery Systems

Nanocarriers can be designed to be triggered when exposed to endogenous or exogenous stimuli at the tumor site. This prevents drug release in the bloodstream, sparing normal tissues and allowing maximum antitumor efficacy [7,109]. X-rays, as other exogenous triggering stimuli, have the advantages of being delivered to a precise region and on demand. As a main limitation, X-rays do not access and treat the metastatic sites of uncertain location [110]. The high clinical translation potential of X-rays is due to its high tissue penetration and the fact that it is already used to treat tumors [69]. The capacity of bond breaking and ROS generation have been explored as means of triggering delivery systems.

The first demonstration of X-ray triggered release from a nanocarrier leading to higher cytotoxicity was published by Starkewolf et al. in 2013 [69]. The nanocarrier consisted of DNA strands attached to gold nanoparticles (AuNP). DXR can be loaded by conjugation to the DNA strands [69,111]. When irradiated with X-rays, the generated ROS break the DNA strands, triggering the release of the DXR. CFA using MCF-7 (human breast cancer) cells was performed to determine the effects of different treatments. When not irradiated, DXR–DNA–AuNP (0.80 cell survivability) and DXR alone (0.81 cell survivability) presented similar toxicity and were more toxic than DNA–AuNP (0.92 cell survivability). Upon 5 Gy irradiation, DXR–DNA–AuNP (0.20 cell survivability) were more toxic than radiation alone (0.32 cell survivability) DXR alone (0.28 cell survivability) and DNA–AuNP (0.30 cell survivability). The extra toxicity of DXR–DNA–AuNP was attributed to the triggering irradiation [69].

Zhang et al. developed bismuth nanoparticles functionalized with S-nitrosothiol (Bi-SNO NPs). When irradiated, the X-ray breaks the S-N bond, triggering the release of large amounts of nitric oxide (NO). NO is a gas signal molecule of vasodilation and can therefore alleviate tumoral hypoxia. The efficacy of this formulation was evaluated in vivo in mice bearing subcutaneous U14 (murine cervical carcinoma) tumors (70 mm^3). At the end of 14 days, animals receiving RT alone (5 Gy) and Bi-SNO NPs presented RTV of ~12.5 and ~14, respectively. The combination of RT (5 Gy) and Bi-SNO NPs led to synergistic activity, and RTV was significantly reduced (~2) [70].

Combining the strategies of co-delivery and X-ray triggering, Fan et al. developed pegylated thioether-hybridized hollow mesoporous organosilica nanoparticles (HMONs) encapsulating tert-butyl hydroperoxide (TBHP) and iron pentacarbonyl (Fe(CO)$_5$). X-ray irradiation of the formulation activates a cascade release of •OH and CO. Upon irradiation, a peroxy bond cleavage takes place within TBHP, generating the highly oxidative •OH radical, for enhanced RT. This radical attacks the Fe(CO)$_5$ releasing CO for gas therapy, leading to mitochondria exhaustion followed by cell apoptosis. The formulation was evaluated in vivo for its efficacy in mice bearing subcutaneous U87MG glioma tumor (~6–8 mm). Animals received either irradiation alone (8 Gy) or different formulations followed by irradiation (8 Gy) 24 h later. Twenty days after the treatments, the RTV was similar (~5.5) for animals receiving either irradiation alone or HMON-Fe(CO)$_5$ followed by irradiation. For animals receiving HMON-TBPH followed by irradiation, the RTV was ~4.5. Treatment with the co-loaded formulation (HMON-TBPH-Fe(CO)$_5$) followed by irradiation was able to cause tumor regression with an RTV close to zero. When administered without irradiation, the HMON-TBPH-Fe(CO)$_5$ formulation was not able to suppress tumor growth (RTV ~9.5) as compared to a PBS control (RTV ~10.5), confirming the synergistic efficacy of co-encapsulated compounds and irradiation [71].

Deng et al. designed liposomes triggered by X-ray irradiation. In this work, a liposomal formulation was embedded with a photosensitizer (verteporfin) and gold nanoparticles. Irradiation induces $^1O_2$ generation by the photosensitizer. Singlet oxygen acts by oxidizing unsaturated lipids, leading to liposomal membrane destabilization and cargo release. The gold nanoparticles interact with X-rays acting as a radiosensitizer. These liposomes were used to encapsulate DXR and evaluated for its activity in xenograft mouse model bearing HCT 116 colorectal cancer. Animals were divided into groups to receive PBS, liposome only, irradiation only (4 Gy), or liposome plus irradiation (4 Gy), and the ability of these treatments to control tumor growth was evaluated. Two weeks post-treatment, the tumor volume increase was verified for animals receiving PBS (3.0-fold), liposome only (2.9-fold), and irradiation only (3.4-fold). On the other hand, treatment with liposome plus irradiation allowed for tumor size reduction (74%) as compared to the PBS control group [72].

Zu et al. developed liposomes encapsulating hemoglobin (Hb) and DXR. In this formulation, Hb alleviates hypoxia, and DXR release is radio-triggered by the action of ROS in the lipid membrane. When evaluated for ROS generation, this was higher in B16 (murine melanoma) tumors after treatment with the formulation plus irradiation as compared to either formulation alone or irradiation alone. Regarding the triggered release of DXR, 10 min after 2 Gy irradiation, up to 6% of content was released. When the irradiation dose was enhanced to 8 Gy, up to 20% of DXR was released. For the nonirradiated formulation, only ~1% of DXR was released in the same time. As expected, when evaluated for antitumor efficacy in a highly radioresistant tumor model (C57BL/6 mice bearing B16), RT alone (8 Gy) was not able to significantly inhibit tumor growth. Combining RT to the formulation co-encapsulating Hb and DXR allowed for significant tumor growth inhibition. This was superior to the combination of RT plus liposomes encapsulating Hb only or RT plus liposomes encapsulating DXR only, confirming the synergistic effects of the combination [73].

Two liposomal formulations designed to be irradiation-triggered were patented by Fologea et al. One formulation consists of pH-sensitive liposomes designed to encapsulate an agent and an organic halogen (such as chloral hydrate, fluoral hydrate, or bromal hydrate). The triggering mechanism relies on the reaction of the organic halogen with water in the vesicle's aqueous interior upon irradiation. This reaction releases H+, leading to a drop in the internal pH and disruption of the pH-sensitive bilayer, releasing the encapsulated content [112]. The other liposomal formulation was designed to contain a nanoscintillator responsive to irradiation, an enzyme capable of hydrolyzing the liposomal membrane, and an enzyme activator in a photolabile molecular cage. Triggered release occurs in a series of events that take place upon irradiation. When the nanoscintillator is irradiated, light is emitted, and the photolabile molecular cage with an enzyme activator is disrupted. The enzyme is then activated to disrupt the liposomal membrane releasing the encapsulated agent [113]. Another patent by Bondurant et al. relates to liposomes composed of a stable forming lipid, an ionizing radiation polymerizable colipid, and a chain transfer agent. Upon irradiation, radical species produced in water can initiate radical chain polymerizations in the polymerizable colipid (e.g., polymerizable phosphatidylcholines), leading to membrane destabilization and content release. The transfer of irradiation-generated free radical ions by the chain transfer agent (such as thiols or esters) increases the polymerization of the radiation polymerizable colipid, enhancing the trigger capacity [114].

7. Microbeam and Minibeam Radiation Therapy to Modulate the EPR Effect

Aiming at the reduction of radiation-induced side effects, many novel RT treatment strategies are arising. Spatially fractionated radiotherapy such as microbeam radiation therapy (MRT) and minibeam radiation therapy (MBRT) have attracted interest in the last years. Figure 3 represents commonly used beam widths for MRT and MBRT.

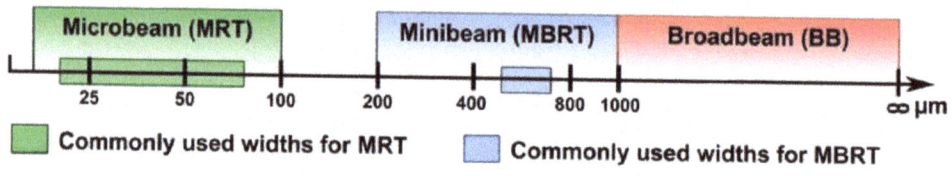

Figure 3. Schematic representation of commonly used widths for microbeam, minibeam, and broadbeam radiotherapy preclinical studies. Reproduced from Brönnimann et al., Nature Publishing Group, 2016 [115].

7.1. Microbeam Radiation Therapy

MRT was proposed by Slatkin and coworkers in 1992 [116]. In MRT, a multislit collimator is used in order to shape an X-ray beam so that the dose deposition profile consists of areas of peaks and valleys, spatially modulated on the micrometer scale (beam width ranging from 25 to 100 µm). On the peak areas, doses might consist of several hundred Grays, while valley regions present doses below the level of tissue tolerance. This distinct dose deposition enables a substantial reduction on toxicity to the normal tissue combined with a tumor control rate similar to that observed with conventional RT. The increased therapeutic index that can be obtained with MRT is of high importance for improved cancer treatment with radiation [117,118]. The mechanisms that underlie the increased antitumor efficacy combined with the sparing of surrounding normal tissues are not yet fully understood. One of the suggested biological mechanisms consists of the fact that MRT damages preferentially the tumor microvasculature in comparison to normal tissue microvasculature. It has been demonstrated that normal tissue mature vessels are highly tolerant against peak (high) doses going through transiently increased permeability only, while immature tumoral vessels undergo complete disruption [119–121].

With this in mind, MRT can be used to modulate the EPR effect. It is true that the EPR effect has been validated in both experimental animal models and different human tumors [3]. However, the importance and extent of the EPR effect in patients is still the focus of intense debate. The EPR effect is known to be more pronounced in small animal models, usually used to evaluate the preclinical efficacy of nanocarriers, as compared to human tumors. This is one explanation for the disbalance between the high amount of promising preclinical nanocarriers and the relative small number of these carriers in the clinical setting [122]. Therefore, a strategy to enhance tumor vessel permeability optimizing the EPR effect is highly desirable.

Sabatasso et al. demonstrated in mice bearing U-87 human glioblastoma that tumor irradiation with MRT (synchrotron generated parallel X-rays in a range of 25–50 µm in width) led to FITC-dextran (~27 nm) extravasation in this area. In nonirradiated animals, administered FITC-dextran remained intravascular with no extravasation to the control tumors. When animals were treated with MRT (150 Gy peak dose), a twofold increase in FITC-dextran transpermeability was observed 45 min postirradiation, as compared to the control. A study with FluoSpheres™ (100 nm microspheres) showed that they remained constrained to MRT paths. This indicates, as expected, a size-dependent transpermeability following MRT. It was possible to conclude from this study that the transient vascular permeability induced by MRT can be a strategy to improve the delivery of nanocarriers to the tumor site [123].

7.2. Minibeam Radiation Therapy

Despite promising preclinical studies for MRT, its production depends on large synchrotron facilities, of which there are currently only a few around the world. In addition to the difficulty to access these facilities, specialized hospitals are rarely close to them, hindering the clinical application of MRT [124]. In order to overcome this problem, efforts are put into using nonsynchrotron irradiators (such as a conventional X-ray tube) to produce microbeams [125]. Another strategy consists of using slightly wider 'minibeams' (beam widths ~500–700 µm), which are more easily produced with custom multislit collimators placed in small animal irradiators, as compared to microbeams [124,126,127]. Minibeam radiation therapy (MBRT) leads to similar radiobiological effects as compared to MRT and is also hypothesized to improve the delivery of nanocarriers. This idea was evaluated by Price et al. on a study of the effects of MBRT on the delivery of liposomal DXR. An in vivo study was performed on mice with syngeneic orthotopic triple-negative breast cancer. Animals were irradiated with either MBRT (28 Gy) or broadbeam radiation therapy (7 Gy) and 24 h later received the liposomal DXR. The delivery of liposomal DXR to the tumor was increased by 7.1-fold for MBRT and 2.7-fold for broadbeam radiation therapy compared to liposomal DXR alone (sham RT) [127].

8. Limitations and Future Directions

Besides the clear advantages of combining nanocarrier-assisted delivery of molecules and RT, which were presented in this review, there are also limitations that must be considered. Among limitations that come from the nanocarriers, it is important to remember that none of them are completely safe and nontoxic. This is affected by the lack of knowledge regarding their distribution and action, controlled by characteristics such as size, charge, degradation, and cancer stage and type, among others [128,129]. The commercial viability and availability of nanocarriers also have to be considered. Some of the most important challenges are: Possible scale-up problems, low production rate, difficulties in separating by-products, lack of quality control system, inconsistencies in reproducibility, and the high cost [130]. These limitations help us understand why the impact of nanocarrier-assisted drug delivery on human patients and clinical outcome has so far been insufficient [131]. For their future wide application, collaborative research efforts with more in vivo studies and clinical trials are necessary [128]. If the developed products are novel, safe, and meet the medical needs with cost effective benefits, the investment in nanocarrier development is likely to increase [130].

RT, in turn, has as its major limitation the damage caused to normal surrounding tissues. In this manner, modern RT and imaging techniques are enhancing the applications of radiation oncology. To the best of our knowledge, the nanocarrier-assisted delivery of molecules has only been evaluated in combination with photon RT, as reviewed herein. Photon RT is also the treatment modality applied to most patients worldwide. However, particle therapy, such as proton and carbon ions, is a promising strategy to be evaluated in combination with nanocarrier drug delivery. These therapy modalities are characterized by steep dose falloff with a minimal exit dose beyond a specified target. This allows for a more accurate and precise treatment, reducing healthy tissue exposure and, therefore, the toxicity [132]. Nevertheless, it is important to have in mind that such techniques have a high cost. So far, their use is concentrated in high-income countries that have centers able to deliver these particles [133].

In addition, the combination of nanocarrier drug delivery and RT has only been evaluated with single RT courses. Fractionated and hypofractionated RT should be evaluated in future in vivo studies [132].

Another important point is the heterogeneity in the RT response observed for tumors of the same histology [134]. Response prediction by means of liquid biopsy and circulating biomarkers allows for a refined treatment with patient stratification by biological parameters. Molecularly designed systems to target specific cancer will lead to future personalized cancer care [132,135].

9. Conclusions

In this review, we present the state of the art of nanocarriers designed to be used in combination with RT. So far, these systems were used to encapsulate one of or a combination of different radiosensitizing molecules such as classic chemotherapeutic drugs, natural products, hypoxic cell radiosensitizers, or DNA repair inhibitors. Nanocarriers have also been successfully designed to encapsulate and deliver oxygen, modulating the hypoxic TME; or to capture and deliver antibodies to antigen-presenting cells, boosting the abscopal effect. X-ray irradiation was shown to be an efficient exogenous trigger to nanoparticles and liposomes, enhancing the therapeutic ratio of these formulations. Finally, we presented how the transient and efficient vascular permeability arising from spatially fractionated RT modalities, such as microbeam and minibeam radiation therapy, can modulate the EPR effect and enhance the passive delivery of nanocarriers to the tumor site. All these different strategies of combining nanocarrier-assisted delivery of molecules and RT were validated in in vitro and/or in vivo studies. Thus, nanotechnology can be used to overcome the limitations of RT and the other way around.

Author Contributions: Conceptualization, M.S.F.; design of Figure 2, M.S.F.; writing—original draft preparation, M.S.F. and E.R.G.; writing—review and editing, M.S.F. and E.R.G. All authors have read and agreed to the published version of the manuscript.

Funding: This research received no external funding.

Acknowledgments: The authors would like to thank Coordenação de Aperfeiçoamento de Pessoal de Nível Superior—CAPES for supporting Eliza Rocha Gomes with a scholarship.

Conflicts of Interest: The authors declare no conflict of interest.

Abbreviations

A2780	platinum-sensitive murine ovarian cancer
A549	human non-small-cell lung cancer cell
C4-2B	human prostatic carcinoma cell
C6	rat glioma cell line
CDDP	cisplatin
CT26	colon carcinoma cell line
CUR	curcumin
DTX	docetaxel
DXR	doxorubicin
ET	etoposide
FaDu	human hypopharyngeal carcinoma cell
HCT 116	human colorectal carcinoma cell line
HT-29	human colorectal adenocarcinoma cell
H1975	human non-small-cell lung cancer cell
H460	human non-small-cell lung cancer cell
K562/ADR	human myelogenous leukemia
LL2	murine Lewis lung carcinoma
MCF-7	human breast cancer cell line with estrogen, progesterone and glucocorticoid receptors

MDA-MB-231	triple-negative breast cancer cell
MMC	mitomycin C
PC3	human prostate adenocarcinoma cell
PMZ	pimonidazole
PTX	paclitaxel
TCG4	human glioma cell line
U14	murine cervical carcinoma
THC	tetahydrocurcumin
TMZ	temozolomide
TPZ	tirapazamine
U87	human primary glioblastoma cell
WTMN	wortmannin
SW480	human colon adenocarcinoma cell
22Rv1	human prostate carcinoma cell
344SQ	human lung cancer cell
4T1	murine mammary carcinoma cell line
5-FU	5-fluorouracil

References

1. Arul, N.; Balachandar, V. Recent advances in radiotherapy and its associated side effects in cancer—A review. *J. Basic Appl. Zoöl.* **2019**, *80*, 14. [CrossRef]
2. Kim, K.; Khang, D. Past, Present, and Future of Anticancer Nanomedicine. *Int. J. Nanomed.* **2020**, *15*, 5719–5743. [CrossRef]
3. Islam, R.; Maeda, H.; Fang, J. Factors affecting the dynamics and heterogeneity of the EPR effect: Pathophysiological and pathoanatomic features, drug formulations and physicochemical factors. *Expert Opin. Drug Deliv.* **2021**, 1–14. [CrossRef]
4. Attia, M.F.; Anton, N.; Wallyn, J.; Omran, Z.; Vandamme, T.F. An overview of active and passive targeting strategies to improve the nanocarriers efficiency to tumour sites. *J. Pharm. Pharmacol.* **2019**, *71*, 1185–1198. [CrossRef]
5. Barenholz, Y. Doxil®—The first FDA-approved nano-drug: Lessons learned. *J. Control. Release* **2012**, *160*, 117–134. [CrossRef]
6. Bazak, R.; Houri, M.; El Achy, S.; Kamel, S.; Officer, H.; Refaat, T.; Medicine, N.; Lurie, R.H. Cancer active targeting by nanoparticles: A comprehensive review of literature. *J. Cancer Res. Clin. Oncol.* **2015**, *141*, 769–784. [CrossRef] [PubMed]
7. Franco, M.S.; Gomes, E.R.; Roque, M.C.; Oliveira, M.C. Triggered Drug Release from Liposomes: Exploiting the Outer and Inner Tumor Environment. *Front. Oncol.* **2021**, *11*, 470. [CrossRef] [PubMed]
8. Labani-Motlagh, A.; Ashja-Mahdavi, M.; Loskog, A. The Tumor Microenvironment: A Milieu Hindering and Obstructing Antitumor Immune Responses. *Front. Immunol.* **2020**, *11*, 940. [CrossRef] [PubMed]
9. Gong, B.-S.; Wang, R.; Xu, H.-X.; Miao, M.-Y.; Yao, Z.-Z. Nanotherapy Targeting the Tumor Microenvironment. *Curr. Cancer Drug Targets* **2019**, *19*, 525–533. [CrossRef]
10. Fernandes, C.; Suares, D.; Yergeri, M.C. Tumor Microenvironment Targeted Nanotherapy. *Front. Pharmacol.* **2018**, *9*, 1230. [CrossRef]
11. Muthu, M.S.; Leong, D.; Mei, L.; Feng, S.-S. Nanotheranostics—Application and Further Development of Nanomedicine Strategies for Advanced Theranostics. *Theranostics* **2014**, *4*, 660–677. [CrossRef]
12. Jo, S.D.; Ku, S.H.; Won, Y.-Y.; Kim, S.H.; Kwon, I.C. Targeted Nanotheranostics for Future Personalized Medicine: Recent Progress in Cancer Therapy. *Theranostics* **2016**, *6*, 1362–1377. [CrossRef] [PubMed]
13. Qi, S.-S.; Sun, J.-H.; Yu, H.-H.; Yu, S.-Q. Co-delivery nanoparticles of anti-cancer drugs for improving chemotherapy efficacy. *Drug Deliv.* **2017**, *24*, 1909–1926. [CrossRef] [PubMed]
14. Franco, M.S.; Oliveira, M.C. Liposomes Co- encapsulating Anticancer Drugs in Synergistic Ratios as an Approach to Promote Increased Efficacy and Greater Safety. *Anti-Cancer Agents Med. Chem.* **2019**, *19*, 17–28. [CrossRef] [PubMed]
15. Franco, M.S.; Oliveira, M.C. Ratiometric drug delivery using non-liposomal nanocarriers as an approach to increase efficacy and safety of combination chemotherapy. *Biomed. Pharmacother.* **2017**, *96*, 584–595. [CrossRef] [PubMed]
16. Caponigro, F.; Cornelia, P.; Budillon, A.; Bryce, J.; Avallone, A.; De Rosa, V.; Ionna, F.; Cornelia, G. Phase I study of Caelyx (doxorubicin HCL, pegylated liposomal) in recurrent or metastatic head and neck cancer. *Ann. Oncol.* **2000**, *11*, 339–342. [CrossRef] [PubMed]
17. Shabason, J.E.; Chen, J.; Apisarnthanarax, S.; Damjanov, N.; Giantonio, B.; Loaiza-Bonilla, A.; O'Dwyer, P.J.; O'Hara, M.; Reiss, K.A.; Teitelbaum, U.; et al. A phase I dose escalation trial of nab-paclitaxel and fixed dose radiation in patients with unresectable or borderline resectable pancreatic cancer. *Cancer Chemother. Pharmacol.* **2018**, *81*, 609–614. [CrossRef] [PubMed]
18. Lammers, P.E.; Lu, B.; Horn, L.; Shyr, Y.; Keedy, V. nab—Paclitaxel in Combination with Weekly Carboplatin with Concurrent Radiotherapy in Stage III Non-Small Cell Lung Cancer. *Oncologist* **2015**, *20*, 491–492. [CrossRef]
19. Sevilla, M.; Bernhard, W. Mechanisms of direct radiation damage to DNA. In *Radiation Chemistry*; EDP Sciences: Les Ulis, France, 2020; pp. 191–202.
20. Desouky, O.; Ding, N.; Zhou, G. Targeted and non-targeted effects of ionizing radiation. *J. Radiat. Res. Appl. Sci.* **2015**, *8*, 247–254. [CrossRef]

21. Gong, L.; Zhang, Y.; Liu, C.; Zhang, M.; Han, S. Application of Radiosensitizers in Cancer Radiotherapy. *Int. J. Nanomed.* **2021**, *16*, 1083–1102. [CrossRef]
22. Dayal, R.; Singh, A.; Pandey, A.; Mishra, K.P. Reactive oxygen species as mediator of tumor radiosensitivity. *J. Cancer Res. Ther.* **2014**, *10*, 811–828. [CrossRef] [PubMed]
23. Kawamura, K.; Qi, F.; Kobayashi, J. Potential relationship between the biological effects of low-dose irradiation and mitochondrial ROS production. *J. Radiat. Res.* **2018**, *59*, ii91–ii97. [CrossRef] [PubMed]
24. Dong, S.; Lyu, X.; Yuan, S.; Wang, S.; Li, W.; Chen, Z.; Yu, H.; Li, F.; Jiang, Q. Oxidative stress: A critical hint in ionizing radiation induced pyroptosis. *Radiat. Med. Prot.* **2020**, *1*, 179–185. [CrossRef]
25. Kim, K.; Lee, S.; Seo, D.; Kang, J.; Seong, K.M.; Youn, H. Cellular Stress Responses in Radiotherapy. *Cells* **2019**, *8*, 1105. [CrossRef]
26. Hur, W.; Yoon, S.K. Molecular Pathogenesis of Radiation-Induced Cell Toxicity in Stem Cells. *Int. J. Mol. Sci.* **2017**, *18*, 2749. [CrossRef] [PubMed]
27. Garibaldi, C.; Jereczek-Fossa, B.A.; Marvaso, G.; Dicuonzo, S.; Rojas, D.P.; Cattani, F.; Starzyńska, A.; Ciardo, D.; Surgo, A.; Leonardi, M.C.; et al. Recent advances in radiation oncology. *Ecancermedicalscience* **2017**, *11*, 785. [CrossRef] [PubMed]
28. Baumann, M.; Krause, M.; Overgaard, J.; Debus, J.; Bentzen, S.M.; Daartz, J.; Richter, C.; Zips, D.; Bortfeld, T. Radiation oncology in the era of precision medicine. *Nat. Cancer* **2016**, *16*, 234–249. [CrossRef]
29. Chen, H.H.W.; Kuo, M.T. Improving radiotherapy in cancer treatment: Promises and challenges. *Oncotarget* **2017**, *8*, 62742–62758. [CrossRef]
30. Begg, A.C.; Stewart, F.A.; Vens, C. Strategies to improve radiotherapy with targeted drugs. *Nat. Cancer* **2011**, *11*, 239–253. [CrossRef]
31. Xie, Y.; Han, Y.; Zhang, X.; Ma, H.; Li, L.; Yu, R.; Liu, H. Application of New Radiosensitizer Based on Nano-Biotechnology in the Treatment of Glioma. *Front. Oncol.* **2021**, *11*, 855. [CrossRef]
32. Lawrence, T.S.; Blackstock, A.; McGinn, C. The mechanism of action of radiosensitization of conventional chemotherapeutic agents. *Semin. Radiat. Oncol.* **2003**, *13*, 13–21. [CrossRef] [PubMed]
33. Wilson, G.; Bentzen, S.M.; Harari, P.M. Biologic Basis for Combining Drugs with Radiation. *Semin. Radiat. Oncol.* **2006**, *16*, 2–9. [CrossRef]
34. Wainford, R.D.; Weaver, R.J.; Stewart, K.N.; Brown, P.; Hawksworth, G.M. Cisplatin nephrotoxicity is mediated by gamma glutamyltranspeptidase, not via a C-S lyase governed biotransformation pathway. *Toxicology* **2008**, *249*, 184–193. [CrossRef]
35. Zhang, X.; Yang, H.; Gu, K.; Chen, J.; Rui, M.; Jiang, G.-L. In vitro and in vivo study of a nanoliposomal cisplatin as a radiosensitizer. *Int. J. Nanomed.* **2011**, *6*, 437–444. [CrossRef]
36. Jung, J.; Jeong, S.-Y.; Park, S.S.; Shin, S.H.; Ju, E.J.; Choi, J.; Park, J.; Lee, J.H.; Kim, I.; Suh, Y.-A.; et al. A cisplatin-incorporated liposome that targets the epidermal growth factor receptor enhances radiotherapeutic efficacy without nephrotoxicity. *Int. J. Oncol.* **2014**, *46*, 1268–1274. [CrossRef]
37. Franken, N.A.P.; Rodermond, H.M.; Stap, J.; Haveman, J.; Van Bree, C. Clonogenic assay of cells in vitro. *Nat. Protoc.* **2006**, *1*, 2315–2319. [CrossRef]
38. Tian, X.; Warner, S.B.; Wagner, K.T.; Caster, J.M.; Zhang, T.; Ohana, P.; Gabizon, A.A.; Wang, A.Z. Preclinical Evaluation of Promitil, a Radiation-Responsive Liposomal Formulation of Mitomycin C Prodrug, in Chemoradiotherapy. *Int. J. Radiat. Oncol.* **2016**, *96*, 547–555. [CrossRef]
39. Tahover, E.; Bar-Shalom, R.; Sapir, E.; Pfeffer, R.; Nemirovsky, I.; Turner, Y.; Gips, M.; Ohana, P.; Corn, B.W.; Wang, A.Z.; et al. Chemo-Radiotherapy of Oligometastases of Colorectal Cancer with Pegylated Liposomal Mitomycin-C Prodrug (Promitil): Mechanistic Basis and Preliminary Clinical Experience. *Front. Oncol.* **2018**, *8*, 544. [CrossRef]
40. Gabizon, A.; Shmeeda, H.; Tahover, E.; Kornev, G.; Patil, Y.; Amitay, Y.; Ohana, P.; Sapir, E.; Zalipsky, S. Development of Promitil®, a lipidic prodrug of mitomycin c in PEGylated liposomes: From bench to bedside. *Adv. Drug Deliv. Rev.* **2020**, *154-155*, 13–26. [CrossRef] [PubMed]
41. Gabizon, A.; Amitay, Y.; Tzemach, D.; Gorin, J.; Shmeeda, H.; Zalipsky, S. Therapeutic efficacy of a lipid-based prodrug of mitomycin C in pegylated liposomes: Studies with human gastro-entero-pancreatic ectopic tumor models. *J. Control. Release* **2012**, *160*, 245–253. [CrossRef]
42. Chastagner, P.; Sudour, H.; Mriouah, J.; Barberi-Heyob, M.; Bernier-Chastagner, V.; Pinel, S. Preclinical Studies of Pegylated- and Non-Pegylated Liposomal Forms of Doxorubicin as Radiosensitizer on Orthotopic High-Grade Glioma Xenografts. *Pharm. Res.* **2014**, *32*, 158–166. [CrossRef] [PubMed]
43. Labussière, M.; Aarnink, A.; Pinel, S.; Taillandier, L.; Escanyé, J.-M.; Barberi-Heyob, M.; Bernier-Chastagner, V.; Plénat, F.; Chastagner, P. Interest of liposomal doxorubicin as a radiosensitizer in malignant glioma xenografts. *Anti-Cancer Drugs* **2008**, *19*, 991–998. [CrossRef]
44. Liu, H.; Xie, Y.; Zhang, Y.; Cai, Y.; Li, B.; Mao, H.; Liu, Y.-G.; Lu, J.; Zhang, L.; Yu, R. Development of a hypoxia-triggered and hypoxic radiosensitized liposome as a doxorubicin carrier to promote synergetic chemo-/radio-therapy for glioma. *Biomaterials* **2017**, *121*, 130–143. [CrossRef] [PubMed]
45. Wei, Q.-C.; Xu, W.-H.; Han, M.; Dong, Q.; Fu, Z.-X.; Diao, Y.-Y.; Liu, H.; Xu, J.; Jiang, H.-L.; Zheng, S.; et al. Doxorubicin-mediated radiosensitivity in multicellular spheroids from a lung cancer cell line is enhanced by composite micelle encapsulation. *Int. J. Nanomed.* **2012**, *7*, 2661–2671. [CrossRef] [PubMed]

46. Minafra, L.; Porcino, N.; Bravatà, V.; Gaglio, D.; Bonanomi, M.; Amore, E.; Cammarata, F.P.; Russo, G.; Militello, C.; Savoca, G.; et al. Radiosensitizing effect of curcumin-loaded lipid nanoparticles in breast cancer cells. *Sci. Rep.* **2019**, *9*, 1–16. [CrossRef]
47. Gao, X.X.; Shi, H.-S.; Li, D.; Zhang, Q.-W.; Wang, Y.-S.; Zheng, Y.; Cai, L.-L.; Zhong, R.-M.; Rui, A.; Li, Z.-Y.; et al. A systemic administration of liposomal curcumin inhibits radiation pneumonitis and sensitizes lung carcinoma to radiation. *Int. J. Nanomed.* **2012**, *7*, 2601–2611. [CrossRef]
48. Silva, V.L.; Ruiz, A.; Ali, A.; Pereira, S.; Seitsonen, J.; Ruokolainen, J.; Furlong, F.; Coulter, J.; Al-Jamal, W.T. Hypoxia-targeted cupric-tirapazamine liposomes potentiate radiotherapy in prostate cancer spheroids. *Int. J. Pharm.* **2021**, *607*, 121018. [CrossRef] [PubMed]
49. Sadeghi, N.; Kok, R.J.; Bos, C.; Zandvliet, M.; Geerts, W.J.C.; Storm, G.; Moonen, C.T.W.; Lammers, T.; Deckers, R. Hyperthermia-triggered release of hypoxic cell radiosensitizers from temperature-sensitive liposomes improves radiotherapy efficacy in vitro. *Nanotechnology* **2019**, *30*, 264001. [CrossRef]
50. Yao, H.; Qiu, H.; Shao, Z.; Wang, G.; Wang, J.; Yao, Y.; Xin, Y.; Zhou, M.; Wang, A.Z.; Zhang, L. Nanoparticle formulation of small DNA molecules, Dbait, improves the sensitivity of hormone-independent prostate cancer to radiotherapy. *Nanomed. Nanotechnol. Biol. Med.* **2016**, *12*, 2261–2271. [CrossRef]
51. Tian, J.; Min, Y.; Rodgers, Z.; Au, K.M.; Hagan, C.T.; Zhang, M.; Roche, K.; Yang, F.; Wagner, K.; Wang, A. Co-delivery of paclitaxel and cisplatin with biocompatible PLGA–PEG nanoparticles enhances chemoradiotherapy in non-small cell lung cancer models. *J. Mater. Chem. B* **2017**, *5*, 6049–6057. [CrossRef]
52. Zhang, M.; Hagan, C.T.; Min, Y.; Foley, H.; Tian, X.; Yang, F.; Mi, Y.; Au, K.M.; Medik, Y.; Roche, K.; et al. Nanoparticle co-delivery of wortmannin and cisplatin synergistically enhances chemoradiotherapy and reverses platinum resistance in ovarian cancer models. *Biomaterials* **2018**, *169*, 1–10. [CrossRef]
53. Zhang, M.; Hagan, C.T.; Foley, H.; Tian, X.; Yang, F.; Au, K.M.; Mi, Y.; Medik, Y.; Roche, K.; Wagner, K.; et al. Co-delivery of etoposide and cisplatin in dual-drug loaded nanoparticles synergistically improves chemoradiotherapy in non-small cell lung cancer models. *Acta Biomater.* **2021**, *124*, 327–335. [CrossRef]
54. Zhang, X.; Zhao, L.; Zhai, G.; Ji, J.; Liu, A. Multifunctional Polyethylene Glycol (PEG)-Poly (Lactic-Co-Glycolic Acid) (PLGA)-Based Nanoparticles Loading Doxorubicin and Tetrahydrocurcumin for Combined Chemoradiotherapy of Glioma. *Med. Sci. Monit.* **2019**, *25*, 9737–9751. [CrossRef]
55. Li, S.; Xu, Q.; Zhao, L.; Ye, C.; Hua, L.; Liang, J.; Yu, R.; Liu, H. Angiopep-2 Modified Cationic Lipid-Poly-Lactic-Co-Glycolic Acid Delivery Temozolomide and DNA Repair Inhibitor Dbait to Achieve Synergetic Chemo-Radiotherapy Against Glioma. *J. Nanosci. Nanotechnol.* **2019**, *19*, 7539–7545. [CrossRef]
56. Liu, N.; Ji, J.; Qiu, H.; Shao, Z.; Wen, X.; Chen, A.; Yao, S.; Zhang, X.; Yao, H.; Zhang, L. Improving radio-chemotherapy efficacy of prostate cancer by co-deliverying docetaxel and dbait with biodegradable nanoparticles. *Artif. Cells Nanomed. Biotechnol.* **2019**, *48*, 305–314. [CrossRef]
57. Yang, C.; Peng, S.; Sun, Y.; Miao, H.; Lyu, M.; Ma, S.; Luo, Y.; Xiong, R.; Xie, C.; Quan, H. Development of a hypoxic nanocomposite containing high-Z element as 5-fluorouracil carrier activated self-amplified chemoradiotherapy co-enhancement. *R. Soc. Open Sci.* **2019**, *6*, 181790. [CrossRef] [PubMed]
58. Hua, L.; Wang, Z.; Zhao, L.; Mao, H.; Wang, G.; Zhang, K.; Liu, X.; Wu, D.; Zheng, Y.; Lu, J.; et al. Hypoxia-responsive lipid-poly-(hypoxic radiosensitized polyprodrug) nanoparticles for glioma chemo- and radiotherapy. *Theranostics* **2018**, *8*, 5088–5105. [CrossRef]
59. Liu, H.; Cai, Y.; Zhang, Y.; Xie, Y.; Qiu, H.; Hua, L.; Liu, X.; Li, Y.; Lu, J.; Zhang, L.; et al. Development of a Hypoxic Radiosensitizer-Prodrug Liposome Delivery DNA Repair Inhibitor Dbait Combination with Radiotherapy for Glioma Therapy. *Adv. Heal. Mater.* **2017**, *6*, 1601377. [CrossRef]
60. Neufeld, M.J.; DuRoss, A.N.; Landry, M.R.; Winter, H.; Goforth, A.M.; Sun, C. Co-delivery of PARP and PI3K inhibitors by nanoscale metal–organic frameworks for enhanced tumor chemoradiation. *Nano Res.* **2019**, *12*, 3003–3017. [CrossRef]
61. Zhou, Z.; Zhang, B.; Wang, H.; Yuan, A.; Hu, Y.; Wu, J. Two-stage oxygen delivery for enhanced radiotherapy by perfluorocarbon nanoparticles. *Theranostics* **2018**, *8*, 4898–4911. [CrossRef]
62. Yao, L.; Feng, L.; Tao, D.; Tao, H.; Zhong, X.; Liang, C.; Zhu, Y.; Hu, B.; Liu, Z.; Zheng, Y. Perfluorocarbon nanodroplets stabilized with cisplatin-prodrug-constructed lipids enable efficient tumor oxygenation and chemo-radiotherapy of cancer. *Nanoscale* **2020**, *12*, 14764–14774. [CrossRef] [PubMed]
63. Song, G.; Liang, C.; Yi, X.; Zhao, Q.; Cheng, L.; Yang, K.; Liu, Z. Perfluorocarbon-Loaded Hollow Bi2Se3Nanoparticles for Timely Supply of Oxygen under Near-Infrared Light to Enhance the Radiotherapy of Cancer. *Adv. Mater.* **2016**, *28*, 2716–2723. [CrossRef] [PubMed]
64. Song, G.; Ji, C.; Liang, C.; Song, X.; Yi, X.; Dong, Z.; Yang, K.; Liu, Z. TaOx decorated perfluorocarbon nanodroplets as oxygen reservoirs to overcome tumor hypoxia and enhance cancer radiotherapy. *Biomaterials* **2016**, *112*, 257–263. [CrossRef]
65. Xu, L.; Qiu, X.; Zhang, Y.; Cao, K.; Zhao, X.; Wu, J.; Hu, Y.; Guo, H. Liposome encapsulated perfluorohexane enhances radiotherapy in mice without additional oxygen supply. *J. Transl. Med.* **2016**, *14*, 268. [CrossRef]
66. Min, Y.; Roche, K.C.; Tian, S.; Eblan, M.J.; McKinnon, K.P.; Caster, J.; Chai, S.; Herring, L.E.; Zhang, L.; Zhang, T.; et al. Antigen-capturing nanoparticles improve the abscopal effect and cancer immunotherapy. *Nat. Nanotechnol.* **2017**, *12*, 877–882. [CrossRef]

67. Yang, K.; Choi, C.; Cho, H.; Ahn, W.; Kim, S.; Shin, S. Antigen-Capturing Mesoporous Silica Nanoparticles Enhance the Radiation-Induced Abscopal Effect in Murine Hepatocellular Carcinoma Hepa1-6 Models. *Pharmaceutics* **2021**, *13*, 1811. [CrossRef]
68. Chen, Y.; Pan, W.; Gao, P.; Shi, M.; Wu, T.; Li, N.; Tang, B. Boosting the abscopal effect of radiotherapy: A smart antigen-capturing radiosensitizer to eradicate metastatic breast tumors. *Chem. Commun.* **2020**, *56*, 10353–10356. [CrossRef]
69. Starkewolf, Z.B.; Miyachi, L.; Wong, J.; Guo, T. X-ray triggered release of doxorubicin from nanoparticle drug carriers for cancer therapy. *Chem. Commun.* **2013**, *49*, 2545–2547. [CrossRef]
70. Zhang, F.; Liu, S.; Zhang, N.; Kuang, Y.; Li, W.; Gai, S.; He, F.; Gulzar, A.; Yang, P. X-ray-triggered NO-released Bi–SNO nanoparticles: All-in-one nano-radiosensitizer with photothermal/gas therapy for enhanced radiotherapy. *Nanoscale* **2020**, *12*, 19293–19307. [CrossRef]
71. Fan, W.; Lu, N.; Shen, Z.; Tang, W.; Shen, B.; Cui, Z.; Shan, L.; Yang, Z.; Wang, Z.; Jacobson, O.; et al. Generic synthesis of small-sized hollow mesoporous organosilica nanoparticles for oxygen-independent X-ray-activated synergistic therapy. *Nat. Commun.* **2019**, *10*, 1241. [CrossRef]
72. Deng, W.; Chen, W.; Clement, S.; Guller, A.; Zhao, Z.; Engel, A.; Goldys, E.M. Controlled gene and drug release from a liposomal delivery platform triggered by X-ray radiation. *Nat. Commun.* **2018**, *9*, 1–11. [CrossRef] [PubMed]
73. Zhu, C.; Guo, X.; Luo, L.; Wu, Z.; Luo, Z.; Jiang, M.; Zhang, J.; Qin, B.; Shi, Y.; Lou, Y.; et al. Extremely Effective Chemoradiotherapy by Inducing Immunogenic Cell Death and Radio-Triggered Drug Release under Hypoxia Alleviation. *ACS Appl. Mater. Interfaces* **2019**, *11*, 46536–46547. [CrossRef]
74. Shafei, A.; El-Bakly, W.; Sobhy, A.; Wagdy, O.; Reda, A.; Aboelenin, O.; Marzouk, A.; El Habak, K.; Mostafa, R.; Ali, M.A.; et al. A review on the efficacy and toxicity of different doxorubicin nanoparticles for targeted therapy in metastatic breast cancer. *Biomed. Pharmacother.* **2017**, *95*, 1209–1218. [CrossRef] [PubMed]
75. Han, M.; Diao, Y.-Y.; Jiang, H.-L.; Ying, X.-Y.; Chen, D.-W.; Liang, W.-Q.; Gao, J.-Q. Molecular mechanism study of chemosensitization of doxorubicin-resistant human myelogenous leukemia cells induced by a composite polymer micelle. *Int. J. Pharm.* **2011**, *420*, 404–411. [CrossRef]
76. Kim, N.; Kim, H.K.; Lee, K.; Hong, Y.; Cho, J.H.; Choi, J.W.; Lee, J.-I.; Suh, Y.-L.; Ku, B.M.; Eum, H.H.; et al. Single-cell RNA sequencing demonstrates the molecular and cellular reprogramming of metastatic lung adenocarcinoma. *Nat. Commun.* **2020**, *11*, 1–15. [CrossRef]
77. Yi, J.J.; Zhu, J.-Q.; Zhao, C.C.; Kang, Q.; Zhang, X.; Suo, K.; Cao, N.; Hao, L.; Lu, J. Potential of natural products as radioprotectors and radiosensitizers: Opportunities and challenges. *Food Funct.* **2021**, *12*, 5204–5218. [CrossRef]
78. Hosseinimehr, S.J. Beneficial effects of natural products on cells during ionizing radiation. *Rev. Environ. Health* **2014**, *29*, 341–353. [CrossRef]
79. Javed, R.; Ghonaim, R.; Shathili, A.; Khalifa, S.A.; El-Seedi, H.R. Phytonanotechnology: A greener approach for biomedical applications. In *Biogenic Nanoparticles for Cancer Theranostics*; Elsevier: Amsterdam, The Netherlands, 2021; pp. 43–86. [CrossRef]
80. Sørensen, B.S.; Horsman, M.R. Tumor Hypoxia: Impact on Radiation Therapy and Molecular Pathways. *Front. Oncol.* **2020**, *10*, 562. [CrossRef]
81. Grimes, D.R.; Partridge, M. A mechanistic investigation of the oxygen fixation hypothesis and oxygen enhancement ratio. *Biomed. Phys. Eng. Express.* **2016**, *1*, 1–22. [CrossRef]
82. Chang, D.S.; Lasley, F.D.; Das, I.J.; Mendonca, M.S.; Dynlacht, J.R. *Basic Radiotherapy Physics and Biology*; Springer: Cham, Switzerland, 2014. [CrossRef]
83. Telarovic, I.; Wenger, R.H.; Pruschy, M. Interfering with Tumor Hypoxia for Radiotherapy Optimization. *J. Exp. Clin. Cancer Res.* **2021**, *40*, 1–26. [CrossRef]
84. Graham, K.; Unger, E. Overcoming tumor hypoxia as a barrier to radiotherapy, chemotherapy and immunotherapy in cancer treatment. *Int. J. Nanomed.* **2018**, *13*, 6049–6058. [CrossRef]
85. Arthur-Baidoo, E.; Ameixa, J.; Ončák, M.; Denifl, S. Ring-Selective Fragmentation in the Tirapazamine Molecule upon Low-Energy Electron Attachment. *Int. J. Mol. Sci.* **2021**, *22*, 3159. [CrossRef]
86. Romero, J.; Maihom, T.; Limão-Vieira, P.; Probst, M. Electronic structure and reactivity of tirapazamine as a radiosensitizer. *J. Mol. Model.* **2021**, *27*, 1–12. [CrossRef] [PubMed]
87. Silva, V.L.; Kaassis, A.; Dehsorkhi, A.; Koffi, C.-R.; Severic, M.; Abdelhamid, M.; Nyimanu, D.; Morris, C.; Al-Jamal, W.T. Enhanced selectivity, cellular uptake, and in vitro activity of an intrinsically fluorescent copper–tirapazamine nanocomplex for hypoxia targeted therapy in prostate cancer. *Biomater. Sci.* **2020**, *8*, 2420–2433. [CrossRef] [PubMed]
88. Bonnet, M.; Hong, C.R.; Wong, W.W.; Liew, L.P.; Shome, A.; Wang, J.; Gu, Y.; Stevenson, R.J.; Qi, W.; Anderson, R.F.; et al. Next-Generation Hypoxic Cell Radiosensitizers: Nitroimidazole Alkylsulfonamides. *J. Med. Chem.* **2018**, *61*, 1241–1254. [CrossRef] [PubMed]
89. Wardman, P. Nitroimidazoles as hypoxic cell radiosensitizers and hypoxia probes: Misonidazole, myths and mistakes. *Br. J. Radiol.* **2018**, *92*, 20170915. [CrossRef] [PubMed]
90. Nickoloff, J.A.; Taylor, L.; Sharma, N.; Kato, T.A. Exploiting DNA repair pathways for tumor sensitization, mitigation of resistance, and normal tissue protection in radiotherapy. *Cancer Drug Resist.* **2021**, *4*, 244–263. [CrossRef]
91. Biau, J.; Chautard, E.; Berthault, N.; De Koning, L.; Court, F.; Pereira, B.; Verrelle, P.; Dutreix, M. Combining the DNA Repair Inhibitor Dbait With Radiotherapy for the Treatment of High Grade Glioma: Efficacy and Protein Biomarkers of Resistance in Preclinical Models. *Front. Oncol.* **2019**, *9*, 549. [CrossRef]

92. Biau, J.; Devun, F.; Verrelle, P.; Dutreix, M. Dbait: Un concept innovant pour inhiber la réparation de l'ADN et contribuer aux traitements des cancers. *Bull Cancer* **2016**, *103*, 227–235. [CrossRef]
93. Wang, H.; Huang, Y. Combination therapy based on nano codelivery for overcoming cancer drug resistance. *Med. Drug Discov.* **2020**, *6*, 100024. [CrossRef]
94. Mokhtari, R.B.; Homayouni, T.S.; Baluch, N.; Morgatskaya, E.; Kumar, S.; Das, B.; Yeger, H. Combination therapy in combating cancer. *Oncotarget* **2017**, *8*, 38022–38043. [CrossRef]
95. Kemp, J.A.; Shim, M.S.; Heo, C.Y.; Kwon, Y.J. "Combo" nanomedicine: Co-delivery of multi-modal therapeutics for efficient, targeted, and safe cancer therapy. *Adv. Drug Deliv. Rev.* **2015**, *98*, 3–18. [CrossRef]
96. Hu, Q.; Sun, W.; Wang, C.; Gu, Z. Recent advances of cocktail chemotherapy by combination drug delivery systems. *Adv. Drug Deliv. Rev.* **2015**, *98*, 19–34. [CrossRef] [PubMed]
97. Marupudi, N.; E Han, J.; Li, K.W.; Renard, V.M.; Tyler, B.M.; Brem, H. Paclitaxel: A review of adverse toxicities and novel delivery strategies. *Expert Opin. Drug Saf.* **2007**, *6*, 609–621. [CrossRef] [PubMed]
98. Choudhury, H.; Pandey, M.; Chin, P.X.; Phang, Y.L.; Cheah, J.Y.; Ooi, S.C.; Mak, K.-K.; Pichika, M.R.; Kesharwani, P.; Hussain, Z.; et al. Transferrin receptors-targeting nanocarriers for efficient targeted delivery and transcytosis of drugs into the brain tumors: A review of recent advancements and emerging trends. *Drug Deliv. Transl. Res.* **2018**, *8*, 1545–1563. [CrossRef]
99. Ho, M.Y.; Mackey, J. Presentation and management of docetaxel-related adverse effects in patients with breast cancer. *Cancer Manag. Res.* **2014**, *6*, 253–259. [CrossRef]
100. Cordier, P.-Y.; Nau, A.; Ciccolini, J.; Oliver, M.; Mercier, C.; Lacarelle, B.; Peytel, E. 5-FU-induced neurotoxicity in cancer patients with profound DPD deficiency syndrome: A report of two cases. *Cancer Chemother. Pharmacol.* **2011**, *68*, 823–826. [CrossRef]
101. Rabus, H.; Gargioni, E.; Li, W.B.; Nettelbeck, H.; Villagrasa, C. Erratum: Determining dose enhancement factors of high-Z nanoparticles from simulations where lateral secondary particle disequilibrium exists. *Phys. Med. Biol.* **2019**, *64*, 155016. [CrossRef]
102. Chen, M.-H.; Hanagata, N.; Ikoma, T.; Huang, J.-Y.; Li, K.-Y.; Lin, C.-P.; Lin, F.-H. Hafnium-doped hydroxyapatite nanoparticles with ionizing radiation for lung cancer treatment. *Acta Biomater.* **2016**, *37*, 165–173. [CrossRef] [PubMed]
103. Chen, Y.; Yang, J.; Fu, S.; Wu, J. Gold Nanoparticles as Radiosensitizers in Cancer Radiotherapy. *Int. J. Nanomed.* **2020**, *15*, 9407–9430. [CrossRef]
104. Cunningham, C.; de Kock, M.; Engelbrecht, M.; Miles, X.; Slabbert, J.; Vandevoorde, C. Radiosensitization Effect of Gold Nanoparticles in Proton Therapy. *Front. Public Health* **2021**, *9*. [CrossRef] [PubMed]
105. Craig, D.J.; Nanavaty, N.S.; Devanaboyina, M.; Stanbery, L.; Hamouda, D.; Edelman, G.; Dworkin, L.; Nemunaitis, J.J. The abscopal effect of radiation therapy. *Futur. Oncol.* **2021**, *17*, 1683–1694. [CrossRef] [PubMed]
106. Daguenet, E.; Louati, S.; Wozny, A.-S.; Vial, N.; Gras, M.; Guy, J.-B.; Vallard, A.; Rodriguez-Lafrasse, C.; Magné, N. Radiation-induced bystander and abscopal effects: Important lessons from preclinical models. *Br. J. Cancer* **2020**, *123*, 339–348. [CrossRef]
107. Morales-Orue, I.; Chicas-Sett, R.; Lara, P.C. Nanoparticles as a promising method to enhance the abscopal effect in the era of new targeted therapies. *Rep. Pr. Oncol. Radiother.* **2019**, *24*, 86–91. [CrossRef]
108. Thanekar, A.M.; Sankaranarayanan, S.A.; Rengan, A.K. Role of nano-sensitizers in radiation therapy of metastatic tumors. *Cancer Treat. Res. Commun.* **2021**, *26*, 100303. [CrossRef]
109. Murugan, B.; Sagadevan, S.; Fatimah, I.; Oh, W.C.; Hossain, M.A.M.; Johan, M.R. Smart stimuli-responsive nanocarriers for the cancer therapy—Nanomedicine. *Nanotechnol. Rev.* **2021**, *10*, 933–953. [CrossRef]
110. Mi, P. Stimuli-responsive nanocarriers for drug delivery, tumor imaging, therapy and theranostics. *Theranostics* **2020**, *10*, 4557–4588. [CrossRef]
111. Guo, T.; Starkewolfe, Z.B. Methods and Compositions for Targeted Release of Molecules from Nanoscale Carriers. U.S. Patent No. 9,993,553, 14 March 2014.
112. Fologea, D.; Henry, R.; Salamo, G.; Mazur, Y.; Borelli, M.J. Methods and Compositions for X-ray Induced Release from Ph Sensitive Liposomes. U.S. Patent No. 9,849,087, 8 November 2012.
113. Fologea, D.; Salamo, G.; Henry, R.; Borelli, M.J. Corry, P.M. Method of Controlled Drug Release from a Liposome Carrier. U.S. Patent No. 8,808,733, 31 March 2010.
114. Bondurant, K.A. Mcgovern, R.M. Sutherland, Radiation Sensitive Liposomes U.S. Patent No. 2009/0304589 A1, 26 September 2008.
115. Brönnimann, D.; Bouchet, A.; Schneider, C.; Potez, M.; Serduc, R.; Bräuer-Krisch, E.; Graber, W.; Von Gunten, S.; Laissue, J.A.; Djonov, V. Synchrotron microbeam irradiation induces neutrophil infiltration, thrombocyte attachment and selective vascular damage in vivo. *Sci. Rep.* **2016**, *6*, 33601. [CrossRef] [PubMed]
116. Slatkin, D.N.; Spanne, P.; Dilmanian, F.A.; Sandborg, M. Microbeam radiation therapy. *Med Phys.* **1992**, *19*, 1395–1400. [CrossRef]
117. Smyth, L.; Donoghue, J.; Ventura, J.A.; Livingstone, J.; Bailey, T.; Day, L.R.J.; Crosbie, J.C.; Rogers, P.A.W. Comparative toxicity of synchrotron and conventional radiation therapy based on total and partial body irradiation in a murine model. *Sci. Rep.* **2018**, *8*, 1–11. [CrossRef]
118. Bartzsch, S.H.; Corde, S.; Crosbie, J.C.; Day, L.R.J.; Donzelli, M.; Krisch, M.; Lerch, M.L.F.; Pellicioli, P.; Smyth, L.M.L.; Tehei, M. Technical advances in X-ray microbeam radiation therapy. *Phys. Med. Biol.* **2019**, *65*, 02TR01. [CrossRef]

119. Bouchet, A.; Lemasson, B.; Christen, T.; Potez, M.; Rome, C.; Coquery, N.; Le Clec'H, C.; Moisan, A.; Bräuer-Krisch, E.; Leduc, G.; et al. Synchrotron microbeam radiation therapy induces hypoxia in intracerebral gliosarcoma but not in the normal brain. *Radiother. Oncol.* **2013**, *108*, 143–148. [CrossRef]
120. Bouchet, A.; Sakakini, N.; El Atifi, M.; Le Clec'H, C.; Brauer, E.; Moisan, A.; Deman, P.; Rihet, P.; Le Duc, G.; Pelletier, L. Early Gene Expression Analysis in 9L Orthotopic Tumor-Bearing Rats Identifies Immune Modulation in Molecular Response to Synchrotron Microbeam Radiation Therapy. *PLoS ONE* **2013**, *8*, e81874. [CrossRef]
121. Bouchet, A.; Lemasson, B.; Le Duc, G.; Maisin, C.; Bräuer-Krisch, E.; Siegbahn, A.; Renaud, L.; Khalil, E.; Rémy, C.; Poillot, C.; et al. Preferential Effect of Synchrotron Microbeam Radiation Therapy on Intracerebral 9L Gliosarcoma Vascular Networks. *Int. J. Radiat. Oncol.* **2010**, *78*, 1503–1512. [CrossRef]
122. Shi, Y.; Van Der Meel, R.; Chen, X.; Lammers, T. The EPR effect and beyond: Strategies to improve tumor targeting and cancer nanomedicine treatment efficacy. *Theranostics* **2020**, *10*, 7921–7924. [CrossRef] [PubMed]
123. Sabatasso, S.; Fernandez-Palomo, C.; Hlushchuk, R.; Fazzari, J.; Tschanz, S.; Pellicioli, P.; Krisch, M.; Laissue, J.; Djonov, V. Transient and Efficient Vascular Permeability Window for Adjuvant Drug Delivery Triggered by Microbeam Radiation. *Cancers* **2021**, *13*, 2103. [CrossRef]
124. Bazyar, S.; Inscoe, C.R.; O'Brian, E.T.; Zhou, O.Z.; Lee, Y.Z.; Iii, E.T.O. Minibeam radiotherapy with small animal irradiators; in vitro and in vivo feasibility studies. *Phys. Med. Biol.* **2017**, *62*, 8924–8942. [CrossRef] [PubMed]
125. Bartzsch, S.; Cummings, C.; Eismann, S.; Oelfke, U. A preclinical microbeam facility with a conventional X-ray tube. *Med. Phys.* **2016**, *43*, 6301–6308. [CrossRef] [PubMed]
126. González, W.; dos Santos, M.; Guardiola, C.; Delorme, R.; Lamirault, C.; Juchaux, M.; Le Dudal, M.; Jouvion, G.; Prezado, Y. Minibeam radiation therapy at a conventional irradiator: Dose-calculation engine and first tumor-bearing animals irradiation. *Phys. Med.* **2020**, *69*, 256–261. [CrossRef]
127. Price, L.S.; Rivera, J.N.; Madden, A.J.; Herity, L.B.; Piscitelli, J.A.; Mageau, S.; Santos, C.M.; Roques, J.R.; Midkiff, B.; Feinberg, N.N.; et al. Minibeam radiation therapy enhanced tumor delivery of PEGylated liposomal doxorubicin in a triple-negative breast cancer mouse model. *Ther. Adv. Med. Oncol.* **2021**, *13*. [CrossRef]
128. Ali, I. Nano Anti-Cancer Drugs: Pros and Cons and Future Perspectives. *Curr. Cancer Drug Targets* **2011**, *11*, 131–134. [CrossRef] [PubMed]
129. Dang, Y.; Guan, J. Nanoparticle-based drug delivery systems for cancer therapy. *Smart Mater. Med.* **2020**, *1*, 10–19. [CrossRef]
130. Ali, E.S.; Sharker, S.M.; Islam, M.T.; Khan, I.N.; Shaw, S.; Rahman, A.; Uddin, S.J.; Shill, M.C.; Rehman, S.; Das, N.; et al. Targeting cancer cells with nanotherapeutics and nanodiagnostics: Current status and future perspectives. *Semin. Cancer Biol.* **2020**, *69*, 52–68. [CrossRef]
131. Yan, S.; Zhao, P.; Yu, T.; Gu, N. Current applications and future prospects of nanotechnology in cancer immunotherapy. *Cancer Biol. Med.* **2019**, *16*, 486–497.
132. A Chandra, R.; Keane, F.K.; Voncken, F.E.M.; Thomas, C.R. Contemporary radiotherapy: Present and future. *Lancet* **2021**, *398*, 171–184. [CrossRef]
133. Durante, M.; Orecchia, R.; Loeffler, J.S. Charged-particle therapy in cancer: Clinical uses and future perspectives. *Nat. Rev. Clin. Oncol.* **2017**, *14*, 483–495. [CrossRef]
134. Baumann, M.; Ebert, N.; Kurth, I.; Bacchus, C.; Overgaard, J. What will radiation oncology look like in 2050? A look at a changing professional landscape in Europe and beyond. *Mol. Oncol.* **2020**, *14*, 1577–1585. [CrossRef] [PubMed]
135. Gomathi, H.; Ayisha Hamna, T.P.; Jijo, A.J.; Saradha Devi, K.M.; Sung, H.; Ferlay, J.; Siegel, R.L.; Laversanne, M.; Soerjomataram, I.; Jemal, A.; et al. Global Cancer Statistics 2020: GLOBOCAN Estimates of Incidence and Mortality Worldwide for 36 Cancers in 185 Countries. *CA Cancer J. Clin.* **2021**, *71*, 209–249. [CrossRef]

MDPI
St. Alban-Anlage 66
4052 Basel
Switzerland
Tel. +41 61 683 77 34
Fax +41 61 302 89 18
www.mdpi.com

Pharmaceutics Editorial Office
E-mail: pharmaceutics@mdpi.com
www.mdpi.com/journal/pharmaceutics

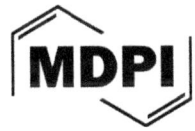

www.ingramcontent.com/pod-product-compliance
Lightning Source LLC
LaVergne TN
LVHW070156100526
838202LV00015B/1953